Nurse's
Quick
Check

Diseases

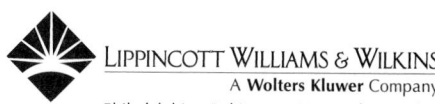

LIPPINCOTT WILLIAMS & WILKINS
A **Wolters Kluwer** Company

Philadelphia • Baltimore • New York • London
Buenos Aires • Hong Kong • Sydney • Tokyo

STAFF

Executive Publisher
Judith A. Schilling McCann, RN, MSN

Editorial Directors
H. Nancy Holmes, William J. Kelly

Clinical Director
Joan M. Robinson, RN, MSN

Senior Art Director
Arlene Putterman

Editorial Project Managers
Ann Houska, William Welsh

Clinical Project Manager
Kate McGovern, RN, MSN, CCRN

Editors
Catherine E. Harold, David P. Lenker, Teresa P. Sussman

Copy Editors
Kimberly Bilotta (supervisor), Tom DeZego,
Heather Ditch, Dona Hightower Perkins, Liz Mooney,
Judith Orioli, Irene Pontarelli, Lisa Stockslager

Designers
Jan Greenberg (project manager),
Will Boehm

Digital Composition Services
Diane Paluba (manager), Joyce Rossi Biletz,
Donna S. Morris

Manufacturing
Patricia K. Dorshaw (director), Beth Janae Orr

Editorial Assistants
Megan L. Aldinger, Tara L. Carter-Bell, Arlene Claffee,
Linda K. Ruhf

Librarian
Wani Z. Larsen

Indexer
Deborah K. Tourtlotte

Library of Congress Cataloging-in-Publication Data
Nurse's quick check : diseases.
        p. ; cm.
Includes index.
        1. Diseases — Handbooks, manuals, etc. 2. Nursing — Handbooks, manuals,etc. I. Lippincott Williams & Wilkins.
        [DNLM: 1. Disease — Handbooks. 2. Nursing Care — Handbooks. 3. Therapeutics — Handbooks.
WY 49 N9742 2004]
RT65.N78 2004
616 — dc22
ISBN 1-58255-305-X (alk. paper)   2003023470

Contents

Contributors
and consultants

Marguerite Ambrose, RN, DNSc, APRN, BC
Adjunct Faculty
Immaculata (Pa.) University

Margaret W. Bellak, RN, MN
Associate Professor
Indiana University of Pennsylvania

Mary Ann Boucher, RN, APRN, BC, ND
Assistant Professor, Nursing
University of Massachusetts Dartmouth

Lillian Craig, RN, MSN, FNP, CS
Family Nurse Practitioner
Veterans Administration Medical Center
Amarillo, Tex.

Peggy A. Davis, RN, MSN, CNS
Assistant Professor of Nursing
The University of Tennessee at Martin

Shelba Durston, RN, MSN, CCRN
Adjunct Faculty
San Joaquin Delta College
Stockton, Calif.
Staff Nurse
San Joaquin General Hospital
French Camp, Calif.

Angela R. Irvin, RN, BSN, FNP student
Clinical Instructor
Western Kentucky University
Bowling Green

Kathy J. Keister, RN, MS
Assistant Professor
Miami University
Middletown, Ohio

Linda Kucher, RN, MSN
Assistant Professor of Nursing
Gordon College
Barnesville, Ga.

Patricia Laing-Arie, RN, BSEd
Coordinator, Practical Nursing
Central Technology Center
Drumright, Okla.

Ellen Marcolongo, RN, MSN, CRNP
Clinical Nurse Specialist
North Philadelphia Health System

Lakshmi McRae, RN,C, BA
Staff Nurse
Doctor's Outpatient Surgical Center
Pasadena, Tex.

Clare Petrotta, RN, PHN, BSN
Nursing Instructor
Pacific College
Costa Mesa, Calif.

Lisa A. Salamon, RNBC, MSN, ET
Clinical Nurse Specialist
Cleveland Clinic Foundation

Barbara K. Scheirer, RN, BS, MSN
Assistant Professor
Grambling (La.) State University

Bruce Austin Scott, RN, MSN, APRN, BC
Instructor
San Joaquin Delta College
Stockton, Calif.
Clinical Nurse
University of California, Davis Medical Center
Sacramento

Sharon Wing, RN, MSN
Assistant Professor
Cleveland State University

Denise York, RNC, CNS, MS, MEd
Associate Professor
Columbus (Ohio) State Community College

Foreword

These days, it seems that nurses are expected to do the impossible — routinely. For starters, they need to cultivate a deep and detailed knowledge of hundreds of disorders, diagnostic procedures, and interventions while providing excellent nursing care in facilities that offer fewer colleagues, less time, more work, and sicker patients. Even meeting this impossible challenge won't be enough, however, given the constantly expanding nature of health-care knowledge.

Keeping up

Experts say each nurse should expect to face a fivefold increase in the body of medical knowledge in her lifetime. Not only are scientists gaining knowledge about the causes and treatments of diseases, but nurses are also facing the emergence of brand-new diseases, the resurgence of diseases thought to be conquered, and an exponential expansion in chronic disease that threatens to greatly reduce our national quality of life.

As caring health professionals, how can Nurses possibly keep up? It takes a lot of heart, and lots of help. That's where this book comes in. In *Nurse's Quick Check: Diseases*, experienced nurses have created brief but detailed reviews of more than 400 disorders, all arranged in A-to-Z order for quick access. No long, garbled sentences to decipher. Just handy bulleted lists of all the most pertinent data you'll need.

Up-to-date information

Each disease entry puts the latest information at your fingertips. You'll find a brief overview of each disease followed by sections outlining the crucial elements of assessment, treatment, nursing care, and patient teaching. Although concise, each section offers complete coverage. For instance, you might expect an overview to contain a mere paragraph to describe a disease. Not so with *Nurse's Quick Check: Diseases*. In this book, each overview outlines pathophysiology, causes, incidence, common characteristics, and complications. Each assessment section covers history, physical findings, and relevant test results, including laboratory tests, imaging

tests, and other diagnostic procedures. Each treatment section includes an array of lifestyle and noninvasive approaches in addition to drug treatments and invasive interventions. Nursing considerations sections include key outcomes, nursing interventions, and monitoring. The patient teaching sections list the most important topics you need to cover with patients at all stages of illness, including discharge.

To help highlight important details, this book also contains special logo features. For instance, an *Alert* logo draws your attention to critical content. An *Age issue* symbol appears beside information pertinent to patients of certain age groups. Plus, you'll notice that the most serious diseases start with the eye-catching *Life-threatening disorder* banner.

Meeting the challenge

Accurate, current, comprehensive, and organized, *Nurse's Quick Check: Diseases* can help you remember the familiar and expand your knowledge. As you use it, you'll find that you have a trusted source where you can quickly get what you need.

Simultaneously managing shrinking time, ballooning information, and sicker patients is the main challenge for every nurse. The risk of errors is growing, and the need to avoid them is paramount. Quickly finding the knowledge you need to deliver the best possible care to patients and their families is a nursing imperative. *Nurse's Quick Check: Diseases* is just the tool to help meet this challenge, and I recommend it.

Gloria F. Donnelly, RN, PhD, FAAN
Dean and Professor
Drexel University
Philadelphia

*Nurse's
Quick
Check*

Diseases

Abortion

Overview

Description

○ Expelled products of conception from the uterus before fetal viability
○ May be spontaneous (miscarriage) (see *Types of spontaneous abortion*)
○ May be therapeutic (elective) to preserve the mother's mental or physical health in cases of rape, unplanned pregnancy, or medical conditions, such as cardiac dysfunction or fetal abnormality

Pathophysiology

○ May result from fetal, placental, or maternal factors

Fetal factors
○ Usually cause abortion to occur between 9 and 12 weeks' gestation
○ Defective embryologic development
○ Faulty implantation of fertilized ovum
○ Failure of the endometrium to accept the fertilized ovum

Placental factors
○ Usually cause abortion to occur around 14 weeks' gestation when the placenta takes over the hormone production necessary to maintain pregnancy
○ Premature separation of a normally implanted placenta
○ Abnormal placental implantation
○ Abnormal platelet function

Maternal factors
○ Usually cause abortion to occur between 11 and 19 weeks' gestation

Causes

Spontaneous abortion
○ Fetal factors
○ Placental factors
○ Maternal infection
○ Severe malnutrition
○ Abnormalities of the reproductive organs
○ Thyroid gland dysfunction
○ Lowered estriol secretion
○ Diabetes mellitus
○ Trauma
○ Surgery that necessitates manipulation of the pelvic organs
○ Blood group incompatibility and Rh isoimmunization
○ Recreational drug use
○ Environmental toxins
○ Incompetent cervix

Incidence

○ Up to 15% of all pregnancies end in miscarriage.
○ About 30% of first pregnancies end in miscarriage.
○ At least 75% of miscarriages occur during the first trimester.

○ Legally induced abortions are increasing in the United States.

Common characteristics

○ Pink discharge for several days before cramping
○ Scant brown discharge for several weeks before cramping
  ○ Abdominal cramps
○ Vaginal bleeding

Complications

○ Infection
○ Hemorrhage
○ Anemia
○ Coagulation defects
○ Disseminated intravascular coagulation
○ Psychological issues of loss and failure

Assessment

History

○ Pink discharge for several days or scant brown discharge for several weeks before onset of cramps and increased vaginal bleeding
○ Cramps that appear for a few hours, intensify, then occur more frequently
○ Continued cramps and bleeding if any uterine contents remain (cramps and bleeding may subside if entire contents expelled)

Physical findings

○ Vaginal bleeding
○ Cervical dilation
○ Passage of nonviable products of conception

Test results

Laboratory
○ Decreased levels of serum human chorionic gonadotropin suggesting spontaneous abortion
○ Evidence of products of conception as shown by cytologic analysis
○ Decreased levels of serum hemoglobin and hematocrit due to blood loss
Imaging
○ Presence or absence of fetal heart tones or empty amniotic sac is revealed by ultrasound examination.

Treatment

General

○ An accurate evaluation of uterine contents is necessary before planning treatment.
○ The progression of spontaneous abortion can't be prevented, except in those cases caused by an incompetent cervix.
○ Hospitalization is necessary to control severe hemorrhage.
○ Bed rest may be required.

Medication

○ Transfusion with packed red blood cells or whole blood (severe bleeding)
○ I.V. oxytocin (stimulates uterine contractions)
○ $Rh_o(D)$ immune globulin for an Rh-negative female with a negative indirect Coombs' test

Induced abortion

○ Ingestion of mifepristone (single oral dosage of 600 mg followed by two 200-mg tablets of misoprostol on day three if abortion hasn't occurred)
○ Injection of hypertonic saline solution into amniotic sac
○ Injection of prostaglandin into the amniotic sac
○ Insertion of a prostaglandin vaginal suppository

Surgery

○ Dilatation and curettage or dilatation and evacuation (D&E), if remnants remain in the uterus
○ D&E, if first-trimester induced abortion
○ Surgical reinforcement of the cervix (cerclage) to prevent abortion

Nursing considerations

Key outcomes

The patient will:
○ exhibit no signs and symptoms of infection
○ communicate feelings about the current situation
○ express feelings of having greater control over the current situation
○ use available support systems, such as family and friends, to aid in coping.

Nursing interventions

○ Do *not* allow bathroom privileges, as the patient may expel uterine contents without knowing it.
○ Inspect bedpan contents carefully for intrauterine material.
○ Save all sanitary pads for evaluation.
○ Give prescribed drugs.
○ Provide perineal care.
○ Provide emotional support and counseling.
○ Encourage expression of feelings.
○ Help the patient develop effective coping strategies.

Monitoring

○ Amount, color, and odor of vaginal bleeding
○ Vital signs
○ Intake and output

Patient teaching

Be sure to cover:
○ the disorder, diagnosis, and treatment
○ vaginal bleeding or spotting
○ bleeding that lasts longer than 8 to 10 days or excessive bleeding
○ importance of reporting signs of bright red blood immediately

Types of spontaneous abortion

Depending on clinical findings, a spontaneous abortion (miscarriage) may be threatened or inevitable, incomplete or complete, or missed, habitual, or septic. Here's how the seven types compare.

Threatened abortion

Bloody vaginal discharge occurs during the first half of pregnancy. About 20% of pregnant women have vaginal spotting or actual bleeding early in pregnancy; of these, about 50% abort.

Inevitable abortion

The membranes rupture and the cervix dilates. As labor continues, the uterus expels the products of conception.

Incomplete abortion

The uterus retains part or all of the placenta. Before 10 weeks' gestation, the fetus and placenta usually are expelled together; after the 10th week, they're expelled separately. Because part of the placenta may adhere to the uterine wall, bleeding continues. Hemorrhage is possible because the uterus doesn't contract and seal the large vessels that fed the placenta.

Complete abortion

The uterus passes all the products of conception. Minimal bleeding usually accompanies complete abortion because the uterus contracts and compresses the maternal blood vessels that fed the placenta.

Missed abortion

The uterus retains the products of conception for 2 months or more after the death of the fetus. Uterine growth ceases; uterine size may even seem to decrease. Prolonged retention of the dead products of conception may cause coagulation defects such as disseminated intravascular coagulation.

Habitual abortion

Spontaneous loss of three or more consecutive pregnancies constitutes habitual abortion.

Septic abortion

Infection accompanies abortion. This may occur with spontaneous abortion, but usually results from an illegal abortion or from the presence of an intrauterine device.

○ signs of infection, such as fever and foul-smelling vaginal discharge
○ gradual increase of daily activities
○ schedule for returning to work (normally within 1 to 4 weeks)
○ abstinence from intercourse for 1 to 2 weeks
○ prevention of spontaneous abortion
○ contraceptive information
○ avoidance of tampons for 1 to 2 weeks
○ follow-up examination.

Discharge planning

○ Refer the patient for professional counseling, if indicated.

Abruptio placentae

Overview

Description
- Premature separation of the placenta from the uterine wall
- Usually occurs after 20 weeks' gestation, most commonly during the third trimester
- Common cause of bleeding during the second half of pregnancy
- Fetal prognosis depends on gestational age and amount of blood lost
- Good maternal prognosis if hemorrhage can be controlled
- Classified according to degree of placental separation and severity of maternal and fetal symptoms (see *Degrees of placental separation in abruptio placentae*)
- Also called *placental abruption*

Pathophysiology
- Spontaneous rupture of blood vessels at the placental bed may be due to lack of resiliency or to abnormal changes in uterine vasculature.
- State may be complicated by hypertension or by an enlarged uterus that can't contract sufficiently to seal off the torn vessels.
- Bleeding continues unchecked, possibly shearing off the placenta partially or completely.

Causes
- Exact cause unknown
- Traumatic injury
- Amniocentesis
- Chronic or pregnancy-induced hypertension
- Multiparity
- Short umbilical cord
- Dietary deficiency
- Smoking
- Advanced maternal age
- Pressure on the vena cava from an enlarged uterus
- Diabetes mellitus

Incidence
- Most common in multigravida women older than age 35, women with pregnancy-induced hypertension, and women who use cocaine

Common characteristics
- Vaginal bleeding
- Abdominal discomfort
- Abdominal tenderness

Complications
- Hemorrhage
- Shock
- Renal failure
- Disseminated intravascular coagulation (DIC)
- Maternal death
- Fetal death

Assessment

History
Mild abruptio placentae (marginal separation)
- Mild to moderate vaginal bleeding
- Vague lower abdominal discomfort
- Mild to moderate abdominal tenderness

Moderate abruptio placentae (about 50% placental separation)
- Continuous abdominal pain
- Moderate dark red vaginal bleeding
- Severe or abrupt onset of symptoms

Severe abruptio placentae (70% placental separation)
- Abrupt onset of agonizing, unremitting uterine pain
- Moderate vaginal bleeding

Physical findings
Mild abruptio placentae
- Fetal monitoring possibly indicating uterine irritability
- Strong and regular fetal heart tones

Moderate abruptio placentae
- Vital signs possibly indicating impending shock
- Tender uterus remaining firm between contractions
- Barely audible or irregular and bradycardic fetal heart tones
- Labor that usually starts within 2 hours and proceeds rapidly

Severe abruptio placentae
- Vital signs that indicate rapidly progressive shock
- Absence of fetal heart tones
- Tender uterus with boardlike rigidity
- Possible increased uterine size in severe concealed abruptions

Test results
Laboratory
- Decreased serum hemoglobin level and platelet count
- Progression of abruptio placentae and detection of DIC as shown by fibrin split products

Imaging
- Pelvic examination under double setup (preparations for an emergency cesarean delivery) and ultrasonography (may rule out placenta previa)

Treatment

General
- Assess, control, and restore amount of blood loss
- Deliver a viable infant
- Prevent coagulation disorders

Degrees of placental separation in abruptio placentae

Mild separation
Internal bleeding between the placenta and uterine wall characterize mild separation.

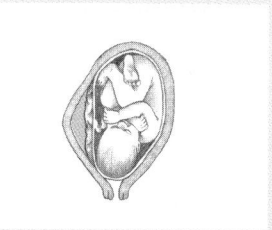

Moderate separation
In moderate separation, external hemorrhage occurs through the vagina.

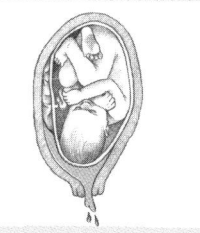

Severe separation
External hemorrhage is also characteristic in severe separation.

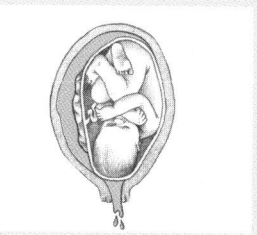

○ If placental separation is severe with no signs of fetal life, vaginal delivery unless contraindicated by uncontrolled hemorrhage or other complications

 Alert

Because of possible fetal blood loss through the placenta, a pediatric team should be ready at delivery to assess and treat the neonate for shock, blood loss, and hypoxia.

 Alert

Complications of abruptio placentae require prompt appropriate treatment. With a complication such as DIC, the patient needs immediate intervention with platelets and whole blood, as ordered, to prevent exsanguination.

○ Nothing to eat or drink until delivery of the fetus
○ Bed rest until delivery of the fetus

Medication

○ I.V. fluid infusion (by large-bore catheter), as ordered

Surgery

○ Cesarean delivery if the fetus is in distress

Nursing considerations

Key outcomes

The patient will:
○ maintain stable vital signs
○ maintain balanced fluid volume
○ express feelings of increased comfort
○ communicate feelings about the situation
○ use available support systems to aid in coping.

Nursing interventions

○ Insert an indwelling urinary catheter.

○ Obtain blood specimens for hemoglobin level and hematocrit, coagulation studies, and type and cross-matching, as ordered.
○ Provide emotional support during labor.
○ Provide information of progress and condition of fetus during labor.
○ Encourage verbalization of feelings.
○ Help develop effective coping strategies.
○ Give I.V. fluids and blood products.

Monitoring

○ Maternal vital signs
○ Central venous pressure
○ Intake and output
○ Vaginal bleeding
○ Fetal heart rate (electronically)
○ Progression of labor

Patient teaching

Be sure to cover:
○ the disorder, diagnosis, and treatment
○ signs of placental abruption
○ possibility of an emergency cesarean delivery
○ possibility of the delivery of a premature infant
○ changes to expect in the postpartum period
○ possibility of neonatal death
○ factors affecting survival of neonate
○ importance of frequent monitoring and prompt management to reduce risk of death.

Discharge planning

○ Refer the patient for professional counseling, if indicated.

Acceleration-deceleration injuries

Overview

Description
- Injury resulting from sharp hyperextension and flexion of the neck that damages muscles, ligaments, disks, and nerve tissue
- Excellent prognosis; symptoms usually subside with symptomatic treatment
- Also called *whiplash*

Pathophysiology
- Unexpected force causes the head to jerk back and then forward.
- The neck bones snap out of position, causing injury.
- Irritated nerves can interfere with blood flow and transmission of nerve impulses.
- Pinched nerves can affect certain body part functions.

Causes
- Motor vehicle accident
- Sports accident
- Fall

Risk factors
- Absence of head restraint in automobile
- Osteoporosis
- Driving under the influence of alcohol or drugs

Incidence
- There are 1,000,000 cases each year in the United States.
- Average age of patient with acceleration-deceleration injury is the late 40's.

Common characteristics
- Nuchal rigidity
- Neck muscle asymmetry

Complications
- Temporomandibular disorder

Assessment

History
- Mechanism of injury
- Pain initially minimal, but increases 12 to 72 hours after the accident
- Dizziness
- Headache
- Back pain
- Shoulder pain
- Vision disturbances
- Tinnitus

Physical findings
- Neck muscle asymmetry
- Reduced neck mobility
- Gait disturbances
- Rigidity or numbness in the arms
- Tenderness at the exact location of the injury
- Decreased active and passive range of motion

Test results
Imaging
- Full cervical spine X-rays (to rule out cervical fracture)

Treatment

General
- Soft cervical collar (see *Applying a cervical collar*)
- Ice packs
- Physical therapy
- Limited activity during the first 72 hours after the injury
- Limited neck movement
- Limited strenuous activities, such as lifting and contact sports, until full recovery has been established (which may take more than 2 years)

Medication
- Oral analgesics (acetaminophen, nonsteroidal anti-inflammatory drugs, opioids)
- Muscle relaxants
- Corticosteroids

Surgery
- Surgical stabilization may be necessary in severe cervical acceleration-deceleration injuries

Nursing considerations

Key outcomes
The patient will:
- identify factors that intensify pain
- modify behavior to limit movement and avoid extended injury
- develop effective coping mechanisms
- attain the highest degree of mobility possible
- state feelings and fears about the injury.

Nursing interventions
- Provide protection of the spine during all care.
- Give prescribed drugs.
- Apply a soft cervical collar.

Monitoring
- Pain control
- Response to medications
- Complications
- Neurologic status

Applying a cervical collar

Cervical collars are used to support an injured or weakened cervical spine and to maintain alignment during healing. The soft cervical collar, made of spongy foam, provides gentler support and reminds the patient to avoid cervical spine motion.

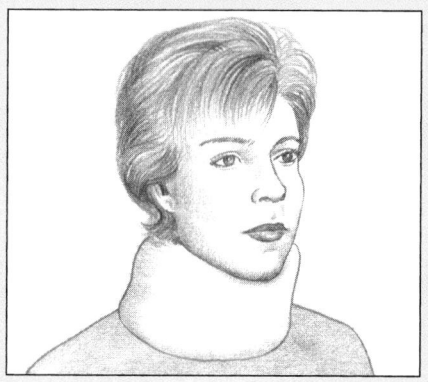

Patient teaching

Be sure to cover:
- activity restrictions
- proper application of soft cervical collar
- all medications, including administration, dosage, and possible adverse effects
- instructions regarding driving and the use of alcohol while on narcotics.

Acne vulgaris

Overview

Description

○ Inflammatory disorder of the sebaceous gland contiguous with a hair follicle (pilosebaceous follicle)
○ Possibly developing in distinctive pilosebaceous units (sebaceous follicles)
○ Acne lesions: inflammatory (pustules, papules, and nodules) and noninflammatory (closed and open comedones) lesions
○ Good prognosis with treatment

Pathophysiology

○ Acne begins with sebum accumulation that obstructs the pilosebaceous unit.
○ The mass of accumulated keratinous sebaceous material and bacteria within the pilosebaceous follicle causes inflammation when it's exposed to the dermis with rupture of a follicle.
○ The *Propionibacterium acnes* bacteria produce substances that promote inflammation.
○ In noninflammatory acne, the comedones are open, called blackheads, or closed, called whiteheads; accumulated material causes distention of the follicle and thinning of follicular canal walls.
○ Inflammatory acne develops in closed comedones when the follicular wall ruptures, expelling sebum into the surrounding dermis and initiating inflammation.
○ Pustules form when the inflammation is close to the surface; papules and cystic nodules can develop when the inflammation is deeper, causing mild to severe scarring.

Causes

○ Exact cause unknown
○ Follicular hyperkeratinization
○ Excessive sebum production
○ Proliferation of *P. acnes*
○ Hormonal dysfunction

Causes of acne flare-ups
○ Menstrual cycle
○ Stress
○ Trauma
○ Tropical climates
○ Rubbing from tight clothing
○ Environmental exposure to coal tar derivatives, certain chemicals, cosmetics, or hair pomades
○ Hormonal contraceptives containing norethindrone and norgestrel; testosterone
○ Anabolic agents
○ Corticotropin, gonadotropins, corticosteroids (prolonged use)
○ Iodine- or bromine-containing drugs
○ Trimethadione
○ Phenytoin
○ Isoniazid
○ Lithium
○ Halothane

Incidence

○ Affects nearly 75% of adolescents, although lesions can appear as young as age 8
○ Affects males more often and more severely
○ Occurs in females at an earlier age and tends to affect them for a longer time, sometimes into adulthood
○ Tends to be familial

Common characteristics

○ Pustules, papules, nodules
○ Closed and open comedones
○ Follicles located primarily on face and upper parts of chest and back

Complications

○ Deep cystic process
○ Gross inflammation
○ Abscess formation
○ Secondary bacterial infection
○ Acne scars

Assessment

History

○ Presence of one or more predisposing factors
○ Seasonal or monthly eruption patterns
○ Pain and tenderness around area of infected follicle

Physical findings

○ Acne lesions, commonly located on the face, neck, shoulders, chest, and upper back
○ Red and swollen area around the infected follicle
○ Acne plugs that appear as closed or open comedones
○ Oily and thickened skin
○ Visible scars

Test results

Laboratory
○ Culture and sensitivity of pustules or abscesses showing causative organism of secondary bacterial infection

Other
○ History and physical examination findings

Treatment

General

○ Treatment of causative factors
○ Well-balanced diet
○ Regular exercise

Medication

○ Antibacterials
○ Anticomedonals
○ Keratinolytic agents

- ○ Anti-inflammatory agents
- ○ Antiandrogens
- ○ Antisebaceous agents
- ○ Tretinoin
- ○ Isotretinoin

Surgery

- ○ Comedo extraction
- ○ Intralesional steroids
- ○ Cryosurgery
- ○ Dermabrasion

 Age issue

Tetracycline is contraindicated during pregnancy and childhood because it may cause permanent discoloration of teeth (in children under age 8), enamel defects, and bone growth retardation. Erythromycin is an alternative for these patients.

 Alert

Because oral tretinoin is known to cause birth defects, the manufacturer, with Food and Drug Administration approval, recommends pregnancy testing before dispensing, dispensing only a 30-day supply, repeat pregnancy testing throughout the treatment period, effective contraception during treatment, and informed consent of the patient or parents regarding the danger of the drug.

Nursing considerations

Key outcomes

The patient will:
- ○ exhibit improved or healed wounds or lesions
- ○ demonstrate the recommended skin care regimen
- ○ verbalize feelings about body image
- ○ verbalize understanding of the condition and treatment.

Nursing interventions

- ○ Give prescribed drugs.
- ○ Assist the patient in identifying and eliminating predisposing factors.
- ○ Encourage good personal hygiene and the use of oil-free skin care products.
- ○ Discourage picking or squeezing the lesions.
- ○ Encourage the patient to verbalize his feelings.
- ○ Encourage the patient to develop interests that support a positive self-image and de-emphasize appearance.

Monitoring

- ○ Liver function studies and serum triglyceride levels with tretinoin use
- ○ Complications
- ○ Sensitivity reactions
- ○ GI disturbances
- ○ Liver dysfunction
- ○ Response to treatment
- ○ Skin and mucous membranes

Patient teaching

Be sure to cover:
- ○ disorder and treatment
- ○ medications and potential adverse reactions
- ○ when to notify the physician
- ○ signs and symptoms of infection
- ○ causative factors associated with acne flare-up
- ○ well-balanced diet
- ○ adequate rest
- ○ stress management.

Acquired immunodeficiency syndrome and human immunodeficiency virus

Overview

Description

○ Human immunodeficiency virus (HIV) type I; retrovirus causing acquired immunodeficiency syndrome (AIDS).
○ Causes patients to become susceptible to opportunistic infections, unusual cancers, and other abnormalities
○ Marked by progressive failure of the immune system
○ Transmitted by contact with infected blood or body fluids and associated with identifiable high-risk behaviors

Pathophysiology

○ HIV strikes helper T cells bearing the CD4 antigen.
○ The antigen serves as a receptor for the retrovirus and lets it enter the cell.
○ After invading a cell, HIV replicates, leading to cell death, or becomes latent.
○ HIV infection leads to profound pathology, either directly, through destruction of CD4+ cells, other immune cells, and neuroglial cells, or indirectly, through the secondary effects of CD4+ T-cell dysfunction and resultant immunosuppression.

Causes

○ Infection with HIV, a retrovirus

Risk factors

○ I.V. drug users who share needles or syringes
○ Unprotected sexual intercourse
○ Placental transmission
○ History of sexually transmitted disease
○ Homosexual lifestyle
○ Contact with infected blood

Incidence

○ The average time between exposure to the virus and diagnosis of AIDS is 8 to 10 years, but shorter and longer incubation times have been recorded.

Common characteristics

○ May produce no symptoms for years
○ Flulike symptoms

Complications

○ Repeated opportunistic infections
○ Neoplasms
○ Premalignant diseases
○ Organ-specific syndrome

Assessment

History

○ After a high-risk exposure and inoculation, a mononucleosis-like syndrome usually develops; then may remain asymptomatic for years
○ In the latent stage, the only sign of HIV infection is laboratory evidence of seroconversion

Physical findings

○ Persistent generalized adenopathy
○ Nonspecific symptoms (weight loss, fatigue, night sweats, fevers)
○ Neurologic symptoms resulting from HIV encephalopathy
○ Opportunistic infection or cancer (Kaposi's sarcoma)

 Age issue

Children show a higher incidence of bacterial infections.

Test results

Laboratory
○ CD4+ T-cell count of at least 200 cells/ml confirms HIV infection.
○ Screening test enzyme-linked immunosorbent assay and confirmatory test (Western blot) detect the presence of HIV antibodies, which indicate HIV infection.

Treatment

General

○ Variety of therapeutic options for opportunistic infections (the leading cause of morbidity and mortality in patients infected with HIV)
○ Disease-specific therapy for a variety of neoplastic and premalignant diseases and organ-specific syndromes
○ Symptom management (fatigue and anemia)
○ Well-balanced diet
○ Regular exercise, as tolerated, with adequate rest periods

Medication

○ Immunomodulatory agents
○ Anti-infective agents
○ Antineoplastic agents
○ Highly active antiretroviral therapy (HAART)
Primary therapy
○ Protease inhibitors
○ Nucleoside reverse transcriptase inhibitors
○ Nonnucleoside reverse transcriptase inhibitors

○ Use precautions in all situations that risk exposure to blood, body fluids, and secretions. Diligently practicing standard precautions can prevent the inadvertent transmission of human immunodeficiency virus (HIV), hepatitis B, and other infectious diseases that are transmitted by similar routes.

○ Teach the patient, his family, sexual partners, and friends about disease transmission and prevention of extending the disease to others.

○ Tell the patient not to donate blood, blood products, organs, tissue, or sperm.

○ If the patient uses I.V. drugs, caution him not to share needles.

○ Inform the patient that high-risk sexual practices for HIV transmission are those that exchange body fluids, such as vaginal or anal intercourse without a condom.

○ Discuss safe sexual practices, such as hugging, petting, mutual masturbation, and protected sexual intercourse. Abstinence is the most effective method to prevent transmission.

○ Advise the female patient of childbearing age to avoid pregnancy. Explain that an infant may become infected before birth, during delivery, or during breast-feeding.

Nursing considerations

Key outcomes

The patient will:

○ achieve management of symptoms of illness

○ demonstrate use of protective measures, including conservation of energy, maintenance of well-balanced diet, and getting adequate rest

○ follow safe sex practices

○ utilize available support systems to assist with coping

○ voice feelings about changes in sexual identity and social response to disease

○ develop no complications of illness

○ comply with the treatment regimen.

Nursing interventions

○ Help the patient to cope with an altered body image, the emotional burden of serious illness, and the threat of death.

○ Avoid glycerin swabs for mucous membranes. Use normal saline or bicarbonate mouthwash for daily oral rinsing.

○ Ensure adequate fluid intake during episodes of diarrhea.

○ Provide meticulous skin care, especially in the debilitated patient.

○ Encourage the patient to maintain as much physical activity as he can tolerate. Make sure his schedule includes time for exercise and rest.

Monitoring

○ Fever, noting any pattern

○ Skin integrity

○ Signs of illness, such as cough, sore throat, or diarrhea

○ Swollen, tender lymph nodes

○ Laboratory values

○ Calorie intake

○ Progression of lesions in Kaposi's sarcoma

○ Opportunistic infections or signs of disease progression

○ Compliance with medication regimen

Patient teaching

Be sure to cover:

○ medication regimens

○ importance of informing potential sexual partners, caregivers, and health care workers of HIV infection (see *Preventing HIV transmission*)

○ signs of impending infection and the importance of seeking immediate medical attention

○ symptoms of AIDS dementia and its stages and progression.

Discharge planning

○ Refer the patient to a local support group.

○ Refer the patient to hospice care, as indicated.

Acute poststreptococcal glomerulonephritis

Overview

Description

- Renal disease in which the glomeruli become inflamed
- Usually associated with a postinfectious state, commonly a streptococcal infection of the respiratory tract or, less commonly, a skin infection such as impetigo
- Up to 95% of children and 70% of adults recover fully
- Elderly patients may progress to chronic renal failure within months
- Relatively common
- Also called *acute glomerulonephritis*

Pathophysiology

- Antigen-antibody complexes are produced in response to group A beta-hemolytic streptococcus infection.
- Entrapment and collection of antigen-antibody complexes occurs in the glomerular capillary membranes.
- Inflammatory damage results, impeding glomerular function.
- Immune complement may further damage the glomerular membrane.
- Damaged and inflamed glomeruli lose the ability to be selectively permeable.
- Red blood cells (RBCs) and proteins then filter through as the glomerular filtration rate decreases.
- Uremic poisoning may result.

Causes

- Untreated group A beta-hemolytic streptococcus infection, especially of the respiratory tract

Risk factors

- Impetigo

Incidence

- Occurs most commonly in boys ages 3 to 7; can occur at any age

Common characteristics

- Oliguria
- Fluid overload
- Periorbital edema

Complications

- Progressive deterioration of renal function

Assessment

History

- Untreated respiratory streptococcal infection 1 to 3 weeks before
- Decreased urination
- Smoky or coffee-colored urine
- Fatigue
- Dyspnea and orthopnea

Physical findings

- Oliguria
- Mild to moderate periorbital edema
- Mild to severe hypertension
- Bibasilar crackles (with heart failure)

Test results

Laboratory

- Electrolyte imbalances
- Elevated blood urea nitrogen (BUN) and creatinine levels
- Decreased serum protein levels
- The presence of RBCs, white blood cells, mixed cell casts, and protein in the urine that indicate renal failure
- High levels of fibrin-degradation products and C3 protein

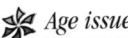 **Age issue**

Proteinuria in an elderly patient usually isn't as pronounced.

- Elevated antistreptolysin-O titers (in 80% of patients), elevated streptozyme and anti-DNase B titers, and low serum complement levels, which verify recent streptococcal infection
- Group A beta-hemolytic streptococci as revealed by throat culture

Imaging

- Kidney-ureter-bladder X-rays reveal bilateral kidney enlargement.

Diagnostic procedures

- Renal biopsy or assessment of renal tissue confirms diagnosis.

Treatment

General

- Correction of electrolyte imbalances (possible dialysis)
- Fluid restriction
- High-calorie, low-protein, low-sodium, low-potassium diet
- Bed rest

Medication

- Antibiotics if appropriate
- Loop diuretics, such as metolazone or furosemide

Nursing considerations

Key outcomes

The patient will:
- avoid or minimize complications
- maintain fluid balance
- maintain urine specific gravity within the designated limits
- report increased comfort
- identify risk factors that exacerbate the condition and modify lifestyle accordingly.

Nursing interventions

- Give prescribed drugs.
- Encourage verbalization.
- Provide support.

Monitoring

- Vital signs
- Electrolyte values, serum creatinine, and BUN levels
- Urine creatinine clearance test results
- Intake and output
- Daily weight

Patient teaching

Be sure to cover:
- the disorder, diagnosis, and treatment
- importance of follow-up examinations to monitor renal function
- medication administration, dosage, and possible adverse effects.

Discharge planning

- Refer the patient to appropriate resources for information and support.

Acute pyelonephritis

Overview

Description

○ Inflammation of the kidney occurring mainly in the interstitial tissue and renal pelvis and occasionally in the renal tubules
○ Affecting one or both kidneys
○ Good prognosis; extensive permanent damage rarely occurs
○ Also called *acute infective tubulointerstitial nephritis*

Pathophysiology

○ Infection spreads from the bladder to ureters to the kidneys, commonly through vesicoureteral reflux.
○ Vesicoureteral reflux may result from congenital weakness at the junction of the ureter and bladder.
○ Bacteria refluxed to intrarenal tissues may create colonies of infection within 24 to 48 hours.
○ Female anatomy allows for higher incidence of infection.

Causes

○ Bacterial infection of the kidneys

Risk factors

○ Renal procedures that involve instrumentation such as cystoscopy
○ Hematogenic infection such as septicemia
○ Sexually active women
○ Pregnant women
○ Neurogenic bladder
○ Obstructive disease
○ Renal diseases

Incidence

○ More common in women than in men
○ Community-acquired cases in 15 per 100,000 annually
○ Hospital-acquired cases in 7 per 10,000 annually

Common characteristics

○ Pain over one or both kidneys
○ Urinary urgency and frequency
○ Dysuria
○ Nocturia

Complications

○ Renal calculi
○ Renal failure
○ Renal abscess
○ Multisystem infection
○ Septic shock
○ Chronic pyelonephritis

Assessment

History

○ Pain over one or both kidneys
○ Urinary urgency and frequency
○ Burning during urination
○ Dysuria, nocturia, hematuria
○ Anorexia, vomiting, diarrhea
○ Fatigue
○ Symptoms that develop rapidly over a few hours or a few days

Physical findings

○ Pain on flank palpation
○ Cloudy urine
○ Ammonia-like or fishy odor to urine
○ Fever of 102° F (38.9° C) or higher
○ Shaking chills

Test results

Laboratory
○ Urinalysis and culture and sensitivity testing reveals pyuria, significant bacteriuria, low specific gravity and osmolality, slightly alkaline urine pH, or proteinuria, glycosuria, and ketonuria (less frequent)
○ Elevated white blood cell count, neutrophil count, and erythrocyte sedimentation rate

Imaging
○ Kidney-ureter-bladder radiography reveals calculi, tumors, or cysts in the kidneys or urinary tract.
○ Excretory urography shows asymmetrical kidneys, possibly indicating a high frequency of infection.

Treatment

General

○ Identification and correction of predisposing factors to infection, such as obstruction or calculi
○ Short courses of therapy for uncomplicated infections
○ Increased fluid intake

Medication

○ Antibiotics
○ Urinary analgesics such as phenazopyridine

Nursing considerations

Key outcomes

The patient will:
○ maintain fluid balance
○ maintain urine specific gravity within the designated limits
○ identify risk factors that exacerbate decreased tissue perfusion and modify lifestyle appropriately
○ report increased comfort.

Nursing interventions

○ Give prescribed drugs.

Monitoring

○ Vital signs
○ Intake and output
○ Characteristics of urine
○ Pattern of urination
○ Daily weight
○ Renal function studies

Patient teaching

Be sure to cover:
○ the disorder, diagnosis, and treatment
○ avoidance of bacterial contamination by following hygienic toileting practices (wiping the perineum from front to back after bowel movements for women)
○ proper technique for collecting a clean-catch urine specimen
○ drug administration, dosage, and possible adverse effects
○ routine checkup with a history of urinary tract infections
○ signs and symptoms of recurrent infection.

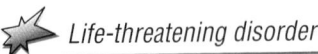 *Life-threatening disorder*

Acute respiratory distress syndrome

Overview

Description

- Severe form of alveolar injury or acute lung injury
- A form of pulmonary edema; may be difficult to recognize
- Hallmark sign includes hypoxemia despite increased supplemental oxygen
- A four-stage syndrome; can rapidly progress to intractable and fatal hypoxemia
- Little or no permanent lung damage occurring in patients who recover
- May coexist with disseminated intravascular coagulation (DIC)
- Also known as *adult respiratory distress syndrome* and *shock, stiff, white, wet,* or *Da Nang lung*

Pathophysiology

- Increased permeability of the alveolocapillary membranes that allows fluid to accumulate in the lung interstitium, alveolar spaces, and small airways, causing the lung to stiffen
- Ventilation that's impaired, reducing oxygenation of pulmonary capillary blood
- Elevated capillary pressure that increases interstitial and alveolar edema
- Alveolar closing pressure that then exceeds pulmonary pressures
- Closure and collapse of the alveoli

Causes

- Indirect or direct lung trauma (most common)
- Anaphylaxis
- Aspiration of gastric contents
- Diffuse pneumonia (especially viral)
- Drug overdose
- Idiosyncratic drug reaction
- Inhalation of noxious gases
- Near-drowning
- Oxygen toxicity
- Coronary artery bypass grafting
- Hemodialysis
- Leukemia
- Acute miliary tuberculosis
- Pancreatitis
- Thrombotic thrombocytopenic purpura
- Uremia
- Venous air embolism

Incidence

- Patients with three concurrent causes have an 85% probability of developing acute respiratory distress syndrome.

Common characteristics

- Shortness of breath
- Dry cough with thick, frothy sputum
- Bloody, sticky secretions

Complications

- Metabolic acidosis
- Respiratory acidosis
- Cardiac arrest
- Multiple organ dysfunction syndrome

Assessment

History

- Causative factor (one or more)
- Dyspnea, especially on exertion

Physical findings

Stage I
- Shortness of breath, especially on exertion
- Normal to increased respiratory and pulse rates
- Diminished breath sounds

Stage II
- Respiratory distress
- Use of accessory muscles for respiration
- Pallor, anxiety, and restlessness
- Dry cough with thick, frothy sputum
- Bloody, sticky secretions
- Cool, clammy skin
- Tachycardia and tachypnea
- Elevated blood pressure
- Basilar crackles

Stage III
- Respiratory rate more than 30 breaths/minute
- Tachycardia with arrhythmias
- Labile blood pressure
- Productive cough
- Pale, cyanotic skin
- Crackles and rhonchi possible

Stage IV
- Acute respiratory failure with severe hypoxia
- Deteriorating mental status (may become comatose)
- Pale, cyanotic skin
- Lack of spontaneous respirations
- Bradycardia with arrhythmias
- Hypotension
- Metabolic and respiratory acidosis

Test results

Laboratory
- Arterial blood gas (ABG) analysis initially showing a reduced partial pressure of arterial oxygen (Pao_2) (less than 60 mm Hg) and a decreased partial pressure of arterial carbon dioxide ($Paco_2$) (less than 35 mm Hg)

- ABG analysis later showing increased $Paco_2$ (more than 45 mm Hg) and decreased bicarbonate levels (less than 22 mEq/L) and decreased Pao_2 despite oxygen therapy
- Gram stain and sputum culture and sensitivity showing infectious organism
- Blood cultures revealing infectious organisms
- Toxicology tests showing drug ingestion in overdose
- Increased serum amylase in pancreatitis

Imaging
- Chest X-rays may show early bilateral infiltrates; in later stages, a ground-glass appearance and, eventually, "whiteouts" of both lung fields.

Diagnostic procedures
- Pulmonary artery catheterization may show a pulmonary artery wedge pressure of 12 to 18 mm Hg.

Treatment

General
- Treatment of the underlying cause
- Correction of electrolyte and acid-base imbalances

For mechanical ventilation
- Target low tidal volumes; use of increased respiratory rates
- Target plateau pressures less than or equal to 40 cm H_2O
- Positive end-expiratory pressure (PEEP) as necessary
- Fluid restriction
- Tube feedings or parenteral nutrition
- Bed rest

Medication
- Humidified oxygen
- Bronchodilators
- Diuretics

For mechanical ventilation
- Sedatives
- Opioids
- Neuromuscular blocking agents
- Short course of high-dose corticosteroids if fatty emboli or chemical injury
- Sodium bicarbonate if severe metabolic acidosis
- Fluids and vasopressors if hypotensive
- Antimicrobials if nonviral infection

Surgery
- Possible tracheostomy

Nursing considerations

Key outcomes
The patient will:
- maintain adequate ventilation
- maintain a patent airway
- use effective coping strategies
- maintain skin integrity
- report feelings of increased comfort.

Nursing interventions
- Give prescribed drugs.
- Maintain a patent airway.
- Perform tracheal suctioning, as necessary.
- Ensure adequate humidification.
- Reposition the patient often.
- Consider prone positioning for alveolar recruitment.
- Administer tube feedings or parenteral nutrition, as ordered.
- Allow periods of uninterrupted sleep.
- Perform passive range-of-motion exercises.
- Provide meticulous skin care.
- Reposition the endotracheal tube per facility policy.
- Provide emotional support.
- Provide alternative communication means.

Monitoring
- Vital signs and pulse oximetry
- Hemodynamics
- Intake and output
- Respiratory status (breath sounds, ABG results)
- Mechanical ventilator settings
- Sputum characteristics
- Level of consciousness
- Daily weight
- Laboratory studies
- Response to treatment
- Complications, such as cardiac arrhythmias, DIC, GI bleeding, infection, malnutrition, or pneumothorax
- Nutritional status

 Alert

Because PEEP may lower cardiac output, check for hypotension, tachycardia, and decreased urine output. To maintain PEEP, suction only as needed.

If the patient requires mechanical ventilation
- Ventilator settings
- Cuff pressure
- Complications of mechanical ventilation
- Endotracheal tube position and patency
- Signs and symptoms of stress ulcer

Patient teaching

Be sure to cover:
- the disorder, diagnosis, and treatment
- medications and potential adverse reactions
- when to notify the physician
- complications, such as GI bleeding, infection, and malnutrition
- recovery time.

Discharge planning
- Refer the patient to a pulmonary rehabilitation program, if indicated.

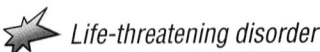
Acute respiratory failure

Overview

Description

○ Inadequate ventilation resulting from the inability of the lungs to adequately maintain arterial oxygenation or eliminate carbon dioxide

Pathophysiology

○ If respiratory failure is primarily hypercapnic, it's the result of inadequate alveolar ventilation.
○ If respiratory failure is primarily hypoxemic, it's the result of inadequate exchange of oxygen between the alveoli and capillaries.
○ Many people have a combined hypercapnic and hypoxemic respiratory failure.

Causes

○ Any condition that increases the work of breathing and decreases the respiratory drive of patients with chronic obstructive pulmonary disease
○ Respiratory tract infection
○ Bronchospasm
○ Accumulated secretions secondary to cough suppression
○ Ventilatory failure
○ Gas exchange failure
○ Central nervous system depression
○ Myocardial infarction (MI)
○ Heart failure
○ Pulmonary emboli
○ Airway irritants
○ Endocrine or metabolic disorders
○ Thoracic abnormalities

Incidence

○ Occurs in patients with hypercapnia and hypoxemia
○ Occurs in patients who have an acute deterioration in arterial blood gas (ABG) values

Common characteristics

○ Rapid breathing
○ Restlessness
○ Anxiety
○ Depression
○ Lethargy
○ Agitation
○ Confusion

Complications

○ Tissue hypoxia
○ Chronic respiratory acidosis
○ Metabolic alkalosis
○ Respiratory and cardiac arrest

Assessment

History

Precipitating events

○ Infection
○ Accumulated pulmonary secretions secondary to cough suppression
○ Trauma
○ MI
○ Heart failure
○ Pulmonary emboli
○ Exposure to irritants (smoke or fumes)
○ Myxedema
○ Metabolic acidosis

Physical findings

○ Cyanosis of the oral mucosa, lips, and nail beds
○ Yawning and use of accessory muscles
○ Pursed-lip breathing
○ Nasal flaring
○ Ashen skin
○ Rapid breathing
○ Cold, clammy skin
○ Asymmetrical chest movement
○ Decreased tactile fremitus over an obstructed bronchi or pleural effusion
○ Increased tactile fremitus over consolidated lung tissue
○ Hyperresonance
○ Diminished or absent breath sounds
○ Wheezes (in asthma)
○ Rhonchi (in bronchitis)
○ Crackles (in pulmonary edema)

Test results

Laboratory

○ ABG analysis revealing hypercapnia and hypoxemia
○ Increased serum white blood cell count in bacterial infections
○ Serum hemoglobin and hematocrit showing decreased oxygen-carrying capacity
○ Serum electrolyte results revealing hypokalemia and hypochloremia
○ Blood cultures, Gram stain, and sputum cultures showing the pathogen (see *Identifying respiratory failure*)

Imaging

○ Chest X-rays may show underlying pulmonary diseases or conditions, such as emphysema, atelectasis, lesions, pneumothorax, infiltrates, and effusions.

Diagnostic procedures

○ Electrocardiography may show arrhythmias, cor pulmonale, and myocardial ischemia.
○ Pulse oximetry may show decreased arterial oxygen saturation.

- Pulmonary artery catheterization may show pulmonary or cardiovascular causes of acute respiratory failure.

Treatment

General

- Mechanical ventilation with an endotracheal or a tracheostomy tube
- High-frequency ventilation, if the patient doesn't respond to conventional mechanical ventilation
- Fluid restriction with heart failure
- Activity as tolerated

Medication

- Cautious oxygen therapy to increase partial pressure of arterial oxygen
- Antacids
- Histamine-receptor antagonists, as ordered
- Antibiotics
- Bronchodilators
- Corticosteroids
- Positive inotropic agents
- Vasopressors
- Diuretics

Surgery

- Possible tracheostomy

Nursing considerations

Key outcomes

The patient will:
- maintain a patent airway
- maintain adequate ventilation
- use a support system to assist with coping
- maintain skin integrity
- express feelings of increased comfort
- modify lifestyle to minimize the risk of decreased tissue perfusion.

Nursing interventions

- Give prescribed drugs.
- Orient the patient frequently.
- Administer oxygen, as ordered.
- Maintain a patent airway.
- Encourage pursed-lip breathing.
- Encourage the use of an incentive spirometer.
- Reposition the patient every 1 to 2 hours.
- Help clear the patient's secretions with postural drainage and chest physiotherapy.
- Assist with or perform oral hygiene.
- Position the patient for comfort and optimal gas exchange.
- Maintain normothermia.
- Schedule care to provide frequent rest periods.

If the patient requires mechanical ventilation

- Obtain blood samples for ABG analysis, as ordered.
- Suction the trachea after hyperoxygenation, as needed.
- Provide humidification.
- Secure the endotracheal (ET) tube per facility policy.
- Prevent infection.
- Prevent tracheal erosion.
- Maintain skin integrity.
- Provide alternative communication means.
- Provide sedation, as necessary.

Monitoring

- Vital signs and pulse oximetry
- Intake and output
- Laboratory studies
- Daily weight
- Cardiac rate and rhythm
- Respiratory status (breath sounds and ABG results)
- Chest X-ray results
- Complications
- Sputum quality, consistency, and color
- Signs and symptoms of infection

If the patient requires mechanical ventilation

- Ventilator settings
- Cuff pressures
- Complications of mechanical ventilation
- ET tube position and patency
- Signs and symptoms of stress ulcers

Patient teaching

Be sure to cover:
- the disorder, diagnosis, and treatment
- drugs and potential adverse reactions
- when to notify the physician
- smoking cessation, if appropriate
- communication techniques, if intubated
- signs and symptoms of respiratory infection.

Discharge planning

- Refer the patient to a smoking-cessation program, if applicable.

Acute tubular necrosis

Overview

Description
- Injury to the nephron's tubular segment resulting from ischemic or nephrotoxic injury and causes renal failure and uremic syndrome
- Also known as *acute tubulointerstitial nephritis*

Pathophysiology
- In ischemic injury, circulatory collapse, severe hypotension, trauma, hemorrhage, dehydration, cardiogenic or septic shock, surgery, anesthetics, and reactions to transfusions may cause disruption of blood flow to the kidneys.
- Nephrotoxic injury may follow ingestion of certain chemical agents, such as contrast medium or antibiotics, or result from a hypersensitive reaction of the kidneys.

Causes
- Diseased tubular epithelium
- Obstructed urine flow
- Ischemic injury to glomerular epithelial cells or vascular endothelium

Incidence
- Accounts for about 75% of acute renal failure cases
- The most common cause of acute renal failure in critically ill patients

Common characteristics
- Decreased urine output
- Hyperkalemia
- Uremic syndrome with oliguria or, rarely, anuria

Complications
- Heart failure
- Uremic pericarditis
- Pulmonary edema
- Uremic lung
- Anemia
- Anorexia, intractable vomiting
- Poor wound healing due to debilitation

 Alert

Fever and chills may signal the onset of an infection, the leading cause of death in acute tubular necrosis.

Assessment

Diagnosis is usually delayed until the condition has progressed to an advanced stage.

History
- Ischemic or nephrotoxic injury
- Low urine output (less than 400 ml/24 hours)
- Fever and chills

Physical findings
- Evidence of bleeding abnormalities, such as petechiae and ecchymosis
- Dry, pruritic skin
- Dry mucous membranes
- Uremic breath
- Cardiac arrhythmia, if hyperkalemic
- Muscle weakness

Test results
Laboratory
- Urinary sediment contains red blood cells (RBCs) and casts
- Low urine specific gravity (1.010)
- Low urine osmolality (less than 400 mOsm/kg)
- High urine sodium level (40 to 60 mEq/L)
- Elevated blood urea nitrogen and serum creatinine levels
- Anemia
- Defects in platelet adherence
- Metabolic acidosis
- Hyperkalemia

Diagnostic procedures
- Electrocardiogram may show arrhythmias and, with hyperkalemia, a widening QRS complex, disappearing P waves, and tall, peaked T waves.

Treatment

General
Acute phase
- Vigorous supportive measures until normal kidney function resumes

Long-term management
- Daily replacement of projected and calculated fluid loss (including insensible loss)
- Peritoneal dialysis or hemodialysis if the patient is catabolic or if hyperkalemia and fluid volume overload aren't controlled by other measures
- Fluid restriction
- Low-sodium, low-potassium diet
- Rest periods when fatigued

Medication
- Diuretics
- Transfusion of packed RBCs
- Epoetin alfa
- Antibiotics
- Emergency I.V. administration of 50% glucose, regular insulin, and sodium bicarbonate (with hyperkalemia)
- Sodium polystyrene sulfonate with sorbitol by mouth or enema (with hyperkalemia)

Nursing considerations

Key outcomes

The patient will:
- maintain fluid balance
- maintain hemodynamic stability
- maintain urine specific gravity within the designated limits
- have improved kidney function.

Nursing interventions

- Give prescribed drugs and blood products.
- Restrict food containing high sodium and potassium levels.
- Use aseptic technique, particularly when handling catheters.
- Perform passive range-of-motion exercises.
- Provide good skin care.

Monitoring

- Intake and output
- Vital signs
- Laboratory studies
- Complications

Patient teaching

Be sure to cover:
- the disorder, diagnosis, and treatment
- signs of infection and when to report them to the physician
- dietary restrictions
- how to set goals that are realistic for the patient's prognosis.

Discharge planning

- Refer the patient to appropriate supportive services or social service.

Adrenal hypofunction

Overview

Description

- Primary adrenal hypofunction or insufficiency (Addison's disease) originating within the adrenal gland and characterized by the decreased secretion of mineralocorticoids, glucocorticoids, and androgens
- Secondary adrenal hypofunction due to a disorder outside the gland such as impaired pituitary secretion of corticotropin; characterized by decreased glucocorticoid secretion
- Adrenal crisis (addisonian crisis), a critical deficiency of mineralocorticoids and glucocorticoids generally following acute stress, sepsis, trauma, surgery, or the omission of steroid therapy in patients who have chronic adrenal insufficiency; adrenal crisis, a medical emergency that needs immediate, vigorous treatment

Pathophysiology

- Results from the partial or complete destruction of the adrenal cortex
- Manifests as a clinical syndrome in which the symptoms are associated with deficient production of the adrenocortical hormones cortisol, aldosterone, and androgen
- High levels of corticotropin and corticotropin-releasing hormone
- Addison's disease: involves all zones of the cortex, causing deficiencies of the adrenocortical secretions, glucocorticoids, androgens, and mineralocorticoids
- Cortisol deficiency: causes decreased liver gluconeogenesis (the formation of glucose from molecules that aren't carbohydrates); resulting low blood glucose levels can become dangerously low in patients who take insulin routinely
- Aldosterone deficiency: causes increased renal sodium loss and enhances potassium reabsorption
- Hypotension due to sodium excretion
- Increased production of angiotensin II due to low plasma volume and arteriolar pressure
- Androgen deficiency: may decrease hair growth in axillary and pubic areas (less noticeable in men) as well as on the extremities of women

Causes

Primary hypofunction
- Autoimmune process in which circulating antibodies react specifically against the adrenal tissue
- Tuberculosis (once the chief cause, now responsible for less than 20% of adult cases)
- Bilateral adrenalectomy
- Hemorrhage into the adrenal gland
- Neoplasms
- Infections (histoplasmosis, cytomegalovirus)

- Family history of autoimmune disease (may predispose the patient to Addison's disease and other endocrinopathies)

Secondary hypofunction
- Hypopituitarism
- Abrupt withdrawal of long-term corticosteroid therapy
- Removal of a corticotropin-secreting tumor

Adrenal crisis
- Exhausted body stores of glucocorticoids in a patient with adrenal hypofunction after trauma, surgery, or other physiologic stress

Incidence

Primary hypofunction
- Relatively uncommon
- Can occur at any age and in both sexes

Autoimmune Addison's disease
- Most common in white females (genetic predisposition is likely)
- More common in patients with a familial predisposition to autoimmune endocrine diseases

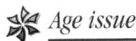 *Age issue*

Most people with Addison's disease are diagnosed in their 20s to 40s.

Common characteristics

Primary hypofunction
- Conspicuous bronze color of the skin
- Darkening of scars, areas of vitiligo (absence of pigmentation), and increased pigmentation of the mucous membranes, especially the buccal mucosa
- Decreased tolerance for even minor stress
- Fasting hypoglycemia
- Craving for salty food

Secondary hypofunction
- Similar to primary hypofunction, but without hyperpigmentation

Addisonian crisis
- Profound weakness and fatigue
- Nausea, vomiting, and dehydration
- Hypotension
- High fever followed by hypothermia (occasionally)

Complications

- Hyperpyrexia
- Psychotic reactions
- Deficient or excessive steroid treatment
- Shock
- Profound hypoglycemia
- Ultimate vascular collapse, renal shutdown, coma, and death (if untreated)

Assessment

History

- Synthetic steroid use, adrenal surgery, or recent infection
- Muscle weakness
- Fatigue
- Weight loss
- Craving for salty food
- Decreased tolerance for stress
- GI disturbances
- Dehydration
- Amenorrhea (in women)
- Impotence (in men)

Physical findings

- Poor coordination
- Decreased axillary and pubic hair (in women)
- Bronze coloration of the skin, darkening of scars
- Areas of vitiligo
- Increased pigmentation of mucous membranes
- Weak irregular pulse
- Hypotension

Test results

Laboratory

- Rapid corticotropin stimulation test: low corticotropin level indicates a secondary disorder; elevated level indicates a primary disorder
- Decreased plasma cortisol level (less than 10 mcg/dl in the morning; less in the evening)
- Decreased serum sodium and fasting blood glucose levels
- Increased serum potassium, calcium, and blood urea nitrogen levels
- Elevated hematocrit; increased lymphocyte and eosinophil counts

Imaging

- Chest X-ray showing small heart
- Computed tomography scan of the abdomen showing adrenal calcification (if the cause is infectious)

Treatment

General

- I.V. fluids
- Periods of rest
- Small, frequent, high-protein meals

Medication

- Lifelong corticosteroid replacement, usually with cortisone or hydrocortisone
- Oral fludrocortisone
- Hydrocortisone
- I.V. saline and glucose solutions (for adrenal crisis)

Nursing considerations

Key outcomes

The patient will:

- maintain stable vital signs
- maintain an adequate fluid balance
- remain free from signs and symptoms of infection
- develop adequate coping skills.

Nursing interventions

- Until onset of mineralocorticoid effect, encourage fluids to replace excessive fluid loss.
- Arrange for a diet that maintains sodium and potassium balances; if the patient is anorexic, suggest six small meals per day to increase caloric intake.
- Observe for cushingoid signs such as fluid retention around the eyes and face.
- Check for petechiae.
- If the patient receives glucocorticoids alone, observe for orthostatic hypotension or electrolyte abnormalities.

Monitoring

- Vital signs
- Signs of shock (decreased level of consciousness and urine output)
- Hyperkalemia before treatment; hypokalemia after treatment
- Cardiac rhythm
- Blood glucose levels
- Daily weight
- Intake and output

Patient teaching

Be sure to cover:

- lifelong steroid therapy requirement
- symptoms of steroid overdose (swelling, weight gain) and steroid underdose (lethargy, weakness)
- dosage may need to be increased during times of stress or illness (when the patient has a cold, for example)
- infection, injury, or profuse sweating in hot weather may precipitate adrenal crisis
- importance of carrying a medical identification card that states the patient is on steroid therapy (name of the drug and its dosage should be included on the card)
- how to give a hydrocortisone injection and to keep an emergency kit containing hydrocortisone in a prepared syringe available for use in times of stress
- stress management techniques.

Discharge planning

- Refer the patient to the National Adrenal Diseases Foundation for support and information.

Adrenogenital syndrome

Overview

Description

○ A group of disorders resulting from hyperplasia of the adrenal cortex
○ May be inherited (congenital adrenal hyperplasia [CAH]) or acquired, usually as a result of an adrenal tumor (adrenal virilism)
○ May cause fatal adrenal crisis in neonates (salt-losing CAH)

Pathophysiology

○ Deficiencies occur in the enzymes needed for adrenocortical secretion of cortisol and, possibly, aldosterone.
○ Compensatory secretion of corticotropin produces varying degrees of adrenal hyperplasia.

Simple virilizing CAH

○ Deficiency of the enzyme 21-hydroxylase results in underproduction of cortisol.
○ This cortisol deficiency stimulates increased secretion of corticotropin, producing large amounts of cortisol precursors and androgens that don't require 21-hydroxylase for synthesis.

Salt-losing CAH

○ 21-hydroxylase is almost completely absent.
○ Corticotropin secretion increases, causing excessive production of cortisol precursors, including salt-wasting compounds.
○ Plasma cortisol and aldosterone levels — both dependent on 21-hydroxylase — fall precipitously and, in combination with the excessive production of salt-wasting compounds, precipitate acute adrenal crisis.
○ Corticotropin hypersecretion stimulates adrenal androgens and produces masculinization.

Causes

○ Transmitted as an autosomal recessive trait

Incidence

○ Acquired adrenal virilism is rare and affects twice as many females as males.

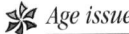 **Age issue**

CAH is the most prevalent adrenal disorder in infants and children; simple virilizing CAH and salt-losing CAH are the most common forms.

Common characteristics

Simple virilizing CAH

○ Ambiguous genitalia but normal genital tract and gonads (Female neonates may present with labioscrotal fusion and an enlarged clitoris with a urethral opening at its base.)

Salt-losing CAH

FEMALES

○ More complete virilization than the simple form
○ Results in development of male external genitalia without testes

MALES

○ No external genital abnormalities
○ Difficult immediate neonatal diagnosis; commonly delayed until the infant develops severe systemic symptoms

Complications

○ Hypertension
○ Hyperkalemic infertility
○ Adrenal tumor
○ Adrenal crisis
○ Altered growth, external genitalia, and sexual maturity

Salt-losing CAH

○ Cardiovascular collapse
○ Cardiac arrest

Assessment

History

Simple virilizing CAH

○ Failure to begin menstruation (in females)
○ Frequent erections at an early age (in males)

Salt-losing CAH

○ Apathy, failure to eat, and diarrhea (in infants)
○ Symptoms of adrenal crisis in the first week of life (vomiting, dehydration from hyponatremia, hyperkalemia)

Physical findings

○ Pseudohermaphroditism in females or precocious puberty in both sexes strongly suggests CAH

Salt-losing CAH

○ Signs of progressive virilization at an early age: early appearance of pubic and axillary hair, deep voice, acne, facial hair
○ Small testes
○ Possibly taller than other children of the same age

Test results

Laboratory

○ Elevated levels of plasma 17-ketosteroids (17-KS), which can be suppressed by administering oral dexamethasone
○ Elevated urinary levels of hormone metabolites, particularly pregnanetriol
○ Elevated plasma 17-hydroxyprogesterone level
○ Normal or decreased urinary levels of 17-hydroxycorticosteroids

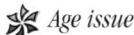 *Age issue*

Diagnostic procedures
○ Gonadal biopsy and chromosomal studies to confirm
hermaphrodism
Other
○ Sex chromatin and karyotype studies: determine the
genetic sex of patients with ambiguous external genitalia

Treatment

General
○ Well-balanced diet
○ No activity restriction

Medication
Simple virilizing CAH
○ Daily administration of cortisone or hydrocortisone
Salt-losing CAH with patient in adrenal crisis
○ Immediate I.V. sodium chloride and glucose infusion
○ Desoxycorticosterone I.M. and hydrocortisone I.V.
○ Maintenance includes mineralocorticoid (desoxycor-
ticosterone, fludrocortisone, or both) and glucocor-
ticoid (cortisone or hydrocortisone) replacement

Surgery
○ Reconstructive surgery based on the determined sex
and external genitalia

Nursing considerations

Key outcomes
The patient will:
○ maintain stable vital signs
○ maintain adequate fluid balance
○ have normal laboratory test results
○ express understanding of the disorder and treatment
modality, as will his family.

Nursing interventions
○ Maintain I.V. access, infuse fluids, and give steroids,
as ordered.
○ Watch for cyanosis, hypotension, tachycardia, tachypnea, and signs of shock.
○ Minimize external stressors.
○ If a child is receiving maintenance therapy with
steroid injections, rotate I.M. injection sites to prevent atrophy; tell the parents to do the same.

Monitoring
○ Body weight
○ Blood pressure
○ Serum electrolyte levels
○ Edema, weakness, and hypertension for the patient
receiving desoxycorticosterone or fludrocortisone

Patient teaching

Be sure to cover:
○ possible adverse effects (cushingoid symptoms) of
long-term therapy (lifelong maintenance therapy with
hydrocortisone, cortisone, or the mineralocorticoid
fludrocortisone is essential)
○ importance of not withdrawing therapeutic drugs
suddenly because potentially fatal adrenal hypofunction will result
○ need to report stress and infection, which require increased steroid dosages
○ importance of carrying a medical identification card
that states the patient is on steroid therapy (name of
the drug and its dosage should be included on the
card).

Discharge planning
○ Refer for psychological counseling to help accept this
disorder.

Age-related macular degeneration

Overview

Description

○ Deterioration of the macular portion of the retina, which is responsible for detailed vision
○ May be atrophic, also called *involutional* or *dry*
○ May be exudative, also called *hemorrhagic* or *wet*
○ No cure for atrophic form
○ Commonly affects both eyes
○ Also known as *AMD*

Pathophysiology

○ Pathologic changes occur primarily in the retinal pigment epithelium, Bruch's membrane, and choriocapillaries in the macular region that result from the hardening and obstruction of retinal arteries.
○ Formation of new blood vessels in the macular area obscures central vision.
○ Visual loss occurs as the retinal pigment epithelium detaches and becomes atrophic.
○ Exudative macular degeneration develops as new blood vessels in the choroid project through abnormalities in Bruch's membrane, invading the potential space underneath the retinal pigment epithelium.
○ The vessels leak, and fluid in the retinal pigment epithelium increases, resulting in blurry vision.

Causes

○ Unknown
○ Genetic in origin

Risk factors

○ Smoking
○ Age
○ Race
○ High blood pressure
○ Vascular disease
○ High intake of saturated fat and cholesterol
○ Farsightedness
○ Exposure to sunlight

Incidence

○ Affects more than 10 million Americans
○ Leading cause of blindness in people older than age 55 in the United States
○ Irreversible central vision loss in at least 10% of elderly people
○ Atrophic form in about 70% of patients
○ More common in whites, but affects all races

Common characteristics

○ Decreased central vision, for near and distance (see *How AMD affects central vision*)
○ Progressive worsening
○ Blind spots

Complications

○ Blindness
○ Nystagmus

How AMD affects central vision

Central vision occurs in the macula and involves the ability to perceive sharp, detailed images. At the center of the macula is the fovea — containing the highest concentration of rods and cones — and the most light-sensitive portion of the macula.

Light entering the cornea and lens are focused on the fovea. If any part of the macula deteriorates, the eye must rely on the less-sensitive, outer portion of the retina, which is responsible for peripheral vision.

With age-related macular degeneration, grayness, haziness, or a blind spot may appear in the area of central vision. Words may be blurred on a page; straight lines may appear to have kinks in them; colors may seem dimmer.

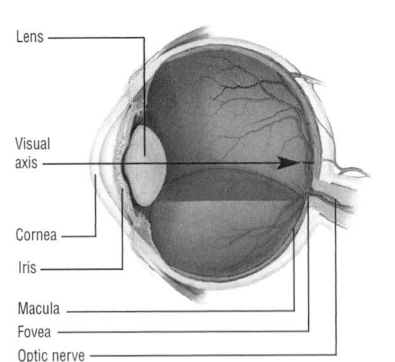

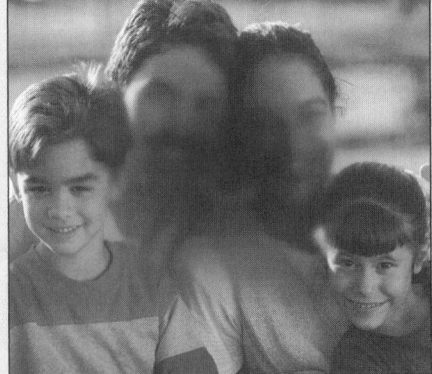

Assessment

History

- Sees blank spot in the center of a page (scotoma) while reading
- Central vision blurs intermittently and has gradually worsened
- Straight lines appear distorted
- Letters appear fragmented

Physical findings

- Tiny yellowish spots (drusen) beneath retina

Test results

Diagnostic procedures

- Indirect ophthalmoscopy may show changes in the macular region of the fundus.
- Fluorescein angiography may show leaking vessels in subretinal neovascular net.
- Amsler grid test may detect visual distortion.

Treatment

General

- Laser treatment, if leaking blood vessels have developed away from the fovea
- Diet high in vitamins A, C, and E; beta-carotene; and zinc
- Activity restrictions based on visual acuity

Medication

- Zinc supplements
- Lutein, vitamins C and E, and beta-carotene (investigational)

Surgery

- In exudative form, argon laser photocoagulation (may slow the progression of severe visual loss)

Nursing considerations

Key outcomes

The patient will:
- express feelings and concerns over diminishing eyesight
- sustain no harm or injury
- verbalize understanding of the condition and treatment
- maintain optimal visual function or adapt as necessary.

Nursing interventions

- Help the patient to obtain optical aids such as magnifiers.
- Offer the patient emotional support.
- Encourage expression of fears and concerns.

Monitoring

- Visual acuity
- Environment (for safety purposes)

Patient teaching

Be sure to cover:
- ways to modify the home environment for safety
- affects on peripheral vision.

Discharge planning

- Refer the patient to the American Foundation for the Blind or Associated Services for the Blind, as indicated.
- Refer the patient to a local support group.

Alcoholism

Overview

Description

- Chronic disorder of uncontrolled intake of alcoholic beverages
- Interferes with physical and mental health, social and familial relationships, and occupational responsibilities

Pathophysiology

- Alcohol is soluble in water and lipids and permeates all body tissues.
- Liver metabolizes 90% of alcohol absorbed and is the most severely affected organ; hepatic steatosis followed by hepatic fibrosis is evident days after heavy drinking.
- Laennec's cirrhosis may develop after inflammatory response (alcoholic hepatitis) or in absence of inflammation, as a consequence of direct activation of lipocytes (Ito cells).
- Lactic acidosis and excess uric acid is promoted; gluconeogenesis, B-oxidation of fatty acids, and the Krebs cycle are opposed; and hypoglycemia and hyperlipidemia develop.
- Toxicity of cells occurs through reduction of mitochondrial oxygenation utilization, depletion of deoxyribonucleic acid, and other actions.

Causes

- Biological factors
- Psychological factors
- Sociocultural factors

Risk factors

- Male gender
- Low socioeconomic status
- Family history
- Depression
- Anxiety
- History of other substance abuse disorders

Incidence

- Affects all social and economic groups
- 10% of the population accounts for 50% of all alcohol consumed
- About 13% of all adults older than age 18 have suffered from alcohol abuse or dependence
- Males are two to five times more likely to abuse alcohol than females
- Occurs at all stages of the life cycle, beginning as early as elementary school age
- Prevalent in 20% of adult hospital inpatients

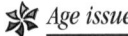 *Age issue*

Prevalence of drinking is highest between ages 21 and 34, but current statistics show that up to 19% of 12- to 17-year-olds have serious drinking problems. Research also suggests that alcoholism affects 2% to 10% of adults older than age 60.

Common characteristics

- Hide or deny addiction
- May temporarily manage to maintain a functional lifestyle

Complications

- Cardiomyopathy
- Pneumonia
- Cirrhosis
- Esophageal varices
- Pancreatitis
- Alcoholic dementia
- Wernicke's encephalopathy
- Seizure disorder
- Depression
- Multiple substance abuse
- Hypoglycemia
- Leg and foot ulcers
- Suicide and homicide
- Death

Assessment

History

- Need for daily or episodic alcohol use for adequate function
- Inability to discontinue or reduce alcohol intake
- Episodes of anesthesia or amnesia during intoxication
- Episodes of violence during intoxication
- Interference with social and familial relationships and occupational responsibilities
- Malaise, dyspepsia, mood swings or depression, and an increased incidence of infection
- Secretive behavior

Physical findings

- Poor personal hygiene
- Unusually high tolerance for sedatives and opioids
- Signs of nutritional deficiency
- Signs of injury
- Withdrawal signs and symptoms
- Major motor seizures

DSM-IV-TR criteria

A diagnosis is confirmed when the patient meets at least three of these signs and symptoms:

- more alcohol ingested than intended
- persistent desire or efforts to diminish alcohol use
- excessive time spent obtaining alcohol
- frequent intoxication or withdrawal symptoms
- impairment of social, occupational, or recreational activities

- continued alcohol consumption despite knowledge of a social, psychological, or physical problem that's caused or exacerbated by alcohol use
- marked tolerance
- characteristic withdrawal symptoms
- alcohol used to relieve or avoid withdrawal symptoms
- persistent symptoms for at least 1 month or recurrence over a longer time.

Test results

Laboratory
- Blood alcohol tests show levels of at least 0.10% weight/volume (200 mg/dl)
- Abnormal serum electrolyte levels
- Increased serum ammonia levels
- Increased serum amylase levels
- Urine toxicology (may show abuses of other drugs)
- Abnormal liver function study results

Other

- CAGE screening test: two affirmative responses make patient 7 times more likely to be alcohol dependent
- Alcohol disorders identification test (AUDIT): score greater than 8 indicates alcohol dependency
- Michigan alcohol screening test (MAST): score greater than 5 indicates alcohol dependency

Treatment

General

Immediate
- Support respiration
- Prevent aspiration of vomitus
- Replace fluids
- Give I.V. glucose
- Correct hypothermia or acidosis
- Treat for trauma, infection, or GI bleeding

Long-term
- Total abstinence
- Detoxification, rehabilitation, and aftercare program
- Supportive counseling
- Individual, group, or family psychotherapy
- Ongoing support groups
- Well-balanced diet
- Safety precautions, including preventing aspiration of vomitus
- Seizure precautions

Medication

- Anticonvulsants
- Antiemetics
- Antidiarrheals
- Tranquilizers, particularly benzodiazepines
- Naltrexone
- Antipsychotics
- Daily oral disulfiram
- Vitamin supplements

Nursing considerations

Key outcomes

The patient (or family) will:
- report feeling safe in hospital environment
- join gradually in self-care and the decision-making process
- engage in appropriate social interaction with others
- demonstrate a decrease in negative self-evaluation verbally and behaviorally
- identify support systems to assist them and participate in mobilizing these systems.

Nursing interventions

- Institute seizure precautions.
- Give prescribed drugs.
- Orient the patient to reality.
- Maintain a calm environment, minimizing noise and shadows.
- Avoid restraints, unless necessary for protection.
- Use a nonthreatening approach.

Monitoring

- Mental status
- Vital signs
- Safety measures
- Nutritional and hydration status
- Intake and output

Patient teaching

Be sure to cover:
- the disorder, diagnosis, and treatment
- alcohol abstinence
- plan for relapse
- drug administration, dosage, and possible adverse effects
- effects of disorder on significant others.

Discharge planning

- Refer the patient to a rehabilitation program.
- Refer the patient to social services.
- Refer the patient to support services.
- Refer the patient to personal and family counseling.

Allergic purpura

Overview

Description

- An acute or chronic vascular inflammation affecting the skin, joints, and GI and genitourinary (GU) tracts, in association with allergy symptoms
- Purpura associated with other conditions such as erythema nodosum
- A nonthrombocytopenic purpura
- Known as *Henoch-Schönlein syndrome* or *anaphylactoid purpura* when it primarily affects the GI tract and is accompanied by joint pain

Pathophysiology

- An autoimmune reaction directed against vascular walls, triggered by a bacterial infection
- An inflammation of the veins and capillaries disrupts the vascular wall, resulting in loss of red blood cells and bleeding and leakage into the skin and mucous membranes

Causes

- Bacterial infection (particularly streptococcal infection)
- Allergic reactions to some drugs and vaccines, insect bites, and foods (such as wheat, eggs, milk, and chocolate)

Incidence

- Affects more males than females
- Most prevalent in children ages 3 to 7

Common characteristics

- Skin lesions that are purple, macular, ecchymotic, and of varying size and are caused by vascular leakage into the skin and mucous membranes (see *Identifying purpuric lesions*)

Identifying purpuric lesions

Lesions of allergic purpura, such as those pictured on the foot and leg below, characteristically vary in size.

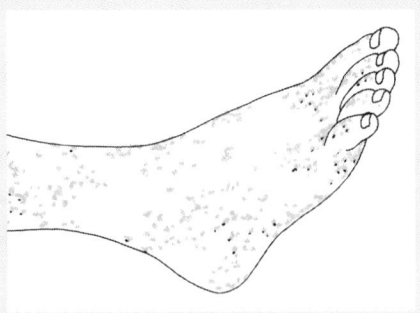

Henoch-Schönlein syndrome

- Transient or severe colic
- Tenesmus (spasmodic contraction of the anal sphincter)
- GI bleeding
- Rheumatoid pains and periarticular effusions, usually affecting the legs and feet

Complications

- Renal disease (renal failure and acute glomerulonephritis)
- Hypertension

Assessment

History

- Bacterial infection or exposure to allergen
- Moderate and irregular fever
- Headache
- Anorexia
- Pruritus and paresthesia in areas of lesions

Physical findings

- Characteristic lesions that usually appear in symmetric patterns on the arms, legs, and buttocks
- In children, urticarial skin lesions that expand and become hemorrhagic
- Possibly scattered petechiae on the legs, buttocks, and perineum
- Localized edema of the hands, feet, or scalp

Test results

Laboratory
- Results of tests for blood in the urine and stool may be positive.
- Increased blood urea nitrogen and creatinine levels may indicate renal involvement.

 Alert

No laboratory test clearly identifies allergic purpura (although white blood cell count and erythrocyte sedimentation rate are elevated).

Imaging
- Small bowel X-rays may reveal areas of transient edema.

Other
- Clinical evaluation

Treatment

General

- Symptomatic

Medication

- Steroids
- Analgesics

Nursing considerations

Key outcomes

The patient will:

○ express feelings of comfort and relief of pain
○ exhibit improved or healed lesions
○ identify precipitating factors with appropriate skin care regimen.

Nursing interventions

○ Encourage maintenance of an elimination diet to help identify specific allergenic foods.
○ Provide analgesics, as needed.
○ Provide passive range-of-motion exercises, if appropriate.
○ Provide emotional support and reassurance, especially if the patient is temporarily disfigured by florid skin lesions.

Monitoring

○ Condition and number of skin lesions
○ Level of pain
○ GI and GU complications

Patient teaching

Be sure to cover:

○ need for the patient to immediately report any recurrence of symptoms (most common about 6 weeks after initial symptoms)
○ importance of returning for follow-up urinalysis as scheduled.

Allergic rhinitis

Overview

Description

○ An immune response of the upper airways triggered by inhaled airborne allergens.
○ Seasonal allergic rhinitis is an immunoglobulin (Ig) E-mediated type I hypersensitivity response to an environmental antigen (allergen) in a genetically susceptible person.
○ In perennial rhinitis, inhaled allergens provoke antigen responses that produce signs and symptoms year-round.

Pathophysiology

○ The body's immune system overresponds to common allergens in the nose.
○ Antibodies attach to mast cells, which release several chemicals, including histamine, which cause dilation of blood vessels, skin redness, and swollen membranes in the nose.

Causes

Seasonal allergic rhinitis
○ Tree pollens (in spring)
○ Grass and weed pollens (in summer)
○ Weed pollens (in fall)
○ Mold spores (occasionally, in summer and fall)
Perennial allergic rhinitis
○ House dust and dust mites
○ Molds
○ Animal dander
○ Tobacco smoke
○ Processed materials or industrial chemicals

Incidence

○ Affects more than 20 million Americans
○ Can affect anyone at any age
○ Most prevalent in young children and adolescents

Common characteristics

○ Swollen nasal membranes

Complications

○ Secondary sinus and middle ear infections
○ Nasal polyps

Assessment

History

Seasonal allergic rhinitis
○ Paroxysmal sneezing, profuse watery rhinorrhea
○ Nasal obstruction or congestion
○ Pruritus of the nose and eyes
○ Headache or sinus pain
○ Itchy throat, malaise, and fever

Perennial allergic rhinitis
○ Chronic and extensive nasal obstruction or stuffiness

Physical findings

Seasonal allergic rhinitis
○ Pale, cyanotic, edematous nasal mucosa
○ Red and edematous eyelids and conjunctivae
○ Excessive lacrimation
Perennial allergic rhinitis
○ Nasal polyps
○ Dark circles under the eyes (allergic shiners)

Test results

Laboratory
○ High number of eosinophils in sputum and nasal secretions
○ Normal or elevated IgE levels, possibly linked to seasonal overproduction of interleukin-4 and -5 (involved in the allergic inflammatory process)

Treatment

General

○ Eliminate environmental antigens, if possible
○ Increased fluid intake to loosen secretions
○ Restrict activities in areas of allergen exposure

Medication

○ Antihistamines
○ Intranasal corticosteroids
○ Nasal decongestants
Long-term management
○ Immunotherapy or desensitization with injections of allergen extracts administered before or during the allergy season or perennially

Nursing considerations

Key outcomes

The patient (or family) will:
○ maintain current health status
○ verbalize feelings and concerns
○ express feelings of increased comfort.

Nursing interventions

○ Implement measures to relieve signs and symptoms and increase the patient's comfort.
○ Encourage increased fluid intake to loosen secretions.
○ Elevate the head of the bed and provide humidification to ease breathing.

 Alert

Before giving a desensitization injection, assess the patient's symptoms. After giving the injection, observe him for 30 minutes to detect adverse reactions, including anaphylaxis and severe localized

erythema. Make sure epinephrine and emergency resuscitation equipment are available.

Monitoring

○ Compliance with the prescribed drug regimen
○ Changes in control of signs and symptoms
○ Indications of drug misuse

Patient teaching

Be sure to cover:
○ importance of calling the physician if the patient experiences a delayed reaction to the desensitizing injections
○ reduction of environmental exposure to airborne allergens
○ skin protectant applications
○ possible lifestyle changes, such as relocation to a pollen-free area either seasonally or year-round, in severe and resistant allergic rhinitis
○ medication dosage, administration, and adverse effects.

Alopecia

Overview

Description

- More commonly known as *hair loss*, typically occurs on the scalp; less common and conspicuous elsewhere on the body
- Can be irreversible because scarring alopecia usually destroys hair follicle
- Nonscarring form (noncicatricial alopecia) can generally regrow hair
- Most common form of nonscarring alopecia known as male-pattern alopecia or androcentric alopecia
- Telogen effluvium: a diffuse alopecia in which numerous hair follicles simultaneously change from the growing anagen phase to the resting telogen phase of the hair growth cycle
- Alopecia areata (idiopathic form): a generally reversible and self-limiting disorder most prevalent in young and middle-aged adults of both sexes
- Genetic predisposition commonly influences time of onset, degree of baldness, speed with which it spreads, and pattern of hair loss
- Poor prognosis for regrowth with hair loss that persists for more than 1 year

Pathophysiology

- In male-pattern alopecia, a genetically predisposed response to androgens causes transformation of the androgen-sensitive follicles into vellus follicles; normal hair is shed and replaced by fine, light, short hair.
- In female-pattern alopecia, there's commonly an elevation in serum adrenal androgen dehydroepiandrosterone sulfate.

Causes

Nonscarring alopecia
- Genetic predisposition
- Androgen response
- Aging
- Radiation
- Chemotherapy
- Drugs (see *Cancer drugs that cause alopecia*)
- Bacterial and fungal infections
- Psoriasis
- Seborrhea
- Endocrine disorders
- Excess vitamin A

Scarring alopecia
- Physical or chemical trauma
- Radiation
- Chemotherapy
- Chronic tension on a hair shaft
- Destructive skin tumors
- Granulomas
- Lupus erythematosus
- Scleroderma
- Follicular lichen planus
- Severe bacterial or viral infections

Incidence

- Affects males more than females
- Occurs most frequently in males older than age 50 in male-pattern alopecia
- Rises with increasing age in male-pattern alopecia
- Occurs to some degree in 37% of postmenopausal women

Common characteristics

- Hair loss

Complications

- Impaired self-image

Assessment

History

Male-pattern alopecia
- Presence of predisposing factors
- Family history of hair loss
- Gradual onset of hair loss
- Typically describes hairline as receding and his crown becoming bald

Female-pattern alopecia
- Typically describes a widening of her part and increasing visibility of her front scalp or crown

Telogen effluvium
- Loss of about 400 hairs per day, which is four to five times greater than the normal daily hair loss

Alopecia areata
- Sudden loss of hair

Physical findings

- Small patches of visible scalp or the entire scalp may be visible (alopecia totalis); hair loss may involve the entire body (alopecia universalis).
- Although mild erythema may occur initially, affected areas of scalp or skin appear normal.
- "Exclamation point" hairs (loose hairs with dark, rough, brushlike tips on narrow, less pigmented shafts) occur at the periphery of new patches.
- Regrowth initially appears as fine, white, downy hair, which is replaced by normal hair.

Test results

Laboratory
- Direct microscopic examination showing structural abnormalities or signs of infection

Diagnostic procedures

TELOGEN EFFLUVIUM
- Pluck or pull test reveals positive results if more than four hairs come out.
- Wood's lamp examination shows presence of fungal infection.
- Trichogram shows abnormal ratio of anagen to telogen hairs.

Cancer drugs that cause alopecia

Certain cancer drugs can cause hair loss ranging from sporadic thinning to complete baldness. Some drugs damage hair follicles and cause hair roots to atrophy.

Mild alopecia
- bleomycin
- carmustine
- fluorouracil
- hydroxyurea
- melphalan

Moderate alopecia
- busulfan
- etoposide
- floxuridine
- methotrexate
- mitomycin

Severe alopecia
- cyclophosphamide
- daunorubicin
- doxorubicin
- vinblastine
- vincristine

- Scalp biopsy shows hair phase and the extent of structural damage.

Treatment

General

- Identification and treatment of underlying cause
- Cosmetic interventions, such as hairpieces, weaving, or bonding
- Occlusive dressing promotes normal hair growth by protecting the site of hair loss (in trichotillomania)
- Cold cap application and scalp tourniquet that reduce the blood supply to the scalp and thereby preserve more hair structure

Medication

- Topical application of minoxidil
- Oral finasteride

 Alert

Finasteride is contraindicated in women of childbearing age.

- Corticosteroids
- Photochemotherapy with methoxsalen and ultraviolet light
- Dermatomucosal agents
- Antibiotics
- Antifungal agents

Surgery

- Surgical redistribution of hair follicles by autografting
- Hair transplantation and tunnel grafting

Nursing considerations

Key outcomes

The patient will:
- express concerns about his condition or treatment
- avoid complications
- verbalize feelings about changed body image.

Nursing interventions

- Give prescribed drugs.

- Reassure the patient with female-pattern alopecia that hair thinning doesn't lead to total baldness. Suggest that she use a wig or hairpiece.
- For the patient undergoing radiation therapy or chemotherapy with drugs that cause alopecia, suggest selecting a hair replacement before treatment.
- Encourage the patient to express his feelings. Help him develop interests that contribute to a positive self-image.

Monitoring

- Complications
- Response to treatment

Patient teaching

Be sure to cover:
- the disorder, diagnosis, and treatment
- medications and potential adverse reactions
- when to notify the physician
- familial link in male-pattern alopecia
- well-balanced diet with adequate protein
- avoidance of excess vitamin A
- myths concerning commercial preparations
- signs and symptoms of skin infection
- possibility that hair may grow back in a different color or type, such as curly or straight.

Alzheimer's disease

Overview

Description

- Degenerative disorder of the cerebral cortex (especially the frontal lobe), which accounts for more than 50% of all cases of dementia
- Poor prognosis
- No cure or definitive treatment

Pathophysiology

- Genetic abnormality on chromosome 21
- Brain damage caused by genetic substance (amyloid)
- Three distinguishing features of brain tissue: neurofibrillary tangles, neuritic plaques, and granulovascular degeneration

Causes

- Unknown

Risk factors

Neurochemical
- Deficiencies of the neurotransmitters

Environmental
- Aluminum and manganese
- Trauma
- Genetic abnormality on chromosome 21
- Slow-growing central nervous system viruses

Incidence

- Severe form in patients over age 65
- Mild to moderate dementia in 12% of patients
- May affect up to 5 million Americans and more than 30 million people worldwide

Common characteristics

- Gradual loss of recent and remote memory
- Loss of sense of smell
- Flattening of affect and personality
- Difficulty with learning new information
- Deterioration in personal hygiene
- Inability to concentrate
- Increasing difficulty with abstraction and judgment
- Impaired communication
- Loss of coordination
- Inability to write or speak
- Nocturnal awakenings
- Signs of anxiety
- Loss of eye contact and fearful look
- Acute confusion, agitation, obsessive-compulsive behavior

Complications

- Injury from violent behavior, wandering, or unsupervised activity
- Pneumonia and other infections
- Malnutrition and dehydration

Assessment

History

- History obtained from a family member or caregiver
- Insidious onset
- Initial changes almost imperceptible
- Forgetfulness and subtle memory loss
- Recent memory loss
- Difficulty learning and remembering new information
- General deterioration in personal hygiene
- Inability to concentrate
- Tendency to perform repetitive actions and experience restlessness
- Negative personality changes (irritability, depression, paranoia, hostility)
- Nocturnal awakening
- Disorientation
- Suspicious and fearful of imaginary people and situations
- Misperceives own environment
- Misidentifies objects and people
- Complains of stolen or misplaced objects
- Emotions may be described as labile
- Mood swings, sudden angry outbursts, and sleep disturbances

Physical findings

- Impaired sense of smell (usually an early symptom)
- Impaired stereognosis
- Gait disorders
- Tremors
- Loss of recent memory
- Positive snout reflex
- Organic brain disease in adults
- Urinary or fecal incontinence
- Seizures

Test results

- Diagnosed by exclusion; tests performed to rule out other diseases.
- Positive diagnosis is made on autopsy.

Imaging
- Position emission tomography reveals metabolic activity of the cerebral cortex.
- Computed tomography scan shows excessive and progressive brain atrophy.
- Magnetic resonance imaging rules out intracranial lesions.
- Cerebral blood flow studies reveal abnormalities in blood flow to the brain.

Diagnostic procedures
- Cerebrospinal fluid analysis shows chronic neurologic infection.
- EEG evaluates the brain's electrical activity and may show slowing of the brain waves in late stages of the disease.

Other
- Neuropsychologic tests may show impaired cognitive ability and reasoning.

Treatment

General

- Behavioral interventions (patient-centered or care-giver training) focused on managing cognitive and behavioral changes
- Well-balanced diet (may need to be monitored)
- Safe activities, as tolerated (may need to be monitored)

Medication

- Cerebral vasodilators
- Psychostimulators
- Antidepressants
- Anxiolytics
- Neurolytics
- Anticonvulsants (experimental)
- Anti-inflammatories (experimental)
- Anticholinesterase agents
- Vitamin E

Nursing considerations

Key outcomes

The patient will:
- perform activities of daily living
- maintain daily calorie requirements
- remain free from signs and symptoms of infection
- perform self-care needs
- use support systems and develop adequate coping behaviors.

Nursing interventions

- Provide an effective communication system.
- Use soft tones and a slow, calm manner when speaking to the patient.
- Allow the patient sufficient time to answer questions.
- Protect the patient from injury.
- Provide rest periods.
- Provide an exercise program.
- Encourage independence.
- Offer frequent toileting.
- Assist with hygiene and dressing.
- Give prescribed drugs.
- Provide familiar objects to help with orientation and behavior control.

Monitoring

- Response to medications
- Fluid intake and nutrition status
- Environment (for safety purposes)

Patient teaching

Be sure to cover:
- disease process
- exercise regimen
- importance of cutting food and providing finger foods, if indicated
- use of plates with rim guards, built-up utensils, and cups with lids
- independence.

Discharge planning

- Refer the patient (and his family or caregivers) to the Alzheimer's Association.
- Refer the patient (and his family or caregivers) to a local support group.
- Refer the patient (and his family or caregivers) to social services for additional support.

Amebiasis

Overview

Description

○ An acute or chronic protozoal infection caused by *Entamoeba histolytica*
○ Produces varying degrees of illness, from no symptoms to mild diarrhea to fulminant dysentery
○ Extraintestinal type can induce hepatic abscess and infections of the lungs, pleural cavity, pericardium, peritoneum and, rarely, the brain
○ Also known as *amebic dysentery*

Pathophysiology

○ *E. histolytica* exists in two forms, as a cyst (which can survive outside the body) and a trophozoite (which can't survive outside the body).
○ The ingested cysts pass through the intestine, where digestive secretions break them down and liberate the motile trophozoites within.
○ The trophozoites multiply and either invade and ulcerate the mucosa of the large intestine or simply feed on intestinal bacteria.
○ As the trophozoites are carried slowly toward the rectum, they're encysted and then excreted in feces.

Causes

○ Ingestion of feces-contaminated food or water

Incidence

○ Occurs worldwide but is most common in the tropics, subtropics, and other areas with poor sanitation and health practices
○ Incidence in the United States between 1% and 3%; may be higher among homosexuals and institutionalized people, in whom fecal-oral contamination is common

Common characteristics

○ The clinical effects of amebiasis vary with the severity of the infestation
Acute amebic dysentery
○ Sudden high temperature of 104° to 105° F (40° to 40.6° C)
○ Profuse, bloody, mucoid diarrhea with tenesmus
Chronic amebic dysentery
○ Intermittent diarrhea that lasts for 1 to 4 weeks and recurs several times per year
Amebic granuloma
○ Blood and mucus in the stool
○ Partial or complete bowel obstruction

Complications

○ Subacute appendicitis
○ Perforation of the intestinal wall with spread to the liver, lungs, pleural cavity, peritoneum, and brain.

Assessment

History

Acute amebic dysentery
○ Fever, chills
○ Abdominal cramping
○ Profuse, bloody, mucoid diarrhea
Chronic amebic dysentery
○ Multiple (4 to 18) foul-smelling mucus- and blood-tinged stools daily
○ Mild fever
○ Vague abdominal cramps
○ Possible weight loss

Physical findings

Acute amebic dysentery
○ Diffuse abdominal tenderness
Chronic amebic dysentery
○ Tenderness over the cecum and ascending colon
○ Hepatomegaly (occasionally)

Test results

Laboratory
○ Stool or aspirates from abscesses, ulcers, or tissue show *E. histolytica*
○ Positive indirect hemagglutination test with current or previous infection
○ Positive complement fixation (usually only during active disease)
Imaging
○ Barium studies to rule out nonamebic causes of diarrhea, such as polyps and cancer
Diagnostic procedures
○ Sigmoidoscopy to detect rectosigmoid ulceration

Treatment

General

○ Small, frequent meals
○ Increased fluid intake
○ Frequent rest periods
○ Avoidance of enemas

Medication

○ Metronidazole
○ Emetine hydrochloride
○ Iodoquinol (diiodohydroxyquin)
○ Chloroquine
○ Tetracycline (in combination with emetine hydrochloride, metronidazole, or paromomycin)

Surgery

○ Exploratory surgery is hazardous; it can lead to peritonitis, perforation, and pericecal abscess

Nursing considerations

Key outcomes

The patient will:
○ maintain or improve weight
○ maintain skin integrity
○ return to a normal elimination pattern
○ express feelings of increased comfort and relief from pain.

Nursing interventions

○ Encourage adequate fluid intake.
○ Give prescribed drugs.
○ Apply perirectal protective cream to prevent excoriation and skin breakdown.

Monitoring

○ Vital signs, especially temperature
○ Fluid and electrolyte balance
○ Daily weight
○ Frequency, amount, and character of stools
○ Skin integrity

Patient teaching

Be sure to cover:
○ need for avoiding alcohol ingestion when taking metronidazole, which can cause nausea, vomiting, and headache
○ importance of returning for follow-up appointments
○ advising family and sexual partners to seek medical attention for amebiasis
○ how to handle infectious material and perform proper hand washing
○ safe sex practices
○ boiling untreated or contaminated water when traveling to endemic areas.

Amenorrhea

Overview

Description

❍ The abnormal absence or suppression of menstruation
❍ Primary amenorrhea: the absence of menarche in an adolescent (age 16 and older)
❍ Secondary amenorrhea: the failure of menstruation for at least 3 months after the normal onset of menarche

Pathophysiology

Primary amenorrhea
❍ The hypothalamic-pituitary-ovarian axis is dysfunctional.
❍ Anatomic defects of the central nervous system cause the ovary not to receive the hormonal signals that normally initiate the development of secondary sex characteristics and the beginning of menstruation.

Secondary amenorrhea
❍ The endometrium is sufficiently scarred and no functional endometrium exists.

Causes

❍ Pregnancy
❍ Hormonal abnormalities
❍ Lack of ovarian response to gonadotropins
❍ Constant presence of progesterone or other endocrine abnormalities
❍ Absence of a uterus
❍ Endometrial damage
❍ Ovarian, adrenal, or pituitary tumors
❍ Emotional disorders
❍ Malnutrition and intense exercise

Incidence

❍ Primary amenorrhea occurs in 0.3% of women.
❍ Secondary amenorrhea is seen in 5% of women.

Common characteristics

❍ Absence of menstruation
❍ Vasomotor flushes, vaginal atrophy, hirsutism (abnormal hairiness), and acne (secondary amenorrhea)

Complications

❍ Infertility
❍ Endometrial adenocarcinoma
❍ Estrogen deficiency syndrome
❍ Osteoporosis

Assessment

History

❍ Failure to menstruate in females age 16 and older
❍ Absence of menstruation for 3 months in a previously established menstrual pattern
❍ Change in menstrual pattern
❍ Dependent on cause: may include headaches, hot flashes, nausea, weight gain or loss, emotional upset, trauma, extreme exercise, prolonged use of hormonal contraceptives

Physical findings

❍ Based on cause of amenorrhea: may include hirsutism, acne, abdominal mass, signs of malnutrition

Test results

Laboratory
❍ Positive pregnancy test (when pregnancy is the cause)
❍ Elevated or low pituitary gonadotropin levels
❍ Abnormal thyroid levels
❍ Abnormal serum progesterone levels
❍ Abnormal serum androgen levels
❍ Elevated urinary 17-ketosteroid levels with excessive androgen secretions
❍ Plasma follicle-stimulating hormone (FSH) level more than 50 IU/L, depending on the laboratory (suggests primary ovarian failure)
❍ Normal or low FSH level (possible hypothalamic or pituitary abnormality, depending on the clinical situation)

Imaging
❍ X-rays to identify ovarian, adrenal, and pituitary tumors

Diagnostic procedures
❍ Ferning of cervical mucus on microscopic examination (an estrogen effect)
❍ Vaginal cytologic examination
❍ Endometrial biopsy

Other
❍ Pelvic examination reveals anatomic abnormalities

Treatment

General

❍ Based on cause
❍ Well-balanced diet
❍ Moderate exercise routine

Medication

❍ Progestational agents (to stimulate menstruation)
❍ Calcium supplement (if cause is hypoestrogenism)
❍ Clomiphene citrate (may induce ovulation in women with amenorrhea caused by gonadotropin deficiency, polycystic ovarian disease, or excessive weight loss or gain)
❍ FSH and human menopausal gonadotropins for women with pituitary disease

Surgery

❍ Removal of tumor or obstruction

Nursing considerations

Key outcomes

The patient will:
○ maintain adequate fluid balance
○ express understanding of disorder
○ communicate feelings about the situation.

Nursing interventions

○ Provide reassurance and emotional support.
○ Give prescribed drugs.

Monitoring

○ Signs and symptoms
○ Intake and output
○ Laboratory test results

Patient teaching

Be sure to cover:
○ the disorder, diagnosis, and treatment
○ how to keep an accurate record of menstrual cycles to aid early detection of recurrent amenorrhea.

Discharge planning

○ Refer the patient for psychological counseling, if appropriate.

Amyotrophic lateral sclerosis

Overview

Description

- Most common motor neuron disease of muscular atrophy
- Chronic, progressive, and debilitating disease that's invariably fatal
- No cure
- Also known as *Lou Gehrig disease*

Pathophysiology

- An excitatory neurotransmitter that accumulates to toxic levels
- Motor units that no longer innervate
- Progressive degeneration of axons that cause loss of myelin
- Progressive degeneration of upper and lower motor neurons
- Progressive degeneration of motor nuclei in the cerebral cortex and corticospinal tracts

Causes

- Exact cause unknown
- 10% of patients inherit as an autosomal dominant trait
- Virus that creates metabolic disturbances in motor neurons
- Immune complexes such as those formed in autoimmune disorders

Precipitating factors that cause acute deterioration
- Severe stress such as myocardial infarction
- Traumatic injury
- Viral infections
- Physical exhaustion

Incidence

- Three times more common in men than in women
- Affects people ages 40 to 70

Common characteristics

- Muscle weakness
- Atrophy
- Fasciculations

Complications

- Respiratory tract infections
- Complications of physical immobility

Assessment

History

- Mental function intact
- Family history of amyotrophic lateral sclerosis (ALS)
- Asymmetrical weakness first noticed in one limb
- Easy fatigue and easy cramping in the affected muscles

Physical findings

- Location of the affected motor neurons
- Severity of the disease
- Fasciculations in the affected muscles
- Progressive weakness in muscles of the arms, legs, and trunk
- Brisk and overactive stretch reflexes
- Difficulty talking, chewing, swallowing, and breathing
- Shortness of breath and occasional drooling

Test results

Laboratory
- Increased protein in cerebrospinal fluid

Imaging
- Computed tomography scan to rule out other disorders

Diagnostic procedures
- Muscle biopsy to disclose atrophic fibers

Other
- EEG to rule out other disorders
- Electromyography showing the electrical abnormalities of involved muscles
- Nerve conduction studies appear normal

Treatment

General

- Rehabilitative measures
- May need tube feedings
- Activity as tolerated

Medication

- Muscle relaxants
- Dantrolene
- Baclofen
- I.V. or intrathecal administration of thyrotropin-releasing hormone
- Riluzole

Nursing considerations

Key outcomes

The patient will:
- maintain a patent airway and adequate ventilation
- maintain joint mobility and range of motion (ROM)
- maintain daily calorie requirements
- seek support systems and exhibit adequate coping behaviors
- remain free from infection.

Nursing interventions

- Provide emotional and psychological support.
- Promote independence.
- Turn and reposition the patient frequently.
- Give prescribed drugs.

To help the patient with amyotrophic lateral sclerosis (ALS) live safely at home, follow these guidelines:

○ Explain basic safety precautions, such as keeping stairs and pathways free from clutter; using nonskid mats in the bathroom and in place of loose throw rugs; keeping stairs well lit; installing handrails in stairwells and the shower, tub, and toilet areas; and removing electrical and telephone cords from traffic areas.

○ Discuss the need for rearranging the furniture, moving items in or out of the patient's care area, and obtaining a hospital bed, a commode, or oxygen equipment.

○ Recommend devices to ease the patient's and caregiver's work, such as extra pillows or a wedge pillow to help the patient sit up, a draw sheet to help him move up in bed, a lap tray for eating, or a bell for calling the caregiver.

○ Help the patient adjust to changes in the environment. Encourage independence.

○ Advise the patient to keep a suction machine handy to reduce the fear of choking due to secretion accumulation and dysphagia. Teach him how to suction himself when necessary.

○ Provide airway and respiratory management.
○ Promote nutrition.
○ Maintain aspiration precautions.

Monitoring

○ Muscle weakness
○ Respiratory status
○ Speech
○ Swallowing ability
○ Skin integrity
○ Nutritional status
○ Environment (for safety purposes)
○ Response to treatment
○ Complications
○ Signs and symptoms of infection

Patient teaching

Be sure to cover:
○ the disorder, diagnosis, and treatment
○ swallowing therapy regimen
○ medications and adverse effects
○ skin care
○ ROM exercises
○ deep-breathing and coughing exercises
○ safety in the home. (See *Modifying the home for a patient with ALS.*)

Discharge planning

○ Refer the patient to a local ALS support group.

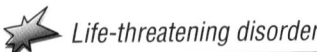

Anaphylaxis

Overview

Description

○ Dramatic, acute atopic reaction to an allergen
○ Marked by sudden onset of rapidly progressive urticaria and respiratory distress
○ More severe the sooner signs and symptoms appear after exposure to the antigen
○ Severe reactions may initiate vascular collapse, leading to systemic shock and, possibly, death

Pathophysiology

○ After initial exposure to an antigen, the immune system produces specific immunoglobulin (Ig) antibodies in the lymph nodes. Helper T cells enhance the process.
○ The antibodies (IgE) then bind to membrane receptors located on mast cells and basophils.
○ After the body re-encounters the antigen, the IgE antibodies, or cross-linked IgE receptors, recognize the antigen as foreign; this activates the release of power chemical mediators.
○ IgG or IgM enters into the reaction and activates the release of complement factors.

Causes

○ Systemic exposure to sensitizing drugs, foods, insect venom, or other specific antigens

Incidence

○ Most common anaphylaxis-causing antigen is penicillin, which induces a reaction in 1 to 4 of every 10,000 patients treated

Common characteristics

○ Apprehension and anxiety
○ Dyspnea
○ Hoarseness
○ Angioedema

Complications

○ Respiratory obstruction
○ Systemic vascular collapse
○ Death

Assessment

History

○ Immediately after exposure, complaints of a feeling of impending doom or fright and exhibiting apprehension, restlessness, cyanosis, cool and clammy skin, erythema, edema, tachypnea, weakness, sweating, sneezing, dyspnea, nasal pruritus, and urticaria

○ A "lump" in the patient's throat caused by angioedema
○ Dyspnea and complaints of chest tightness

Physical findings

○ Hives
○ Hoarseness or stridor, wheezing
○ Severe abdominal cramps, nausea, diarrhea
○ Urinary urgency and incontinence
○ Dizziness, drowsiness, headache, restlessness, and seizures
○ Hypotension, shock; sometimes, angina and cardiac arrhythmias
○ Angioedema

Test results

○ No tests are required to identify anaphylaxis. The patient's history and signs and symptoms establish the diagnosis.
Laboratory
○ Skin testing may help to identify a specific allergen.

Treatment

General

○ Patent airway (establish and maintain)
○ Cardiopulmonary resuscitation, if cardiac arrest occurs
○ Nothing by mouth, until stable
○ Bed rest, until stable

Medication

○ *Immediate* injection of epinephrine 1:1,000 aqueous solution, 0.1 to 0.5 ml S.C. or I.V.
○ Corticosteroids
○ Diphenhydramine I.V.
○ Volume expander infusions, as needed
○ Vasopressors
○ Norepinephrine
○ Dopamine
○ Aminophylline I.V.
○ Antihistamines

Nursing considerations

Key outcomes

The patient will:
○ maintain a patent airway
○ maintain adequate ventilation
○ express feelings of increased comfort and decreased pain
○ maintain normal cardiac output and normal heart rate
○ identify causative allergen.

Nursing interventions

○ Provide supplemental oxygen and prepare to assist with insertion of an endotracheal tube, if necessary.
○ Insert a peripheral I.V. line.

○ Continually reassure the patient, and explain all tests and treatments.
○ If the patient undergoes skin or scratch testing, monitor for signs of a serious allergic response. Keep emergency resuscitation equipment readily available.

 Alert

If a patient must receive a drug to which he's allergic, prevent a severe reaction by making sure he receives careful desensitization with gradually increasing doses of the antigen or with advance administration of corticosteroids. Closely monitor the patient during testing and have resuscitation equipment and epinephrine readily available.

Monitoring

○ Vital signs
○ Adverse reactions from radiographic contrast media
○ Respiratory status
○ Serious allergic response after skin or scratch testing
○ Neurologic status
○ Response to treatment
○ Complications
○ Degree of edema

Patient teaching

Be sure to cover:
○ risk for delayed symptoms and importance of reporting them immediately
○ avoidance of exposure to known allergens
○ importance of carrying and becoming familiar with an anaphylaxis kit and learning to use it before the need arises
○ need for medical identification jewelry to identify allergy.

Anemia, aplastic

Overview

Description

○ Potentially fatal marrow failure syndrome resulting from injury to or destruction of stem cells in bone marrow or the bone marrow matrix
○ Causes pancytopenia (anemia, leukopenia, thrombocytopenia) and bone marrow hypoplasia

Pathophysiology

○ Usually develops when damaged or destroyed stem cells inhibit red blood cell (RBC) production
○ Less commonly, develops when damaged bone marrow microvasculature creates an unfavorable environment for cell growth and maturation

Causes

○ Result of adverse drug reaction
○ Immunologic factors; severe disease, especially hepatitis; viral infection, especially in children; and preleukemic and neoplastic infiltration of bone marrow
○ Congenital hypoplastic anemia, also known as *anemia of Blackfan and Diamond*, which develops between ages 2 and 3 months and *Fanconi's syndrome*, between birth and age 10
○ May be idiopathic

Incidence

○ More common in children and young adults

Common characteristics

○ Pallor and ecchymoses

Complications

○ Hemorrhage
○ Infection
○ Heart failure

Assessment

History

○ Fatigue
○ Weakness
○ Weight loss
○ Dizziness
○ Syncope
○ Bruising
○ Nosebleeds
○ Shortness of breath

Physical findings

○ Pallor, ecchymosis, petechiae, or retinal hemorrhage
○ Alterations in level of consciousness, weakness, fatigue
○ Bibasilar crackles, tachycardia, and a gallop murmur

○ Fever, oral and rectal ulcers, and sore throat
○ Nausea
○ Decreased hair and skin quality
○ Petechial rash

Test results

Laboratory

○ RBC count of 1 million/mm^3 or less, usually with normochromic and normocytic cells; very low absolute reticulocyte count
○ Elevated serum iron levels (unless bleeding occurs), but normal or slightly reduced total iron-binding capacity
○ Decreased serum platelet and white blood cell counts

Diagnostic procedures

○ Bone marrow biopsies performed at several sites may yield a dry tap or show severely hypocellular or aplastic marrow, with a varying amount of fat, fibrous tissue, or gelatinous replacement; absence of tagged iron and megakaryocytes; and depression of erythroid elements.

Treatment

General

○ Effective treatment must eliminate any identifiable cause
○ Vigorous supportive measures, such as packed RBCs, platelets, and experimental histocompatibility antigen-matched leukocyte transfusions
○ Respiratory support with oxygen
○ Prevention of infection ranging from frequent hand washing to filtered airflow
○ Well-balanced diet
○ Neutropenic precautions, if appropriate

Medication

○ Antibiotics
○ Corticosteroids
○ Marrow-stimulating agents such as androgens, anti-lymphocyte globulin (experimental), and immunosuppressant agents
○ Granulocyte colony-stimulating factor, granulocyte-macrophage colony-stimulating factor, and erythropoietic-stimulating factor

Surgery

○ Bone marrow transplantation (for severe aplasia and patients who need constant RBC transfusions)

Nursing considerations

Key outcomes

The patient will:
○ state the need to increase activity level gradually
○ maintain vital signs within prescribed limits during activity
○ maintain normal cardiac output

- exhibit adequate ventilation
- express feelings of increased comfort and decreased pain.

Nursing interventions

- Help the patient to prevent or manage hemorrhage, infection, adverse effects of drug therapy, and blood transfusion reaction.
- If the patient's platelet count is low (less than 20,000/mm³), prevent hemorrhage by avoiding I.M. injections, and suggesting the use of an electric razor and a soft toothbrush. Apply pressure to venipuncture sites until bleeding stops.
- Follow neutropenic precautions.
- Make sure throat, urine, nasal, stool, and blood cultures are done regularly and correctly to check for infection.
- Schedule frequent rest periods.
- Administer oxygen therapy.
- Ensure a comfortable environmental temperature.
- If blood transfusions are necessary, administer according to facility policy and assess for transfusion reactions.

Monitoring

- Blood studies in patients receiving anemia-inducing drugs
- Early detection of bleeding

Patient teaching

Be sure to cover:
- avoidance of contact with potential sources of infection, such as crowds, soil, and standing water that can harbor organisms
- disorder and its treatment
- prescribed drugs and possible adverse reactions and when to report them
- normal lifestyle with appropriate restrictions until remission occurs (for the patient who doesn't require hospitalization).

Discharge planning

- Refer the patient to the Aplastic Anemia Foundation of America for additional information, assistance, and support.

Anemia, folic acid (folate) deficiency

Overview

Description
- A common, slowly progressive megaloblastic anemia
- Caused by a deficiency of the vitamin folate

Pathophysiology
- When folic acid stores in the body are low or diet is deficient in folic acid, the bone marrow produces large red blood cells or megaloblasts resulting in anemia.

Causes
- Alcohol abuse
- Poor diet
- Impaired absorption from small intestine
- Bacteria competing for available folic acid
- Excessive cooking of foods, which destroys the available nutrient
- Limited storage capacity in infants
- Prolonged drug therapy with such drugs as anticonvulsants, estrogens, and methotrexate
- Increased folic acid requirements during pregnancy, rapid growth periods in infancy, childhood and adolescence, and in patients with neoplastic diseases or some skin diseases such as exfoliative dermatitis

Incidence
- Most prevalent in infants, adolescents, pregnant and lactating women, alcoholics, elderly people, and people with malignant or intestinal diseases

Common characteristics
- Progressive fatigue
- Systemic signs of anemia

Complications
- Pregnant women deficient in folic acid have an increased risk for giving birth to a neonate with a neural tube defect.

Assessment

History
- Severe, progressive fatigue, the hallmark of folic acid deficiency
- Diarrhea
- Nausea
- Anorexia
- Headaches
- Forgetfulness
- Irritability

Physical findings
- Shortness of breath
- Palpitations
- Weakness and light-headedness
- Generalized pallor and jaundice
- Wasted or malnourished appearance
- Possible cheilosis and glossitis
- Red, swollen, smooth, shiny, and tender tongue (glossitis)
- Reduced sense of taste

Test results

Laboratory
- Folic acid deficiency anemia and pernicious anemia distinguished by the Schilling test and a therapeutic trial of vitamin B_{12} injections
- Macrocytosis, decreased reticulocyte count, increased mean corpuscular volume, abnormal platelets, and serum folate levels less than 4 mg/ml

Treatment

General
- Elimination of contributing causes
- Well-balanced diet high in folic acid (see *Foods high in folic acid*)
- Frequent rest periods during activity, as needed

Medication
- Folic acid supplements
- Vitamin supplementation (women planning to become pregnant should begin at least 3 months before conception)
- Blood transfusions in severe cases

Nursing considerations

Key outcomes
The patient will:
- state the need to increase activity level gradually
- maintain vital signs within prescribed limits during activity
- remain hemodynamically stable
- have normal bowel movements
- experience no further weight loss.

Nursing interventions
- Plan activities, rest periods, and necessary diagnostic tests to conserve energy.
- Advise the patient to report signs and symptoms of decreased perfusion to vital organs (dyspnea, chest pain, dizziness).
- If the patient has glossitis, emphasize the importance of good oral hygiene.
- Ask the dietitian to give the patient nonirritating foods because a sore mouth and tongue make eating painful. If these symptoms make talking difficult, supply a pad and pencil or some other aid to facilitate communication.

Foods high in folic acid

The body needs folic acid to develop healthy red blood cells and synthesize deoxyribonucleic acid. Although body stores are comparatively small (about 70 mg), this vitamin is plentiful in most well-balanced diets. But because folic acid is water-soluble and heat-labile, it's easily destroyed by cooking. Also, about 20% of folic acid intake is excreted unabsorbed. Daily folic acid intake less than 50 mcg/day usually induces folic acid deficiency within 4 months. At the top of the next column is a list of foods high in folic acid.

Food	mcg/100 g
Asparagus spears	109
Beef liver	294
Broccoli spears	54
Collards (cooked)	102
Mushrooms	24
Oatmeal	33
Peanut butter	57
Red beans	180
Wheat germ	305

○ To ensure accurate Schilling test results, make sure that all urine excreted over a 24-hour period is collected and that the specimens remain uncontaminated by bacteria.
○ Provide a well-balanced diet, including foods high in folate, such as dark green leafy vegetables, organ meats, eggs, milk, oranges, bananas, dry beans, and whole-grain breads.

Monitoring

○ Vital signs
○ Fluid and electrolyte balance

Patient teaching

Be sure to cover:
○ importance of a well-balanced diet high in folic acid
○ use of commercially prepared formulas for mothers who aren't breast-feeding
○ daily folic acid requirements and the need to keep taking the supplements even when he begins to feel better
○ importance of guarding against infections and reporting signs of infection promptly.

Anemia, iron deficiency

Overview

Description

○ Decreased total iron body content diminishing erythropoiesis
○ Produces smaller (microcytic) cells with less color on staining (hypochromia)

Pathophysiology

○ Body stores of iron, including plasma iron, decrease.
○ Transferrin, which binds with and transports iron, also decreases.
○ Insufficient body stores of iron lead to a depleted red blood cell mass and to a decreased hemoglobin concentration.
○ Results in decreased oxygen-carrying capacity of the blood. (See *Iron absorption and storage.*)

Causes

○ Inadequate dietary intake of iron
○ Iron malabsorption
○ Blood loss secondary to drug-induced GI bleeding or due to heavy menses, hemorrhage from trauma, GI ulcers, malignant tumors, and varices
○ Pregnancy
○ Intravascular hemolysis-induced hemoglobinuria or paroxysmal nocturnal hemoglobinuria
○ Mechanical erythrocyte trauma caused by a prosthetic heart valve or vena cava filter
○ Can be related to lead poisoning in children

Incidence

○ Common worldwide
○ Affects 10% to 30% of the adult population of the United States
○ Most prevalent among premenopausal women, infants, children, adolescents, alcoholics, and elderly people

Iron absorption and storage

Found in abundance throughout the body, iron is needed for erythropoiesis. Two-thirds of total-body iron is found in hemoglobin; the other third, mostly in the reticuloendothelial system (liver, spleen, and bone marrow), with small amounts in muscle, serum, and body cells.

Adequate iron in the diet and recirculation of iron released from disintegrating red blood cells maintain iron supplies. The duodenum and upper part of the small intestine absorb dietary iron. Such absorption depends on gastric acid content, the amount of reducing substances (ascorbic acid, for example) present in the alimentary canal, and amount of iron intake. If iron intake is deficient, the body gradually depletes its iron stores, causing decreased hemoglobin levels and, eventually, signs and symptoms of iron deficiency anemia.

Common characteristics

○ Fatigue
○ Systemic signs of anemia

Complications

○ Infection
○ Pneumonia
○ Overreplacement of oral or I.M. iron supplements, which can affect the liver, heart, pituitary glands, and joints

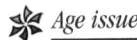 **Age issue**

In a child, iron deficiency anemia can cause pica, which may lead to eating lead-based paint resulting in lead poisoning.

Assessment

History

○ Can persist for years without signs and symptoms
○ Fatigue
○ Inability to concentrate
○ Headache, shortness of breath (especially on exertion)
○ Increased frequency of infections
○ Pica, an uncontrollable urge to eat strange things, such as clay, starch, ice and, in children, lead
○ Menorrhagia
○ Dysphagia
○ Vasomotor disturbances
○ Numbness and tingling of the extremities
○ Neuralgic pain

Physical findings

○ Red, swollen, smooth, shiny, and tender tongue (glossitis)
○ Corners of the mouth may be eroded, tender, and swollen (angular stomatitis)
○ Spoon-shaped, brittle nails
○ Tachycardia

Test results

Laboratory

○ Decreased serum hemoglobin (males, less than 12 g/dl; females, less than 10 g/dl) or decreased mean corpuscular hemoglobin in severe anemia
○ Decreased serum hematocrit (males, less than 47 ml/dl; females, less than 42 ml/dl)
○ Decreased serum iron levels with high binding capacity
○ Decreased serum ferritin levels
○ Decreased serum RBC count with microcytic and hypochromic cells (in early stages, RBC count may be normal, except in infants and children)

- Bone marrow studies reveal depleted or absent iron stores (done by staining) as well as normoblastic hyperplasia.
- GI studies, such as guaiac stool tests, barium swallow and enema, endoscopy, and sigmoidoscopy, rule out or confirm the diagnosis of bleeding causing the iron deficiency.

Treatment

General

- Underlying cause must first be determined
- Nutritious, nonirritating foods
- Planned rest periods during activity

Medication

- Oral preparation of iron or a combination of iron and ascorbic acid
- I.M. iron in rare cases
- Total-dose I.V. infusions of supplemental iron for pregnant and elderly patients with severe disease

Nursing considerations

Key outcomes

The patient will:
- maintain weight without further loss
- maintain vital signs within prescribed limits during activity
- express feelings of increased energy
- express feelings of increased comfort and decreased pain.

Nursing interventions

- Note the patient's signs or symptoms of decreased perfusion to vital organs.
- Provide oxygen therapy, as necessary.
- Assess the family's dietary habits for iron intake, noting the influence of childhood eating patterns, cultural food preferences, and family income on adequate nutrition.
- Ask the dietitian to give the patient nonirritating foods.
- Give prescribed analgesics for headache and other discomfort.
- Evaluate the patient's drug history. Certain drugs, such as pancreatic enzymes and vitamin E, can interfere with iron metabolism and absorption; aspirin, steroids, and other drugs can cause GI bleeding.
- Provide frequent rest periods.
- If the patient receives iron I.V., monitor the infusion rate carefully and observe for an allergic reaction.
- Use the Z-track injection method when administering iron I.M. to prevent skin discoloration, scarring, and irritating iron deposits in the skin.
- Provide good nutrition and meticulous care of I.V. sites.

Recognizing iron overdose

Excessive iron replacement may produce signs and symptoms, such as diarrhea, fever, severe stomach pain, nausea, and vomiting.

When these signs and symptoms occur, notify the physician and give prescribed treatment, which may include chelation therapy, vigorous I.V. fluid replacement, gastric lavage, whole-bowel irrigation, and supplemental oxygen.

Monitoring

- Vital signs
- Compliance with prescribed iron supplement therapy
- Iron replacement overdose (see *Recognizing iron overdose*)

Patient teaching

Be sure to cover:
- the disorder, diagnosis, and treatment
- dangers of lead poisoning, especially if the patient reports pica
- importance of continuing therapy, even after the patient begins to feel better
- absorption interference with milk or antacid of iron supplementation
- increased absorption with vitamin C
- avoidance of staining teeth by drinking liquid supplemental iron through a straw
- when to report adverse effects of iron therapy
- basics of a nutritionally balanced diet
- importance of avoiding infection and when to report signs of infection
- need for regular checkups
- compliance with prescribed treatment.

Anemia, pernicious

Overview

Description

- Deficiency of vitamin B_{12} causing serious neurologic, psychological, gastric, and intestinal abnormalities
- Characterized by decreased gastric production of hydrochloric acid and deficiency of intrinsic factor, essential for vitamin B_{12} absorption
- Also known as *Addison's anemia*

Pathophysiology

- An inherited autoimmune response may cause gastric mucosal atrophy and resultant decreased hydrochloric acid and intrinsic factor production, a substance normally secreted by the parietal cells of the gastric mucosa.
- Intrinsic factor deficiency impairs vitamin B_{12} absorption.
- Vitamin B_{12} deficiency inhibits the growth of all cells, particularly red blood cells (RBCs), leading to insufficient and deformed RBCs with poor oxygen-carrying capacity.

Causes

- Genetic predisposition
- Secondary pernicious anemia results from partial removal of the stomach
- Chronic gastric inflammation

Incidence

- In the United States, most common in New England and the Great Lakes region because of ethnic concentration
- Common in Northern Europeans of fair complexion
- Rare in children, Blacks, and Asians
- Onset typically between ages 50 and 60; incidence increases with advancing age

Common characteristics

- Weakness
- Beefy red, sore tongue
- Systemic signs of anemia

Complications

- Heart failure with severe anemia
- Myocardial ischemia
- Paralysis
- Psychotic behavior
- Loss of sphincter control of bowel and bladder
- Peptic ulcer disease

Assessment

History

- Characteristic triad of symptoms: weakness; a beefy red, sore tongue; and numbness and tingling in the extremities
- GI disturbance: nausea, vomiting, anorexia, weight loss, flatulence, diarrhea, and constipation
- Peripheral numbness and paresthesia
- Light-headedness
- Headache
- Diplopia and blurred vision
- Loss of taste
- Tinnitus

Physical findings

- Smooth, beefy red, painful tongue
- Slightly jaundiced sclera and pale to bright yellow skin
- Tachycardia
- Systolic murmur
- Enlarged liver and spleen
- Weakness in the extremities
- Disturbed position sense
- Lack of coordination
- Impaired fine finger movement
- Loss of bowel and bladder control
- Impotence (in males)
- Irritable, depressed, delirious, and ataxic
- Memory loss
- Positive Babinski's and Romberg's signs
- Optic muscle atrophy

Test results

Laboratory

- Decreased hemoglobin level (4 to 5 g/dl)
- Decreased RBC count
- Increased mean corpuscular volume (under 120 mm^3); increased mean corpuscular hemoglobin concentration
- Possibly decreased white blood cell and platelet counts and large, malformed platelets
- Serum vitamin B_{12} tests may show levels less than 0.1 µg/ml
- Elevated serum lactate dehydrogenase levels

Diagnostic procedures

- Bone marrow studies reveal erythroid hyperplasia with increased numbers of megaloblasts but few normally developing RBCs.
- Gastric analysis shows an absence of free hydrochloric acid after histamine or pentagastrin injection.
- The Schilling test may reveal a urinary excretion of less than 3% in the first 24 hours in patients with pernicious anemia; may reveal normal excretion of vitamin B_{12} when repeated with intrinsic factor added.

Treatment

General

○ Based on underlying cause
○ Well-balanced diet, including foods high in vitamin B_{12}
○ Sodium and fluid restriction for heart failure
○ If anemia causes extreme fatigue, bed rest until hemoglobin increases

Medication

○ Early I.M. vitamin B_{12} replacement
○ Maintenance levels (monthly) of vitamin B_{12} doses, after the patient's condition improves

Nursing considerations

Key outcomes

The patient will:
○ state his understanding of the need to increase activity level gradually
○ modify lifestyle to minimize risk for decreased tissue perfusion
○ maintain normal hemoglobin level and hematocrit
○ maintain normal coagulation profile.

Nursing interventions

○ If the patient has severe anemia, plan activities, rest periods, and necessary diagnostic tests to conserve his energy.
○ To ensure accurate Schilling test results, make sure that all urine excreted over a 24-hour period is collected.
○ Provide a well-balanced diet, including foods high in vitamin B_{12}.
○ Institute safety precautions to prevent falls.

Monitoring

○ Vital signs
○ Mental and neurologic status
○ Environment (for safety purposes)

Patient teaching

Be sure to cover:
○ protection against infections and when to report signs of infection
○ when to report signs and symptoms of decreased perfusion to vital organs and symptoms of neuropathy
○ avoidance of irritating foods
○ avoidance of exposure to extreme heat or cold on the extremities
○ continuation of vitamin B_{12} replacement even after symptoms subside
○ proper injection techniques

○ observance of and when to report confusion and irritability
○ prevention of pernicious anemia, by taking vitamin B_{12} supplements, in patients who have had extensive gastric resections or who follow strict vegetarian diets.

Anemia, sickle cell

Overview

Description

○ Congenital hemolytic disease that results from a defective hemoglobin (Hb) molecule (HbS) that causes red blood cells (RBCs) to become sickle shaped
○ Sickle-shaped cells impair circulation, resulting in chronic ill health (fatigue, dyspnea on exertion, swollen joints), periodic crises, long-term complications, and premature death
○ No cure

Pathophysiology

○ The abnormal HbS found in the patient's RBCs becomes insoluble whenever hypoxia occurs.
○ The RBCs become rigid, rough, and elongated, forming a crescent or sickle shape.
○ Sickling can produce hemolysis (cell destruction).
○ The altered cells accumulate in capillaries and smaller blood vessels, making the blood more viscous.
○ Normal circulation is impaired, causing pain, tissue infarctions, and swelling.

Causes

○ Homozygous inheritance of the HbS-producing gene (defective Hb gene from each parent)

Incidence

○ Most common in tropical Africans and in people of African descent
○ About 1 in 10 blacks carry the abnormal gene; if two such carriers have offspring, each child has a 1-in-4 chance of developing the disease
○ One in every 500 blacks in the United States has sickle cell anemia
○ Also occurs in Puerto Rico, Turkey, India, the Middle East, and the Mediterranean area

Common characteristics

○ Chronic fatigue
○ Intense pain due to vascular occlusion in a sickling episode
○ Frequent bacterial infections due to involvement of spleen
○ Systemic signs of anemia

Complications

○ Chronic obstructive pulmonary disease
○ Heart failure
○ Retinopathy
○ Nephropathy

Assessment

History

○ Signs and symptoms usually don't develop until after age 6 months
○ Chronic fatigue
○ Unexplained dyspnea or dyspnea on exertion
○ Joint swelling
○ Aching bones
○ Chest pain
○ Ischemic leg ulcers
○ Increased susceptibility to infection
○ Pulmonary infarctions and cardiomegaly

Physical findings

○ Jaundice or pallor
○ May appear small in stature for age
○ Delayed growth and puberty
○ Spiderlike body build (narrow shoulders and hips, long extremities, curved spine, and barrel chest) in adult
○ Tachycardia
○ Hepatomegaly and, in children, splenomegaly
○ Systolic and diastolic murmurs
○ Sleepiness with difficulty awakening
○ Hematuria
○ Pale lips, tongue, palms, and nail beds
○ Body temperature over 104° F (40° C) or a temperature of 100° F (37.8° C) that persists for 2 or more days

In painful crisis
○ Most common crisis and the hallmark of the disease, usually appears periodically after age 5, characterized by severe abdominal, thoracic, muscle, or bone pain and, possibly, increased jaundice, dark urine, and a low-grade fever

In aplastic crisis
○ Pallor, lethargy, sleepiness, dyspnea, possible coma, markedly decreased bone marrow activity, and RBC hemolysis

In acute sequestration crisis
○ Occurs in infants between ages 8 months and 2 years, causes lethargy and pallor and, if untreated, progresses to hypovolemic shock and death

In hemolytic crisis
○ Liver congestion and hepatomegaly

Test results

Laboratory
○ Stained blood smear showing sickle cells and Hb electrophoresis showing HbS (Electrophoresis should be done on umbilical cord blood samples at birth to provide sickle cell disease screening for all neonates at risk.)
○ Decreased RBC counts, elevated white blood cell and platelet counts, decreased erythrocyte sedimentation rate, increased serum iron levels
○ Decreased RBC survival and reticulocytosis; normal or low Hb levels

Imaging
❍ A lateral chest X-ray detects the characteristic "Lincoln log" deformity. (This spinal abnormality develops in many adults and some adolescents with sickle cell anemia, leaving the vertebrae resembling logs that form the corner of a cabin.)

Diagnostic procedures
❍ Ophthalmoscopic examination revealing corkscrew or comma-shaped vessels in the conjunctivae

Treatment

General
❍ Avoidance of extreme temperatures
❍ Avoidance of stress
❍ Well-balanced diet
❍ Adequate amounts of folic acid-rich foods
❍ Adequate fluid intake
❍ Bed rest with crises
❍ Activity, as tolerated

Medication
❍ Vaccines, such as polyvalent pneumococcal vaccine and *Haemophilus influenzae* B vaccine
❍ Anti-infectives
❍ Analgesics
❍ Iron supplements
❍ Transfusion of packed RBCs, if Hb level decreases suddenly or if condition deteriorates rapidly
❍ Sedation and administration of analgesics, blood transfusion, oxygen therapy, and large amounts of oral or I.V. fluids, in an acute sequestration crisis

Nursing considerations

Key outcomes
The patient will:
❍ demonstrate age-appropriate skills and behaviors to the extent possible
❍ exhibit adequate ventilation
❍ maintain collateral circulation
❍ maintain balanced fluid volume where input will equal output
❍ express feelings of increased comfort and decreased pain
❍ maintain normal peripheral pulses
❍ maintain normal skin color and temperature.

Nursing interventions
❍ Encourage the patient to talk about his fears and concerns.
❍ If a male patient develops sudden, painful priapism, reassure him that such episodes are common and have no permanent harmful effects.
❍ Ensure that the patient receives adequate amounts of folic acid-rich foods such as green leafy vegetables.
❍ Encourage adequate fluid intake.

❍ Apply warm compresses, warmed thermal blankets, and warming pads or mattresses to painful areas of the patient's body, unless he has neuropathy.
❍ Administer analgesics and antipyretics, as necessary.
❍ When cultures demonstrate the presence of infection, give prescribed antibiotics.
❍ Give prescribed prophylactic antibiotics.
❍ Use strict sterile technique when performing treatments.
❍ Encourage bed rest with the head of the bed elevated to decrease tissue oxygen demand.
❍ Administer oxygen, as needed.
❍ Administer blood transfusions.
❍ If the patient requires general anesthesia for surgery, help ensure that he receives adequate ventilation to prevent hypoxic crisis.

Monitoring
❍ Vital signs
❍ Intake and output
❍ CBC and other laboratory study results

Patient teaching

Be sure to cover:
❍ avoidance of tight clothing that restricts circulation
❍ conditions that provoke hypoxia, such as strenuous exercise, vasoconstricting medications, cold temperatures, unpressurized aircraft, and high altitude
❍ importance of normal childhood immunizations, meticulous wound care, good oral hygiene, regular dental checkups, and a balanced diet as safeguards against infection
❍ need for prompt treatment of infection
❍ need to increase fluid intake to prevent dehydration, which can cause increased blood viscosity
❍ symptoms of vaso-occlusive crisis
❍ need for hospitalization in a vaso-occlusive crisis in which I.V. fluids, parenteral analgesics, oxygen therapy, and blood transfusions may be necessary
❍ need to inform all health care providers that the patient has this disease before undergoing any treatment, especially major surgery
❍ pregnancy and the disease
❍ balanced diet, including folic acid supplements during pregnancy.

Discharge planning
❍ Refer parents of children with sickle cell anemia for genetic counseling to answer their questions about the risk to future offspring.
❍ Refer other family members for genetic counseling to determine if they're heterozygote carriers.
❍ If necessary, refer the patient for psychological counseling to help him cope.
❍ Refer women with sickle cell anemia for birth control counseling.

Anemia, sideroblastic

Overview

Description
- A group of heterogenous disorders with a common defect that causes failure to use iron in hemoglobin synthesis despite the availability of adequate iron stores
- Can be acquired or hereditary; the acquired form, in turn, can be primary or secondary

Pathophysiology
- Normoblasts fail to use iron to synthesize hemoglobin.
- Iron is deposited in the mitochondria of normoblasts, rather than in the hemoglobin molecules.
- Iron toxicity can cause organ damage.

Causes
- Hereditary; may be due to a rare genetic defect on the X chromosome
- Acquired form may be secondary to ingestion of or exposure to toxins, such as alcohol and lead, or to drugs, such as isoniazid and chloramphenicol
- Complication of neoplastic and inflammatory diseases, such as lymphoma, rheumatoid arthritis, lupus erythematosus, multiple myeloma, tuberculosis, and severe infections
- Primary acquired form cause unknown

Incidence
- Most prevalent in young males
- Appears to be transmitted by X-linked inheritance; females are carriers and usually show no signs of this disorder
- Primary acquired form most common in elderly people, but occasionally develops in young people

Common characteristics
- Anorexia and fatigue
- Systemic signs of anemia

Complications
- Severe cardiac, hepatic, splenic, and pancreatic disease
- Acute myelogenous leukemia

Assessment

History
- Anorexia
- Fatigue
- Weakness
- Dizziness
- Dyspnea

Physical findings
- Pale skin and oral mucous membranes
- Slight jaundice
- Petechiae or bruises
- Enlarged lymph nodes
- Hepatosplenomegaly

Test results
Laboratory
- Red blood cell (RBC) indices that are revealed by microscopic examination of blood show erythrocytes to be hypochromic or normochromic and slightly macrocytic; RBC precursors that may be megaloblastic, with anisocytosis (abnormal variation in RBC size) and poikilocytosis (abnormal variation in RBC shape)
- Vitamin B_{12} and folic acid levels that are normal unless combined anemias are present
- Serum reticulocyte count that's low because young cells die in the marrow

Diagnostic procedures
- Ringed sideroblasts on microscopic examination of bone marrow aspirate stained with Prussian blue dye confirms the diagnosis. (See *Ringed sideroblast.*)

Treatment

General
- Underlying cause determines the course of treatment (for example, in acquired secondary form, the causative drug or toxin is removed)
- Phlebotomy may be indicated
- Nutritious diet
- Frequent rest periods

Medication
In hereditary sideroblastic anemia
- High doses of pyridoxine
In primary acquired anemia
- Transfusion or high doses of androgens
In chronic iron overload
- Deferoxamine

Nursing considerations

Key outcomes
The patient will:
- express feelings of increased energy
- maintain skin integrity
- not develop infection
- show improvement or healing in his lesions or wounds
- express feelings of increased comfort and decreased pain.

Nursing interventions

○ Provide frequent rest periods. Plan activities and diagnostic tests so the patient can rest in between.
○ Institute safety measures to prevent falls.
○ Give prescribed drugs.
○ Provide comfort measures; have the patient perform relaxation techniques to facilitate coping.
○ Administer blood transfusions. Notify the physician if signs of a transfusion reaction occur.
○ If the patient has jaundice or pruritus, provide meticulous skin care.
○ Inquire about possible exposure to lead in the home (especially for children) or on the job.

Monitoring

○ Vital signs
○ Complications
○ Response to treatment
○ Signs and symptoms of neuropathy
○ Signs and symptoms of decreased perfusion

Patient teaching

Be sure to cover:
○ prescribed treatment and possible complications
○ importance of continuing prescribed therapy, even after the patient begins to feel better
○ precautions for parents about house paint and not allowing children to eat paint chips because of the possibility of lead
○ recognition of and when to report adrenergic adverse effects, if androgens are used as part of the treatment
○ phlebotomy (if scheduled)
○ recognition of and when to report signs and symptoms of heart failure
○ need for proper hygiene and other measures to guard against infections and when to report signs and symptoms of infection.

Discharge planning

○ Identify patients who abuse alcohol and refer them for appropriate therapy.

Ringed sideroblast

Electron micocroscopy shows large iron deposits in the mitochondria that surround the nucleus, forming the characteristic ringed sideroblast.

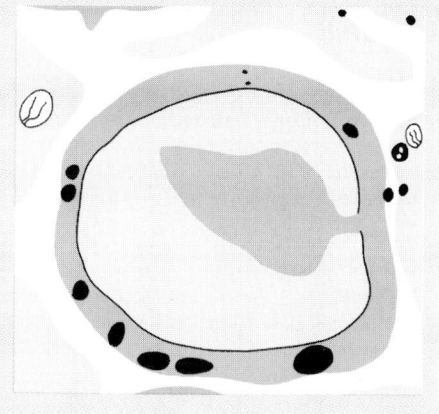

Aneurysm, abdominal aortic

Overview

Description
- Abnormal dilation in the arterial wall of the aorta, commonly between the renal arteries and iliac branches
- Can be fusiform (spindle-shaped), saccular (pouch-like), or dissecting

Pathophysiology
- Focal weakness in the tunica media layer of the aorta due to degenerative changes, which allows the tunica intima and tunica adventitia layers to stretch outward
- Blood pressure within the aorta that progressively weakens vessel walls and enlarges aneurysm

Causes
- Arteriosclerosis or atherosclerosis (95%)
- Trauma
- Syphilis; other infections

Incidence
- Seven times more common in hypertensive men than in women
- Most common in whites ages 50 to 80

Common characteristics
- 98% are located in the infrarenal aorta
- Most develop at bifurcations in the vessels

Complications
- Hemorrhage
- Shock
- Dissection

Assessment

History
- Asymptomatic until the aneurysm enlarges and compresses surrounding tissue
- Syncope when aneurysm ruptures
- When clot forms and bleeding stops, the patient may again be asymptomatic or have abdominal pain because of bleeding into the peritoneum

Physical findings
Intact aneurysm
- Gnawing, generalized, steady abdominal pain
- Lower back pain unaffected by movement
- Gastric or abdominal fullness
- Sudden onset of severe abdominal pain or lumbar pain with radiation to flank and groin
- May note a pulsating mass in the periumbilical area: don't palpate

Ruptured aneurysm
- Into the peritoneal cavity, severe, persistent abdominal and back pain
- Into the duodenum, GI bleeding with massive hematemesis and melena
- Mottled skin; poor distal perfusion
- Absent peripheral pulses distally
- Decreased level of consciousness
- Diaphoresis
- Hypotension
- Tachycardia
- Oliguria
- Distended abdomen
- Ecchymosis or hematoma in the abdominal, flank, or groin area
- Paraplegia if aneurysm rupture reduces blood flow to the spine
- Systolic bruit over the aorta
- Tenderness over affected area

Test results
Imaging
- Abdominal ultrasonography or echocardiography determines the size, shape, and location of the aneurysm.
- Anteroposterior and lateral abdominal X-rays detects aortic calcification, which outlines the mass, at least 75% of the time.
- Computed tomography scan can visualize aneurysm's effect on nearby organs.
- Aortography shows condition of vessels proximal and distal to the aneurysm and extent of aneurysm; aneurysm diameter may be underestimated because it shows only the flow channel and not the surrounding clot.

Treatment

General
- If the aneurysm is small and asymptomatic, surgery may be delayed
- Careful control of hypertension
- Fluid and blood replacement
- Weight reduction, if appropriate
- Low-fat diet
- Activity, as tolerated

Medication
- Beta-adrenergic blockers
- Antihypertensives
- Analgesics
- Antibiotics

Surgery
- Endovascular grafting or resection of large aneurysms or those that produce symptoms (see *Endovascular grafting for AAA*)
- Bypass procedures for poor perfusion distal to aneurysm
- Repair of ruptured aneurysm with a graft replacement

Endovascular grafting is a minimally invasive procedure for the patient who requires repair of an abdominal aortic aneurysm (AAA). Endovascular grafting reinforces the walls of the aorta to prevent rupture and prevents expansion of the size of the aneurysm.

The procedure is performed with fluoroscopic guidance, whereby a delivery catheter with an attached compressed graft is inserted through a small incision into the femoral or iliac artery over a guidewire. The delivery catheter is advanced into the aorta, where it's positioned across the aneurysm. A balloon on the catheter expands the graft and affixes it to the vessel wall. The procedure usually takes 2 to 3 hours to perform. Patients are instructed to walk the first day after surgery and are discharged from the hospital in 1 to 3 days.

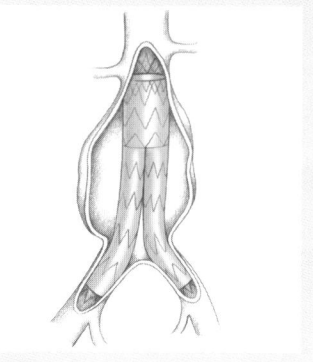

Nursing considerations

Key outcomes

The patient will:
○ maintain adequate cardiac output
○ maintain hemodynamic stability
○ maintain palpable pulses distal to the aneurysm site
○ maintain adequate urine output (output equivalent to intake)
○ express feelings of increased comfort and decreased pain.

Nursing interventions

In a nonacute situation
○ Allow the patient to express his fears and concerns and identify effective coping strategies.
○ Offer the patient and his family psychological support.
○ Before elective surgery, weigh the patient, insert an indwelling urinary catheter and an I.V. line, and assist with insertion of the arterial line and pulmonary artery catheter to monitor hemodynamic balance.
○ Give prescribed preventive antibiotics.
In an acute situation
○ Insert an I.V. line with at least a 14G needle to facilitate blood replacement.
○ Obtain blood samples for laboratory tests, as ordered.
○ Give prescribed drugs.

 Alert

Be alert for signs of rupture, which may be immediately fatal. If rupture does occur, surgery needs to be immediate. Medical antishock trousers may be used while transporting the patient to surgery.

After surgery
○ Assess peripheral pulses for graft failure or occlusion.
○ Watch for signs of bleeding retroperitoneally from the graft site.

○ Maintain blood pressure in prescribed range with fluids and medications.

 Alert

Assess the patient for severe back pain, which can indicate that the graft is tearing.

○ Have the patient cough, or suction the endotracheal tube, as needed.
○ Provide frequent turning, and assist with ambulation as soon as the patient is able.

Monitoring

○ Cardiac rhythm and hemodynamics
○ Vital signs, intake and output hourly, neurologic status, and pulse oximetry
○ Respirations and breath sounds at least every hour
○ Arterial blood gas values, as ordered
○ Daily weight
○ Fluid status
○ Nasogastric intubation for patency, amount, and type of drainage
○ Laboratory studies
○ Abdominal dressings
○ Wound site for infection

Patient teaching

Be sure to cover:
○ surgical procedure and the expected postoperative care
○ importance of taking all medications as prescribed and carrying a list of medications at all times, in case of an emergency
○ physical activity restrictions until medically cleared by the physician
○ need for regular examination and ultrasound checks to monitor progression of the aneurysm, if surgery wasn't performed.

Aneurysm, femoral and popliteal

Overview

Description

- Progressive atherosclerotic changes occurring in the walls (medial layer) of the femoral and popliteal arteries resulting in a dilation or outpouching (see *Arteries of the leg*)
- May be fusiform (spindle-shaped) or saccular (pouchlike)
- Usually progressive, eventually ending in thrombosis, embolization, and gangrene

Pathophysiology

- Atherosclerotic plaque formation or loss of elastin and collagen in the vessel wall causes localized outpouching or dilation of a weakened arterial wall.

Causes

- Atherosclerosis
- Congenital weakness in the arterial wall (rare)
- Trauma (blunt or penetrating)
- Bacterial infection
- Peripheral vascular reconstructive surgery (which causes *suture line* or *false aneurysms,* whereby a blood clot forms a second lumen)

Incidence

- Most common in men over age 50

Common characteristics

- Pain
- Edema and venous distention
- Symptoms of severe ischemia in the leg or foot

Complications

- Gangrene

Assessment

History

- Pain in affected extremity

Physical findings

- Loss of pulse and color, coldness in the affected leg or foot
- Distal petechial hemorrhages (from aneurysmal emboli)
- Pulsating mass above or below the inguinal ligament
- Firm, nonpulsating mass above or below the inguinal ligament when thrombosis has occurred

Test results

Diagnostic procedures
- Arteriography or ultrasonography reveals aneurysm.

Other
- Physical examination reveals signs and symptoms of aneurysm.

Treatment

General

- Nothing by mouth before surgery
- Limited movement of the affected extremity

Medication

- Analgesics
- Antibiotics (before surgery)
- Anticoagulants

Surgery

- Surgical bypass and reconstruction of the artery, usually with an autogenous saphenous vein graft replacement
- Leg amputation if arterial occlusion causes severe ischemia and gangrene

Nursing considerations

Key outcomes

The patient will:
- maintain pulses and adequate circulation to damaged aneurysm site
- express feelings of increased comfort and decreased pain
- carry out activities of daily living without excess fatigue or exhaustion.

Nursing interventions

Before corrective surgery, perform the following:
- Evaluate the patient's circulatory status, noting the location and quality of peripheral pulses in the affected arm or leg.
- Administer a prophylactic antibiotic or anticoagulant, as needed.
- Discuss expected postoperative procedures with the patient, and review the surgical procedure.

After arterial surgery, perform the following:
- Correlate condition of extremity with preoperative circulatory assessment. Mark the sites on the patient's skin where pulses are palpable, to facilitate repeated checks.
- Help the patient walk soon after surgery, to prevent venostasis and thrombus formation.

Monitoring

- Neurovascular condition of affected extremity (pulse, temperature, sensation, color)
- Vital signs
- Pain control

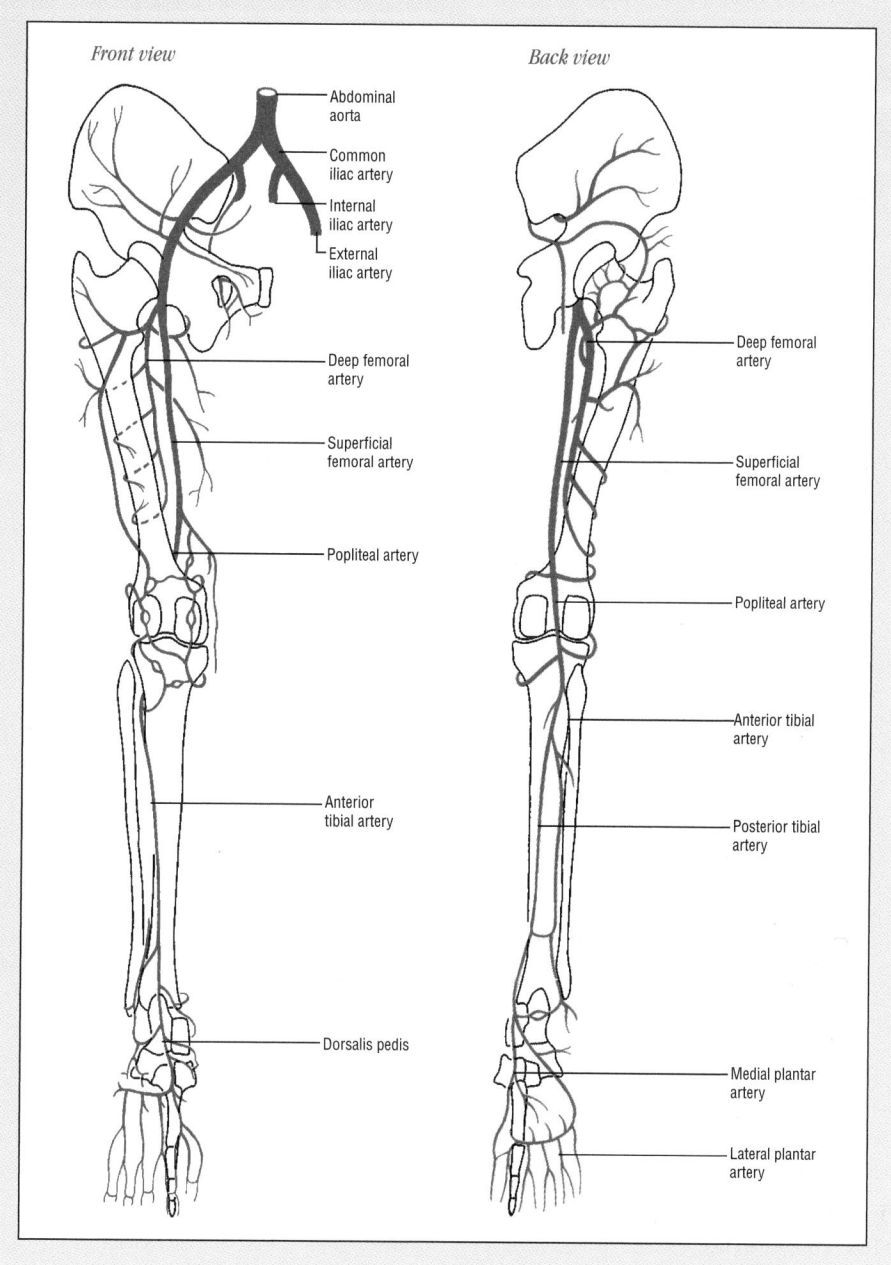

Front view

- Abdominal aorta
- Common iliac artery
- Internal iliac artery
- External iliac artery
- Deep femoral artery
- Superficial femoral artery
- Popliteal artery
- Anterior tibial artery
- Dorsalis pedis

Back view

- Deep femoral artery
- Superficial femoral artery
- Popliteal artery
- Anterior tibial artery
- Posterior tibial artery
- Medial plantar artery
- Lateral plantar artery

Patient teaching

Be sure to cover:
- importance of immediately informing the physician of any recurrence of symptoms
- how to apply antiembolism stockings (Warn the patient against wearing constrictive clothing.)
- measures to prevent bleeding (if an anticoagulant is prescribed) such as using an electric razor
- importance of reporting signs of bleeding immediately (bleeding gums, easy bruising, or black, tarry stools)
- importance of follow-up blood studies to monitor anticoagulant therapy.

Aneurysm, intracranial

Overview

Description

○ Weakness in the wall of a cerebral artery that causes localized dilation
○ Most common form is the berry aneurysm, a saclike outpouching in a cerebral artery
○ Usually occurs at an arterial junction in the Circle of Willis, the circular anastomosis forming the major cerebral arteries at the base of the brain
○ Often rupture and cause subarachnoid hemorrhage

Pathophysiology

○ Blood flow exerts pressure against a congenitally weak arterial wall, stretching it like an overblown balloon and making it likely to rupture.
○ Such a rupture is followed by a subarachnoid hemorrhage, in which blood spills into the space normally occupied by cerebrospinal fluid.
○ Blood spills into brain tissue, where a clot can cause potentially fatal increased intracranial pressure and brain tissue damage.

Causes

○ Congenital defect
○ Degenerative process
○ Combination of congenital defect and degenerative process
○ Trauma

Incidence

○ Slightly higher in women than in men, especially those in their late 40s or early- to mid-50s
○ May occur at any age in either sex

Common characteristics

○ Headache
○ Nuchal rigidity
○ Stiff back and legs
With rupture
○ Sudden severe headache
○ Altered level of consciousness

Complications

○ Neurologic deficits
○ Rebleeding
○ Vasospasm
○ Death

Assessment

History

○ Headache
○ Intermittent nausea
○ Seizure
○ Photophobia
○ Blurred vision

Physical findings

Typically, the severity of a ruptured intracranial aneurysm is graded according to the patient's signs and symptoms. (See *Determining severity of an intracranial aneurysm rupture.*)
○ Nuchal rigidity
○ Back and leg pain
○ Fever
○ Restlessness
○ Irritability
○ Hemiparesis
○ Hemisensory defects
○ Dysphagia
○ Visual defects (diplopia, ptosis, dilated pupil, and inability to rotate the eye caused by compression on the oculomotor nerve if aneurysm is near the internal carotid artery)

Test results

Imaging
○ Computed tomography scan reveals subarachnoid or ventricular bleeding with blood in subarachnoid space and displaced midline structures.
○ Magnetic resonance imaging shows a cerebral blood flow void.
○ Skull X-rays may reveal calcified wall of the aneurysm and areas of bone erosion.
Diagnostic procedures
○ Cerebral angiography reveals altered cerebral blood flow, vessel lumen dilation, and differences in arterial filling.

Treatment

General

○ Bed rest in a quiet, darkened room with minimal stimulation
○ Avoidance of coffee, other stimulants, and aspirin

Medication

○ Analgesics
○ Antihypertensive agents
○ Sedatives
○ Calcium channel blockers
○ Corticosteroids
○ Anticonvulsants
○ Aminocaproic acid

The severity of symptoms varies from patient to patient, depending on the site and amount of bleeding. Five grades characterize a ruptured cerebral aneurysm:

○ *Grade I: minimal bleeding*—The patient is alert with no neurologic deficit; he may have a slight headache and nuchal rigidity.

○ *Grade II: mild bleeding*—The patient is alert, with a mild to severe headache and nuchal rigidity; he may have third-nerve palsy.

○ *Grade III: moderate bleeding*—The patient is confused or drowsy, with nuchal rigidity and, possibly, a mild focal deficit.

○ *Grade IV: severe bleeding*—The patient is stuporous, with nuchal rigidity and, possibly, mild to severe hemiparesis.

○ *Grade V: moribund (often fatal)* —If the rupture is nonfatal, the patient is in a deep coma or decerebrate.

Surgery

○ Surgical repair by clipping, ligation, or wrapping (before or after rupture)

Nursing considerations

Key outcomes

The patient will:
○ maintain adequate ventilation
○ maintain or improve level of consciousness
○ maintain hemodynamic stability.

Nursing interventions

○ Establish and maintain a patent airway.
○ Position the patient to promote pulmonary drainage and prevent upper airway obstruction.
○ Impose aneurysm precautions (bed rest in a quiet, darkened room, keeping the head of the bed flat or less than 30 degrees, as ordered; limited visitation; avoidance of strenuous physical activity and straining with bowel movements; and restricted fluid intake).
○ Assist with active range-of-motion (ROM) exercises; if the patient is paralyzed, perform regular passive ROM exercises.
○ If the patient has facial weakness, assess the gag reflex and assist him during meals, placing food in the unaffected side of his mouth. If he can't swallow, insert a nasogastric tube, as ordered, and administer tube feedings.
○ If the patient can't speak, establish a simple means of communication or use cards or a notepad. Encourage his family to speak to him in a normal tone, even if he doesn't seem to respond.
○ Provide emotional support, and include the patient's family in his care as much as possible. Encourage family members to adopt a realistic attitude, but don't discourage hope.

Monitoring

○ Vital signs
○ Neurologic status
○ Arterial blood gases
○ Intake and output

Patient teaching

Be sure to cover:
○ the disorder, diagnosis, and treatment
○ how to recognize signs of rebleeding.

Discharge planning

○ Refer the patient to a visiting nurse or a rehabilitation center when necessary.

Aneurysm, thoracic aortic

Overview

Description

- Abnormal widening of the ascending, transverse, or descending part of the aorta
- May be saccular (outpouching), fusiform (spindle-shaped), or dissecting

Pathophysiology

- Circumferential or transverse tear of the aortic wall intima, usually within the medial layer
- Occurs in about 60% of patients; usually an emergency; poor prognosis

Causes

- Atherosclerosis
- Blunt chest trauma
- Bacterial infections, usually at an atherosclerotic plaque
- Coarctation of the aorta
- Syphilis infection
- Rheumatic vasculitis
- Marfan syndrome

Risk factors

- Cigarette smoking
- Hypertension

Incidence

- Ascending thoracic aorta most common site
- Occurs predominantly in men younger than age 60 who have coexisting hypertension
- Descending thoracic aortic aneurysms most common in younger patients who have had chest trauma

Common characteristics

- Asymptomatic until dissection

Complications

- Cardiac tamponade
- Dissection

Assessment

History

- Without signs and symptoms until aneurysm expands and begins to dissect
- Sudden pain and possibly syncope

Physical findings

- Pallor
- Diaphoresis
- Dyspnea
- Cyanosis
- Leg weakness
- Transient paralysis
- Abrupt onset of intermittent neurologic deficits
- Abrupt loss of radial and femoral pulses and right and left carotid pulses
- Increasing area of flatness over the heart, suggesting cardiac tamponade and hemopericardium

In dissecting ascending aneurysm

- Pain with a boring, tearing, or ripping sensation in the thorax or the right anterior chest; may extend to the neck, shoulders, lower back, and abdomen
- Pain most intense at onset
- Murmur of aortic insufficiency, a diastolic murmur
- Pericardial friction rub (if hemopericardium present)
- Blood pressure may be normal or significantly elevated, with a large difference in systolic blood pressure between the right and left arms

In dissecting descending aneurysm

- Sharp, tearing pain located between the shoulder blades that usually radiates to the chest
- Carotid and radial pulses present and equal bilaterally
- Systolic blood pressure is equal
- May detect bilateral crackles and rhonchi if pulmonary edema is present

In dissecting transverse aneurysm

- Sharp, boring, and tearing pain that radiates to the shoulders
- Hoarseness
- Dyspnea
- Throat pain
- Dysphagia
- Dry cough

Test results

Laboratory

- Normal or decreased hemoglobin levels from blood loss caused by a leaking aneurysm

Imaging

- Posteroanterior and oblique chest X-rays show widening of the aorta and mediastinum.
- Aortography shows lumen of the aneurysm and its size and location.
- Magnetic resonance imaging and computed tomography scan help confirm and locate the presence of aortic dissection.

Diagnostic procedures

- Electrocardiography helps rule out the presence of myocardial infarction.
- Echocardiography may help identify dissecting aneurysm of the aortic root.
- Transesophageal echocardiography can be used to measure the aneurysm in the ascending and descending aorta.

Treatment

General
- I.V. fluids and whole blood transfusions, if needed
- Weight reduction, if appropriate
- Low-fat diet
- No activity restrictions unless surgery

Medication
- Beta-adrenergic blockers
- Antihypertensives
- Negative inotropic agents
- Analgesics
- Antibiotics

Surgery
- Surgical resection with a Dacron or Teflon graft replacement

Nursing considerations

Key outcomes
The patient will:
- maintain adequate cardiac output and hemodynamic stability
- maintain adequate ventilation
- express feelings of increased comfort and decreased pain
- show no signs or symptoms of infection
- maintain adequate fluid volume.

Nursing interventions
- In a nonemergency situation, allow the patient to express his fears and concerns and identify and use effective coping strategies.
- Offer the patient and his family psychological support.
- Give prescribed analgesics to relieve pain.

After repair of thoracic aneurysm
- Maintain blood pressure in prescribed range with fluids and medications.
- Give prescribed analgesics.
- After stabilization of vital signs, encourage and assist the patient in turning, coughing, and deep breathing.
- Help the patient walk as soon as he's able.
- Assist the patient with range-of-motion leg exercises.

Monitoring
- Vital signs and hemodynamics
- Chest tube drainage
- Heart and lung sounds
- Laboratory results
- Distal pulses
- Level of consciousness and pain
- Signs of infection
- I.V. therapy and intake and output

 Alert

After surgical repair, monitor for signs that resemble those of the initial dissecting aneurysm, suggesting a tear at the graft site.

Patient teaching

Be sure to cover:
- diagnosis
- procedure and expected postoperative care, if surgery is scheduled
- compliance with antihypertensive therapy, including the need for such drugs and the expected adverse effects
- monitoring of blood pressure
- when to call the physician if the patient has any sharp pain in the chest or back of the neck.

Discharge planning
- Refer the patient to a smoking-cessation program, if indicated.

Aneurysm, ventricular

Overview

Description

- An outpouching, almost always of the left ventricle, that produces ventricular wall dysfunction
- May develop within days to weeks after myocardial infarction (MI) or may be delayed for years

Pathophysiology

- When MI destroys a large muscular section of the left ventricle, necrosis reduces the ventricular wall to a thin sheath of fibrous tissue.
- Under intracardiac pressure, the thin sheath stretches and forms a separate noncontractile sac (aneurysm).
- Abnormal muscle wall movement accompanies ventricular aneurysm.
- During systolic ejection, the abnormal muscle wall movements cause the remaining normally functioning myocardial fibers to increase the force of contraction to maintain stroke volume and cardiac output.
- At the same time, a portion of the stroke volume is lost to passive distention of the noncontractile sac.

Causes

- MI

Incidence

- Occurs in about 20% of patients after MI

Common characteristics

- Occurs after MI

Complications

- Ventricular arrhythmias
- Cerebral embolization
- Heart failure

Assessment

History

- Previous MI
- Dyspnea
- Fatigue

Physical findings

- Edema
- Visible or palpable systolic precordial bulge
- Distended jugular veins, if heart failure is present
- Irregular peripheral pulse rhythm
- Arrhythmias such as premature ventricular contractions
- Pulsus alternans
- Double, diffuse, or displaced apical impulse
- Gallop rhythm
- Crackles and rhonchi

Test results

Imaging
- Two-dimensional echocardiography demonstrates abnormal motion in the left ventricular wall.
- Left ventriculography reveals left ventricular enlargement, with an area of akinesia or dyskinesia (during cineangiography) and diminished cardiac function.
- Chest X-rays may disclose an abnormal bulge distorting the heart's contour if the aneurysm is large; X-rays may be normal if the aneurysm is small.
- Noninvasive nuclear cardiology scan may indicate the site of infarction and suggest the area of aneurysm.

Diagnostic procedures
- Electrocardiography may show persistent ST-T wave elevations.

Treatment

General

- Depends on the size of the aneurysm and the presence of complications
- May require only routine medical examination to follow the patient's condition
- May require aggressive measures, such as cardioversion, defibrillation, and endotracheal intubation
- Weight reduction, if appropriate
- Low-fat diet
- No activity restrictions, unless surgery

Medication

- Antiarrhythmics
- Cardiac glycosides
- Diuretics
- Fluid and electrolyte replacement
- Analgesics
- Antihypertensives
- Nitrates
- Anticoagulation

Surgery

- Embolectomy
- Aneurysmectomy with myocardial revascularization

Nursing considerations

Key outcomes

The patient will:
- maintain adequate cardiac output
- maintain hemodynamic stability
- maintain adequate fluid balance
- express feelings of increased energy and decreased fatigue
- express feelings of decreased anxiety.

Nursing interventions
○ Give prescribed drugs.
○ Prepare for surgery, if indicated.

 Alert

Be alert for sudden changes in sensorium that may indicate cerebral embolization and for any signs that suggest renal failure or MI.

○ Provide psychological support for the patient and his family.

Monitoring
Heart failure
○ Vital signs and heart sounds
○ Cardiac rhythm, especially for ventricular arrhythmias
○ Intake and output; and fluid and electrolyte balance
○ Blood urea nitrogen and serum creatinine levels
After surgery
○ Pulmonary artery catheter pressures
○ Signs and symptoms of infection
○ Type and amount of chest tube drainage

Patient teaching

Be sure to cover:
○ the disorder, diagnosis, and treatment
○ medications and potential adverse reactions
○ when to notify the physician
○ expected postoperative care, if the patient is scheduled to undergo resection
○ monitoring pulse irregularity and rate changes.

Discharge planning
○ Refer the patient (or his family) to a community-based cardiopulmonary resuscitation training program.
○ Refer the patient to a weight-reduction program, if indicated.
○ Refer the patient to a smoking-cessation program, if indicated.

Ankylosing spondylitis

Overview

Description

○ Rheumatoid disease primarily affecting sacroiliac, apophyseal, and costocervical joints and adjacent ligamentous or tendinous attachments to bone
○ Usually occurs as a primary disorder; may occur secondary to Reiter's syndrome, psoriatic arthritis, or inflammatory bowel disease
○ Also called *rheumatoid spondylitis* or *Marie-Strümpell disease*

Pathophysiology

○ Begins in the sacroiliac; gradually progresses to the lumbar, thoracic, and cervical spine
○ Bone and cartilage deterioration that leads to fibrous tissue formation and eventual fusion of the spine or peripheral joints

Causes

○ Unknown
○ Familial tendency
○ Initial inflammation may result from immune system activation by bacterial infection

Incidence

○ Affects men two to three times more often than women
○ Well recognized in men but commonly overlooked or missed in women
○ Women have more peripheral joint involvement

Common characteristics

○ Symptoms can unpredictably remit, exacerbate, or arrest at any stage

Complications

○ Atlantoaxial subluxation
○ Deposits of amyloid material in the kidneys, which may lead to renal impairment or failure

---

Detecting ankylosing spondylitis in women

Ankylosing spondylitis seldom occurs in women, which is why if a woman's symptoms include pelvic pain diagnosticians typically overlook ankylosing spondylitis and suspect pelvic imflammatory disease. However, it's important to assess a female patient with apparent pelvic disease carefully — especially if culture results identify no apparent cause of her discomfort. Otherwise, misdiagnosis can lead to unwarranted invasive tests and treatments and cause the patient needless anxiety related to contracting a sexually transmitted disease. Asking the patient if there's a family history of ankylosing spondylitis and the performance of a thorough health and social history is advisable.

Assessment

History

○ Intermittent lower back pain most severe in the morning or after inactivity and relieved by exercise
○ Mild fatigue, fever, anorexia, and weight loss
○ May describe pain in shoulders, hips, knees, and ankles
○ Pain over the symphysis pubis, which may lead to its being mistaken for pelvic inflammatory disease (see *Detecting ankylosing spondylitis in women*)

Physical findings

○ Stiffness or limited motion of the lumbar spine
○ Pain and limited chest expansion
○ Kyphosis
○ Iritis
○ Warmth, swelling, or tenderness of affected joints
○ Small joints such as toes may become sausage-shaped
○ Aortic murmur caused by regurgitation
○ Cardiomegaly
○ Upper lobe pulmonary fibrosis, which mimics tuberculosis, that may reduce vital capacity to 70% or less of predicted volume

Test results

○ Diagnosis of primary ankylosing spondylitis requires meeting established criteria. (See *Diagnosing primary ankylosing spondylitis.*)
Laboratory
○ HLA antigen typing test showing serum findings that include HLA-B27 in about 95% of patients with primary ankylosing spondylitis and up to 80% of patients with secondary disease
○ Serum rheumatoid factor tests showing the absence of rheumatoid factor, which helps to rule out rheumatoid arthritis, which has similar symptoms
○ Serum alkaline phosphate and creatine kinase tests showing slightly elevated erythrocyte sedimentation rate, serum alkaline phosphate levels, and creatine kinase levels in active disease
○ Serum immunoglobulin profile showing elevated serum IgA levels
Imaging
○ X-ray studies define characteristic changes, such as bilateral sacroiliac involvement (the hallmark of the disease); blurring of the joints' bony margins in early disease; patchy sclerosis with superficial bony erosions; eventual squaring of vertebral bodies; and "bamboo spine" with complete ankylosis.

Treatment

General

○ Good posture; stretching and deep-breathing exercises
○ Braces and lightweight supports, if appropriate

○ Heat, warm showers, baths, and ice
○ Nerve stimulation
○ Nutritious diet
○ Encourage activity, as tolerated

Medication

○ Nonsteroidal anti-inflammatory drugs

Surgery

○ Hip replacement surgery with severe hip involvement
○ Spinal wedge osteotomy with severe spinal involvement

Nursing considerations

Key outcomes

The patient will:
○ express feelings of increased comfort and decreased pain
○ express feelings of increased energy
○ recognize limitations imposed by illness and express feelings about these limitations
○ identify factors that increase the potential for injury.

Nursing interventions

○ Keep in mind the patient's limited range of motion (ROM) when planning self-care tasks and activities.
○ Offer support and reassurance.
○ Give prescribed analgesics.
○ Apply heat locally and massage, as indicated.
○ Have the patient perform active ROM exercises.
○ Pace periods of exercise and rest to help the patient achieve comfortable energy levels and lung oxygenation.
○ If treatment includes surgery, ensure proper body alignment and positioning.
○ Involve other caregivers, such as a social worker, visiting nurse, and dietitian.

Monitoring

○ Mobility and comfort level
○ Respiratory status
○ Heart sounds

Patient teaching

Be sure to cover:
○ avoidance of physical activity that places stress on the back such as lifting heavy objects
○ importance of standing upright; sitting upright in a high, straight-back chair; and avoiding leaning over a desk
○ importance of sleeping in a prone position on a hard mattress and avoiding using pillows under the neck or knees
○ avoidance of prolonged walking, standing, sitting, or driving
○ regular stretching and deep-breathing exercises; swimming on a regular basis, if possible

Diagnosing primary ankylosing spondylitis

For a reliable diagnosis, the patient must meet:
○ criterion 7 and any one of criteria 1 through 5, or
○ any five of criteria 1 through 6 if he doesn't have criterion 7.

Seven criteria
1. Axial skeleton stiffness for at least 3 months that's relieved by exercise
2. Lumbar pain that persists at rest
3. Thoracic cage pain of at least 3 months' duration that persists at rest
4. Past or current iritis
5. Decreased lumbar range of motion
6. Decreased chest expansion (age-related)
7. Bilateral, symmetrical sacroiliitis demonstrated by radiographic studies

○ measurement of patient's height every 3 to 4 months to detect kyphosis
○ nutrition and weight maintenance.

Discharge planning

○ Refer the patient to physical therapy, as needed.
○ Refer the patient the Spondylitis Association of America or the Arthritis Foundation for additional support and information.

Anorexia nervosa

Overview

Description

- Psychological disorder of self-imposed starvation resulting from a distorted body image and an intense and irrational fear of gaining weight
- Actual loss of appetite, which is rare
- May occur simultaneously with bulimia nervosa

Pathophysiology

- Decreased calorie intake depletes body fat and protein stores.
- Estrogen deficiency occurs (in women) due to lack of lipid substrate for synthesis, causing amenorrhea.
- Testosterone levels fluctuate (in men) and decreased erectile function and sperm count occurs.
- Ketoacidosis occurs from increased use of fat as energy fuel.

Causes

- Exact cause unknown
- Social attitudes that equate slimness with beauty
- Subconscious effort to exert personal control over life or to protect oneself from dealing with issues surrounding sexuality
- Elaborate food preparation and eating rituals
- Achievement pressure
- Dependence and independence issues
- Stress caused by multiple responsibilities
- History of sexual abuse

Risk factors

- Low self-esteem
- Compulsive personality
- High achievement goals

Incidence

- 5% to 10% of the population; more than 90% of those affected are females

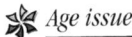 *Age issue*

Anorexia nervosa occurs primarily in adolescents and young adults but also may affect older women and, occasionally, males.

Common characteristics

- Preoccupation with body size
- Tendency to describe self as "fat"
- Dissatisfaction with a particular aspect of physical appearance
- Compulsive exercising
- Self-induced vomiting
- Laxative or diuretic abuse
- Limits or restricts food intake; eats small portions (see *Criteria for hospitalizing a patient with anorexia nervosa*)

Complications

- Death
- Suicide
- Electrolyte imbalances
- Malnutrition
- Dehydration
- Esophageal erosion, ulcers, tears, and bleeding
- Tooth and gum erosion and dental caries
- Decreased left ventricular muscle mass and chamber size
- Decreased cardiac output
- Hypotension
- Electrocardiogram (ECG) changes
- Heart failure
- Increased susceptibility to infection
- Amenorrhea
- Anemia

Assessment

History

- 15% or greater weight loss for no organic reason
- Morbid fear of being fat
- Compulsion to be thin
- Angry disposition
- Tendency to minimize weight loss
- Ritualistic
- Amenorrhea
- Infertility
- Loss of libido
- Fatigue
- Sleep alterations
- Intolerance to cold
- Constipation or diarrhea

Physical findings

- Hypotension
- Bradycardia
- Emaciated appearance
- Skeletal muscle atrophy
- Loss of fatty tissue
- Atrophy of breast tissue
- Blotchy or sallow skin
- Lanugo on the face and body
- Dryness or loss of scalp hair
- Calluses of the knuckles
- Abrasions and scars on the dorsum of the hand
- Dental caries
- Oral or pharyngeal abrasions
- Painless salivary gland enlargement
- Bowel distention
- Slowed reflexes

DSM-IV-TR criteria

These criteria must be documented:
○ Refusal to maintain or achieve normal weight for age and height
○ Intense fear of gaining weight or becoming fat, even though underweight
○ Disturbance in perception of body weight, size, or shape
○ Absence of at least three consecutive menstrual cycles when otherwise expected to occur (in females).

Test results

Laboratory
○ Decreased hemoglobin level, platelet count, and white blood cell count
○ Prolonged bleeding time
○ Decreased erythrocyte sedimentation rate
○ Decreased levels of serum creatinine, blood urea nitrogen, uric acid, cholesterol, total protein, albumin, sodium, potassium, chloride, calcium, and fasting blood glucose
○ Elevated levels of alanine aminotransferase and aspartate aminotransferase in severe starvation states
○ Elevated serum amylase levels
○ In females, decreased levels of serum luteinizing hormone and follicle-stimulating hormone
○ Decreased triiodothyronine levels
○ Urinalysis that shows dilute urine

Diagnostic procedures
○ ECG may show nonspecific ST interval, T-wave changes, and prolonged PR interval; ventricular arrhythmias may also be present.

Treatment

General

○ Behavior modification
○ Curtailed activity for cardiac arrhythmias
○ Group, family, or individual psychotherapy
○ Balanced diet with a normal eating pattern
○ Parenteral nutrition, if necessary
○ Gradual increase in physical activity when weight gain and stabilization occur

Medication

○ Vitamin and mineral supplements

Nursing considerations

Key outcomes

The patient will:
○ acknowledge change in body image
○ express positive feelings about self
○ achieve and maintain expected body weight
○ achieve expected state of wellness.

Nursing interventions

○ Support the patient's efforts to achieve target weight.
○ Negotiate an adequate food intake with the patient.

Criteria for hospitalizing a patient with anorexia nervosa

A patient with anorexia nervosa can be successfully treated on an outpatient basis. However, if the patient displays any of the signs listed here, hospitalization is mandatory:
○ rapid weight loss equal to 15% or more of normal body mass
○ persistent bradycardia (50 beats/minute or less)
○ hypotension with a systolic reading less than or equal to 90 mm Hg
○ hypothermia (core body temperature less than or equal to 97° F (36.1° C)
○ presence of medical complications, suicidal ideation
○ persistent sabotage or disruption of outpatient treatment — resolute denial of condition and the need for treatment.

○ Supervise the patient one-on-one during meals and for 1 hour afterward.

Monitoring

○ Vital signs
○ Intake and output
○ Electrolyte and complete blood count levels
○ Weight on a regular schedule
○ Activity for compulsive exercise

 Alert

Monitor the patient for 1 hour after meals to ensure no self-induced vomiting.

Patient teaching

Be sure to cover:
○ nutrition
○ importance of keeping a food journal
○ avoidance of discussions about food between the patient and her family.

Discharge planning

○ Refer the patient to support services.

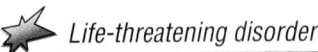

Life-threatening disorder

Anthrax

Overview

Description

○ An acute bacterial infection occuring most commonly in herbivorous animals; the natural resistance of humans to anthrax is greater than that of these animals
○ Also known as a potential agent for use in bioterrorism and biological warfare; it's classified as a Category A biological disease
○ Human cases of anthrax are classified as either agricultural or industrial
○ In humans, anthrax occurs in three forms, depending on the mode of transmission: cutaneous, inhalation (woolsorters' disease), and GI
○ Cutaneous anthrax is the most common form of anthrax
○ Without treatment, mortality rate from cutaneous anthrax is 20%; mortality rate less than 1% with treatment
○ Even with treatment, inhalation anthrax usually fatal
○ With treatment, death occurs in 25% to 60% of cases of GI anthrax
○ There is no screening test for anthrax

Pathophysiology

○ *Bacillus anthracis* is an encapsulated, chain-forming, aerobic, gram-positive rod that forms oval spores; spores are hardy and can survive for years under adverse conditions.
○ *B. anthracis,* an extracellular pathogen, evades phagocytosis, invades the bloodstream, and multiplies rapidly.
○ In cutaneous anthrax, spores enter the body through abraded or broken skin or by biting flies; the spores germinate within hours, the vegetative cells multiply and anthrax toxin is produced.
○ In inhalation anthrax, spores are deposited directly into the alveoli and phagocytized by macrophages; some are carried to and germinate in mediastinal nodes. This may result in overwhelming bacteremia, hemorrhagic mediastinitis, and secondary pneumonia.
○ In GI anthrax, primary infection can occur in the intestine by organisms that survive passage through the stomach; acute inflammation of the intestinal tract results.

Causes

○ Bacterial infection with *B. anthracis*
Human cases
○ Contact with infected animals or contaminated animal products
○ Insect bites
○ Inhalation
○ Ingestion
Agricultural cases
○ Contact with animals that have anthrax
○ Bites of contaminated or infected flies
○ Consumption of contaminated meat
Industrial cases
○ Animal hides
○ Goat's hair
○ Wool
○ Bones

Risk factors

○ Laboratory and industrial workers at risk for occupational exposure

Incidence

○ Occurs worldwide
○ Most common in developing countries
○ Most common in domestic herbivores, including sheep, cattle, horses, and goats, and wild herbivores
○ Estimates of 20,000 to 100,000 cases per year (Approximately 95% of human anthrax are the cutaneous form; about 5% are the inhalation form; GI anthrax is rare.)

Common characteristics

○ History of exposure to *B. anthracis* spores
○ Clinical manifestation will depend upon the form of anthrax
Cutaneous anthrax
○ Painless ulcers associated with vesicles and edema
○ Contact with animals or animal products

Complications

○ Septicemia
○ Hemorrhagic mediastinitis
○ Pneumonia
○ Respiratory failure
○ Hemorrhagic thoracic lymphadenitis
○ Meningitis
○ Death

Assessment

History

Cutaneous anthrax
○ Contact with animals or animal products
○ Painless ulcer
○ Mild or no constitutional symptoms
Inhalational anthrax
○ Initial prodromal flulike symptoms:
 – Malaise; dry cough
 – Mild fever; chills
 – Headache; myalgia
 – Severe respiratory distress
 – Chest pain
GI anthrax
○ Nausea; vomiting

- Decreased appetite
- Fever
- Abdominal pain
- Vomiting blood
- Severe bloody diarrhea

Physical findings

Cutaneous anthrax
- Initially, a small, papular, pruritic lesion that resembles an insect bite
- Lesion that develops into a vesicle in 1 to 2 days
- Lesion that finally becomes a small, painless ulcer with a necrotic center, surrounded by nonpitting edema
- Smaller secondary vesicles that may surround some lesions
- Lesions that are generally located on exposed areas of the skin
- Painful, regional, nonspecific lymphadenitis

Inhalational anthrax
- Increasing fever
- Dyspnea, stridor
- Hypoxia; cyanosis
- Hypotension; shock

GI anthrax
- Fever
- Rapidly developing ascites

Test results

Laboratory
- Gram stain, direct fluorescent antibody staining, and culture showing presence of *B. anthracis*
- Blood cultures showing presence of *B. anthracis*
- Cerebrospinal fluid analysis revealing presence of *B. anthracis*
- Complete blood count showing polymorphonuclear leukocytosis in severe disease
- Serum antibody tests revealing the presence of the specific antibody to *B. anthracis*

Imaging
- Chest X-ray showing symmetric mediastinal widening in hemorrhagic mediastinitis

Treatment

General

- Treatment initiated as soon as exposure to anthrax is suspected (Essential to preventing anthrax infection; early treatment may also help prevent death.)
- No dietary restrictions
- Adequate fluid intake
- Physical activity, as tolerated

Medication

- Antibiotics
- Oxygen, as needed

Surgery

- May be necessary for complications such as hemorrhagic mediastinitis

Nursing considerations

Key outcomes

The patient will:
- maintain adequate nutrition and hydration
- verbalize feelings of fear and anxiety
- demonstrate effective coping mechanisms
- maintain tissue perfusion and cellular oxygenation
- maintain effective ventilation.

Nursing interventions

- Give prescribed drugs.
- Maintain patent airway and adequate ventilation.
- Report any case of anthrax in either livestock or humans to the local board of health.
- Maintain standard precautions.
- Encourage verbalization of fears and concerns.
- Provide adequate hydration.
- Provide a well-balanced diet.
- Assist the patient in the development of effective coping mechanisms.
- Provide adequate rest periods.

Monitoring

- Vital signs
- Intake and output
- Respiratory status
- Neurologic status
- Cardiovascular status
- Skin lesions
- GI status
- Complications
- Response to treatment
- Progression of infection

Patient teaching

Be sure to cover:
- the disorder, diagnosis, and treatment
- medications and potential adverse reactions
- when to notify the physician
- anthrax prevention.

 Alert

An anthrax vaccine is available, but because of limited supplies, it's now given only to U.S. military personnel and isn't for routine civilian use.

Aortic insufficiency

Overview

Description

- A heart condition in which blood flows back into the left ventricle, causing excess fluid volume
- Also called *aortic regurgitation*

Pathophysiology

- Blood flows back into the left ventricle during diastole, causing increased left ventricular diastolic pressure
- Results in volume overload, dilation and, eventually, hypertrophy of the left ventricle
- Excess fluid volume also eventually results in increased left atrial pressure and increased pulmonary vascular pressure

Causes

- Rheumatic fever
- Primary disease of the aortic valve leaflets, the wall or the aortic root, or both
- Hypertension
- Infective endocarditis
- Trauma
- Idiopathic valve calcification
- Aortic dissection
- Aortic aneurysm
- Connective tissue diseases

Incidence

- Occurs most commonly among males
- When associated with mitral valve disease, it's more common among females

Common characteristics

- Typically asymptomatic until the fourth or fifth decade of life
- Orthopnea
- Paroxysmal nocturnal dyspnea
- Exertional dyspnea

Complications

- Left-sided heart failure
- Pulmonary edema
- Myocardial ischemia

Assessment

History

- Exertional dyspnea, orthopnea, paroxysmal nocturnal dyspnea
- Sensation of a forceful heartbeat, especially in supine position
- Angina, especially nocturnal
- Fatigue
- Palpitations, head pounding
- Symptoms of heart failure, in late stages

Physical findings

- Corrigan's pulse
- Bisferious pulse
- Water-hammer pulse
- Pulsating nail beds and Quincke's sign
- Wide pulse pressure
- Diffuse, hyperdynamic apical impulse, displaced laterally and inferiorly
- Systolic thrill at base or suprasternal notch
- S_3 gallop with increased left ventricular end-diastolic pressure
- High frequency, blowing early-peaking, diastolic decrescendo murmur best heard with the patient sitting leaning forward and in deep fixed expiration (see *Identifying the murmur of aortic insufficiency*)
- Austin Flint murmur
- Head bobbing with each heartbeat
- Tachycardia, peripheral vasoconstriction, and pulmonary edema if severe aortic insufficiency

Test results

Imaging
- Chest X-rays may show left ventricular enlargement and pulmonary vein congestion.
- Echocardiography may show left ventricular enlargement, increased motion of the septum and posterior wall, thickening of valve cusps, prolapse of the valve, flail leaflet, vegetations, or dilation of the aortic root.

Diagnostic procedures
- Electrocardiography shows sinus tachycardia, left axis deviation, left ventricular hypertrophy, and left atrial hypertrophy in severe disease.
- Cardiac catheterization shows presence and degree of aortic insufficiency, left ventricular dilation and function, and coexisting coronary artery disease.

Treatment

General

- Periodic noninvasive monitoring of aortic insufficiency and left ventricular function with echocardiogram
- Medical control of hypertension
- Low-sodium diet
- Planned periodic rest periods to avoid fatigue

Medication

- Cardiac glycosides
- Diuretics
- Vasodilators
- Antihypertensives
- Antiarrhythmics
- Infective endocarditis prophylaxis

Avoid using beta-adrenergic blockers due to their negative inotropic effects.

Surgery

○ Valve replacement

Nursing considerations

Key outcomes

The patient will:
○ carry out activities of daily living without excess fatigue or decreased energy
○ maintain cardiac output, demonstrate hemodynamic stability, and not develop arrhythmias
○ maintain adequate fluid balance
○ maintain adequate ventilation.

Nursing interventions

○ Give prescribed drugs.
○ If the patient needs bed rest, stress its importance; provide a bedside commode.
○ Alternate periods of activity and rest.
○ Allow the patient to express his concerns about the effects of activity restrictions on his responsibilities and routines.
○ Keep the patient's legs elevated while he sits in a chair.
○ Place the patient in an upright position, if necessary, and administer oxygen.
○ Keep the patient on a low-sodium diet. Consult a dietitian.
○ Following surgery, watch for hypotension, arrhythmias, and thrombus formation.

Monitoring

○ Signs and symptoms of heart failure
○ Pulmonary edema
○ Adverse reactions to drug therapy
○ Complications
After surgery
○ Vital signs and cardiac rhythm
○ Heart sounds
○ Chest tube drainage
○ Neurologic status
○ Arterial blood gas levels
○ Intake and output; daily weight
○ Blood chemistry studies, prothrombin time, and International Normalized Ratio values
○ Chest X-ray results
○ Pulmonary artery catheter pressures

Identifying the murmur of aortic insufficiency

A high-pitched, blowing decrescendo murmur that radiates from the aortic valve area to the left sternal border characterizes aortic insufficiency.

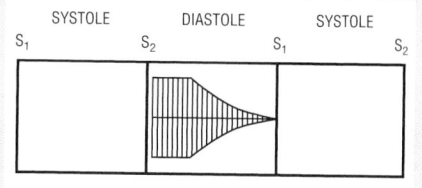

Patient teaching

Be sure to cover:
○ the disorder, diagnosis, and treatment
○ medications and potential adverse reactions
○ when to notify the physician
○ periodic rest periods in the patient's daily routine
○ leg elevation whenever the patient sits
○ dietary restrictions
○ signs and symptoms of heart failure
○ importance of consistent follow-up care
○ monitoring of pulse rate and rhythm
○ blood pressure control.

Discharge planning

○ Refer the patient to an outpatient cardiac rehabilitation program, if indicated.
○ Refer the patient to a smoking-cessation program, if indicated.
○ Refer the patient to a weight-reduction program, if indicated.

Aortic stenosis

Overview

Description

- Narrowing of the aortic valve that affects blood flow in the heart
- Classified as either acquired or rheumatic

Pathophysiology

- Stenosis of the aortic valve results in impedance to forward blood flow.
- The left ventricle requires greater pressure to open the aortic valve.
- Added workload increases myocardial oxygen demands.
- Diminished cardiac output reduces coronary artery blood flow.
- Left ventricular hypertrophy and failure result.

Causes

- Idiopathic fibrosis and calcification
- Congenital aortic bicuspid valve
- Rheumatic fever
- Atherosclerosis

Risk factors

- Diabetes mellitus
- Hypercholesterolemia

Incidence

- Symptoms may not appear until ages 50 to 70, even though stenosis has been present since childhood
- About 80% of patients are male

Common characteristics

- Long latent period
- Classic triad of angina pectoris, syncope, and dyspnea

Complications

- Left-sided heart failure
- Right-sided heart failure
- Infective endocarditis
- Cardiac arrhythmias, especially atrial fibrillation
- Sudden death
- Left ventricular hypertrophy

Assessment

History

- May be asymptomatic
- Dyspnea on exertion
- Angina
- Exertional syncope
- Fatigue
- Palpitations
- Paroxysmal nocturnal dyspnea

Physical findings

- Small, sustained arterial pulses that rise slowly
- Distinct lag between carotid artery pulse and apical pulse
- Orthopnea
- Prominent jugular vein *a* waves
- Peripheral edema
- Diminished carotid pulses with delayed upstroke
- Apex of the heart may be displaced inferiorly and laterally
- Suprasternal thrill

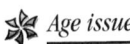 *Age issue*

An early systolic ejection murmur may be present in children and adolescents who have noncalcified valves. The murmur is low-pitched, rough, and rasping and is loudest at the base in the second intercostal space.

- Split S_2 develops as stenosis becomes more severe
- Prominent S_4
- Harsh, rasping, mid- to late-peaking systolic murmur that's best heard at the base and commonly radiates to carotids and apex (see *Identifying the murmur of aortic stenosis*)

Test results

Imaging
- Chest X-ray shows valvular calcification, left ventricular enlargement, pulmonary vein congestion and, in later stages, left atrial, pulmonary artery, right atrial, and right ventricular enlargement.
- Echocardiography shows decreased valve area, increased gradient, and increased left ventricular wall thickness.

Diagnostic procedures
- Cardiac catheterization shows increased pressure gradient across the aortic valve, increased left ventricular pressures, and presence of coronary artery disease.

Other
- Electrocardiography may show left ventricular hypertrophy, atrial fibrillation, or other arrhythmia.

Treatment

General

- Periodic noninvasive evaluation of the severity of valve narrowing
- Lifelong treatment and management of congenital aortic stenosis
- Low-sodium, low-fat, low-cholesterol diet
- Planned rest periods

Medication

- Cardiac glycosides
- Antibiotic infective endocarditis prophylaxis

Alert

The use of diuretics and vasodilators may lead to hypotension and inadequate stroke volume.

Surgery

○ In adults, valve replacement after they become symptomatic with hemodynamic evidence of severe obstruction
○ Percutaneous balloon aortic valvuloplasty
○ In children without calcified valves, simple commissurotomy under direct visualization
○ Ross procedure may be performed in patients younger than age 5

Nursing considerations

Key outcomes

The patient will:
○ perform activities of daily living without excess fatigue or exhaustion
○ avoid complications
○ maintain cardiac output
○ demonstrate hemodynamic stability
○ maintain balanced fluid status
○ maintain joint mobility and range of motion
○ develop and demonstrate adequate coping skills.

Nursing interventions

○ Give prescribed drugs.
○ Maintain a low-sodium diet. Consult with a dietitian.
○ If the patient requires bed rest, stress its importance. Provide a bedside commode.
○ Alternate periods of activity and rest.
○ Allow the patient to voice concerns about the effects of activity restrictions.
○ Keep the patient's legs elevated while he sits in a chair.
○ Place the patient in an upright position and administer oxygen, as needed.
○ Allow the patient to express his fears and concerns.

Monitoring

○ Vital signs
○ Intake and output
○ Signs and symptoms of heart failure
○ Signs and symptoms of progressive aortic stenosis
○ Daily weight
○ Arrhythmias
○ Respiratory status
If the patient has surgery
○ Signs and symptoms of thrombus formation
○ Hemodynamics
○ Arterial blood gas results
○ Blood chemistry results
○ Chest X-ray results

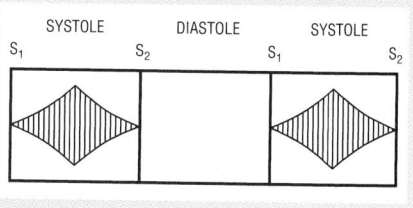
Patient teaching

Be sure to cover:
○ the disorder, diagnosis, and treatment
○ medications and potential adverse reactions
○ when to notify the physician
○ periodic rest in the patient's daily routine
○ leg elevation whenever the patient sits
○ dietary and fluid restrictions
○ importance of consistent follow-up care
○ signs and symptoms of heart failure
○ infective endocarditis prophylaxis
○ pulse rate and rhythm
○ monitoring for atrial fibrillation and other arrhythmias.

Discharge planning

○ Refer the patient to a weight-reduction program, if indicated.
○ Refer the patient to a smoking-cessation program, if indicated.

Appendicitis

Overview

Description

- ⭘ Inflammation of the vermiform appendix
- ⭘ Most common major abdominal surgical disease
- ⭘ Fatal if left untreated; gangrene and perforation develop within 36 hours

Pathophysiology

- ⭘ Mucosal ulceration triggers inflammation, which temporarily obstructs the appendix.
- ⭘ Obstruction causes mucus outflow, increasing pressure in the distended appendix; the appendix then contracts.
- ⭘ Bacteria multiply and inflammation and pressure increase, restricting blood flow and causing thrombus and abdominal pain.

Causes

- ⭘ Foreign body
- ⭘ Neoplasm
- ⭘ Mucosal ulceration
- ⭘ Fecal mass
- ⭘ Stricture
- ⭘ Barium ingestion
- ⭘ Viral infection

Risk factors

- ⭘ Adolescent male

Incidence

- ⭘ Can occur at any age; however, the majority of cases occur between ages 11 and 20
- ⭘ Affects both sexes; however, between puberty and age 25, more prevalent in men

Common characteristics

- ⭘ Abdominal pain
- ⭘ Anorexia
- ⭘ Vomiting

Complications

- ⭘ Wound infection
- ⭘ Intra-abdominal infection
- ⭘ Fecal fistula
- ⭘ Intestinal obstruction
- ⭘ Incisional hernia
- ⭘ Peritonitis (most common)
- ⭘ Death

Assessment

History

- ⭘ Abdominal pain that's initially generalized, then localizes in the right lower abdomen (McBurney's point)
- ⭘ Anorexia
- ⭘ Nausea, vomiting

Physical findings

- ⭘ Low-grade fever, tachycardia
- ⭘ Adjusts posture to decrease pain
- ⭘ Guarding
- ⭘ Normoactive bowel sounds, with possible constipation or diarrhea
- ⭘ Rebound tenderness and spasm of the abdominal muscles
- ⭘ Rovsing's sign (pain in right lower quadrant that occurs with palpation of left lower quadrant)
- ⭘ Psoas sign (abdominal pain that occurs when the patient flexes his hip with pressure applied to his knee)
- ⭘ Obturator sign (abdominal pain that occurs when the hip is rotated)
- ⭘ Absent abdominal tenderness or flank tenderness with retrocele or pelvic appendix

Test results

Laboratory
- ⭘ White blood cell count moderately elevated, with increased numbers of immature cells

Imaging
- ⭘ Abdominal or transvaginal ultrasound shows appendiceal inflammation.
- ⭘ Barium enema reveals nonfilling appendix.
- ⭘ Abdominal computed tomography scan demonstrates suspected perforation or abscess.

Treatment

General

- ⭘ Delaying surgery until antibiotic therapy has been initiated, if an abscess is suspected
- ⭘ Nothing by mouth until after surgery, then gradual return to regular diet
- ⭘ Early postoperative ambulation
- ⭘ Incentive spirometry

Medication

- ⭘ I.V. fluids
- ⭘ Analgesics
- ⭘ Antibiotics preoperatively and if peritonitis develops

Surgery

- ⭘ Appendectomy

Nursing considerations

Key outcomes

The patient will:
- ⭘ express feelings of increased comfort
- ⭘ avoid complications
- ⭘ exhibit no signs of infection
- ⭘ maintain calorie requirement
- ⭘ maintain normal fluid volume.

Nursing interventions

○ Maintain nothing-by-mouth status until surgery is performed.
○ Administer I.V. fluids
○ Avoid administering analgesics until the diagnosis is confirmed.
○ Avoid administering cathartics or enemas that may rupture the appendix.
○ Place the patient in Fowler's position to decrease pain.

 Alert

Never apply heat to the right lower abdomen; this can cause the appendix to rupture.

○ Administer prescribed preoperative drugs.

Monitoring

After surgery
○ Vital signs
○ Intake and output
○ Pain control
○ Bowel sounds, passing of flatus, or bowel movements
○ Wound healing

Patient teaching

Be sure to cover:
○ appendicitis
○ preoperative teaching
○ possible complications
○ appropriate wound care
○ prescribed medications, administration, and possible adverse reactions
○ postoperative activity limitations.

Arterial occlusive disease

Overview

Description

- An obstruction or narrowing of the lumen of the aorta and its major branches
- May affect arteries, including the carotid, vertebral, innominate, subclavian, femoral, iliac, renal, mesenteric, and celiac
- Prognosis depends on location of the occlusion and development of collateral circulation that counteracts reduced blood flow

Pathophysiology

- Narrowing of vessel that leads to interrupted blood flow, usually to the legs and feet
- During times of increased activity or exercise, blood flow to surrounding muscles can't meet the metabolic demand
- Results in pain in affected areas

Causes

- Atherosclerosis
- Immune arteritis
- Embolism
- Thrombosis
- Thromboangiitis obliterans
- Raynaud's disease
- Fibromuscular disease
- Atheromatous debris (plaques)
- Indwelling arterial catheter
- Direct blunt or penetrating trauma

Risk factors

- Smoking
- Hypertension
- Dyslipidemia
- Diabetes mellitus
- Advanced age

Incidence

- More common in males than in females
- Usually occurs in people older than age 50
- Higher incidence in patients with diabetes
- Arteries in the legs more commonly affected

Common characteristics

- Intermittent claudication
- Decreased temperature in arms and legs
- Numbness or paresthesias

Complications

- Severe ischemia
- Skin ulceration
- Gangrene
- Limb loss

Assessment

History

- One or more risk factors
- Family history of vascular disease
- Intermittent claudication
- Rest pain
- Poor healing wounds or ulcers
- Impotence
- Dizziness or near syncope
- Transient ischemic attack symptoms

Physical findings

- Trophic changes of involved arm or leg
- Diminished or absent pulses in arm or leg
- Presence of ischemic ulcers
- Pallor with elevation of arm or leg
- Dependent rubor
- Arterial bruit
- Hypertension
- Pain
- Pallor
- Pulselessness distal to the occlusion
- Paralysis and paresthesia occurring in the affected arm or leg
- Poikilothermy

Test results

Imaging

- Arteriography shows type, location, and degree of obstruction, and the establishment of collateral circulation.
- Ultrasonography and plethysmography show decreased blood flow distal to the occlusion.
- Doppler ultrasonography shows a relatively low-pitched sound and a monophasic waveform.
- Electroencephalography and computed tomography scan may show the presence of brain lesions.

Other

- Segmental limb pressures and pulse volume measurements show the location and extent of the occlusion.
- Ophthalmodynamometry shows the degree of obstruction in the internal carotid artery.
- Electrocardiogram may show presence of cardiovascular disease.

Treatment

General

- Smoking cessation
- Hypertension, diabetes, and dyslipidemia control
- Foot and leg care
- Weight control
- Low-fat, low-cholesterol, high-fiber diet
- Regular walking program

Medication

○ Antiplatelets
○ Lipid-lowering agents
○ Hypoglycemic agents
○ Antihypertensives
○ Thrombolytics
○ Anticoagulation
○ Niacin or vitamin B complex

Surgery

○ Embolectomy
○ Endarterectomy
○ Atherectomy
○ Laser angioplasty
○ Endovascular stent placement
○ Percutaneous transluminal angioplasty
○ Laser surgery
○ Patch grafting
○ Bypass graft
○ Lumbar sympathectomy
○ Amputation
○ Bowel resection

Nursing considerations

Key outcomes

The patient will:
○ report increased comfort and decreased pain
○ maintain palpable pulses and collateral circulation
○ maintain skin integrity
○ maintain joint mobility and range of motion
○ develop no signs or symptoms of infection.

Nursing interventions

For chronic arterial occlusive disease

○ Use preventive measures, such as minimal pressure mattresses, heel protectors, a foot cradle, or a footboard.
○ Avoid using restrictive clothing such as antiembolism stockings.
○ Give prescribed drugs.
○ Allow the patient to express fears and concerns.

For preoperative care during an acute episode

○ Assess the patient's circulatory status.
○ Give prescribed analgesics.
○ Give prescribed heparin or thrombolytics.
○ Wrap the patient's affected foot in soft cotton batting, and reposition it frequently to prevent pressure on any one area.
○ Strictly avoid elevating or applying heat to the affected leg.

For postoperative care

○ Watch the patient closely for signs of hemorrhage.
○ In mesenteric artery occlusion, connect a nasogastric tube to low intermittent suction.
○ Give prescribed analgesics.
○ Assist with early ambulation, but don't allow the patient to sit for an extended period.

○ If amputation has occurred, check the stump carefully for drainage and note and record its color and amount and the time.
○ Elevate the stump, as ordered.

Monitoring

○ Signs and symptoms of fluid or electrolyte imbalance or renal failure
○ Signs and symptoms of stroke
○ Vital signs
○ Intake and output
○ Distal pulses
○ Neurologic status
○ Bowel sounds

Patient teaching

Be sure to cover:
○ the disorder, diagnosis, and treatment
○ medications and potential adverse reactions
○ when to notify the physician
○ dietary restrictions
○ regular exercise program
○ foot care
○ signs and symptoms of graft occlusion
○ signs and symptoms of arterial insufficiency and occlusion
○ avoidance of wearing constrictive clothing, crossing legs, or wearing garters
○ risk factor modification
○ avoidance of temperature extremes.

Discharge planning

○ Refer the patient to a physical and occupational therapist, as indicated.
○ Refer the patient to a podiatrist for foot care, as needed.
○ Refer the patient to an endocrinologist for glucose control, as indicated.
○ Refer the patient to a smoking-cessation program, as indicated.

Arteriovenous malformations

Overview

Description

- Tangled masses of thin-walled, dilated blood vessels between arteries and veins that don't connect by capillaries
- Common in the brain, primarily in the posterior portion of the cerebral hemispheres
- Adequate perfusion of brain tissue prevented due to abnormal channels between arterial and venous system mixing oxygenated and unoxygenated blood
- Range in size from a few millimeters to large malformations extending from the cerebral cortex to the ventricles
- Commonly more than one arteriovenous malformation (AVM) present

Pathophysiology

- Typical structural characteristics of the blood vessels aren't present.
- Vessels of an AVM are very thin. (One or more arteries feed into the AVM, causing it to appear dilated and torturous.)
- Typically, high-pressured arterial flow moves into the venous system through the connecting channels to increase venous pressure, engorging and dilating the venous structures.
- If the AVM is large enough, the shunting can deprive the surrounding tissue of adequate blood flow.
- Thin-walled vessels may ooze small amounts of blood or actually rupture, causing hemorrhage into the brain or subarachnoid space.

Causes

- Congenital (hereditary)
- Penetrating injuries such as trauma

Incidence

- Males and females are affected equally.
- Evidence exists that AVMs run in families.
- Most AVMs are present at birth; however, symptoms typically don't occur until ages 10 to 20.

Common characteristics

- Chronic mild headache and confusion
- Seizures
- Systolic bruit over carotid artery, mastoid process, or orbit
- Focal neurologic deficits (depending on the location of the AVM) resulting from compression and diminished perfusion

- Symptoms of intracranial (intracerebral, subarachnoid, or subdural) hemorrhage, including sudden severe headache, seizures, confusion, lethargy, and meningeal irritation
- Hydrocephalus

Complications

- Aneurysm development and subsequent rupture
- Hemorrhage (intracerebral, subarachnoid, or subdural, depending on the location of the AVM)
- Hydrocephalus

Assessment

History

- Chronic headache
- Seizures
- Change in mental status

Physical findings

- Systolic carotid bruit
- Neurologic deficits

Test results

Diagnostic procedures

- Cerebral arteriogram confirms the presence of AVMs and evaluates blood flow.
- Doppler ultrasonography of cerebrovascular system indicates abnormal, turbulent blood flow.

Treatment

General

- Support measures, including aneurysm precautions to prevent possible rupture
- Nothing by mouth, if scheduled for surgery
- Limited activity
- Quiet atmosphere

Medication

- I.V. fluid
- Analgesics
- Sedatives
- Stool softener

Surgery

- Block dissection, laser, or ligation to repair the communicating channels and remove the feeding vessels
- Embolization or radiation therapy, if surgery isn't possible, to close the communicating channels and feeder vessels and thus reduce the blood flow to the AVM

Nursing considerations

Key outcomes

The patient will:
- maintain stable vital signs
- maintain stable neurologic status
- express an understanding of the disorder and treatment.

Nursing interventions

- Control hypertension and seizure activity.
- Maintain a quiet atmosphere and provide relaxation techniques.
- If the AVM has ruptured, work to control elevated intracranial pressure and intracranial hemorrhage.

Monitoring

- Vital signs
- Neurologic status

Patient teaching

Be sure to cover:
- the disorder, diagnosis, and treatment
- importance of reporting any signs of intracranial bleeding immediately (sudden severe headache, vision changes, decreased movement in extremities, change in level of consciousness).

Discharge planning

- Refer patient to social service for support services if neurologic deficits have occurred from a ruptured AVM.

Asbestosis

Overview

Description

- Lung disease characterized by diffuse interstitial pulmonary fibrosis resulting from prolonged exposure to airborne asbestos particles
- May develop many years (about 15 to 20) after regular exposure to asbestos ceases
- Exposure causes pleural plaques and mesotheliomas of the pleura and the peritoneum
- A form of pneumoconiosis
- Also known as *mesothelioma*

Pathophysiology

- Inhaled asbestos fibers travel down the airway and penetrate respiratory bronchioles and alveolar walls.
- Mucus production and goblet cells are stimulated to protect the airway and aid in expectoration.
- Fibers become encased in a brown, iron-rich, proteinlike sheath, called asbestosis bodies.
- Chronic irritation by the fibers continues, causing edema of the airways.
- Fibrosis develops in response to the chronic irritation.

Causes

- Prolonged inhalation of asbestos fibers from industries, such as mining and milling, construction, fireproofing, and textile
- Production of paints, plastics, and brake and clutch linings
- Exposure to fibrous dust shaken off workers' clothing
- Exposure to fibrous dust or waste piles from nearby asbestos plants

Incidence

- Commonly occurs between ages 40 and 75
- Affects males more commonly than females

Common characteristics

- Exposure to asbestos fibers
- Exertional or rest dyspnea
- Dry cough
- Chest pain ———
- Recurrent respiratory tract infections

Complications

- Pulmonary fibrosis
- Respiratory failure
- Pulmonary hypertension
- Cor pulmonale

Assessment

History

- Exposure to asbestos fibers
- Exertional or rest dyspnea
- Cough
- Chest pain
- Recurrent respiratory tract infections

Physical findings

- Tachypnea
- Clubbing of the fingers
- Characteristic dry crackles in the lung bases

Test results

Laboratory
- Arterial blood gas analysis showing decreased partial pressures of arterial oxygen and carbon dioxide

Imaging
- Chest X-rays may show fine, irregular, and linear diffuse infiltrates; a honeycomb or ground-glass appearance to lungs; and pleural thickening and pleural calcification, bilateral obliteration of costophrenic angles, and an enlarged heart with "shaggy" border.

Other
- Pulmonary function tests may show decreased vital capacity, forced vital capacity (FVC), and total lung capacity; decreased or normal forced expiratory volume in 1 second (FEV_1) a normal ratio of FEV_1 to FVC; and reduced diffusing capacity for carbon monoxide.

Treatment

General

- Controlled coughing and postural drainage with chest percussion and vibration
- At least 3 qt (3 L) of fluids daily
- High-calorie, high-protein, low-sodium diet
- Activity, as tolerated

Medication

- Inhaled mucolytics
- Supplemental oxygen
- Diuretics
- Cardiac glycosides
- Antibiotics

Surgery

- Lung transplantation, in severe cases

Nursing considerations

Key outcomes

The patient will:
- maintain adequate ventilation
- maintain adequate calorie intake

- express understanding of the illness
- identify measures to prevent or reduce fatigue.

Nursing interventions
- Give prescribed drugs.
- Provide supportive care.
- Provide chest physiotherapy.
- Provide high-calorie, high-protein, low-sodium foods in small, frequent meals.
- Encourage oral fluid intake.
- Provide frequent rest periods.

Monitoring
- Vital signs
- Intake and output
- Daily weight
- Respiratory status (breath sounds, arterial blood gas results)
- Sputum production
- Mentation
- Complications

Patient teaching

Be sure to cover:
- the disorder, diagnosis, and treatment
- medications and potential adverse reactions
- transtracheal catheter care, if applicable
- prevention of infection
- signs and symptoms of infection
- influenza and pneumococcus immunizations
- home oxygen therapy, if required
- importance of follow-up care
- chest physiotherapy
- high-calorie, high-protein, low-sodium diet
- adequate oral fluid intake
- energy conservation techniques.

Discharge planning
- Refer the patient to a smoking-cessation program, if indicated.

Ascariasis

Overview

Description

- Intestinal infection caused by the parasitic worm *Ascaris lumbricoides,* a large roundworm resembling an earthworm
- Never passes directly from person to person
- Also known as *roundworm infection*

Pathophysiology

- After ingestion, *A. lumbricoides* ova hatch and release larvae, which penetrate the intestinal wall and reach the lungs through the bloodstream.
- After about 10 days in pulmonary capillaries and alveoli, the larvae migrate to the bronchioles, bronchi, trachea, and epiglottis.
- From the epiglottis, the larvae are swallowed and return to the intestine to mature into worms.

Causes

- Ingestion of food, drink, or soil contaminated with *A. lumbricoides* ova

Incidence

- Occurs worldwide but is most common in tropical areas with poor sanitation and in Asia, where farmers use human stool as fertilizer
- In the United States, more prevalent in the South, particularly among younger children

Common characteristics

- Stomach discomfort
- Vomiting

Complications

- Intestinal obstruction
- Pneumonitis

Assessment

History

- Stomach discomfort or pain
- Nausea and vomiting
- Recent travel to endemic area
- Restlessness
- Disturbed sleep

Physical findings

- Abdominal tenderness
- Dehydration
- Rales, wheezing, and tachypnea (if migrated to the lungs)

Test results

Laboratory

- Microscopic identification of ova in the stool or observation of adult worm in emesis
- Complete blood count: shows eosinophilia

Imaging

- Abdominal X-rays show whirlpool pattern of intraluminal worms (Intestinal obstruction may be noted.)
- Chest X-rays show characteristic bronchovascular markings — infiltrates, patchy areas of pneumonitis, and widening of hilar shadows (if migrated to lungs)

Treatment

General

- Nasogastric suctioning (with intestinal obstruction)
- Nothing by mouth until stable
- Rest as needed

Medication

- I.V. fluids
- Mebendazole and albendazole
- Anthelmintic therapy (pyrantel or piperazine) (avoid use if intestinal obstruction is present)

 Alert

Piperazine is contraindicated in patients with seizure disorders and may cause stomach upset, dizziness, and urticaria. Pyrantel produces red stool and vomitus and may cause stomach upset, headache, dizziness, and rash. Albendazole and mebendazole may cause abdominal pain and diarrhea.

Surgery

- Intestinal surgery to relieve obstruction, if necessary

Nursing considerations

Key outcomes

The patient will:
- maintain adequate fluid balance
- regain normal intestinal function
- express understanding of proper sanitation of food and hands.

Nursing interventions

- Isolation is unnecessary; proper disposal of stool and soiled linen, using standard precautions, should be adequate.
- If the patient is receiving nasogastric suctioning, provide good mouth care.

Monitoring

- Vital signs
- Intake and output
- Appearance of stools (for worms)

Patient teaching

Be sure to cover:

○ proper hand washing, especially before eating and after defecating

○ bathing and changing underwear and bed linens daily

○ adverse effects of medications prescribed for the patient.

Discharge planning

○ Refer the patient to social services if living conditions are questionable regarding cleanliness.

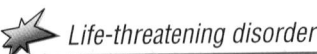 *Life-threatening disorder*

Aspergillosis

Overview

Description

- An opportunistic, sometimes life-threatening infection, growth, or allergic response caused by fungi of the genus *Aspergillus,* usually *A. fumigatus, A. flavus,* or *A. niger.* It occurs in four major forms:
  - Aspergilloma produces a fungus ball in the lungs (called a mycetoma).
  - Allergic aspergillosis is a hypersensitive asthmatic reaction to Aspergillus antigens.
  - Aspergillosis endophthalmitis is an infection of the anterior and posterior chambers of the eye that can lead to blindness.
  - Invasive aspergillosis is an acute infection that produces septicemia, thrombosis, and infarction of virtually any organ, especially the heart, lungs, brain, and kidneys.
- The prognosis varies with each form. Occasionally, aspergilloma causes fatal hemoptysis.

Pathophysiology

- Conidia (asexual spores) travel into the alveoli via inhalation or, in aspergillosis endophthalmitis, through a wound or other tissue injury.
- Pulmonary macrophages may or may not be able to kill the conidia.
- The alternative complement pathway is activated, resulting in recruitment of neutrophils and monocytes.
- The disease may be accompanied by hyphal invasion of the blood vessels in the involved tissues.
- In aspergilloma, colonization of the bronchial tree with *Aspergillus* produces plugs and atelectasis and forms a tangled ball of hyphae (fungal filaments), fibrin, and exudate in a cavity left by a previous illness such as tuberculosis.

Causes

- Contact with *Aspergillus,* which is commonly found growing on dry leaves, stored grain, compost piles, or decaying vegetation

Risk factors

- Excessive or prolonged use of antibiotics, glucocorticoids, or other immunosuppressants
- Radiation therapy
- Acquired immunodeficiency syndrome
- Hodgkin's disease
- Leukemia
- Azotemia
- Alcoholism
- Sarcoidosis
- Bronchitis and bronchiectasis
- Organ transplants
- Tuberculosis or another cavitary lung disease (in aspergilloma)

Incidence

- *Aspergillus* is found worldwide, commonly in fermenting compost piles and damp hay.

Common characteristics

Aspergilloma
- May produce no symptoms
- Mimics tuberculosis, causing a productive cough and purulent or blood-tinged sputum, dyspnea, empyema, and lung abscesses

Allergic aspergillosis
- Wheezing
- Dyspnea
- Cough with some sputum production
- Pleural pain
- Fever

Aspergillosis endophthalmitis
- Usually appears 2 to 3 weeks after an eye injury or surgery
- Clouded vision
- Eye pain
- Reddened conjunctivae

Invasive aspergillosis
- Thrombosis
- Infarctions
- Sepsis

Complications

- Infection of the ear (otomycosis), cornea (mycotic keratitis), or prosthetic heart valve (endocarditis)
- Pneumonia (especially in those receiving an immunosuppressant such as an antineoplastic drug or high-dose steroid therapy)
- Sinusitis
- Brain abscesses
- Life-threatening hemoptysis
- Septicemia

Assessment

History

Aspergilloma and allergic aspergillosis
- Immunosuppression
- Dyspnea
- Cough with sputum production

Aspergillosis endophthalmitis
- Eye pain
- Vision changes
- Recent eye injury or surgery

Invasive aspergillosis
- History based on infected organ

Physical findings

Aspergilloma and allergic aspergillosis
- Diminished breath sounds
- Adventitious breath sounds
- Cough with sputum production

Aspergillosis endophthalmitis
- Reddened conjunctivae
- Blurred vision

Invasive aspergillosis
- Findings based on infected organ

Test results

Laboratory
ASPERGILLOMA
- Serum positive for anti-*Aspergillus* antibodies

ALLERGIC ASPERGILLOSIS
- Sputum culture reveals hyphae that grow *Aspergillus* and eosinophils
- Serum positive for immunoglobulin (Ig) E and IgG anti-*Aspergillus* antibodies

ASPERGILLOSIS ENDOPHTHALMITIS
- Eye culture or exudate shows *Aspergillus*

Diagnostic procedures
INVASIVE ASPERGILLOSIS
- Bronchoscopy and open lung biopsy to obtain tissue sample that confirm diagnosis

Imaging
ASPERGILLOMA
- Chest X-ray shows a round to oval mass with a radiolucent crescent over the upper portion of the mass (Monod's sign)

Treatment

General
- Supportive therapy

Medication

Allergic aspergillosis
- Desensitization
- Steroids

Aspergillosis endophthalmitis
- Amphotericin B

Invasive aspergillosis
- Antifungal therapy

Surgery

Aspergilloma
- Local excision of the lesion
- Lobectomy

Nursing considerations

Key outcomes
The patient will:
- maintain adequate ventilation
- maintain stable vital signs
- express understanding of the disorder and treatment.

Nursing interventions
- Perform chest physiotherapy every 2 hours.
- Encourage coughing and deep breathing every hour.

Monitoring
- Vital signs
- Sputum production, amount, color and character

Patient teaching

Be sure to cover:
- the disorder, diagnosis, and treatment
- adverse effects of medications.

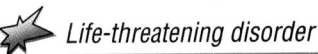

Asphyxia

Overview

Description

- ○ A condition of insufficient oxygen and accumulating carbon dioxide in the blood and tissues
- ○ Leads to cardiopulmonary arrest and is fatal without prompt treatment

Pathophysiology

- ○ An interference with respiration, causing insufficient oxygen intake
- ○ Accumulation of carbon dioxide
- ○ Hypoxemia
- ○ Inadequate tissue perfusion

Causes

- ○ Opioid abuse
- ○ Respiratory muscle paralysis
- ○ Airway obstruction
- ○ Aspiration
- ○ Pulmonary edema
- ○ Near drowning
- ○ Tumor
- ○ Strangulation
- ○ Trauma to airway
- ○ Carbon monoxide poisoning
- ○ Smoke inhalation

Incidence

- ○ Can occur at any age

Common characteristics

- ○ Altered respirations
- ○ Changes in level of consciousness
- ○ Cardiac arrest

Complications

- ○ Neurologic damage
- ○ Death

Assessment

History

- ○ Cause of the asphyxia may be apparent.
- ○ Causes of signs and symptoms vary.

Physical findings

- ○ Anxiousness or agitation
- ○ Confusion
- ○ Dyspnea
- ○ Prominent neck muscles
- ○ Wheezing and stridor
- ○ Altered respiratory rate
- ○ Little or no air movement
- ○ Intercostal rib retractions
- ○ Pale skin
- ○ Cyanosis in mucous membranes, lips, and nail beds
- ○ Erythema and petechiae on the upper chest (trauma)
- ○ Cherry-red mucous membranes (carbon monoxide poisoning)
- ○ Decreased or absent breath sounds

Test results

Laboratory

- ○ Decreased partial pressure of arterial oxygen (less than 60 mm Hg) and increased partial pressure of arterial carbon dioxide (more than 50 mm Hg) indicated by arterial blood gas (ABG) analysis
- ○ Toxicology tests showing drugs, chemicals, or abnormal hemoglobin level

Imaging

- ○ Chest X-rays may detect a foreign body, pulmonary edema, or atelectasis.
- ○ Pulmonary function tests may indicate respiratory muscle weakness.
- ○ Bronchoscopy can locate foreign body.

Treatment

General

- ○ Establish airway and ventilation
- ○ Treat the underlying cause
- ○ Nothing by mouth until able to protect airway
- ○ Activity based on outcome of interventions

Medication

- ○ Oxygen
- ○ Narcan (if caused by opioid abuse)

Surgery

- ○ Tumor removal

Nursing considerations

Key outcomes

The patient will:

- ○ maintain a patent airway
- ○ maintain adequate ventilation
- ○ maintain acceptable cardiac output
- ○ demonstrate knowledge of safety measures to prevent suffocation.

Nursing interventions

- ○ Perform abdominal thrust, if obstruction is present.
- ○ Maintain patent airway.
- ○ Begin cardiopulmonary resuscitation, if necessary.
- ○ Insert a nasogastric tube or an Ewald tube for lavage (for opioid abuse).
- ○ Give prescribed drugs.
- ○ Reassure the patient and his family.
- ○ Ensure I.V. access.

Monitoring
○ ABG levels, pulse oximetry
○ Respiratory status
○ Cardiac status
○ Vital signs
○ Neurologic status

Patient teaching

Be sure to cover:
○ cause of asphyxia (with patient and family members, discuss measures to prevent recurrence, if appropriate)
○ safety measures if the victim is a child.

Discharge planning
○ Refer the patient to the proper authorities, if criminal intent was involved.
○ Refer the patient to resource and support services, if appropriate.

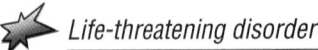
Life-threatening disorder

Asthma

Overview

Description

○ A chronic reactive airway disorder involving episodic, reversible airway obstruction resulting from bronchospasms, increased mucus secretions, and mucosal edema
○ Signs and symptoms that range from mild wheezing and dyspnea to life-threatening respiratory failure
○ Signs and symptoms of bronchial airway obstruction that may persist between acute episodes

Pathophysiology

○ Tracheal and bronchial linings overreact to various stimuli, causing episodic smooth-muscle spasms that severely constrict the airways.
○ Mucosal edema and thickened secretions further block the airways.
○ Immunoglobulin (Ig) E antibodies, attached to histamine-containing mast cells and receptors on cell membranes, initiate intrinsic asthma attacks.
○ When exposed to an antigen such as pollen, the IgE antibody combines with the antigen. On subsequent exposure to the antigen, mast cells degranulate and release mediators.
○ The mediators cause the bronchoconstriction and edema of an asthma attack.
○ During an asthma attack, expiratory airflow decreases, trapping gas in the airways and causing alveolar hyperinflation.
○ Atelectasis may develop in some lung regions.
○ The increased airway resistance initiates labored breathing.

Causes

○ Sensitivity to specific external allergens or from internal, nonallergenic factors
Extrinsic asthma (atopic asthma)
○ Pollen
○ Animal dander
○ House dust or mold
○ Kapok or feather pillows
○ Food additives containing sulfites and any other sensitizing substance
Intrinsic asthma (nonatopic asthma)
○ Emotional stress
○ Genetic factors
Bronchoconstriction
○ Hereditary predisposition
○ Sensitivity to allergens or irritants such as pollutants
○ Viral infections
○ Drugs, such as aspirin, beta-adrenergic blockers, and nonsteroidal anti-inflammatory drugs
○ Tartrazine

○ Psychological stress
○ Cold air
○ Exercise

Incidence

○ Can occur at any age; about 50% of all patients with asthma are under age 10; affects twice as many boys as girls
○ About one-third of patients experience onset between ages 10 and 30
○ About one-third share the disease with at least one immediate family member
○ Can coexist (intrinsic and extrinsic asthma) in many asthmatics

Common characteristics

○ Wheezing
○ Shortness of breath, feelings of suffocation
○ Tightness in chest
○ Extrinsic asthma begins in children; commonly accompanied by other manifestations of atopy

Complications

○ Status asthmaticus
○ Respiratory failure
○ Death

Assessment

History

○ Intrinsic asthma is often preceded by severe respiratory tract infections, especially in adults.
○ Irritants, emotional stress, fatigue, endocrine changes, temperature and humidity variations, and exposure to noxious fumes may aggravate intrinsic asthma attacks.
○ An asthma attack may begin dramatically, with simultaneous onset of severe, multiple symptoms, or insidiously, with gradually increasing respiratory distress.
○ Exposure to a particular allergen is followed by a sudden onset of dyspnea and wheezing and by tightness in the chest accompanied by a cough that produces thick, clear, or yellow sputum.

Physical findings

○ Visibly dyspneic
○ Ability to speak only a few words before pausing for breath
○ Use of accessory respiratory muscles
○ Diaphoresis
○ Increased anteroposterior thoracic diameter
○ Hyperresonance
○ Tachycardia; tachypnea; mild systolic hypertension
○ Inspiratory and expiratory wheezes
○ Prolonged expiratory phase of respiration
○ Diminished breath sounds
○ Cyanosis, confusion, and lethargy indicate the onset of life-threatening status asthmaticus and respiratory failure

Test results

Laboratory
- Arterial blood gas (ABG) analysis revealing hypoxemia
- Increased serum IgE levels from an allergic reaction
- Complete blood count with differential showing increased eosinophil count

Imaging
- Chest X-rays may show hyperinflation with areas of focal atelectasis.

Diagnostic procedures
- Pulmonary function studies may show decreased peak flows and forced expiratory volume in 1 second, low-normal or decreased vital capacity, and increased total lung and residual capacities.
- Skin testing may identify specific allergens.
- Bronchial challenge testing shows the clinical significance of allergens identified by skin testing.

Other
- Pulse oximetry measurements may show decreased oxygen saturation.

Treatment

General
- Identification and avoidance of precipitating factors
- Desensitization to specific antigens
- Establishment and maintenance of patent airway
- Fluid replacement
- Activity as tolerated

Medication
- Bronchodilators
- Corticosteroids
- Histamine antagonists
- Leukotriene antagonists
- Anticholinergic bronchodilators
- Low-flow oxygen
- Antibiotics
- Heliox trial (before intubation)
- I.V. magnesium sulfate (controversial)

 Alert

The patient with increasingly severe asthma that doesn't respond to drug therapy is usually admitted for treatment with corticosteroids, epinephrine, and sympathomimetic aerosol sprays. He may require endotracheal intubation and mechanical ventilation.

Nursing considerations

Key outcomes
The patient will:
- maintain adequate ventilation
- maintain a patent airway
- use effective coping strategies
- report feelings of comfort
- maintain skin integrity.

Nursing interventions
- Give prescribed drugs.
- Place the patient in high Fowler's position.
- Encourage pursed-lip and diaphragmatic breathing.
- Administer prescribed humidified oxygen.
- Adjust oxygen according to the patient's vital signs and ABG values.
- Assist with intubation and mechanical ventilation, if appropriate.
- Perform postural drainage and chest percussion, if tolerated.
- Suction an intubated patient, as needed.
- Treat the patient's dehydration with I.V. or oral fluids, as tolerated.
- Anticipate bronchoscopy or bronchial lavage.
- Keep the room temperature comfortable.
- Use an air conditioner or a fan in hot, humid weather.

Monitoring
- Vital signs
- Intake and output
- Response to treatment
- Signs and symptoms of theophylline toxicity
- Breath sounds
- ABG results
- Pulmonary function test results
- Pulse oximetry
- Complications of corticosteroids
- Level of anxiety

Patient teaching

Be sure to cover:
- the disorder, diagnosis, and treatment
- medications and potential adverse reactions
- when to notify the physician
- avoidance of known allergens and irritants
- metered-dose inhaler or dry powder inhaler use
- pursed-lip and diaphragmatic breathing
- use of peak flow meter
- effective coughing techniques
- maintaining adequate hydration.

Discharge planning
- Refer the patient to a local asthma support group.

Atelectasis

Overview

Description

- Incomplete expansion of alveolar clusters or lung segments leading to partial or complete lung collapse
- May be chronic or acute
- Good prognosis with prompt removal of any airway obstruction, relief of hypoxia, and re-expansion of the collapsed lung

Pathophysiology

- Due to incomplete expansion, certain regions of the lung are removed from gas exchange.
- Unoxygenated blood passes unchanged through these regions and produces hypoxia.
- Alveolar surfactant causes increased surface tension, permitting complete alveolar deflation.

Causes

- Bronchial occlusion
- Bronchiectasis
- Cystic fibrosis
- Bed rest in a supine position
- General anesthesia
- Pleural effusion
- Pulmonary embolism
- Sarcoidosis
- Bronchogenic carcinoma
- Inflammatory lung disease
- Idiopathic respiratory distress syndrome of the neonate
- Oxygen toxicity
- Pulmonary edema
- External compression

Incidence

- Common in patients after upper abdominal or thoracic surgery
- More common in patients with prolonged immobility, on mechanical ventilation, or with central nervous system (CNS) depression
- Increased predisposition in patients who smoke and those with chronic obstructive pulmonary disease (COPD)

Common characteristics

- Shortness of breath
- Chest pain
- Anxiety

Complications

- Hypoxemia
- Acute respiratory failure
- Pneumonia

Assessment

History

- Recent abdominal surgery
- Prolonged immobility
- Mechanical ventilation
- CNS depression
- Smoking
- COPD
- Rib fractures, tight chest dressings

Physical findings

- Decreased chest wall movement
- Cyanosis
- Diaphoresis
- Substernal or intercostal retractions
- Anxiety
- Decreased fremitus
- Mediastinal shift to the affected side
- Dullness or flatness over lung fields
- End-inspiration crackles
- Decreased (or absent) breath sounds
- Tachycardia

Test results

Laboratory
- Arterial blood gas analysis showing hypoxia

Imaging
- Chest X-rays show characteristic horizontal lines in the lower lung zones and characteristic dense shadows.

Diagnostic procedures
- Bronchoscopy may show an obstructing neoplasm, foreign body, or pneumonia.
- Pulse oximetry shows decreased oxygen saturation.

Treatment

General

- Incentive spirometry
- Chest percussion
- Postural drainage
- Frequent coughing and deep-breathing exercises
- Bronchoscopy if above measures fail
- Humidity
- Intermittent positive-pressure breathing therapy
- Radiation may be required for obstructing neoplasm
- Diet based on patient's condition, as tolerated
- Increased fluids
- Activity as tolerated; discourage bed rest

Medication

- Bronchodilators
- Analgesics after surgery

Surgery

- May be required if obstructing neoplasm present

Nursing considerations

Key outcomes

The patient will:
- ○ maintain a patent airway
- ○ maintain adequate ventilation
- ○ report feelings of increased comfort
- ○ use support systems to assist with anxiety and fear.

Nursing interventions

- ○ Give prescribed drugs.
- ○ Encourage coughing and deep breathing.
- ○ Reposition the patient often.
- ○ Encourage and assist with ambulation as soon as possible.
- ○ Help the patient use an incentive spirometer.
- ○ Humidify inspired air.
- ○ Encourage adequate fluid intake.
- ○ Loosen secretions with postural drainage and chest percussion.
- ○ Provide suctioning, as needed.
- ○ Offer the patient reassurance and emotional support.

Monitoring

- ○ Vital signs
- ○ Intake and output
- ○ Pulse oximetry
- ○ Respiratory status (breath sounds, arterial blood gas results)

Patient teaching

Be sure to cover:
- ○ use of incentive spirometer
- ○ postural drainage and percussion
- ○ coughing and deep-breathing exercises
- ○ importance of splinting incisions
- ○ energy-conservation techniques
- ○ stress-reduction strategies
- ○ importance of mobilization.

Discharge planning

- ○ Refer the patient to a smoking-cessation program, if indicated.
- ○ Refer the patient to a weight-reduction program, if indicated.

Atopic dermatitis

Overview

Description

❍ A chronic skin disorder characterized by superficial skin inflammation and intense itching

Pathophysiology

❍ The allergic mechanism of hypersensitivity results in a release of inflammatory mediators through sensitized antibodies of the immunoglobulin (Ig) E class.
❍ Histamine and other cytokines induce acute inflammation.
❍ Abnormally dry skin and a decreased threshold for itching set up the "itch-scratch-itch" cycle, which eventually causes lesions (excoriations, lichenification).

Causes

❍ The exact etiology of atopic dermatitis is unknown; however, a genetic predisposition is likely.
❍ Possible contributing factors include:
   – food allergy
   – infection
   – chemical irritants
   – extremes of temperature and humidity
   – psychological stress or strong emotions.

 Alert

About 10% of juvenile cases of atopic dermatitis are caused by allergic reactions to certain foods, especially eggs, peanuts, milk, and wheat.

Factors contributing to atopy

❍ Changes associated with industrialization, such as exposure to new chemicals like diesel fumes, have proven to increase the antigenicity of common pollens.
❍ Increased exposure to antigens, such as dust mites (in wall-to-wall carpets), especially at an early age, contributes to a predisposition to developing allergies.
❍ Dietary changes, such as increased fat intake and an earlier weaning from human breast milk, may be contributing factors.
❍ Vaccination may cause a shift in T-cell function away from the normal helper T cell (Th1) response to the Th2 allergic response by limiting early bacterial and viral infections.
❍ Lack of exposure to intestinal parasites may contribute to a similar shift in T-cell functioning.
❍ Frequent use of antibiotics, especially in early childhood, may decrease normal intestinal flora and further contribute to the shift.

Incidence

❍ May appear at any age but typically begins during infancy or early childhood (may then subside spontaneously, followed by exacerbations in late childhood, adolescence, or early adulthood)
❍ Affects less than 1% of the population

Common characteristics

❍ Erythematous, weeping lesions, usually located in areas of flexion and extension, such as the neck, antecubital fossa, popliteal folds, and behind the ears
In children with atopic dermatitis
❍ Pink pigmentation and swelling of the upper eyelid and a double fold under the lower lid (Morgan's line or Dennie's sign)

Complications

❍ Scarring
❍ Severe viral infections
❍ Bacterial and fungal skin infections
❍ Ocular disorders
❍ Allergic contact dermatitis

Assessment

History

❍ Atopy, such as asthma, hay fever, or urticaria (or similar family history) (see *Factors contributing to atopy*)
❍ Exposure to allergen
❍ Pruritus

Physical findings

❍ Erythematous, weeping lesions (see *Signs of atopic dermatitis*)
❍ Pink pigmentation and swelling of the upper eyelid and a double fold under the lower lid

Test results

Laboratory
❍ Eosinophilia
❍ Elevated serum IgE levels
Other
❍ Physical examination findings

Treatment

General

❍ Meticulous skin care
❍ Environmental control of offending allergens
❍ Nonirritating topical lubricants

Medications

❍ Corticosteroids
❍ Antipruritics
❍ Antihistamines
❍ Antibiotics if secondary infection develops

Nursing considerations

Key outcomes

The patient will:
○ express relief from itching and pain
○ demonstrate improved skin condition
○ remain free from infection.

Nursing interventions

○ Offer support to help the patient and his family cope with this chronic disorder.
○ Dissuade the patient from scratching during urticaria to help prevent infection.
○ Apply prescribed topical medications.

Monitoring

○ Compliance with drug therapy
○ Treatment of lesions
○ Nutritional status

Patient teaching

Be sure to cover:
○ when and how to apply topical corticosteroids
○ importance of regular personal hygiene using only water with little soap
○ signs and symptoms of secondary infection
○ avoidance of laundry additives, such as fragrances and dyes
○ avoidance of allergens.

Signs of atopic dermatitis

This illustration shows the typical lesions involved in atopic dermatitis

Edema, crusting, and scaling

Erythematous areas on dry skin

Atrial fibrillation

Overview

Description

- ◯ Rhythm disturbance of the atria
- ◯ Characterized by an irregularly irregular cardiac rate and rhythm (see *Recognizing atrial fibrillation*)

Pathophysiology

- ◯ Rapid discharges from numerous ectopic foci in the atria
- ◯ Leads to erratic and uncoordinated atrial rhythm

Causes

- ◯ Hypertension
- ◯ Myocardial infarction (MI)
- ◯ Pulmonary embolism
- ◯ Heart failure
- ◯ Cardiomyopathy
- ◯ Hypersympathetic state associated with acute alcohol ingestion
- ◯ Pericarditis
- ◯ Hyperthyroidism
- ◯ Valvular disease
- ◯ Cardiothoracic surgery
- ◯ Atrial fibrosis

Incidence

- ◯ Seen more commonly in patients older than age 70
- ◯ Men affected more than women

Common characteristics

- ◯ Cardiac rhythm is irregularly irregular

Complications

- ◯ Transient ischemic attack
- ◯ Stroke
- ◯ Heart failure
- ◯ Thromboembolism

Assessment

History

- ◯ Palpitations
- ◯ Fatigue
- ◯ Dyspnea
- ◯ Chest pain
- ◯ Syncope

Physical findings

- ◯ Irregular pulse
- ◯ Possible tachycardia
- ◯ Hypotension
- ◯ Signs of heart failure
- ◯ Respiratory distress

Test results

Laboratory
- ◯ Cardiac enzymes showing myocardial damage (with MI)
- ◯ Thyroid function studies revealing hyperthyroidism
- ◯ Complete blood count, if history of recent blood loss

Imaging
- ◯ Chest X-ray may determine if pulmonary edema is present.
- ◯ Echocardiogram or transesophageal echocardiography may help to identify valvular disease, left ventricular dysfunction, or atrial clots.

Diagnostic procedures
- ◯ Electrocardiogram may indicate irregular rhythm.
- ◯ Holter monitor may diagnose paroxysmal atrial fibrillation.

Treatment

General

- ◯ Possible electrical cardioversion
- ◯ Atrial fibrillation suppression pacemaker
- ◯ Ablation
- ◯ Low-fat, low-sodium diet
- ◯ Fluid restriction, if indicated
- ◯ Planned rest periods, as needed

Recognizing atrial fibrillation

The following rhythm strip shows atrial fibrillation.

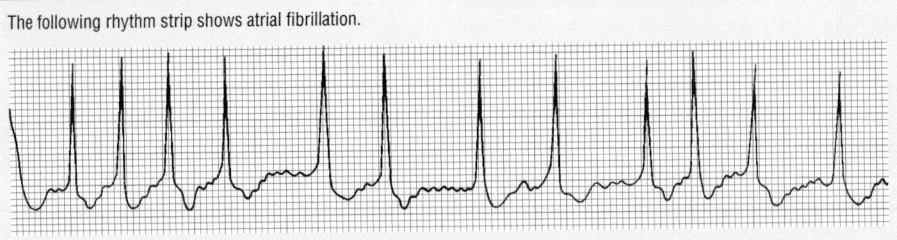

- ◯ Rhythm: irregular
- ◯ Rate: atrial — indiscernible; ventricular — 130 beats/minute
- ◯ P wave: absent; replaced by fine fibrillatory waves
- ◯ PR interval: indiscernible
- ◯ QRS complex: 0.08 second
- ◯ T wave: indiscernible
- ◯ QT interval: unmeasurable
- ◯ Other: none

Medication

○ Calcium channel blockers
○ Beta-adrenergic blockers
○ Antiarrhythmics
○ Cardiac glycosides
○ Anticoagulants

Nursing considerations

Key outcomes

The patient will:
○ report ways to reduce activity intolerance
○ identify effective coping mechanisms to manage anxiety
○ discuss the causes of fatigue
○ verbalize understanding of medication regimen.

Nursing interventions

○ Give prescribed drugs.
○ Encourage the patient and his family to talk about feelings and concerns.
○ Plan rest periods.

Monitoring

○ Vital signs at rest and after physical activity
○ Signs and symptoms of embolism
○ Intake and output
○ Daily weight
○ Abnormal bleeding

Patient teaching

Be sure to cover:
○ the disorder, diagnosis, and treatment
○ medications and potential adverse reactions
○ when to notify the physician
○ instructions on how to monitor pulse
○ anticoagulation precautions
○ abnormal bleeding
○ signs and symptoms of embolic events.

Discharge planning

○ Refer the patient to programs such as "Coumadin Clinic" to monitor anticoagulant therapy.

Atrial septal defect

Overview

Description

- An acyanotic congenital heart defect featuring an opening between the left and right atria that allows blood to flow from left to right, resulting in ineffective pumping of the heart, thus increasing the risk of heart failure
- Three types:
  - Ostium secundum defect, the most common type, occurs in the region of the fossa ovalis and, occasionally, extends inferiorly, close to the vena cava.
  - Sinus venosus defect occurs in the superior-posterior portion of the atrial septum, sometimes extending into the vena cava, and is almost always associated with abnormal drainage of pulmonary veins into the right atrium.
  - Ostium primum defect occurs in the inferior portion of the septum primum and is usually associated with atrioventricular valve abnormalities (cleft mitral valve) and conduction defects.

Pathophysiology

- Blood shunts from the left atrium to the right atrium because the left atrial pressure is normally slightly higher than the right atrial pressure.
- This pressure difference forces large amounts of blood through a defect.
- This shunt results in right heart volume overload, affecting the right atrium, right ventricle, and pulmonary arteries.
- Eventually, the right atrium enlarges, and the right ventricle dilates to accommodate the increased blood volume.
- If pulmonary artery hypertension develops, increased pulmonary vascular resistance and right ventricular hypertrophy follow.
- Irreversible pulmonary artery hypertension causes reversal of the shunt direction in some adults, which results in unoxygenated blood entering the systemic circulation, causing cyanosis.

Causes

- No known cause
- Ostium primum defects commonly occur in patients with Down syndrome

Incidence

- Accounts for about 10% of congenital heart defects
- Appears almost twice as often in females than in males, with a strong familial tendency
- Usually benign defect during infancy and childhood (Delayed development of symptoms and complications makes it one of the most common congenital heart defects diagnosed in adults.)

Common characteristics

- Fatigue after exertion
- Early to midsystolic murmur at the second or third left intercostal space
- Low-pitched diastolic murmur at the left lower sternal border; more pronounced on inspiration
- Fixed, widely split S_2
- Systolic click or late systolic murmur at the apex
- Clubbing and cyanosis, if a right-to-left shunt develops

 Alert

An infant may be cyanotic because he has a cardiac or pulmonary disorder. Cyanosis that worsens with crying most likely has a cardiac cause because crying increases pulmonary flow, resulting in an increased right-to-left shunt. Cyanosis that improves with crying most likely has a pulmonary cause because deep breathing improves tidal volume.

Complications

- Physical underdevelopment
- Respiratory infections
- Heart failure
- Atrial arrhythmias
- Mitral valve prolapse

Assessment

History

- Increasing fatigue
- Chest pain
- Dyspnea
- Coughing
- Dizziness or syncope

Physical findings

- Early to midsystolic murmur at the second or third left intercostal space
- Low-pitched diastolic murmur at the left lower sternal border, more pronounced on inspiration
- Fixed, widely split S_2
- Systolic click or late systolic murmur at the apex
- Peripheral edema
- Cyanosis
- Distended jugular veins

Test results

Imaging
- Chest X-ray shows an enlarged right atrium and right ventricle, a prominent pulmonary artery, and increased pulmonary vascular markings.

Diagnostic procedures
- Electrocardiography results may be normal, but commonly show right axis deviation, a prolonged PR interval, varying degrees of right bundle branch

block, right ventricular hypertrophy, atrial fibrillation (particularly in severe cases in patients older than age 30) and, in ostium primum defect, left axis deviation.

○ Echocardiography measures right ventricular enlargement, may locate the defect, and shows volume overload in the right side of the heart. It may reveal right ventricular and pulmonary artery dilation.

○ Two-dimensional echocardiography with color Doppler flow, contrast echocardiography, or both has supplanted cardiac catheterization as the confirming test for atrial septal defects (ASDs). Cardiac catheterization is used if inconsistencies exist in the clinical data or if significant pulmonary hypertension is suspected.

Treatment

General

○ Activity, as tolerated
○ Low fat, low cholesterol diet

Medication

○ Diuretics
○ Antibiotics
○ Analgesics

Surgery

○ Minimally invasive heart surgery may be required for the patient with an uncomplicated ASD with evidence of significant left-to-right shunting.
○ A large defect may need immediate surgical closure with sutures or a patch graft.
○ Cardiac catheterization closure, inserting an umbrella-like patch or septal occluder through a cardiac catheter, may be performed.

Nursing considerations

Key outcomes

The patient will:
○ maintain an optimal cardiac output
○ maintain hemodynamic stability
○ experience no cardiac arrhythmias.

Nursing interventions

○ Encourage the child to engage in any activity he can tolerate.
○ Give prescribed drugs.

Monitoring

○ Vital signs
○ Central venous and intra-arterial pressures
○ Intake and output
○ Cardiac rhythm
○ Oxygenation

Patient teaching

Be sure to cover:
○ pretest and posttest procedures to the child and his parents (If possible, use drawings or other visual aids to explain it to the child.)
○ postoperative procedures, tubes, dressings, and monitoring equipment
○ antibiotic prophylaxis to prevent infective endocarditis.

Attention deficit hyperactivity disorder

Overview

Description

❍ A behavioral problem characterized by difficulty with inattention, impulsivity, hyperactivity, and boredom
❍ Also called *ADHD* and *ADD*

Pathophysiology

❍ Alleles of dopamine genes may alter dopamine transmission in the neural networks.
❍ During fetal development, bouts of hypoxia and hypotension could selectively damage neurons located in some of the critical regions of the anatomical networks.

Causes

❍ Underlying cause unknown
❍ Limited evidence of a genetic component
❍ Some studies indicate that it may result from altered neurotransmitter levels in the brain

Risk factors

❍ Family history
❍ History of learning disability
❍ Mood or conduct disorder

Incidence

❍ Present at birth, but diagnosis before age 4 or 5 is difficult; some patients aren't diagnosed until adulthood
❍ Occurs in 3% to 5% of school-age children
❍ Affects males three times more than females

Common characteristics

❍ Impulsive behavior
❍ Inattentiveness
❍ Disorganization in school
❍ Tendency to jump quickly from one partly completed project, thought, or task to another
❍ Difficulty meeting deadlines and keeping track of school or work tools and materials

Complications

❍ Emotional and social complications
❍ Poor nutrition

Assessment

History

❍ Characterized as a fidgeter and a daydreamer
❍ Appears inattentive and lazy
❍ Performs sporadically at school or work

Physical findings

Symptoms of inattention
❍ Makes careless mistakes
❍ Struggles to sustain attention
❍ Fails to finish activities
❍ Difficulty with organization
❍ Avoids tasks that require sustained mental effort
❍ Distracted or forgetful
Symptoms of hyperactivity
❍ Fidgets
❍ Can't sit still for sustained period
❍ Difficulty playing quietly
❍ Talks excessively
Symptoms of impulsivity
❍ Interrupts
❍ Can't wait patiently

DSM-IV-TR criteria

These criteria confirm a diagnosis:
❍ six symptoms or more from the inattention or hyperactivity-impulsivity categories
❍ symptoms present for at least 6 months
❍ symptoms evident before age 7
❍ impairment present in two or more settings
❍ symptoms aren't accounted for by another mental disorder.

Test results

❍ Complete psychological, medical, and neurologic evaluations rule out other problems; specific tests include continuous performance test, behavior rating scales, and learning disability.

Treatment

General

❍ Education regarding the nature and effect of the disorder
❍ Behavior modification
❍ External structure
❍ Supportive psychotherapy
❍ Elimination of sugar, dyes, and additives from diet
❍ Monitor activity (for safety purposes)

Medication

❍ Stimulants
❍ Tricyclic antidepressants
❍ Mood stabilizers
❍ Beta-adrenergic blockers

Nursing considerations

Key outcomes

The patient (or family) will:
❍ demonstrate effective social interaction skills in one-on-one and group settings
❍ report improvement in family and social interactions
❍ demonstrate effective coping behavior.

Nursing interventions

○ Set realistic expectations and limits to avoid frustrating the patient.
○ Maintain a calm and consistent manner.
○ Keep all instructions short and simple — make one-step requests.
○ Provide praise, rewards, and positive feedback whenever possible.
○ Provide diversional activities suited to a short attention span.

Monitoring

○ Activity level
○ Nutritional status
○ Adverse drug reactions
○ Response to treatment
○ Complications
○ Activity (for safety purposes)

Patient teaching

Be sure to cover:
○ behavior therapy
○ reinforcement of good behavior
○ realistic expectations
○ medication regimen and possible adverse reactions
○ nutrition.

Discharge planning

○ Refer the patient to family therapy.

Autistic disorder

Overview

Description

○ A severe, pervasive developmental disorder
○ Degree of impairment varies
○ Usually apparent before age 3
○ Poor prognosis
○ Sometimes called *Kanner's autism*

Pathophysiology

○ Defects in the central nervous system (CNS) that may arise from prenatal complications.

Causes

○ Exact cause unknown
○ Defects in CNS from prenatal complications such as rubella
○ Nutritional deficiency
○ Disease caused or triggered by immunizations

Risk factors

○ High-risk pregnancy

Incidence

○ Affects 4 to 5 children per 10,000 births
○ Four to five times more likely in males than in females, usually the firstborn male

Common characteristics

○ Unresponsive to social contact
○ Gross deficit in intelligence and language development
○ Ritualistic and compulsive behavior
○ Restricted capacity for developmentally appropriate activities and interests
○ Bizarre response to the environment

Complications

○ Epileptic seizures
○ Depression
During stress
○ Catatonic phenomena
○ Undifferentiated psychotic state

Assessment

History

○ Becomes rigid or flaccid when held
○ Cries when touched
○ Shows little or no interest in human contact

Physical findings

○ Delayed smiling response
○ Severe language impairment
○ Lack of socialization and imaginative play
○ Echolalia

○ Pronoun reversal
○ Bizarre or self-destructive behavior
○ Extreme compulsion for sameness
○ Abnormal reaction to sensory stimuli
○ Cognitive impairment
○ Eating, drinking, and sleeping problems
○ Mood disorders

DSM-IV-TR criteria

At least 6 of these 12 characteristics must be present, including at least 2 items from the first section, 1 from the second, and 1 from the third.
○ Qualitative impairment in social interaction:
  – Impaired nonverbal behavior
  – Absence of peer relationships
  – Failure to seek or share enjoyment, interests, or achievements
  – Lack of social or emotional reciprocity
○ Qualitative impairment in communication:
  – Delay or lack of language development
  – Inability to initiate or sustain conversation
  – Idiosyncratic or repetitive language
  – Lack of appropriate imaginative play
○ Restricted repetitive and stereotyped patterns of behavior, interests, and activities:
  – Abnormal preoccupation with a restricted pattern of interest
  – Inflexible routines or rituals
  – Repetitive motor mannerisms
  – Preoccupation with parts of objects
○ The diagnostic criteria also include delays or abnormal functioning in at least one of these areas before age 3:
  – Social interaction and language skills
  – Symbolic or imaginative play

Treatment

General

○ Structured treatment plan
○ Behavioral techniques
○ Pleasurable sensory and motor stimulation
○ Monitor activities (for safety purposes)

Medication

○ Haloperidol

Nursing considerations

Key outcomes

The patient (or family) will:
○ identify and contact available resources, as needed
○ openly share feelings about the present situation
○ as much as possible, demonstrate age-appropriate skills and behaviors
○ practice safety measures and take safety precautions in the home
○ interact with family or friends.

Nursing interventions

○ Institute safety measures when appropriate.
○ Provide positive reinforcement.
○ Encourage development of self-esteem.
○ Encourage self-care.
○ Prepare the child for change by telling him about it.
○ Assist family members to develop strong one-on-one relationships with the patient.

Monitoring

○ Response to treatment
○ Complications
○ Adverse drug reactions
○ Patterns of behavior
○ Nutritional status
○ Social interaction
○ Communication skills
○ Activity

Patient teaching

Be sure to cover:
○ physical care for the child's needs
○ importance of identifying signs of excessive stress and coping skills.

Discharge planning

○ Refer the parents to resource and support services.

Basal cell carcinoma

Overview

Description

- Slow-growing, destructive cancerous skin tumor
- Two major types: noduloulcerative and superficial
- Most common malignant tumor that affects whites (see *Identifying basal cell carcinoma*)

Pathophysiology

- Although the pathogenesis is uncertain, some experts hypothesize that it originates when undifferentiated basal cells become carcinomatous instead of differentiating into sweat glands, sebum, and hair.

Causes

- Prolonged sun exposure (90% of tumors occur on sun-exposed areas of the body)

Risk factors

- Arsenic ingestion
- Radiation exposure
- Burns
- Immunosuppression
- Vaccinations (a rare possibility)
- History of previous nonmelanoma skin cancer

Incidence

- Usually occurs in people over age 40
- Most prevalent in blond, fair-skinned men

Common characteristics

- Lesion found on face, head, neck, and back
- Five warning signs, including:
    - an open sore
    - a reddish patch
    - a shiny bump
    - a pink growth
    - a scarlike area.

Complications

- Disfiguring lesions of the eyes, nose, and cheeks

Assessment

History

- Odd-looking skin lesion
- Prolonged exposure to the sun
- Nonhealing sore of varying duration

Physical findings

- Lesions characterized as small, smooth, pinkish, and translucent papules (early-stage noduloulcerative)
- Telangiectatic vessels cross the surface and the lesions may be pigmented
- Lesions become enlarged with depressed centers and firm and elevated borders (also called *rodent ulcers*)
- Multiple oval or irregularly shaped, lightly pigmented plaques on chest or back
- Head and neck may show waxy, sclerotic, yellow to white plaques without distinct borders

Test results

Diagnostic procedures
- Incisional or excisional biopsy and histologic study may help to determine the tumor type and histologic subtype.

Other
- All types of basal cell carcinomas are diagnosed by clinical appearance.

Treatment

General

- Depending on the size, location, and depth of the lesion
- Irradiation, if the tumor location requires it; preferred for elderly or debilitated patients who might not tolerate surgery
- Cryotherapy (liquid nitrogen that freezes the cells and kills them)
- Well-balanced diet; no restrictions
- Avoid sun exposure

Medications

- Chemotherapy, such as topical fluorouracil and topical corticosteroids

Surgery

- Curettage and electrodesiccation
- Microscopically controlled surgical excision carefully removes recurrent lesions until a tumor-free plane is achieved (after removal of large lesions, skin grafting may be required)

Identifying basal cell carcinoma

This illustration shows an enlarged nasal nodule in basal cell carcinoma. Note its depressed center and firm, elevated border.

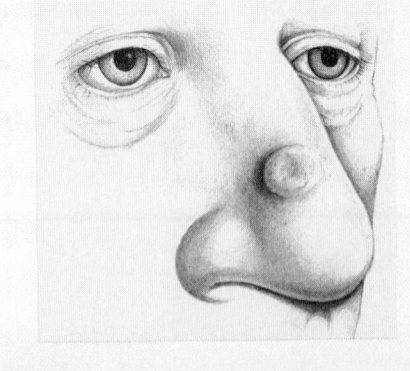

○ Chemosurgery

Nursing considerations

Key outcomes

The patient will:
○ express positive feelings about self
○ express feelings of increased comfort
○ exhibit improved or healed lesions or wounds
○ demonstrate effective coping mechanisms.

Nursing interventions

○ Encourage verbalization and provide support.
○ Provide appropriate wound care.

Monitoring

○ Complications of treatment
○ Response to treatment
○ Signs and symptoms of infection
○ Wound healing
○ Skin surveillance for additional lesions

Patient teaching

Be sure to cover:
○ the disorder, diagnosis, and treatment
○ appropriate skin care.

Discharge planning

○ Tell the patient to avoid excessive sun exposure and
to use a strong sunscreen or sunshade to protect the
skin.
○ Refer the patient to resource and support services.

Bell's palsy

Overview

Description

- Condition in which the impulses from the seventh cranial nerve are blocked, causing muscle weakness or paralysis
- Rapid onset
- Subsides spontaneously in 80% to 90% of patients
- Complete recovery in 1 to 8 weeks
- Recovery may be delayed in elderly people
- Partial recovery: contractures may develop on the paralyzed side of the face
- May recur on the same or the opposite side of the face

Pathophysiology

- Inflammatory reaction around the seventh cranial nerve (motor innervation of the facial muscles)
- Inflammation usually at the internal auditory meatus
- Unilateral facial weakness or paralysis results

Causes

- Unknown
- Ischemia
- Viral disease, such as herpes simplex or herpes zoster
- Local traumatic injury

Facial paralysis in Bell's palsy

Unilateral facial paralysis characterizes Bell's palsy. The paralysis produces a distorted appearance and an inability to wrinkle the forehead, close the eyelid, smile, show the teeth, or puff out the cheek.

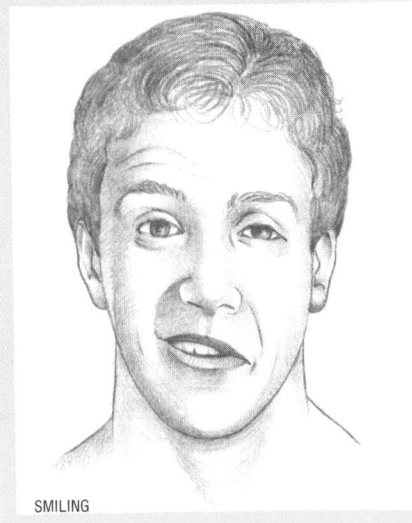

SMILING

- Autoimmune disease
- Lyme disease
- Tumor
- Bacterial infections such as meningitis

Incidence

- Affects all age-groups
- Most common between ages 20 and 60
- Affects males and females equally

Common characteristics

- Unilateral face weakness
- Aching at jaw angle
- Drooping mouth
- Distorted and loss of taste
- Impaired ability to fully close eye on affected side
- Tinnitus

Complications

- Corneal ulceration and blindness
- Impaired nutrition secondary to paralysis of the lower face
- Long-term psychosocial problems

Assessment

History

- Pain on the affected side around the angle of the jaw or behind the ear for a few hours or days before onset of weakness
- Difficulty chewing on the affected side
- Difficulty speaking clearly

Physical findings

- Mouth droops on the affected side (see *Facial paralysis in Bell's palsy*)
- Smooth forehead
- Distorted taste perception
- Inability to raise eyebrow, smile, show teeth, or puff out cheek
- Impaired ability to close eye on the weak side
- Eye rolls upward (Bell's phenomenon) when attempting to close the eye
- Excessive tearing

Test results

- Diagnosis is based on clinical presentation.
Imaging
- Magnetic resonance imaging rules out tumor.

Treatment

General

- Eliminating the source of damage to the nerve immediately
- Oral hygiene maintenance
- Eye protection such as sunglasses
- Hearing protection

- Moist heat
- Diet, as tolerated
- Activity, as tolerated

Medications

- Oral corticosteroids
- Analgesics
- Antiviral agent

Surgery

- Exploration of the facial nerve may be necessary
- Facial reanimation, such as direct facial nerve repair or facial nerve grafting

Nursing considerations

Key outcomes

The patient will:
- experience increased comfort and relief from pain
- consume an adequate number of calories daily
- express positive feelings about self
- express understanding of the condition and treatment regimen.
- exhibit improvement in facial muscle movement.

Nursing interventions

- Provide psychological support.
- Apply moist heat to the affected side of the face.
- Massage the patient's face with a gentle upward motion.
- Provide a facial sling.
- If the patient had surgery, provide preoperative and postoperative care.
- Administer medication, as ordered.

Monitoring

- Response to medications
- Signs and symptoms of peptic ulceration, pancreatitis, or other GI adverse effects of prednisone
- Nutritional status
- Facial muscle movement

Patient teaching

Be sure to cover:
- the disorder
- medication and adverse effects
- protection of affected eye
- exercises of the facial muscles
- nutritional management program.

Benign prostatic hyperplasia

Overview

Description

- Prostate gland enlarges sufficiently to compress urethra, causing overt urinary obstruction
- May be treated surgically or symptomatically, depending on the size of prostate, age and health of patient, and extent of obstruction
- Referred to as *BPH*

Pathophysiology

- Changes occur in periurethral glandular tissue.
- Prostate enlarges; may extend into bladder.
- Compression or distortion of prostatic urethra obstructs urine outflow.
- BPH may cause a diverticulum musculature, retaining urine.

Causes

- Unknown
- Recent evidence suggests a link with hormonal activity

Risk factors

- Age
- Intact testes

Incidence

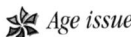 *Age issue*

BPH occurs in 80% of all men older than age 40, and in 95% of all men older than age 80.

Common characteristics

- Changes in voiding patterns and urine stream

Complications

- Urinary stasis, urinary tract infection (UTI), or renal calculi
- Bladder wall trabeculation
- Detrusor muscle hypertrophy
- Bladder diverticula and saccules
- Urethral stenosis
- Hydronephrosis
- Paradoxical (overflow) incontinence
- Acute or chronic renal failure
- Acute postobstructive diuresis

Assessment

History

- Decreased urine stream caliber and force
- Interrupted urinary stream
- Urinary hesitancy and frequency
- Difficulty initiating urination
- Nocturia, hematuria
- Dribbling, incontinence
- Urine retention

Physical findings

- Visible midline mass above the symphysis pubis
- Distended bladder
- Enlarged prostate on digital rectal examination

Test results

Laboratory
- Elevated blood urea nitrogen and serum creatinine levels suggesting impaired renal function
- Bacterial count that exceeds $100,000/mm^3$ revealing hematuria, pyuria, and UTI

Imaging
- Excretory urography may indicate urinary tract obstruction, hydronephrosis, calculi or tumors, and bladder filling and emptying defects.

Diagnostic procedures
- Cystourethroscopy determines the best surgical intervention and shows prostate enlargement, bladder wall changes, calculi, and raised bladder.

Other
- International Prostate Symptom Score classifies disorder's severity

Treatment

General

- Prostatic massage
- Short-term fluid restriction (prevents bladder distention)
- Avoidance of lifting, performing strenuous exercises, and taking long automobile rides for at least 1 month after surgery
- Regular sexual intercourse (if surgery not indicated)
- No sexual intercourse for several weeks after surgery

Medications

- Antibiotics, if infection present
- Alpha-1-adrenergic blockers such as terazosin
- 5-Alpha-reductase inhibitors such as finasteride

Surgery

- For relief of acute urine retention, hydronephrosis, severe hematuria, and recurrent UTI or for palliative relief of intolerable symptoms
- Suprapubic (transvesical) prostatectomy
- Perineal prostatectomy
- Retropubic (extravesical) prostatectomy
- Transurethral resection
- Balloon dilatation, ultrasound needle ablation, and use of stents

Nursing considerations

Key outcomes

The patient will:
- express feelings of increased comfort
- express understanding of disorder and treatment
- demonstrate skill in managing urinary elimination
- express feelings about potential or actual changes in sexual activity.

Nursing interventions

- Give prescribed drugs.
- Avoid giving tranquilizers, alcohol, antidepressants, or anticholinergics (which can worsen the obstruction).
- Provide I.V. therapy, as ordered.

Monitoring

- Vital signs
- Intake and output
- Daily weight

 Alert

Watch for signs of postobstructive diuresis, characterized by polyuria exceeding 2 L in 8 hours and excessive electrolyte losses. Although usually self-limiting, it can result in vascular collapse and death if not promptly treated.

After prostatic surgery
- Pain control
- Catheter function and drainage
- Signs of infection

Patient teaching

Be sure to cover:
- the disorder, diagnosis, and treatment
- signs of UTI that should be reported
- when to seek medical care (fever, unable to void, or passing bloody urine).

Bipolar disorder

Overview

Description

- An affective disorder marked by severe pathologic mood swings from hyperactivity and euphoria to sadness and depression
- In cyclothymia, a variant of bipolar disorder, numerous episodes of hypomania and depressive symptoms are too mild to meet the criteria for major depression or bipolar disorder (see *Cyclothymic disorder*)
- Manic episodes emerge over a period of days to weeks, but onset within hours is possible
- Untreated episodes can last weeks or as long as 8 to 12 months, with some having an unremitting course
- Rapid cycling occurs when four or more episodes of either depression or mania occur in a given year and occurs in 15% of all patients, almost all women
- Approximately half of all patients with this disorder have difficulties in work performance and psychosocial functioning

Pathophysiology

- Autosomal dominant inheritance has been found in genetic studies
- Linked to an X chromosome disorder
- Mood swings may involve membrane changes in sodium- and potassium-activated adenosine triphosphatase involving disordered intracellular signals

Causes

- Exact cause unclear
- Autosomal dominant inheritance found in genetic studies
- Some evidence that it's linked to an X chromosome disorder
- May be triggered by death, separation, or divorce
- Imbalances in the biochemistry that controls food (biochemical) imbalances

Risk factors

- Family history
- Substance abuse

Incidence

- Affects 3 million people in the United States
- Equally common in women and men
- Women are likely to have more depressive episodes
- Men experience more manic episodes in a lifetime
- Higher among relatives of affected patients than in the general population

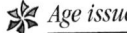 *Age issue*

Age of onset is usually between ages 20 and 35, but 35% of patients experience onset between ages 35 and 60.

Common characteristics

Manic phase
- Accelerated speech
- Frequent changes of topic
- Flight of ideas

Depressive phase
- Loss of self-esteem
- Overwhelming inertia
- Social withdrawal
- Feelings of hopelessness
- Apathy or self-reproach
- Suicidal thoughts

Bipolar II disorder
- Meets all the diagnostic criteria for a manic episode
- May experience recurrent depressions, separated by periods of mild activation and increased energy

Complications

- Emotional and social consequences
- Sexually transmitted disease
- Exhaustion
- Nutritional deficits
- Sleep disturbances
- Suicide

Assessment

History

- Sleeping and eating disturbances
- Exhibits expansive, grandiose, sometimes irritable mood alternating with symptoms of depression

Physical findings

Mania
- Increased psychomotor activity
- Excessive social extroversion
- Impulsive actions
- Impaired judgment
- Delusions
- Paranoid thinking
- Limited attention span
- Inflated sense of self-esteem
- Rapid responses to external stimuli

Depression
- Slow speech and response
- No obvious disorientation or intellectual impairment
- Psychomotor retardation
- Lethargy
- Low muscle tone
- Weight loss
- Slowed gait

DSM-IV-TR criteria

A diagnosis is confirmed when the patient meets the criteria established for a manic or hypomanic episode:
- experiences a distinct period of abnormally and persistently elevated, expansive, or irritable mood
- during the mood disturbance, at least three of these symptoms must persist (four, if the mood is only irritable) and be present to a significant degree:

- inflated self-esteem or grandiosity
- decreased need for sleep
- excessive talking
- flight of ideas
- easily distracted
- psychomotor agitation
- excessive involvement in dangerous activities
- symptoms don't meet criteria for a mixed episode
- impairment in occupational function, usual social activities, or relations with others severe enough to require hospitalization to prevent harm to self or others
- substance use or medical conditions aren't present.

Treatment

General

❍ Group and individual therapy
❍ Monitoring of activity when in manic phase
❍ No dietary restrictions

Medications

❍ Lithium
❍ Antipsychotics
❍ Valproic acid
❍ Carbamazepine
❍ Antidepressants

Nursing considerations

Key outcomes

The patient will:
❍ identify effective coping techniques
❍ recognize symptoms and comply with medication regimen
❍ express feelings related to self-esteem
❍ join gradually in self-care and the decision-making processes.

Nursing interventions

For the manic patient
❍ Encourage activities that require gross motor movements.
❍ Assist with personal hygiene; encourage responsibility for personal care.
❍ Protect from overstimulation.
❍ Set realistic goals and limits for the patient's behavior.
❍ Provide diversional activities suited to a short attention span.
❍ Reorient to reality.
❍ Avoid power struggles.
For the depressed patient
❍ Avoid overwhelming expectations.
❍ Allow increased time for activities and responses.
❍ Provide a structured routine.
❍ Promote interaction with others.
❍ Encourage verbalization; provide support.

Cyclothymic disorder

A chronic mood disturbance of at least 2 years' duration, cyclothymic disorder involves numerous episodes of hypomania or depressive symptoms that aren't of sufficient severity or duration to qualify as a major depressive episode.

In the hypomanic phase, the patient may experience insomnia; hyperactivity; inflated self-esteem; increased productivity and creativity; overinvolvement in pleasurable activities, including an increased sexual drive; physical restlessness; and rapid speech. Depressive symptoms may include insomnia, feelings of inadequacy, decreased productivity, social withdrawal, loss of libido, loss of interest in pleasurable activities, lethargy, depressed speech, and crying.

A number of medical disorders (for example, endocrinopathies, such as Cushing's disease, stroke, brain tumors, head trauma, and drug overdose) can produce a similar pattern of mood alteration. These organic causes must be ruled out before making a diagnosis of cyclothymic disorder.

❍ Institute safety measures.
❍ Encourage physical activity.

Monitoring

❍ Patterns of behavior
❍ Response to treatment
❍ Social interaction
❍ Complications
❍ Adverse drug reactions
❍ Nutritional status

Patient teaching

Be sure to cover:
❍ the disorder, diagnosis, and treatment
❍ medication administration, dosage, and possible adverse effects
❍ importance of continuing the prescribed medication regimen.

Discharge planning

❍ Refer the patient for psychological counseling.
❍ Refer the patient to support services.

Bladder cancer

Overview

Description

- Malignant tumor that develops on the bladder wall surface or grows within the wall and quickly invades underlying muscles
- Less common bladder tumors include adenocarcinomas, epidermoid carcinomas, squamous cell carcinomas, sarcomas, tumors in bladder diverticula, and carcinoma in situ
- Most common cancer of the urinary tract

Pathophysiology

- About 90% of bladder cancers are transitional cell carcinomas, arising from the transitional epithelium of mucous membranes. (They may result from malignant transformation of benign papillomas.)

Causes

- Exact cause unknown
- Associated with chronic bladder irritation and infection in people with renal calculi, indwelling urinary catheters, chemical cystitis caused by cyclophosphamide, or pelvic irradiation

Risk factors

- Certain environmental carcinogens, such as 2-naphthylamine, tobacco, nitrates, and coffee
- Occupational exposure to carcinogens

Incidence

- Bladder tumors most prevalent in people older than age 50
- More common in men than in women
- Occurs more commonly in densely populated industrial areas

Common characteristics

- Asymptomatic in early stages for 25% of patients
- First sign is gross, painless, intermittent hematuria, with or without clots
- Suprapubic pain after voiding most often associated with invasive lesions
- Bladder irritability
- Urinary frequency
- Nocturia
- Dribbling

Complications

- Bone metastasis
- Problems resulting from tumor invasion of contiguous viscera

Assessment

History

- Gross, painless, intermittent hematuria, usually with clots
- Suprapubic pain after voiding, which suggests invasive lesions
- Bladder irritability, urinary frequency, nocturia, and dribbling
- Flank pain that may indicate an obstructed ureter

Physical findings

- Gross hematuria
- Flank tenderness if ureteral obstruction present

Test results

Laboratory
- Complete blood count helping to detect anemia
- Urinalysis detecting blood and malignant cells in the urine

Imaging
- Excretory urography can identify a large, early-stage tumor or an infiltrating tumor; delineate functional problems in the upper urinary tract; assess hydronephrosis; and detect rigid deformity of the bladder wall.
- Retrograde cystography evaluates bladder structure and integrity; it also helps confirm a bladder cancer diagnosis.
- Bone scan can detect metastasis.
- Computed tomography scan defines the thickness of the involved bladder wall and discloses enlarged retroperitoneal lymph nodes.
- Ultrasonography reveals metastases in tissues beyond the bladder and can distinguish a bladder cyst from a bladder tumor.

Diagnostic procedures
- Cystoscopy and biopsy confirm bladder cancer diagnosis; if the test results show cancer cells, further studies will determine the cancer stage and treatment.

Other
- Bimanual examination may be performed during a cystoscopy if the patient has received an anesthetic; this helps to determine whether the bladder is fixed to the pelvic wall.

Treatment

General

- Cancer's stage, patient's lifestyle, other health problems, and mental outlook influence selection of therapy
- Initially postoperatively, avoid heavy lifting and contact sports
- After recovery, no activity restrictions

Medications

○ Intravesical chemotherapy, such as thiotepa, doxorubicin, and mitomycin
○ Attenuated bacille Calmette-Guérin vaccine live

Surgery

○ Transurethral resection (cystoscopic approach) and fulguration (electrically)
○ Segmental bladder
○ Radical cystectomy
○ Ureterostomy, nephrostomy, continent vesicostomy (Kock pouch), ileal bladder, and ureterosigmoidostomy

Nursing considerations

Key outcomes

The patient will:
○ maintain adequate fluid balance
○ express feelings of increased comfort and decreased pain
○ exhibit adequate coping mechanisms
○ express feelings about potential or actual changes in sexual activity.

Nursing interventions

○ Provide support and encourage verbalization.
○ Give prescribed drugs.
○ Provide preoperative teaching; discuss procedure and postoperative course.

Monitoring

○ Wound site
○ Postoperative complications
○ Intake and output
○ Pain control

Patient teaching

Be sure to cover:
○ the disorder, diagnosis, and treatment
○ stoma care
○ skin care and evaluation
○ avoidance of heavy lifting and contact sports (postoperatively with a urinary stoma)
○ encouragement of participation in usual athletic and physical activities.

Discharge planning

○ Refer the patient to resource and support services.
○ Before discharge, arrange for follow-up home nursing care.
○ Refer the patient to an enterostomal therapist and for services provided by the therapist.

Blastomycosis

Overview

Description
- Fungal infection that usually affects the lungs and produces bronchopneumonia
- May develop into extrapulmonary disease
- Also called *Gilchrist's disease*

Pathophysiology
- Inhalation of aerosolized conidial forms of the fungus from its natural soil habitat
- Transformation of the conidia to the yeast phase at body temperature (thermal dimorphism)
- Inflammatory response evoked by multiplication of organism
- Possible dissemination through the blood and lymphatics to other organs

Causes
- Inhalation of the yeastlike fungus *Blastomyces dermatitidis*

Incidence
- Generally found in North America, where *B. dermatitidis* normally inhabits the soil
- Endemic to the southeastern United States
- More common in men than women
- Onset most common between ages 30 and 50, but can occur at any age

Common characteristics
- Signs and symptoms of a viral upper respiratory tract infection
- Small, painless, nonpruritic, and nondistinctive macules or papules on exposed body parts

Complications
- Osteomyelitis
- Central nervous system, skin, and genital disorders
- Addison's disease (adrenal insufficiency)
- Pericarditis
- Arthritis

Assessment

History
- Fever, chills
- Dry, hacking, productive cough
- Weight loss
- Night sweats
- Pleuritic chest pain
- Malaise
- Mylagia

Physical findings
- Thick sputum (may contain blood)
- Bronchial breath sounds; dullness on chest percussion
- Decreased breath sounds
- Tachypnea
- Decreased pulse oximetry
- Raised and reddened lesions
- Chest pain
- Dyspnea

Extrapulmonary findings
- Skin lesions
- Osteolytic lesions
- Joint swelling

Test results
Laboratory
- Culture of *B. dermatitidis* from skin lesions, pus, sputum, or pulmonary secretions
- Increased white blood cell count and erythrocyte sedimentation rate
- Slightly increased serum globulin levels, mild normochromic anemia
- Increased alkaline phosphatase level (with bone lesions)

Imaging
- Chest X-ray may show pulmonary infiltrates.

Diagnostic procedures
- Biopsy of tissue from the skin or lungs or of bronchial washings, sputum, or pus shows infecting organism.

Other
- Immunodiffusion testing detects antibodies for the A and B antigens of blastomycosis.

Treatment

General
- Increased fluid intake
- Respiratory treatments
- Rest periods, as needed

Medications
- Amphotericin B
- Oral itraconazole
- Fluconazole
- Antipyretic

Nursing considerations

Key outcomes
The patient will:
- maintain adequate oxygenation
- improve skin integrity
- report increased comfort and decreased pain.

Nursing interventions

○ Provide a cool room; if the patient is feverish, administer a tepid sponge bath.
○ Elevate painful joints and apply heat.
○ Provide appropriate skin care.
○ Give prescribed drugs.

Monitoring

○ Vital signs
○ Pulse oximetry
○ Laboratory tests
○ Sputum production for hemoptysis
○ Level of consciousness pupil response
○ Hematuria
○ Lesion healing

Patient teaching

Be sure to cover:
○ the disorder, diagnosis, and treatment
○ proper administration of medications
○ skin care.

Discharge planning

○ Stress appropriate follow-up care.

Blepharitis

Overview

Description
○ Common inflammation of eyelash follicles and meibomian glands of the upper or lower eyelids
○ May affect both eyes
○ May affect upper and lower eyelids
○ Ulcerative type may coexist with seborrheic blepharitis

Pathophysiology
○ Inflammatory responses of the eyelids to bacteria or seborrheic dermatitis

Causes
Seborrheic blepharitis
○ Generally results from seborrhea of the scalp, eyebrows, and ears
Ulcerative blepharitis
○ Generally results from a *Staphylococcus aureus* infection
○ Pediculosis

Incidence
○ More common in elderly people
○ Most common ocular disease

Common characteristics
○ Eye drainage
○ Burning, itching, and swelling of eyes
○ Tends to recur
○ May become chronic

Complications
○ Ocular involvement
○ Keratitis

Assessment

History
○ Eyelids itch or burn
○ Feeling of foreign body
○ Crusty eyelids, which stick together when awakening
○ Loss of eyelashes

Physical findings
○ Continual blinking
○ Red-rimmed appearance to the eyelid margins
○ Swelling of eyelids
Seborrheic blepharitis
○ Scales along eyelids, especially upon awakening
○ Dandruff on scalp and eyebrows

Ulcerative blepharitis
○ Flaky scales on eyelashes, especially in morning
○ Missing eyelashes
○ Ulcerations on eyelid margins

Test results
Laboratory
○ Culture of the ulcerated eyelid margin revealing *S. aureus* in ulcerative blepharitis

Treatment

General
○ Early treatment to prevent recurrence or complications
○ Daily shampooing (using a mild shampoo on a cotton-tipped applicator or washcloth) to remove scales from eyelid margins
○ Warm eye compresses
○ Removal of nits with forceps for blepharitis from pediculosis
○ Avoidance of eye makeup
○ Avoidance of contact lens use until resolved

Medications
○ Sulfonamide or appropriate antibiotic eye ointment for ulcerative blepharitis
○ Ophthalmic physostigmine or other insecticidal ointment for blepharitis from pediculosis

Nursing considerations

Key outcomes
The patient will:
○ sustain no harm or injury
○ verbalize feelings and concerns
○ identify available health resources
○ demonstrate appropriate coping skills
○ maintain current visual acuity.

Nursing interventions
○ Provide eyelid care at least twice daily.
○ Apply warm compresses, four times daily.
○ Give prescribed drugs.
○ Apply ointments, as ordered. (See *Applying an ophthalmic ointment.*)

Monitoring
○ Response to treatment
○ Adverse reactions to medication
○ Complications

Applying an ophthalmic ointment

Follow these directions to apply an ophthalmic ointment cleanly and quickly:

○ Tilt the patient's head backward and ask him to look toward the ceiling.
○ Gently pull the lower eyelid down and squeeze a small ribbon of ointment along the edge of the conjunctival sac from the inner to the outer canthus.
○ Take care to avoid touching the eye with the tip of the ointment tube.
○ Repeat this procedure for the other eye, if ordered.

Patient teaching

Be sure to cover:
○ the disorder and treatment
○ daily eyelid care
○ removal of scales from eyelids
○ application of warm compresses
○ medications and potential adverse reactions
○ potential complications.

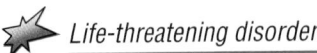 *Life-threatening disorder*

Blood transfusion reaction

Overview

Description

- ○ A hemolytic reaction following the transfusion of mismatched blood
- ○ Accompanies or follows I.V. administration of blood components
- ○ Mediated by immune or nonimmune factors
- ○ Severity varies from mild to severe

Pathophysiology

- ○ Recipient's antibodies, immunoglobulin (Ig) G or IgM, attach to donor red blood cells (RBCs), leading to widespread clumping and destruction of recipient's RBCs.
- ○ Transfusion with Rh-incompatible blood triggers a less serious reaction, known as Rh isoimmunization, within several days to 2 weeks. (See *Understanding the Rh system*.)
- ○ A febrile nonhemolytic reaction — the most common type of reaction — develops when cytotoxic or agglutinating antibodies in the recipient's plasma attack antigens on transfused lymphocytes, granulocytes, or plasma cells.

Causes

- ○ Transfusion with incompatible blood

Understanding the Rh system

The Rh system contains more than 30 antibodies and antigens. Of the world's population, about 85% are Rh positive, which means that their red blood cells carry the D or Rh antigen. The rest of the population are Rh negative and don't have this antigen.

Effects of sensitization

When an Rh-negative person receives Rh-positive blood for the first time, he becomes sensitized to the D antigen but shows no immediate reaction to it. If he receives Rh-positive blood a second time, he experiences a massive hemolytic reaction.

For example, an Rh-negative mother who delivers an Rh-positive baby is sensitized by the baby's Rh-positive blood. During her next Rh-positive pregnancy, her sensitized blood will cause a hemolytic reaction in the fetal circulation.

Preventing sensitization

To prevent the formation of antibodies against Rh-positive blood, an Rh-negative mother should receive $Rh_0(D)$ immune globulin (human) (RhoGAM) I.M. within 72 hours after delivering an Rh-positive baby.

Incidence

- ○ Mild reactions occur in 1% to 2% of transfusions

Common characteristics

- ○ Mild to severe fever within the first 15 minutes of transfusion or within 2 hours after its completion
- ○ Chills
- ○ Urticaria
- ○ Shortness of breath

Complications

- ○ Bronchospasm
- ○ Acute tubular necrosis leading to acute renal failure
- ○ Anaphylactic shock
- ○ Vascular collapse
- ○ Disseminated intravascular coagulation

Assessment

History

- ○ Transfusion of blood product
- ○ Chills, nausea, vomiting, chest tightness, or chest and back pain

Physical findings

- ○ Fever, tachycardia, and hypotension
- ○ Dyspnea and apprehension
- ○ Urticaria and angioedema
- ○ Wheezing
- ○ In a surgical patient, blood oozing from mucous membranes or the incision site
- ○ In a hemolytic reaction: fever, an unexpected decrease in serum hemoglobin level, frank blood in urine, and jaundice

Test results

Laboratory

- ○ Decreased serum hemoglobin levels
- ○ Elevated serum bilirubin levels and indirect bilirubin levels
- ○ Urinalysis revealing hemoglobinuria
- ○ Indirect Coombs' test or serum antibody screen positive for serum anti-A or anti-B antibodies
- ○ Increased prothrombin time and decreased fibrinogen level
- ○ Increased blood urea nitrogen and serum creatinine levels

Treatment

General

- ○ Immediate halt of transfusion
- ○ Dialysis (may be necessary if acute tubular necrosis occurs)
- ○ Diet, as tolerated
- ○ Bed rest

Medications

- ○ Osmotic or loop diuretics

- I.V. normal saline solution
- I.V. vasopressors
- Epinephrine
- Diphenhydramine
- Corticosteroids
- Antipyretics

Nursing considerations

Key outcomes

The patient will:
- maintain hemodynamic stability
- show no signs of active bleeding
- maintain adequate ventilation
- express understanding of disorder.

Nursing interventions

- Stop blood transfusion.
- Maintain a patent I.V. line with normal saline solution.
- Insert an indwelling urinary catheter.
- Report early signs of complications.
- Cover the patient with blankets to ease chills.
- Administer supplemental oxygen, as needed.
- Document the transfusion reaction on the patient's chart, noting the duration of the transfusion and the amount of blood absorbed.
- Follow your facility's blood transfusion policy and procedure.

 Alert

Double-check the patient's name, identification number, blood type, and Rh status before administering blood. If you find any discrepancy, don't administer the blood. Notify the blood bank immediately and return the unopened unit.

Monitoring

- Vital signs
- Intake and output
- Signs of shock
- Laboratory results

Patient teaching

Be sure to cover:
- signs and symptoms of transfusion reaction
- type of transfusion after recovery.

Bone tumors, primary malignant

Overview

Description

- Rare type of bone cancer (less than 1% of all malignant tumors)
- Also known as *osteoblastoma*

Pathophysiology

- Proliferation of cancerous cells that clump together to form a tumor
- Able to spread beyond the original site
- Osseous bone tumors
  - arise from the bony structure itself
  - include osteogenic sarcoma (most common), parosteal osteogenic sarcoma, chondrosarcoma (chondroblastic), and malignant giant cell tumor
- Nonosseous bone tumors
  - arise from hematopoietic, vascular, and neural tissues
  - include Ewing's sarcoma, fibrosarcoma (fibroblastic), and chordoma

Causes

- No immediately apparent cause in most cases
- Genetic abnormalities (retinoblastoma, Rothmund Thomson syndrome)
- Exposure to carcinogens
- Heredity, trauma, and excessive radiation therapy, according to theories

Incidence

- Account for less than 0.2% of all cancers
- More common in males than females
- Higher incidence in children and adolescents, although some types do occur in patients between ages 35 and 60 (see *Types of primary malignant bone tumors*)

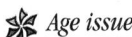 **Age issue**

Osteogenic and Ewing's sarcomas are the most common bone tumors in children.

Common characteristics

- Localized, dull bone pain
- Usually more intense at night

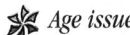 **Age issue**

Limb pain, refusal to walk, and limited range of motion are common findings in children with bone tumors.

- Presence of a mass or tumor

Complications

- Infection
- Hemorrhage
- Local recurrence

Assessment

History

- Localized dull bone pain
- Weight loss
- Impaired mobility
- Pathological fracture

Physical findings

- Palpable mass
- Cachectic appearance
- Abnormal gait

Test results

Laboratory

- Elevated serum alkaline phosphatase levels (with sarcoma)

Imaging

- Bone X-rays and radioisotope bone and computed tomography (CT) scans show tumor size.
- Bone scans and CT scans of the lungs reveal metastatic disease.

Diagnostic procedures

- Incision or aspiration biopsy confirms primary malignancy.

Treatment

General

- High-protein, high-calorie diet
- Rest periods, as needed
- Physical therapy

Medications

- Chemotherapy
- Analgesics

Surgery

- Excision of the tumor
- Radical surgery, such as hemipelvectomy or interscapulothoracic amputation

Nursing considerations

Key outcomes

The patient will:
- maintain weight within an acceptable range
- maintain joint mobility and range of motion
- express feelings of comfort and decreased pain
- express feelings and fears.

Types of primary malignant bone tumors

Type	Clinical features	Treatment
OSSEOUS ORIGIN		
Chondrosarcoma	• Develops from cartilage • Painless; grows slowly, but is locally recurrent and invasive • Occurs most commonly in pelvis, proximal femur, ribs, and shoulder girdle • Usually in men ages 30 to 50	• Hemipelvectomy, surgical resection (ribs) • Radiation (palliative) • Chemotherapy
Malignant giant cell tumor	• Arises from benign giant cell tumor • Found most commonly in long bones, especially in the knee area • Usually in women ages 18 to 50	• Curettage • Total excision • Radiation for recurrent disease
Osteogenic sarcoma	• Osteoid tumor present in specimen • Tumor arises from bone-forming osteoblast and bone-digesting osteoclast • Occurs most commonly in femur, but also tibia and humerus; occasionally, in fibula, ileum, vertebra, or mandible • Usually in men ages 10 to 30	• Surgery (tumor resection, high thigh amputation, hemipelvectomy, interscapulothoracic surgery) • Chemotherapy
Parosteal osteogenic sarcoma	• Develops on surface of bone instead of interior • Progresses slowly • Occurs most commonly in distal femur, but also in tibia, humerus, and ulna • Usually in women ages 30 to 40	• Surgery (tumor resection, possible amputation, interscapulothoracic surgery, hemipelvectomy) • Chemotherapy • Combination of the above
NONOSSEOUS ORIGIN		
Chordoma	• Derived from embryonic remnants of notochord • Progresses slowly • Usually found at end of spinal column and in spheno-occipital, sacrococcygeal, and vertebral areas • Characterized by constipation and visual disturbances • Usually in men ages 50 to 60	• Surgical resection (often resulting in neural defects) • Radiation (palliative, or when surgery not applicable, as in occipital area)
Ewing's sarcoma	• Originates in bone marrow and invades shafts of long and flat bones • Usually affects lower extremities, most commonly femur, innominate bones, ribs, tibia, humerus, vertebra, and fibula; may metastasize to lungs • Pain increasingly sever and persistent • Usually in men ages 10 to 20 • Prognosis poor	• High-voltage radiation (tumor is radiosensitive) • Chemotherapy to slow growth • Amputation only if there's no evidence of metastasis
Fibrosarcoma	• Relatively rare • Originates in fibrous tissue of bone • Invades long or flat bones (femur, tibia, mandible) but also involves periosteum and overlying muscle • Usually in men ages 30 to 40	• Amputation • Radiation • Chemotherapy • Bone grafts (with low-grade fibrosarcoma)

Nursing interventions

○ Encourage communication, and help the patient set realistic goals.
○ Give prescribed I.V. infusions and drugs.
○ Elevate the foot of the bed or place the affected stump on a pillow for the first 24 hours. (Be careful not to leave the stump elevated for more than 48 hours because this may lead to contractures.)

Monitoring

○ Vital signs
○ Circulation to the affected extremity
○ Wound dressings

Patient teaching

Be sure to cover:
○ use of assistive devices
○ wound care
○ reporting new pain or masses
○ the need for antibiotic prophylaxis when undergoing dental procedures (with bone grafts or prosthetic implants).

Discharge planning

○ Refer the patient to the American Cancer Society for information and support.

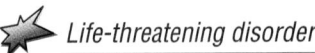 *Life-threatening disorder*

Botulism

Overview

Description

- Life-threatening paralytic illness
- Results from an exotoxin produced by the gram-positive, anaerobic bacillus *Clostridium botulinum*
- Occurs as botulism food poisoning, wound botulism, and infant botulism (see *Infant botulism*)
- Mortality about 25%, with death most commonly caused by respiratory failure during the first week of illness
- Onset within 24 hours signals critical and potentially fatal illness

Pathophysiology

- Endotoxin acts at the neuromuscular junction of skeletal muscle, preventing acetylcholine release and blocking neural transmission, eventually resulting in paralysis.

Causes

- *Clostridium botulinum* bacteria

Risk factors

- Eating improperly preserved foods
- Use of injectable street drugs

Incidence

- Occurs worldwide
- Average yearly occurrence of about 110 cases in the United States
- Affects adults more than children

Infant botulism

Infant botulism, which usually afflicts neonates and infants between 3 and 20 weeks old, is often caused by ingesting the spores of botulinum bacteria, which then grow in the intestines and release toxin. This disorder can produce floppy infant syndrome, characterized by constipation, a feeble cry, a depressed gag reflex, and an inability to suck. The infant also exhibits a flaccid facial expression, ptosis, and ophthalmoplegia — the result of cranial nerve deficits.

As the disease progresses, the infant develops generalized weakness, hypotonia, areflexia, and sometimes a striking loss of head control. Almost 50% of affected infants develop respiratory arrest.

Intensive supportive care allows most infants to recover completely. Antitoxin therapy isn't recommended because of the risk of anaphylaxis.

Common characteristics

- Signs appear 18 to 30 hours after ingestion of contaminated food, but there may be a delay of up to 10 days before symptoms appear
- Signs range in severity and can mimic other illnesses, especially neurologic disorders

Complications

- Respiratory failure
- Paralytic ileus
- Death

Assessment

History

- Consumption of home-canned food 18 to 30 hours before onset of symptoms
- Vertigo
- Sore throat
- Weakness
- Nausea and vomiting
- Constipation or diarrhea
- Diplopia
- Blurred vision
- Dysarthria
- Dysphagia
- Dyspnea
- Heroin use

Physical findings

- Ptosis
- Dilated, nonreactive pupils
- Appearance of dry, red, and crusted oral mucous membranes
- Abdominal distention with absent bowel sounds
- Descending weakness or paralysis of muscles in the extremities or trunk
- Deep tendon reflexes may be intact, diminished, or absent
- Unexplained postural hypotension
- Urinary retention
- Photophobia
- Slurred speech

Test results

Laboratory
- Mouse bioassay detects toxin that's found in the patient's serum, stool, or gastric contents.

Diagnostic procedures
- Electromyogram shows diminished muscle action potential after a single supramaximal nerve stimulus.

Treatment

General

- Supportive measures
- Early tracheotomy and ventilatory assistance in respiratory failure

---

○ Nasogastric suctioning
○ Total parenteral nutrition
○ Bed rest

Medications

○ I.V. or I.M. botulinum antitoxin

Surgery

○ Debridement of wounds to remove source of toxin-producing bacteria

Nursing considerations

Key outcomes

The patient will:
○ maintain tissue perfusion and cellular oxygenation
○ maintain adequate ventilation
○ maintain stable neurologic status.

Nursing interventions

○ Obtain history of food intake for the past several days.
○ Obtain family history of similar symptoms and food intake.
○ Administer I.V. fluids, as ordered.
○ Administer oxygen as needed.
○ Perform nasogastric suctioning as needed.

 Alert

Immediately report all cases of botulism to the local board of health.

Monitoring

○ Neurologic status
○ Cardiac and respiratory function
○ Cough and gag reflexes
○ Input and output
○ Arterial blood gas levels

Patient teaching

Be sure to cover:
○ the disorder, diagnosis, and treatment
○ proper techniques in processing and preserving foods
○ never tasting food from a bulging can or one with a peculiar odor
○ sterilizing utensils by boiling what came in contact with suspected contaminated food
○ not feeding honey to infants (can be fatal if contaminated).

Brain tumor, malignant

Overview

Description
- Abnormal growth among cells within the intracranial space
- May affect brain tissue, meninges, pituitary gland, and blood vessels
- In adults, the most common tumor types are gliomas and meningiomas, which usually occur above the covering of the cerebellum, or supratentorial tumors
- In children, the most common tumor types are astrocytomas, medulloblastomas, ependymomas, and brain stem gliomas

Pathophysiology
- Classified based on histology or grade of cell malignancy
- Central nervous system changes by cancer cells invading and destroying tissues and by secondary effect—mainly compression of the brain, cranial nerves, and cerebral vessels; cerebral edema; and increased intracranial pressure (ICP)

Causes
- Unknown

Risk factors
- Preexisting cancer

Incidence
- Slightly more common in men than in women
- Gliomas, meningiomas, and schwannomas have an overall incidence of 4.5 per 100,000
- Can occur at any age, but most occur in children before age 1 or between ages 2 and 12
- In adults, incidence is highest between ages 40 and 60

Common characteristics
- Increased ICP
- Headache
- Decreased motor strength and coordination
- Seizures
- Altered vital signs
- Nausea and vomiting
- Papilledema

Complications
- Radiation encephalopathy

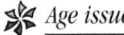 **Age issue**

Brain tumors are the most common cause of cancer death in children.

Life-threatening complications from increased ICP
- Coma
- Respiratory or cardiac arrest
- Brain herniation

Assessment

History
- Insidious onset
- Headache
- Nausea and vomiting

Physical findings
Signs and symptoms of increased ICP
- Vision disturbances
- Weakness, paralysis
- Aphasia, dysphagia
- Ataxia, incoordination
- Seizure

Test results
Imaging
- Skull X-rays confirming presence of tumor
- Brain scan confirming presence of tumor
- Computed tomography scan confirming presence of tumor
- Magnetic resonance imaging confirming presence of tumor
- Cerebral angiography confirming presence of tumor
- Positron emission tomography confirming presence of tumor

Diagnostic procedures
- Tissue biopsy confirming type of tumor

Other
- Lumbar puncture showing increased cerebrospinal fluid (CSF) pressure, which reflects ICP, increased protein levels, decreased glucose levels and, occasionally, tumor cells in CSF

Treatment

General
- Specific treatments vary with the tumor's histologic type, radiosensitivity, and location.
- No dietary restrictions unless swallowing impaired
- Possibly altered physical ability based on neurologic status

Medications
- Chemotherapy such as nitrosoureas
- Steroids
- Antacids and histamine-receptor antagonists
- Anticonvulsants

Surgery
For glioma
- Resection by craniotomy
- Radiation therapy and chemotherapy follow resection

For low-grade cystic cerebellar astrocytoma
○ Surgical resection
For astrocytoma
○ Repeated surgeries, radiation therapy, and shunting of fluid from obstructed CSF pathways
For oligodendroglioma and ependymoma
○ Surgical resection and radiation therapy
For medulloblastoma
○ Surgical resection
○ Possibly, intrathecal infusion and methotrexate or another antineoplastic drug
For meningioma
○ Surgical resection, including dura mater and bone
For schwannoma
○ Microsurgical technique

Nursing considerations

Key outcomes

The patient will:
○ recognize limitations imposed by illness and express feelings about them
○ continue to function in usual roles as much as possible
○ enlist support from available sources
○ express feelings of increased comfort.

Nursing interventions

○ Maintain a patent airway.
○ Take steps to protect the patient's safety.
○ Give prescribed drugs.
○ After supratentorial craniotomy, elevate the head of the bed about 30 degrees.
○ After infratentorial craniotomy, keep the patient flat for 48 hours.
○ As appropriate, instruct the patient to avoid Valsalva's maneuver and isometric muscle contractions when moving or sitting up in bed.
○ Consult with occupational, speech, and physical therapists.
○ Provide emotional support.

Monitoring

○ Neurologic status
○ Vital signs
○ Wound site
○ Postoperative complications

Patient teaching

Be sure to cover:
○ the disease process, diagnosis, and treatment
○ signs of infection or bleeding that may result from chemotherapy
○ adverse effects of chemotherapy and other treatments and actions that may alleviate them
○ early signs of tumor recurrence.

Discharge planning

○ Consult with occupational and physical therapy staff for postdischarge care plan.
○ Refer the patient to resource and support services.

Breast cancer

Overview

Description

○ Malignant proliferation of epithelial cells lining the ducts or lobules of the breast
○ Early detection and treatment influences the prognosis considerably.

 Alert

The most reliable detection method of breast cancer is regular breast self-examination, followed by an immediate professional evaluation of any abnormality. (Theoretically, slow-growing breast cancer may take up to 8 years to become palpable at 1 cm.)

○ With adjunctive therapy, 70% to 75% of women with negative nodes survive 10 years or more, compared to 20% to 25% of women with positive nodes.

Pathophysiology

○ Breast cancer spreads by way of the lymphatic system and the bloodstream through the right side of the heart to the lungs and to the other breast, chest wall, liver, bone, and brain.

Classification

○ Adenocarcinoma (ductal) — arising from the epithelium
○ Intraductal — developing within the ducts (includes Paget's disease)
○ Infiltrating — occurring in the breast's parenchymal tissue
○ Inflammatory (rare) — growing rapidly and causing overlying skin to become edematous, inflamed, and indurated
○ Lobular carcinoma in situ — involving the lobes of glandular tissue
○ Medullary or circumscribed — enlarging tumor with rapid growth rate

Causes

○ Unknown

Risk factors

○ Family history of breast cancer, particularly first-degree relatives, including mother, sister, maternal grandmother, and maternal aunt
○ Positive tests for genetic mutations (BRCA 1)
○ A woman older than age 45 and premenopausal
○ Long menstrual cycles
○ Early onset of menses, late menopause
○ Nulliparous or first pregnancy after age 30
○ High-fat diet
○ Endometrial or ovarian cancer
○ History of unilateral breast cancer
○ Radiation exposure
○ Estrogen therapy
○ Antihypertensive therapy
○ Alcohol and tobacco use
○ Preexisting fibrocystic disease

Incidence

○ A woman living in the United States to age 80 has a 1-in-9 chance of developing invasive breast cancer sometime during her life.
○ Breast cancer is the second-leading cause of cancer death in women after lung cancer.
○ Although breast cancer may develop anytime after puberty, it's most common after age 50.

 Age issue

Breast cancer is the leading cause of cancer deaths among women ages 35 to 54.

○ The disease seldom occurs in men.

Common characteristics

○ Lump or mass in the breast (see *Breast tumor sources and sites*)
○ Breast pain
○ Change in symmetry or size of breast
○ Change in skin, such as thickening, scaly skin around the nipple, dimpling, edema, or ulceration
○ Nipple discharge

Complications

○ Distant metastasis
○ Infection
○ Central nervous system effects
○ Respiratory effects

Assessment

History

○ Detection of a painless lump or mass in the breast
○ Change in breast tissue
○ History of risk factors

Physical findings

○ Clear, milky, or bloody nipple discharge, nipple retraction, scaly skin around the nipple, and skin changes, such as dimpling or inflammation
○ Arm edema
○ Hard lump, mass, or thickening of breast tissue
○ Lymphadenopathy

Test results

Laboratory

○ Alkaline phosphatase levels and liver function revealing distant metastases
○ Hormonal receptor assay determining whether the tumor is estrogen- or progesterone-dependent; also guides decisions to use therapy that blocks the action of the estrogen hormone that supports tumor growth

Imaging

- Mammography can reveal a tumor that's too small to palpate.
- Ultrasonography can distinguish between a fluid-filled cyst and solid mass.
- Chest X-rays can pinpoint metastases in the chest.
- Scans of the bone, brain, liver, and other organs can detect distant metastases.

Diagnostic procedures

- Fine-needle aspiration and excisional biopsy provide cells for histologic examination that may confirm the diagnosis.

Treatment

General

- The choice of treatment usually depends on the stage and type of disease, the woman's age and menopausal status, and any disfiguring effects of surgery.
- Therapy may include any combination of surgery, radiation, chemotherapy, and hormone therapy.
- The patient may need arm-stretching exercises after surgery.
- Primary radiation therapy
- Preoperative breast irradiation

Medications

- Chemotherapy such as a combination of drugs including cyclophosphamide, fluorouracil, methotrexate, doxorubicin, vincristine, paclitaxel, and prednisone
- Regimen of cyclophosphamide, methotrexate, and fluorouracil, which is used in premenopausal and postmenopausal women
- Antiestrogen therapy such as tamoxifen
- Hormonal therapy, including estrogen, progesterone, androgen, or antiandrogen aminoglutethimide therapy

Surgery

- Lumpectomy
- Partial, total, or modified radical mastectomy

Nursing considerations

Key outcomes

The patient will:
- recognize limitations imposed by illness and express feelings about these limitations
- express positive feelings about self
- report feelings of comfort
- express increased sense of well-being
- use situational supports to reduce fear.

Nursing interventions

- Provide information about the disease process, diagnostic tests, and treatment.
- Give prescribed drugs.
- Provide emotional support.

Breast tumor sources and sites

About 90% of all breast tumors arise from the epithelial cells lining the ducts. About half of all breast cancers develop in the breast's upper outer quadrant—the section containing the most glandular tissue.

The second most common cancer site is the nipple, where all the breast ducts converge.

The next most common site is the upper inner quadrant, followed by the lower outer quadrant and, finally, the lower inner quadrant.

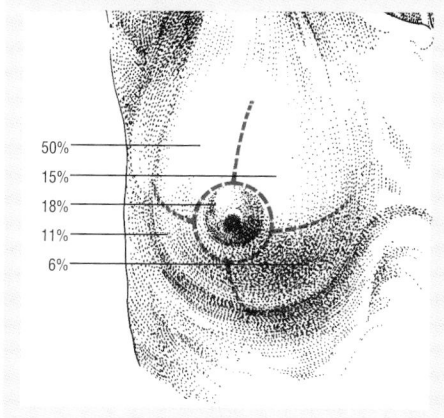

50%
15%
18%
11%
6%

Monitoring

- Wound site
- Postoperative complications
- Vital signs
- Intake and output
- White blood cell count
- Pain control
- Psychological status

Patient teaching

Be sure to cover:
- all procedures and treatments
- activities or exercises that promote healing
- breast self-examination
- risks and signs and symptoms of recurrence
- avoidance of venipuncture or blood pressure monitoring on the affected arm.

Discharge planning

- Refer the patient to local and national support groups.

Bronchiectasis

Overview

Description

- Lung disease characterized by abnormal dilation of the bronchi and destruction of the bronchial walls
- Results from conditions associated with repeated damage to bronchial walls and with abnormal mucociliary clearance, causing a breakdown of supporting tissue adjacent to the airways
- Can occur throughout the tracheobronchial tree, or may be confined to one segment or lobe
- Usually bilateral and involves the basilar segments of the lower lobes
- Occurs in three forms: cylindrical (fusiform), varicose, and saccular (cystic)

Pathophysiology

- Hyperplastic squamous epithelium, denuded of cilia, replaces ulcerated columnar epithelia.
- Abscess formation occurs, involving all layers of the bronchial walls, which produces inflammatory cells and fibrous tissues, resulting in dilation and narrowing of the airways.
- Sputum stagnates in the dilated bronchi and leads to secondary infection, characterized by inflammation and leukocytic accumulations.
- Additional debris collects in the bronchi and occludes them.
- Building pressure from the retained secretions induces mucosal injury.
- Extensive vascular proliferation of bronchial circulation occurs and produces frequent hemoptysis.

Causes

- Mucoviscidosis
- Immune disorders
- Recurrent bacterial respiratory tract infections
- Complications of measles, pneumonia, pertussis, or influenza
- Obstruction with recurrent infection
- Inhalation of corrosive gas
- Repeated aspiration of gastric juices
- Congenital anomalies (rare) such as bronchomalacia
- Various rare disorders such as immotile cilia syndrome

Incidence

- Affects people of both sexes and of all ages
- Dramatically decreased incidence over the past 20 years due to the availability of antibiotics to treat acute respiratory infections
- Incidence highest among Inuit populations in the northern hemisphere and the Maoris of New Zealand

Common characteristics

- Chronic cough productive for copious, foul-smelling, mucopurulent secretions
- Dyspnea
- Weight loss
- Malaise

Complications

- Chronic malnutrition
- Amyloidosis
- Right-sided heart failure
- Cor pulmonale

Assessment

History

- Frequent bouts of pneumonia
- Coughing up of blood or blood-tinged sputum
- Chronic cough that produces copious, foul-smelling, mucopurulent secretions
- Dyspnea
- Weight loss
- Malaise

Physical findings

- Sputum may show a cloudy top layer, a central layer of clear saliva, and a heavy, thick, purulent bottom layer
- Clubbed fingers and toes
- Cyanotic nail beds
- Dullness over affected lung fields, if pneumonia or atelectasis present
- Diminished breath sounds
- Inspiratory crackles during inspiration over affected area
- Occasional wheezes

Test results

Laboratory
- Sputum culture and Gram stain showing predominant pathogens
- Complete blood count revealing anemia and leukocytosis

Imaging
- Computed tomography scan shows bronchiectasis.
- Bronchography shows location and extent of disease.
- Chest X-rays show peribronchial thickening, atelectatic areas, and scattered cystic changes.

Diagnostic procedures
- Bronchoscopy may show the source of secretions or the bleeding site in hemoptysis.
- Pulmonary function studies show decreased vital capacity, expiratory flow, and hypoxemia.

Other
- A sweat electrolyte test may show cystic fibrosis as the underlying cause.

Treatment

General

- Postural drainage and chest percussion
- Bronchoscopy to remove secretions

○ Well-balanced, high-calorie diet
○ Adequate hydration
○ Activity, as tolerated

Medication

○ Antibiotics
○ Bronchodilators
○ Oxygen

Surgery

For poor pulmonary function
○ Segmental resection
○ Bronchial artery embolization
○ Lobectomy
○ Surgical removal of the affected lung portion

○ postural drainage and percussion
○ coughing and deep-breathing techniques
○ avoidance of air pollutants and people with known upper respiratory tract infections
○ immunizations
○ balanced, high-protein diet
○ avoidance of milk products
○ adequate hydration.

Discharge planning

○ Refer the patient to a smoking-cessation program, if indicated.

Nursing considerations

Key outcomes

The patient will:
○ maintain a patent airway
○ maintain adequate ventilation
○ utilize energy conservation techniques
○ demonstrate effective coping mechanisms.

Nursing interventions

○ Give prescribed drugs.
○ Provide supportive care.
○ Administer oxygen, as needed.
○ Perform chest physiotherapy.
○ Provide a warm, quiet, comfortable environment.
○ Alternate rest and activity periods.
○ Provide well-balanced, high-calorie meals.
○ Offer small, frequent meals.
○ Provide adequate hydration.
○ Provide frequent mouth care.

Monitoring

○ Vital signs
○ Intake and output
○ Respiratory status
○ Breath sounds
○ Sputum production
○ Pulse oximetry
○ Arterial blood gas results
○ Complications
○ Chest tube drainage after surgery

Patient teaching

Be sure to cover:
○ the disorder, diagnosis, and treatment
○ medications and potential adverse reactions
○ when to notify the physician
○ proper disposal of secretions
○ infection control techniques
○ frequent rest periods
○ preoperative and postoperative instructions, if surgery is required

Bronchitis, chronic

Overview

Description

- An inflammation of the lining of the bronchial tubes
- Form of chronic obstructive pulmonary disease
- Characterized by excessive production of tracheo-bronchial mucus with a cough for at least 3 months each year for 2 consecutive years
- Severity linked to the amount of cigarette smoke or other pollutants inhaled and inhalation duration
- Respiratory tract infections that typically exacerbate the cough and related symptoms
- Development of significant airway obstruction seen in few patients with chronic bronchitis

Pathophysiology

- Hypertrophy and hyperplasia of the bronchial mucous glands, increased goblet cells, ciliary damage, squamous metaplasia of the columnar epithelium, and chronic leukocytic and lymphocytic infiltration of bronchial walls
- Additional effects: widespread inflammation, airway narrowing, and mucus within the airways — all producing resistance in the small airways and, in turn, a severe ventilation-perfusion imbalance (see *What happens in chronic bronchitis*)

Causes

- Cigarette smoking
- Possible genetic predisposition
- Environmental pollution
- Organic or inorganic dusts and noxious gas exposure

Incidence

- About 20% of men have chronic bronchitis.
- More than 8.8 million people in the United States are diagnosed with chronic bronchitis annually.
- More prevalent in females than in males.
- Children of parents who smoke are at higher risk for contracting chronic bronchitis than children of parents who don't smoke.

Common characteristics

- Longtime smoker
- Frequent upper respiratory tract infections
- Productive cough
- Exertional dyspnea

Complications

- Cor pulmonale
- Pulmonary hypertension
- Right ventricular hypertrophy
- Acute respiratory failure

Assessment

History

- Longtime smoker
- Frequent upper respiratory tract infections
- Productive cough
- Exertional dyspnea
- Cough, initially prevalent in winter, but gradually becoming year-round
- Increasingly severe coughing episodes
- Worsening dyspnea

Physical findings

- Cough producing copious gray, white, or yellow sputum
- Cyanosis
- Accessory respiratory muscle use
- Tachypnea
- Substantial weight gain
- Pedal edema
- Neck vein distention
- Wheezing
- Prolonged expiratory time
- Rhonchi

Test results

Laboratory

- Arterial blood gas analysis showing decreased partial pressure of oxygen and normal or increased partial pressure of carbon dioxide
- Sputum culture revealing how many microorganisms and neutrophils

Imaging

- Chest X-ray may show hyperinflation and increased bronchovascular markings.

Diagnostic procedures

- Pulmonary function tests show increased residual volume, decreased vital capacity and forced expiratory flow, and normal static compliance and diffusing capacity.

Other

- Electrocardiography may show atrial arrhythmias; peaked P waves in leads II, III, and aV_F; and right ventricular hypertrophy.

Treatment

General

- Smoking cessation
- Avoidance of air pollutants
- Chest physiotherapy
- Ultrasonic or mechanical nebulizer treatments
- Adequate fluid intake
- High-calorie, protein-rich diet
- Activity, as tolerated with frequent rest periods

Medications

- Oxygen
- Antibiotics

In chronic bronchitis, irritants inhaled for a prolonged period inflame the tracheobronchial tree. The inflammation leads to increased mucus production and a narrowed or blocked airway.

As inflammation continues, the mucus-producing goblet cells undergo hypertrophy, as do the ciliated epithelial cells that line the respiratory tract. Hypersecretion from the goblet cells blocks the free movement of the cilia, which normally sweep dust, irritants, and mucus from the airways.

As a result, the airway stays blocked, and mucus and debris accumulate in the respiratory tract.

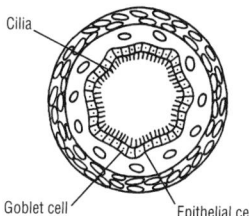

CROSS SECTION OF THE NORMAL BRONCHIAL TREE

Cilia

Goblet cell   Epithelial cell

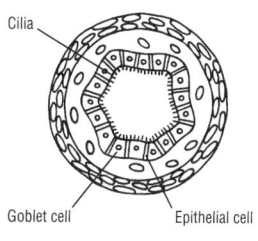

NARROWED BRONCHIAL TUBE IN CHRONIC BRONCHITIS

Cilia

Goblet cell   Epithelial cell

○ Bronchodilators
○ Corticosteroids
○ Diuretics

Surgery

○ Tracheostomy in advanced disease

Nursing considerations

Key outcomes

The patient will:
○ maintain adequate ventilation
○ identify measures to prevent or reduce fatigue
○ express understanding of the illness
○ maintain a patent airway.

Nursing interventions

○ Give prescribed drugs.
○ Encourage expression of fears and concerns.
○ Include the patient and his family in care decisions.
○ Perform chest physiotherapy.
○ Provide a high-calorie, protein-rich diet.
○ Offer small, frequent meals.
○ Encourage energy-conservation techniques.
○ Ensure adequate oral fluid intake.
○ Provide frequent mouth care.
○ Encourage daily activity.
○ Provide diversional activities, as appropriate.
○ Provide frequent rest periods.

Monitoring

○ Vital signs
○ Intake and output
○ Sputum production
○ Respiratory status
○ Breath sounds
○ Daily weight
○ Edema
○ Response to treatment

Patient teaching

Be sure to cover:
○ the disorder, diagnosis, and treatment
○ medications and possible adverse reactions
○ when to notify the physician
○ infection control practices
○ influenza and pneumococcus immunizations
○ home oxygen therapy, if required
○ postural drainage and chest percussion
○ coughing and deep-breathing exercises
○ inhaler use
○ high-calorie, protein-rich meals
○ adequate hydration
○ avoidance of inhaled irritants
○ prevention of bronchospasm.

Discharge planning

○ Refer the patient to a smoking-cessation program, if indicated.
○ Refer the patient to the American Lung Association for information and support.

Brucellosis

Overview

Description
- An acute febrile illness transmitted to humans from animals
- Also known as *undulant fever, Malta fever,* or *Bang's disease*

Pathophysiology
- Transmitted through the consumption of unpasteurized dairy products or uncooked or undercooked contaminated meat, and through contact with infected animals or their secretions or excretions

Causes
- The nonmotile, nonspore-forming, gram-negative coccobacilli of the genus *Brucella,* notably *B. suis* (found in swine), *B. melitensis* (in goats), *B. abortus* (in cattle), and *B. canis* (in dogs)

Incidence
- Most common among farmers, stock handlers, butchers, and veterinarians
- Six times more common in men than in women
- Less common in children
- People with chlorhydria particularly susceptible because hydrochloric acid in gastric juices kills *Brucella* bacteria
- Most prevalent in the Middle East, Africa, the former Soviet Union, India, South America, and Europe; uncommon in the United States

Common characteristics
Acute phase
- Fever
- Chills
- Profuse sweating
- Fatigue
- Headache
- Backache
- Enlarged lymph nodes
- Hepatosplenomegaly
- Weight loss
- Abscess and granuloma formulation in subcutaneous tissues, lymph nodes, liver, and spleen

Chronic phase
- Recurrent depression
- Sleep disturbances
- Fatigue
- Headache
- Sweating
- Sexual impotence
- Hepatosplenomegaly
- Enlarged lymph nodes

Complications
- Abscesses in the testes, ovaries, kidneys, and brain (meningitis and encephalitis)
- Osteomyelitis
- Orchitis
- Subacute bacterial endocarditis
- Pleural effusions
- Pneumothorax
- Eczematous rashes, petechiae, purpura

Assessment

History
- Direct exposure to animals
- Ingestion of unpasteurized dairy products
- Recent travel to an endemic area
- Fatigue
- Headache
- Intermittent fever
- Profuse sweating
- Anxiety
- General aching

Physical findings
- Excessive perspiration
- Chills
- Weakness
- Lymphadenopathy
- Hepatosplenomegaly
- Tenderness in the right upper quadrant

Test results
Laboratory
- Agglutinin titers of 1:160 or more
- Definitive diagnosis provided by three to six cultures of blood and bone marrow and biopsies of infected tissue (for example, the spleen)
- Increased erythrocyte sedimentation rate
- Normal or reduced white blood cell count

Treatment

General
- Bed rest during the acute phase
- High-calorie, high-protein diet
- Secretion precautions until lesions stop draining

Medications
- Antibiotics
- Antipyretics
- Corticosteroids

Nursing considerations

Key outcomes
The patient will:
- be free from signs and symptoms of infection
- attain relief from immediate symptoms

○ experience feelings of comfort or absence of pain
○ regain or maintain skin integrity.

Nursing interventions

○ Keep suppurative granulomas and abscesses dry.
○ Double-bag and properly dispose of all secretions and soiled dressings.
○ Reassure the patient that this infection is curable.

Monitoring

○ Temperature
○ Complications
○ Depression and disturbed sleep pattern
○ Lesion healing

Patient teaching

Be sure to cover:
○ continuing medication for the prescribed duration
○ preventing recurrence by cooking meat thoroughly and avoiding unpasteurized milk.
○ warning meat packers and other people at risk of occupational exposure to wear rubber gloves and goggles.

Buerger's disease

Overview

Description

○ An inflammatory, nonatheromatous occlusive condition that impairs circulation to the legs, feet and, occasionally, hands
○ Sometimes called *thromboangiitis obliterans*

Pathophysiology

○ Polymorphonuclear leukocytes infiltrate the walls of small and medium-sized arteries and veins.
○ Thrombus develops in the vascular lumen, eventually occluding and obliterating portions of the small vessels, resulting in decreased blood flow to the feet and legs.
○ This diminished blood flow may produce ulceration and, eventually, gangrene.

Causes

○ Unknown
○ Linked to smoking (suggesting a hypersensitivity reaction to nicotine)

Incidence

○ More common in males than females
○ Most patients age 20 to 45
○ Affects natives of India, Japan, and Korea and Ashkenazic Jews

Common characteristics

○ Intermittent claudication of the instep, aggravated by exercise and relieved by rest
○ Initially, coldness, cyanosis, and numbness in feet during exposure to low temperature; later, redness, heat, and tingling
○ Impaired peripheral pulses and migratory superficial thrombophlebitis

Complications

○ Ulceration
○ Muscle atrophy
○ Gangrene

Assessment

History

○ Exposure to secondhand smoke
○ Use of nicotine patch
○ Use of chewing tobacco
○ Smoking
○ Painful, intermittent claudication of the instep, aggravated by exercise and relieved by rest

Physical findings

○ Feet become cold, numb, and cyanotic when exposed to low temperatures

○ Digital ischemia
○ Trophic nail changes
○ Absent or diminished radial, ulnar, or tibial pulses
○ Ischemic ulcers on the toes, feet, or fingers
○ Superficial thrombophlebitis

Test results

Imaging
○ Doppler ultrasonography showing diminished circulation in the peripheral vessels
○ Arteriography to locate lesions and rule out atherosclerosis
Diagnostic procedures
○ Plethysmography helping to detect decreased circulation in the peripheral vessels
Other
○ Abnormal Allen test results (See *Performing Allen's Test*)

Treatment

General

○ Smoking cessation
○ Nothing by mouth, if surgery is needed
○ Exercise program that uses gravity to fill and drain the blood vessels

Medications

○ Antibiotics for secondary infection
○ Analgesics

Surgery

○ In severe disease, a lumbar sympathectomy to increase blood supply to the skin
○ Amputation for nonhealing ulcers, intractable pain, or gangrene

Nursing considerations

Key outcomes

The patient will:
○ express feelings of increased comfort and decreased pain
○ maintain tissue integrity
○ carry out previous roles without the limitations of the disease process
○ develop adequate coping mechanisms.

Nursing interventions

○ Provide a padded footboard or bed cradle to prevent pressure from bed linens.
○ Protect the feet with soft padding.
○ Provide emotional support.

Monitoring

○ Skin integrity
○ Peripheral circulation
○ Infection

Performing Allen's test

Don't obtain an arterial blood gas specimen from the radial artery until you assess collateral arterial blood supply using the Allen's test.

Direct the patient to close his hand while you occlude his radial and ulnar arteries for 10 to 30 seconds, watching for the hand to blanch.

Tell the patient to open his hand.

Release pressure on the ulnar artery. Color should return to the patient's hand in 15 seconds. If the color doesn't return, select another site for an arterial puncture.

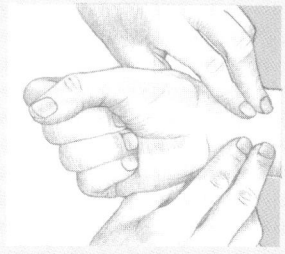 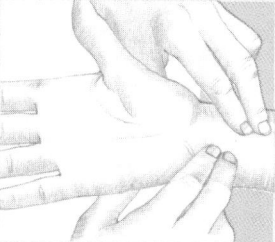 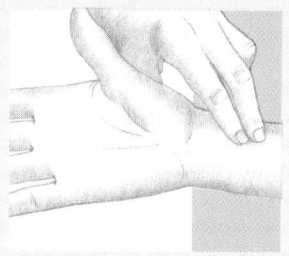

Patient teaching

Be sure to cover:
○ avoiding precipitating factors, such as emotional stress, exposure to extreme temperatures, and trauma
○ proper foot care, especially the importance of wearing well-fitting shoes and cotton or wool socks.

Discharge planning

○ Refer the patient to a self-help group to help him stop smoking.
○ Refer the patient for psychological counseling, if needed.
○ If the patient has undergone amputation, refer him to physical therapists, occupational therapists, and social service agencies, as needed.

Bulimia nervosa

Overview

Description

- Behavioral disorder characterized by eating binges followed by feelings of guilt, humiliation, and self-deprecation
- Self-induced vomiting, the use of laxatives or diuretics, or strict dieting or fasting to overcome the effects of the binges
- Seldom incapacitating

Pathophysiology

- Decreased caloric intake depletes body fat and protein stores.
- Estrogen deficiency occurs in women due to lack of lipid substrate for synthesis, causing amenorrhea.
- Testosterone levels fluctuate in men, causing decreased erectile function and sperm count.
- Ketoacidosis occurs from increased use of fat as energy fuel.

Causes

- Exact cause unknown
- Family disturbance or conflict
- Sexual abuse
- Maladaptive learned behavior
- Struggle for control or self-identity
- Cultural overemphasis on physical appearance
- Parental obesity

Incidence

- Affects nine females for every one male
- Between 1% and 3% of adolescent and young women meet the diagnostic criteria; 5% to 15% have some symptoms of the disorder

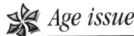 *Age issue*

Bulimia has been found to begin in adolescence or early adulthood.

Common characteristics

- Strongly associated with depression
- Can occur simultaneously with anorexia nervosa
- More prone to psychoactive substance abuse
- Hyperactivity
- Peculiar eating habits or rituals
- Frequent weighing
- Perceived by others as a "perfect" student, mother, or career woman
- Distinguished for participation in competitive activities

Complications

- Dental caries
- Erosion of tooth enamel
- Parotitis
- Gum infections
- Electrolyte imbalances
- Dehydration
- Arrhythmias
- Cardiac failure
- Sudden death
- Esophageal tears
- Gastric ruptures
- Mucosal damage to intestine
- Suicide

Assessment

History

- Episodic binge eating
- Continues eating until abdominal pain, sleep, or the presence of another person interrupts it
- Preferred food usually sweet, soft, and high in calories and carbohydrate content
- Exaggerated sense of guilt
- Depression
- Childhood trauma
- Parental obesity
- Unsatisfactory sexual relationships

Physical findings

- Thin or slightly overweight
- Use of diuretics, laxatives, vomiting, and exercise
- Abdominal and epigastric pain
- Amenorrhea
- Painless swelling of the salivary glands
- Unusual swelling of checks or jaw area
- Hoarseness
- Throat irritation or lacerations
- Calluses of the knuckles or abrasions and scars on the dorsum of the hand

DSM-IV-TR criteria

Diagnosis of bulimia nervosa can be confirmed when these criteria are met, on average, twice a week for 3 months:
- recurrent episodes of binge eating
- repeated inappropriate behaviors to prevent weight gain.

Test results

Laboratory
- Serum electrolyte studies showing elevated bicarbonate, decreased potassium, and decreased sodium levels

Other
- The Beck Depression Inventory may identify coexisting depression.

Treatment

General

- Inpatient or outpatient psychotherapy
- Self-help groups
- Drug rehabilitation
- Balanced diet
- Monitoring of eating pattern
- Monitoring of activity

Medications

- Antidepressants

Nursing considerations

Key outcomes

The patient will:
- acknowledge change in body image
- participate in decision-making about her case
- express positive feelings about self
- achieve expected state of wellness.

Nursing interventions

- Supervise mealtime and for a specified period after meals, usually up to 1 hour.
- Set a time limit for each meal.
- Provide a pleasant, relaxed environment for eating.
- Use behavior modification techniques.
- Establish a food contract, specifying the amount and type of food to be eaten at each meal.
- Encourage verbalization and provide support.

Monitoring

- Suicide potential
- Elimination patterns
- Eating patterns
- Complications
- Response to treatment
- Activity

Patient teaching

Be sure to cover:
- importance of keeping a food journal
- risks of laxative, emetic, and diuretic abuse
- assertiveness training
- prescribed medications, administration, dosage, and possible adverse effects.

Discharge planning

- Refer the patient to support services or specialized in-patient care.
- Refer the patient for psychological counseling.

Burns

Overview

Description

○ Heat or chemical injury to tissue
○ May be permanently disfiguring and incapacitating
○ May be partial thickness or full thickness

Pathophysiology

First-degree burns (superficial, partial thickness)
○ Localized injury to epidermis
○ Not life-threatening

Second-degree burns (deep, partial thickness)
○ Destruction of epidermis and some dermis
○ Thin-walled and fluid-filled blisters
○ Nerve endings exposed to air as blisters break
○ Pain develops when blisters are exposed to air
○ Barrier function of the skin is lost

Third- and fourth-degree burns (full thickness)
○ Affect every body system and organ
○ Extend into the subcutaneous tissue layer
○ Damage muscle, bone, and interstitial tissues
○ Interstitial fluids result in edema
○ Immediate immunologic response occurs
○ Threat of wound sepsis
○ Painless

Causes

○ Residential fires
○ Motor vehicle accidents
○ Improper use or handling of matches
○ Improperly stored gasoline
○ Space heater or electrical malfunctions
○ Improper handling of firecrackers
○ Scalding accidents
○ Child or elder abuse
○ Contact, ingestion, inhalation, or injection of acids, alkali, or vesicants
○ Contact with faulty electrical wiring
○ Contact with high-voltage power lines
○ Chewing electric cords
○ Friction or abrasion
○ Sun exposure

Incidence

○ Affects more than 2 million people each year
○ 70,000 hospitalizations
○ 20,000 specialized burn unit admissions

Common characteristics

First-degree burns
○ Localized pain
○ Erythema
○ Blanching
○ Chills
○ Headache

○ Nausea and vomiting

Second-degree burns
○ Thin-walled, fluid-filled blisters
○ Mild to moderate pain
○ White, waxy appearance of damaged area

Third- and fourth-degree burns
○ Pale, white, brown, or black leathery tissue
○ Visible thrombosed vessels
○ No blister formation
○ Painless

Electrical burns
○ Silver colored, raised area at contact site
○ Smoke inhalation and pulmonary damage
○ Singed nasal hair

Mucosal burns
○ Sores in mouth or nose
○ Voice changes
○ Coughing, wheezing
○ Darkened sputum

Complications

○ Respiratory complications
○ Sepsis
○ Hypovolemic shock
○ Anemia
○ Malnutrition
○ Multiple organ dysfunction syndrome

Assessment

History

○ Cause of the burn revealed
○ Preexisting medical conditions

Physical findings

○ Depth and size of the burn assessed
○ Severity of the burn estimated
○ Major — more than 10% of the patient's body surface area (BSA); more than 20% of a child's BSA
○ Moderate — 3% to 10% of a patient's BSA; 10% to 20% of a child's BSA
○ Minor — less than 3% of a patient's BSA; less than 10% of a child's BSA
○ Respiratory distress and cyanosis
○ Edema
○ Alteration in pulse rate, strength, and regularity
○ Stridor, wheezing, crackles, and rhonchi
○ S_3 or S_4
○ Hypotension

Test results

Laboratory
○ Arterial blood gas levels showing evidence of smoke inhalation; may show decreased alveolar function, hypoxia
○ Complete blood count showing decreased hemoglobin level and hematocrit, if blood loss occurs
○ Abnormal electrolytes due to fluid losses and shifts
○ Increased blood urea nitrogen with fluid losses

- Decreased glucose in children because of limited glycogen storage
- Urinalysis showing myoglobinuria and hemoglobinuria
- Increased carboxyhemoglobin

Diagnostic procedures
- Electrocardiogram may show myocardial ischemia, injury, or arrhythmias, especially in electrical burns.
- Fiber-optic bronchoscopy may show edema of the airways.

Treatment

General

- Stopping the burn source
- Airway secured
- Preventing hypoxia
- Giving I.V. fluids through a large-bore I.V. line (see *Fluid replacement after a burn*)
  - Adult: maintain urine output of 30 to 50 ml/hour.
  - Child under 66 lb (30 kg): maintain urine output of 1 ml/kg/hour.
- Nasogastric tube and urinary catheter insertion
- Wound care
- Nothing by mouth until severity of burn is established, then high-protein, high-calorie diet
- Increased hydration with high-calorie, high-protein drinks, not free water
- Total parenteral nutrition if unable to take food by mouth
- Activity limitation based on extent and location of burn
- Physical therapy

Medications

- Booster of tetanus toxoid
- Analgesics
- Antibiotics
- Antianxiety agents

Surgery

- Loose tissue and blister debridement
- Escharotomy
- Skin grafting

Nursing considerations

Key outcomes

The patient will:
- report increased comfort and decreased pain
- attain the highest degree of mobility
- maintain fluid balance within the acceptable range
- maintain a patent airway
- demonstrate effective coping techniques.

Nursing interventions

- Apply immediate, aggressive burn treatment.
- Use strict sterile technique.
- Remove clothing that's still smoldering.

Fluid replacement after a burn

To replace fluid in an adult with a burn, use one of the following formulas:

First 24 hours
Evans
- 1 ml × patient's weight in kg × % total body surface area (TBSA) burn (0.9% normal saline solution)
- 1 ml × patient's weight in kg × % TBSA burn (colloid solution)

Brooke
- 1.5 ml × patient's weight in kg × % TBSA burn (lactated ringer's solution)
- 0.5 ml × patient's weight in kg × % TBSA burn (colloid solution)

Parkland
- 4 ml × patient's weight in kg × % TBSA burn (lactated ringers solution). Give one-half of volume in first 8 minutes; then infuse remainder over 16 minutes.

Second 24 hours
Evans
- 50% of first 24-hour replacement (0.9% normal saline solution)
- 2,000 ml (dextrose 5% in water [D_5W])

Brooke
- 50% to 75% of first 24-hour replacement (lactated ringer's solution)
- 2,000 ml (D_5W)

Parkland
- 30% to 60% of calculated plasma volume (25% albumin)
- Volume to maintain desired urine output (D_5W)

- Remove constricting items.
- Perform appropriate wound care.
- Provide adequate hydration.
- Weigh the patient daily.
- Encourage verbalization and provide support.

Monitoring

- Vital signs
- Respiratory status
- Signs of infection
- Intake and output
- Hydration and nutritional status

Patient teaching

Be sure to cover:
- the injury, diagnosis, and treatment
- appropriate wound care
- all medications, including administration, dosage, and possible adverse effects
- developing a dietary plan
- signs and symptoms of complications.

Discharge planning

- Refer the patient to rehabilitation, if appropriate.
- Refer the patient to psychological counseling, if needed.
- Refer the patient to resource and support services.

Campylobacteriosis

Overview

Description

- In humans and animals, intestinal infection caused by the *Campylobacter* organism, a spiral-shaped bacteria
- Signs and symptoms usually develop 2 to 5 days after exposure to *Campylobacter*
- May spread to the bloodstream in persons with compromised immune systems, causing a life-threatening infection

Pathophysiology

- Organism invades and destroys the epithelial cells of the jejunum, ileum, and colon
- Produces an increase in motility and secretions that results in diarrhea

Causes

- Ingestion of contaminated food or water or unpasteurized milk
- Occasionally from infected pets or wild animals
- Contact with an infected person's stool

Risk factors

- Occupational exposure to cattle, sheep, and other farm animals
- Laboratory worker
- Homosexual men

Incidence

- Most common bacterial cause of diarrheal illness in the United States

---

Contact precautions

In addition to standard precautions, follow these precautions:

- Place the patient in a private room. If a private room isn't available, consult with infection control personnel. As an alternative, he may be placed in a room with a patient who has an active infection with the same microorganism.
- Wear gloves whenever you enter the patient's room. Always change them after contact with infected material. Remove them before leaving the room. Wash your hands immediately with an antimicrobial soap, or rub them with a waterless antiseptic. Then avoid touching contaminated surfaces.
- Wear a gown when entering the patient's room if you think your clothing will have extensive contact with him or anything in his room or if he has diarrhea or is incontinent. Remove the gown before leaving the room.
- Limit the patient's movement from the room, and check with infection control personnel whenever he must leave it.

- More common in the summer months

Common characteristics

- Mild or severe diarrhea
- Abdominal cramps
- Malaise

Complications

- Bacteremia
- Severe dehydration and electrolyte disturbances
- Guillain-Barré syndrome
- Reiter's syndrome

Assessment

History

- Exposure to contaminated food or water
- Acute onset of diarrhea
- Recent close contact with a person who has diarrhea

Physical findings

- Cramping abdominal pain
- Nausea and vomiting
- Fever
- Traces of blood in the stool

Test results

Laboratory
- Stool culture identifying *Campylobacter*

Treatment

General

- Enteric and contact precautions (see *Contact precautions*)
- Correction of fluid and electrolyte imbalances
- Increased fluid intake
- Activity as tolerated

Medications

- Oral antibiotics

Nursing considerations

Key outcomes

The patient will:
- regain or maintain normal fluid and electrolyte balance
- have an elimination pattern that returns to normal.

Nursing interventions

- Follow contact precautions for those with active diarrhea.
- Isolate a patient who can't practice good hygiene.
- Give prescribed drugs.
- Replace lost fluids and electrolytes through diet or I.V. fluids.

Monitoring

○ Intake and output
○ Vital signs
○ Signs of dehydration
○ Electrolytes
○ Amount and characteristics of stool

Patient teaching

Be sure to cover:
○ the disorder, diagnosis, and treatment
○ proper hand-washing technique
○ proper food-handling practices
○ medications and potential adverse effects
○ complications and when to notify the physician
○ preventive measures.

Candidiasis

Overview

Description

- Mild, superficial fungal infection
- Can lead to severe disseminated infections and fungemia in immunocompromised patient, transplant recipient, burn patient, low-birth-weight neonate, or patient on hyperalimentation
- Prognosis varies, depending on patient's resistance
- Also known as candidosis and moniliasis

Pathophysiology

- Change in the patient's resistance to infection, his immunocompromised state, and antibiotic use permits the sudden proliferation of *Candida albicans.*

Causes

- In most cases, infection with *C. albicans* or *C. tropicalis*

Risk factors

- Maternal vaginitis present during vaginal delivery
- Preexisting diabetes mellitus, cancer, or immunosuppressant illness
- Immunosuppressant drug use
- Radiation
- Aging
- Irritation from dentures
- I.V. or urinary catheterization
- Drug abuse

Identifying thrush

Candidiasis of the oropharyngeal mucosa (thrush) causes cream-colored or bluish white pseudomembranous patches on the tongue, mouth, or pharynx (as shown). Fungal invasion may extend to circumoral tissues.

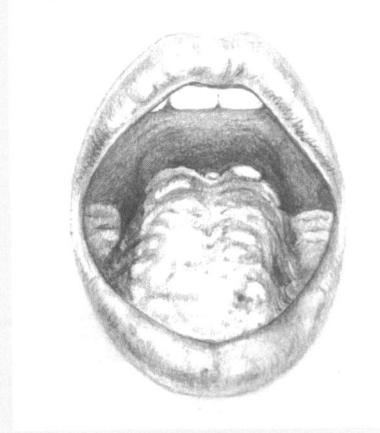

- Total parenteral nutrition
- Surgery
- Use of antibiotic agents

Incidence

- Affects 14% of immunocompromised patients
- Affects men and women equally
- Can occur at any age

Common characteristics

- Causative fungi infect the nails (paronychia), skin (diaper rash), or mucous membranes, especially the oropharynx (thrush), vagina (vaginitis), esophagus, and GI tract. (See *Identifying thrush.*)
- Systemic infection predominates among drug abusers and diabetic and immunosuppressed patients.

Complications

- Dissemination with organ failure of the kidneys, brain, GI tract, eyes, lungs, and heart

Assessment

History

- Underlying illness
- Recent course of antibiotic or antineoplastic therapy
- Drug abuse
- Hyperalimentation

Physical findings

- Scaly, erythematous, papular rash, possibly covered with exudate and erupting in breast folds, between fingers, and at the axillae, groin, and umbilicus
- Red, swollen, darkened nailbeds; occasionally, purulent discharge; possibly nail separation from the nailbed
- Scales in the mouth and throat
- White or yellow vaginal discharge, with local excoriation; white or gray raised patches on vaginal walls, with local inflammation
- Cream-colored or bluish white lacelike patches of exudate on the tongue, mouth, or pharynx that reveal bloody engorgement when scraped
- Hemoptysis, cough; coarse breath sounds in the infected lung fields
- Flank pain, dysuria, hematuria, cloudy urine with casts
- Headache, nuchal rigidity, seizures, focal neurologic deficits
- Blurred vision, orbital or periorbital pain, eye exudate, floating scotomata, and lesions with a white, cotton-ball appearance seen during ophthalmoscopy
- Chest pain and arrhythmias
- Septic shock

Test results

Laboratory

- Fungal serological panel showing the presence of the candidal organism

Treatment

General

○ Treat predisposing condition
○ No dietary restrictions unless oral infection
○ With oral infection, spicy food only as tolerated
○ Activity as tolerated

Medications

○ Antifungals
○ Amphotericin B
○ Topical anesthetics

Surgery

○ Abscess drainage; surgically or percutaneously

Nursing considerations

Key outcomes

The patient will:
○ express increased comfort
○ avoid or have minimal complications
○ maintain skin integrity
○ express understanding of disorder and treatment.

Nursing interventions

○ Follow standard precautions.
○ Give prescribed drugs.
○ Provide a nonirritating mouthwash to loosen tenacious secretions and a soft toothbrush to avoid irritation.
○ Observe high-risk patients daily for patchy areas, irritation, sore throat, oral and gingival bleeding, and other signs of superinfection.
○ Assess the patient for underlying systemic causes.

Monitoring

○ Vital signs
○ Intake and output
○ Blood urea nitrogen, serum creatinine, and urine blood and protein levels
○ Potassium levels

Patient teaching

Be sure to cover:
○ the disorder, diagnosis, and treatment
○ good oral hygiene practices
○ (for a woman in her third trimester of pregnancy) the need for examination for vaginitis to protect her neonate from thrush infection at birth.

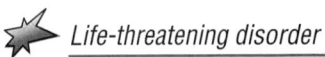 *Life-threatening disorder*

Cardiac tamponade

Overview

Description
○ Rapid increase in intrapericardial pressure caused by fluid accumulation in the pericardial sac
○ Impaired diastolic filling of the heart

Pathophysiology
○ Progressive accumulation of fluid in the pericardial sac causes compression of the heart chambers.
○ Compression of the heart chambers obstructs blood flow into the ventricles and reduces the amount of blood pumped out with each contraction.
○ With each contraction more fluid accumulates, decreasing cardiac output. (See *Understanding cardiac tamponade.*)

Causes
○ May be idiopathic
○ Effusion in cancer, bacterial infections, tuberculosis and, rarely, acute rheumatic fever
○ Trauma
○ Hemorrhage from nontraumatic cause
○ Viral, postirradiation, or idiopathic pericarditis
○ Acute myocardial infarction
○ Chronic renal failure
○ Drug reaction
○ Connective tissue disorders
○ Cardiac catheterization
○ Cardiac surgery

Incidence
○ More common in males than in females
○ Occurs with 2% of penetrating chest traumas

Common characteristics
○ Systemic hypotension
○ Muffled heart sounds
○ Jugular vein distention

Complications
○ Cardiogenic shock
○ Death

Assessment

History
○ Presence of one or more causes
○ Dyspnea
○ Shortness of breath
○ Chest pain

Physical findings
○ Vary with volume of fluid and speed of fluid accumulation
○ Diaphoresis
○ Anxiety and restlessness
○ Pallor or cyanosis
○ Neck vein distention
○ Edema
○ Rapid, weak pulses
○ Hepatomegaly
○ Decreased arterial blood pressure
○ Increased central venous pressure
○ Pulsus paradoxus
○ Narrow pulse pressure
○ Muffled heart sounds

Test results
Imaging
○ Chest X-rays show slightly widened mediastinum and enlargement of the cardiac silhouette.
Diagnostic procedures
○ Electrocardiography may show low voltage complexes in the precordial leads.
○ Hemodynamic monitoring shows equalization of mean right atrial, right ventricular diastolic, pulmonary artery wedge, and left ventricular diastolic pressures.
○ Echocardiography may show an echo-free space, indicating fluid accumulation in the pericardial sac.

Treatment

General
○ Pericardiocentesis, if necessary
○ Diet, as tolerated
○ Bed rest

Medications
○ Intravascular volume expansion
○ Inotropic agents
○ Oxygen

Surgery
○ Pericardiocentesis
○ Pericardial window
○ Subxiphoid pericardiotomy
○ Complete pericardectomy
○ Thoracotomy

Nursing considerations

Key outcomes
The patient will:
○ maintain hemodynamic stability
○ maintain adequate cardiac output
○ not develop arrhythmias
○ express understanding of disorder and treatment.

The pericardial sac, which surrounds and protects the heart, is composed of several layers. The fibrous pericardium is the tough outermost membrane; the inner membrane, called the *serous membrane,* consists of the visceral and parietal layers. The visceral layer clings to the heart and is also known as the *epicardial layer* of the heart. The parietal layer lies between the visceral layer and the fibrous pericardium. The pericardial space — between the visceral and parietal layers — contains 10 to 30 ml of pericardial fluid. This fluid lubricates the layers and minimizes friction when the heart contracts.

In cardiac tamponade, blood or fluid fills the pericardial space, compressing the heart chambers, increasing intracardiac pressure, and obstructing venous return. As blood flow into the ventricles falls, so does cardiac output. Without prompt treatment, low cardiac output can be fatal.

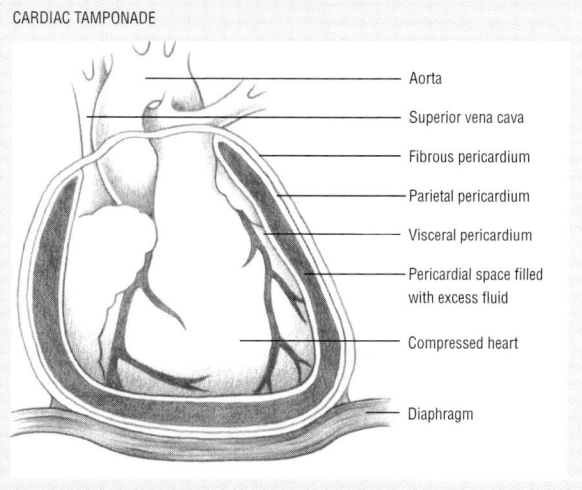

NORMAL HEART AND AND PERICARDIUM

- Aorta
- Superior vena cava
- Parietal pericardium
- Visceral pericardium
- Fibrous pericardium
- Pericardial space
- Attachment of fibrous pericardium to diaphragm
- Diaphragm

CARDIAC TAMPONADE

- Aorta
- Superior vena cava
- Fibrous pericardium
- Parietal pericardium
- Visceral pericardium
- Pericardial space filled with excess fluid
- Compressed heart
- Diaphragm

Nursing interventions

○ Give prescribed drugs.
○ Provide reassurance.
○ Assist with pericardiocentesis, if necessary.
○ Infuse I.V. solutions, as ordered.
○ Administer oxygen therapy, as needed.
○ Maintain the chest drainage system, if used.

Monitoring

○ Vital signs
○ Intake and output
○ Signs and symptoms of increasing tamponade
○ Cardiac rhythm
○ Hemodynamics
○ Arterial blood gas levels
○ Heart and breath sounds
○ Complications

Patient teaching

Be sure to cover:
○ the disorder, diagnosis, and treatment
○ medications and potential adverse reactions
○ when to notify the physician
○ preoperative and postoperative care
○ emergency procedures.

Cardiomyopathy, dilated

Overview

Description
- Disease of the heart muscle fibers
- Also called *congestive cardiomyopathy*

Pathophysiology
- Extensively damaged myocardial muscle fibers reduce contractility of left ventricle.
- As systolic function declines, cardiac output falls.
- The sympathetic nervous system is stimulated to increase heart rate and contractility.
- When compensatory mechanisms can no longer maintain cardiac output, the heart begins to fail. (See *Understanding dilated cardiomyopathy.*)

Causes
- Viral or bacterial infections
- Hypertension
- Peripartum syndrome related to toxemia
- Ischemic heart disease
- Valvular disease
- Drug hypersensitivity
- Chemotherapy
- Cardiotoxic effects of drugs or alcohol

Incidence
- Most commonly affects middle-aged men but can occur in any age group

Common characteristics
- Dyspnea on exertion
- Dry cough at night

Understanding dilated cardiomyopathy

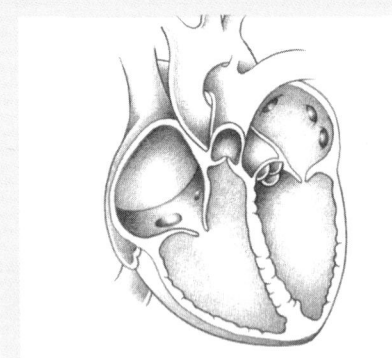

- Greatly increased chamber size
- Thinning of left ventricular muscle
- Increased atrial chamber size
- Increased myocardial mass
- Normal ventricular inflow resistance
- Decreased contractility

Complications
- Intractable heart failure
- Arrhythmias
- Emboli

Assessment

History
- Possible history of a disorder that can cause cardiomyopathy
- Gradual onset of shortness of breath, orthopnea, dyspnea on exertion, paroxysmal nocturnal dyspnea, fatigue, dry cough at night, palpitations, and vague chest pain

Physical findings
- Peripheral edema
- Jugular vein distention
- Ascites
- Peripheral cyanosis
- Tachycardia even at rest and pulsus alternans in late stages
- Hepatomegaly and splenomegaly
- Narrow pulse pressure
- Irregular rhythms, diffuse apical impulses, pansystolic murmur
- S_3 and S_4 gallop rhythms
- Pulmonary crackles

 Alert

Dilated cardiomyopathy may need to be differentiated from other types of cardiomyopathy. (See Assessment findings in cardiomyopathies.)

Test results

Imaging
- Angiography results rule out ischemic heart disease.
- Chest X-rays demonstrate moderate to marked cardiomegaly and possible pulmonary edema.
- Echocardiography may reveal ventricular thrombi, global hypokinesis, and the degrees of left ventricular dilation and systolic dysfunction.
- Gallium scans may identify patients with dilated cardiomyopathy and myocarditis.

Diagnostic procedures
- Cardiac catheterization can show left ventricular dilation and dysfunction, elevated left ventricular and, often, right ventricular filling pressures, and diminished cardiac output.
- Transvenous endomyocardial biopsy may be useful in determining the underlying disorder in some patients.
- Electrocardiography evaluates ischemic heart disease and identifies arrhythmias and intraventricular conduction defects.

Assessment findings in cardiomyopathies

Type	Assessment findings
Dilated cardiomyopathy	• Generalized weakness, fatigue • Chest pain, palpitations • Syncope • Tachycardia • Narrow pulse pressure • Pulmonary congestion, pleural effusions • Jugular vein distention, peripheral edema • Paroxysmal nocturnal dyspnea, orthopnea, dyspnea on exertion
Hypertrophic cardiomyopathy	• Angina, palpitations • Syncope • Orthopnea, dyspnea with exertion • Pulmonary congestion • Loud systolic murmur • Life-threatening arrhythmias • Sudden cardiac arrest
Restrictive cardiomyopathy	• Generalized weakness, fatigue • Bradycardia • Dyspnea • Jugular vein distention, peripheral edema • Liver congestion, abdominal ascites

Treatment

General

○ No ingestion of alcohol if cardiomyopathy caused by alcoholism
○ Low-sodium diet supplemented by vitamin therapy
○ Rest periods

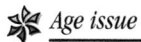 *Age issue*

A woman of childbearing age with dilated cardiomyopathy should avoid pregnancy.

Medications

○ Cardiac glycosides
○ Diuretics
○ Angiotensin-converting enzyme inhibitors
○ Oxygen
○ Anticoagulants
○ Vasodilators
○ Antiarrhythmics
○ Beta-adrenergic blockers

Surgery

○ Heart transplantation
○ Possible cardiomyoplasty

Nursing considerations

Key outcomes

The patient will:
○ maintain adequate cardiac output and hemodynamic stability
○ maintain adequate ventilation
○ develop no complications of excess fluid volume
○ recognize and accept limitations of chronic illness
○ express feelings of increased energy and decreased fatigue.

Nursing interventions

○ Alternate periods of rest with required activities of daily living.
○ Provide active or passive range-of-motion exercises.
○ Consult with the dietitian to provide a low-sodium diet.
○ Administer oxygen, as needed.
○ Check serum potassium levels for hypokalemia, especially if therapy includes cardiac glycosides.
○ Offer support and let the patient express his feelings.
○ Allow the patient and his family to express their fears and concerns and help them identify effective coping strategies.

Monitoring

○ Vital signs
○ Hemodynamics
○ Intake and output
○ Daily weights
○ Signs and symptoms of progressive heart failure

Patient teaching

Be sure to cover:
○ the disorder, diagnosis, and treatment
○ medications and potential adverse reactions
○ when to notify the physician
○ sodium and fluid restrictions
○ signs and symptoms of worsening heart failure.

Discharge planning

○ Refer family members to community cardiopulmonary resuscitation classes.

Cardiomyopathy, hypertrophic

Overview

Description

- ○ Primary disease of cardiac muscle characterized by left ventricular hypertrophy
- ○ Also known as *idiopathic hypertrophic subaortic stenosis, hypertrophic obstructive cardiomyopathy,* and *muscular aortic stenosis*

Pathophysiology

- ○ The hypertrophied ventricle becomes stiff, noncompliant, and unable to relax during ventricular filling.
- ○ Ventricular filling time is reduced as compensation to tachycardia.
- ○ Reduced ventricular filling leads to low cardiac output. (See *Understanding hypertrophic cardiomyopathy.*)

Causes

- ○ Transmission by autosomal dominant trait (about one-half of all cases)
- ○ Associated with hypertension

Incidence

- ○ More common in men than women
- ○ Affects 5 to 8 people per 100,000 in the United States
- ○ More common in blacks

Understanding hypertrophic cardiomyopathy

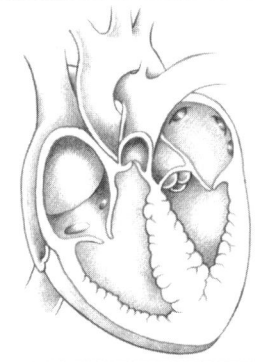

- ○ Normal right and decreased left chamber size
- ○ Left ventricular hypertrophy
- ○ Thickened interventricular septum (hypertrophic obstructive cardiomyopathy)
- ○ Atrial chamber size increased on left
- ○ Increased myocardial mass
- ○ Increased ventricular inflow resistance
- ○ Increased or decreased contractility

Common characteristics

- ○ Dyspnea
- ○ Fatigue
- ○ Signs of heart failure

Complications

- ○ Pulmonary hypertension
- ○ Heart failure
- ○ Ventricular arrhythmias

Assessment

History

- ○ Generally, no visible clinical features until disease is well advanced
- ○ Blood flow to left ventricle abruptly reduced by atrial dilation and, sometimes, atrial fibrillation
- ○ Possible family history of hypertrophic cardiomyopathy
- ○ Orthopnea
- ○ Dyspnea on exertion
- ○ Anginal pain
- ○ Fatigue
- ○ Syncope, even at rest

Physical findings

- ○ Rapidly rising carotid arterial pulse possible
- ○ Pulsus biferiens
- ○ Double or triple apical impulse, possibly displaced laterally
- ○ Bibasilar crackles if heart failure is present
- ○ Harsh systolic murmur heard after S_1 at the apex near the left sternal border
- ○ Possible S_4

 Alert

Hypertrophic cardiomyopathy may need to be differentiated from other types of cardiomyopathy. (See Assessment findings in cardiomyopathies, *page 149.)*

Test results

Imaging

- ○ Chest X-rays may show a mild to moderate increase in heart size.
- ○ Thallium scan usually reveals myocardial perfusion defects.
- ○ Angiography reveals a dilated, diffusely hypokinetic left ventricle.

Diagnostic procedures

- ○ Echocardiography shows left ventricular hypertrophy and a thick, asymmetrical intraventricular septum in obstructive hypertrophic cardiomyopathy, whereas hypertrophy affects various ventricular areas in nonobstructive hypertrophic cardiomyopathy.

○ Cardiac catheterization reveals elevated left ventricular end-diastolic pressure and, possibly, mitral insufficiency.
○ Electrocardiography usually shows left ventricular hypertrophy, ST-segment and T-wave abnormalities, Q waves in leads II, III, aV_F, and in V_4 to V_6 (because of hypertrophy, not infarction), left anterior hemiblock, left axis deviation, and ventricular and atrial arrhythmias.

Treatment

General

○ Cardioversion for atrial fibrillation
○ Low-fat, low-salt diet
○ Fluid restrictions
○ Avoidance of alcohol
○ Activity limitations individualized
○ Bed rest, if necessary

Medications

○ Beta-adrenergic blockers
○ Calcium channel blockers
○ Amiodarone, unless atrioventricular block exists
○ Antibiotic prophylaxis

 Alert

Angiotensin-converting enzyme inhibitors, nitrates, other beta-adrenergic blockers, and digoxin are contraindicated in hypertrophic cardiomyopathy.

Surgery

○ Ventricular myotomy alone or combined with mitral valve replacement
○ Heart transplantation

Nursing considerations

Key outcomes

The patient will:
○ maintain adequate cardiac output and hemodynamic stability
○ develop no complications of excess fluid volume
○ carry out activities of daily living (ADLs) without excess fatigue or decreased energy
○ express feelings of comfort and decreased pain
○ develop adequate coping mechanisms.

Nursing interventions

○ Alternate periods of rest with required ADLs and treatments.
○ Provide personal care, as needed, to prevent fatigue.
○ Provide active or passive range-of-motion exercises.

 Alert

If propranolol is to be discontinued, don't stop the drug abruptly; doing so may cause rebound effects, resulting in myocardial infarction or sudden death.

○ Offer support and let the patient express his feelings.
○ Allow the patient and his family to express their fears and concerns and identify effective coping strategies.

Monitoring

○ Vital signs
○ Hemodynamics
○ Intake and output

Patient teaching

Be sure to cover:
○ that propranolol can cause depression and the need to notify the physician if symptoms occur
○ instructions to take medication as ordered
○ the need to notify any physician caring for the patient that he shouldn't be given nitroglycerin, digoxin, or diuretics because they can worsen obstruction
○ the need for antibiotic prophylaxis before dental work or surgery to prevent infective endocarditis
○ warnings against strenuous activity, which may precipitate syncope or sudden death
○ the need to avoid Valsalva's maneuver or sudden position changes.

Discharge planning

○ Refer family members to community cardiopulmonary resuscitation classes.

Cardiomyopathy, restrictive

Overview

Description

- Disease of the heart muscle fibers that results in restrictive filling and reduced diastolic volume of either one or both ventricles
- Irreversible if severe

Pathophysiology

- Stiffness of the ventricle is caused by left ventricular hypertrophy and endocardial fibrosis and thickening, thus reducing the ventricle's ability to relax and fill during diastole.
- Failure of the rigid myocardium to contract completely during systole causes decreased cardiac output. (See *Understanding restrictive cardiomyopathy.*)

Causes

- Idiopathic or associated with other disease (for example, amyloidosis or endomyocardial fibrosis)
- Heart transplant
- Mediastinal radiation
- Carcinoid heart disease

Incidence

- Rare; accounts for 5% of all cases of primary heart disease
- Occurs equally in men and women

Understanding restrictive cardiomyopathy

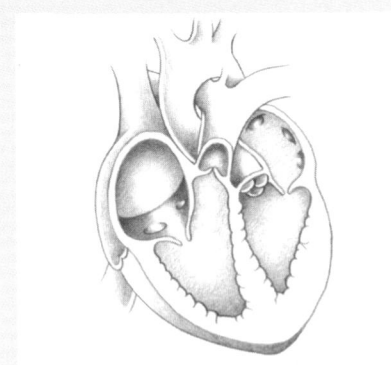

- Decreased ventricular chamber size
- Left ventricular hypertrophy
- Increased atrial chamber size
- Normal myocardial mass
- Increased ventricular inflow resistance
- Decreased contractility

Common characteristics

- Fatigue
- Dyspnea
- Orthopnea
- Chest pain
- Edema
- Systolic murmurs

Complications

- Heart failure
- Arrhythmias
- Systemic or pulmonary embolization
- Sudden death

Assessment

History

- Fatigue
- Viral infection
- Dyspnea
- Chest pain

Physical findings

- Peripheral edema
- Liver engorgement
- Peripheral cyanosis
- Pallor
- S_3 or S_4 gallop rhythms (due to heart failure)
- Systolic murmurs

 Alert

Restricted cardiomyopathy may need to be differentiated from other types of cardiomyopathy. (See Assessment findings in cardiomyopathies, *page 149.)*

Test results

Laboratory
- Complete blood count reveals eosinophilia.

Imaging
- Chest X-ray may reveal cardiomegaly.
- Echocardiography may reveal left ventricular muscle mass, normal or reduced left ventricular cavity size, and decreased systolic function.

Diagnostic procedures
- Electrocardiography may reveal low-voltage hypertrophy, arterioventricular conduction defects, and arrhythmias.
- Cardiac catheterization shows reduced systolic function and myocardial infiltration and increased left ventricular end-diastolic pressures.

Treatment

General

- Treatment of underlying cause
- Low-sodium diet
- Initially, bed rest, then activity, as tolerated

Medications

○ Digoxin
○ Diuretics
○ Vasodilators
○ Angiotensin-converting enzyme inhibitors
○ Anticoagulants
○ Corticosteroids

Surgery

○ Permanent pacemaker
○ Heart transplantation

Nursing considerations

Key outcomes

The patient will:
○ maintain adequate cardiac output and hemodynamic stability
○ express understanding of the disorder
○ recognize and accept limitations of chronic illness
○ seek support and establish coping mechanisms.

Nursing interventions

○ Give prescribed drugs.
○ Provide psychological support.
○ Provide appropriate diversionary activities for the patient restricted to prolonged bed rest.

Monitoring

○ Heart rhythm and rate
○ Vital signs
○ Intake and output
○ Pulmonary artery pressure
○ Daily weight

Patient teaching

Be sure to cover:
○ signs of digoxin toxicity
○ importance of recording daily weight and reporting weight gain of 2 lb (0.9 kg) or more
○ dietary restrictions.

Discharge planning

○ Refer for psychosocial counseling, as necessary, for assistance in coping with restricted lifestyle.

Carpal tunnel syndrome

Overview

Description

○ Compression of the median nerve in the wrist
○ Most common nerve entrapment syndrome
○ May pose a serious occupational health problem

The carpal tunnel

The carpal tunnel is clearly visible in this palmar view and cross section of a right hand. Note the median nerve, flexor tendons of fingers, and blood vessels passing through the tunnel on their way from the forearm to the hand.

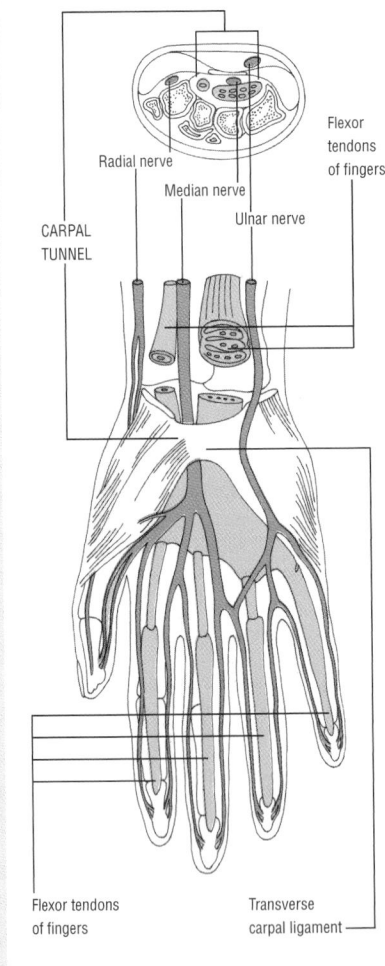

Radial nerve

Median nerve

CARPAL
TUNNEL

Ulnar nerve

Flexor
tendons
of fingers

Flexor tendons
of fingers

Transverse
carpal ligament

Pathophysiology

○ Space-occupying lesion or direct pressure within the carpal canal increases pressure on the median nerve, resulting in compression.
○ Compression of the median nerve interrupts normal function. (See *The carpal tunnel.*)

Causes

○ Exact cause unknown
○ Repetitive wrist motions involving excessive flexion or extension
○ Dislocation
○ Acute sprain that may damage the median nerve
○ Tumors
○ Gout
○ Amyloidosis
○ Edema-producing conditions

Risk factors

○ Diabetes
○ Pregnancy
○ Alcoholism
○ Hypothyroidism
○ Renal failure

Incidence

○ Most common in women between ages 30 and 60
○ Occurs in people who move their wrists continuously

Common characteristics

○ Weakness, pain, burning, numbness, tingling in the hand
○ Thumb, forefinger, middle finger, and half of fourth finger affected by paresthesia
○ Inability to clench fist
○ Atrophic nails
○ Dry and shiny skin

Complications

○ Tendon inflammation
○ Compression
○ Neural ischemia
○ Permanent nerve damage with loss of movement and sensation

Assessment

History

○ Occupation or hobby requiring strenuous or repetitive use of the hands
○ Condition that causes swelling in carpal tunnel structures
○ Weakness, pain, burning, numbness, or tingling that occurs in one or both hands
○ Paresthesia that worsens at night and in the morning
○ Pain that spreads to the forearm and, in severe cases, as far as the shoulder
○ Pain can be relieved by:
  – shaking hands vigorously
  – dangling the arms at sides

Physical findings

○ Inability to make a fist
○ Fingernails may be atrophied, with surrounding dry, shiny skin

Test results

Imaging

○ Electromyography shows a median nerve motor conduction delay of more than 5 milliseconds.
○ Digital electrical stimulation shows median nerve compression by measuring the length and intensity of stimulation from the fingers to the median nerve in the wrist.

Other

○ Compression test result supports the diagnosis.

Treatment

General

○ Conservative initially:
  − Splinting the wrist for 1 to 2 weeks
  − Possible occupational changes
  − Correction of any underlying disorder
○ Activity, as tolerated

Medications

○ Nonsteroidal anti-inflammatory drugs (NSAIDs)
○ Corticosteroids
○ Vitamin B complex

Surgery

○ Decompression of the nerve
○ Neurolysis

Nursing considerations

Key outcomes

The patient will:
○ express feelings of increased comfort and pain relief
○ maintain muscle strength
○ maintain joint mobility and range of motion
○ perform activities of daily living.

Nursing interventions

○ Promote self-care.
○ Give prescribed analgesics.

Monitoring

○ Response to analgesia
○ After surgery, vital signs
○ Color, sensation, and motion of the affected hand

Patient teaching

Be sure to cover:
○ splint application
○ hand exercises in warm water
○ the prescribed medication regimen

○ adverse reactions to drugs
○ avoidance of NSAIDs in pregnancy.

Discharge planning

○ Refer the patient for occupational counseling if a job change is necessary.

Cataract

Overview

Description

- Opacity of the lens or lens capsule of the eye
- Common cause of gradual vision loss
- Commonly affects both eyes
- Traumatic cataracts usually unilateral

Pathophysiology

- The clouded lens blocks light shining through the cornea.
- Images cast onto the retina are blurred.
- A hazy image is interpreted by the brain.

Causes

- Classified according to cause

Senile cataracts
- Chemical changes in lens proteins in elderly patients

Congenital cataracts
- Inborn errors of metabolism
- Maternal rubella infection during the first trimester
- Congenital anomaly
- Genetic causes (usually autosomal dominant)
- Recessive cataracts may be sex-linked

Traumatic cataracts
- Foreign bodies causing aqueous or vitreous humor to enter lens capsule

Complicated cataracts
- Uveitis
- Glaucoma
- Retinitis pigmentosa
- Retinal detachment
- Diabetes
- Hypoparathyroidism
- Atopic dermatitis
- Ionizing radiation or infrared rays

Toxic cataracts
- Drug or chemical toxicity:
  - ergot
  - dinitrophenol
  - naphthalene
  - phenothiazines

Incidence

- Most prevalent in people older than age 70

Common characteristics

- Painless, gradual vision loss
- Glare
- Milky white pupil

Complications

- Complete vision loss

Possible complications of surgery
- Loss of vitreous
- Wound dehiscence
- Hyphema
- Pupillary block glaucoma
- Retinal detachment
- Infection

Assessment

History

- Painless, gradual vision loss
- Blinding glare from headlights with night driving
- Poor reading vision
- Annoying glare
- Poor vision in bright sunlight
- Better vision in dim light than in bright light (central opacity)

Physical findings

- Milky white pupil on inspection with a penlight
- Grayish white area behind the pupil (advanced cataract)
- Red reflex lost (mature cataract)

Test results

Diagnostic procedures
- Indirect ophthalmoscopy reveals a dark area in the normally homogeneous red reflex.
- Slit-lamp examination confirms lens opacity.
- Visual acuity test result establishes the degree of vision loss.

Treatment

General

- Before surgery, eyeglasses and contact lenses that may help to improve vision
- Sunglasses in bright light and lamps that provide reflected lighting rather than direct lighting, decreasing glare and aiding vision
- Restricted activity according to vision loss

Medications

For cataract removal
- Nonsteroidal anti-inflammatory drugs
- Short-acting local anesthetic

Surgery

- Lens extraction and implantation of intraocular lens (see *Comparing methods of cataract removal*)
- Extracapsular cataract extraction
- Intracapsular cataract extraction
- Phacoemulsification

Nursing considerations

Key outcomes

The patient will:
- maintain current health status

Comparing methods of cataract removal

Cataracts can be removed by intracapsular or extracapsular techniques.

Intracapsular cataract extraction
In this technique, the surgeon makes a partial incision at the superior limbus arc. He then removes the lens using specially designed forceps or a cryoprobe, which freezes and adheres to the lens to facilitate its removal.

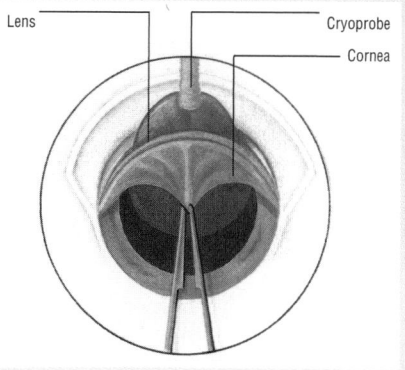

Lens — Cryoprobe — Cornea

Extracapsular cataract extraction
In this technique, the surgeon may use irrigation and aspiration or phacoemulsification. In the former approach, the surgeon makes an incision at the limbus, opens the anterior lens capsule with a cystotome, and exerts pressure from below to express the lens. He then irrigates and suctions the remaining lens cortex.

In phacoemulsification, he uses an ultrasonic probe to break the lens into minute particles, which are aspirated by the probe.

IRRIGATION AND ASPIRATION

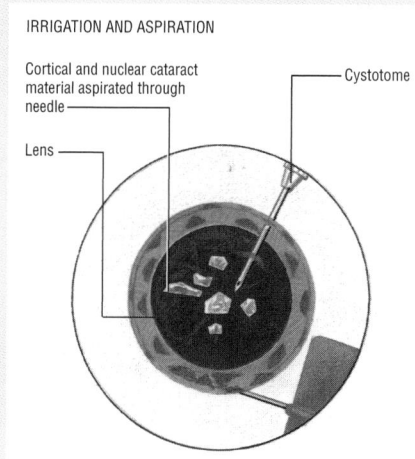

Cortical and nuclear cataract material aspirated through needle — Cystotome
Lens —

PHACOEMULSIFICATION

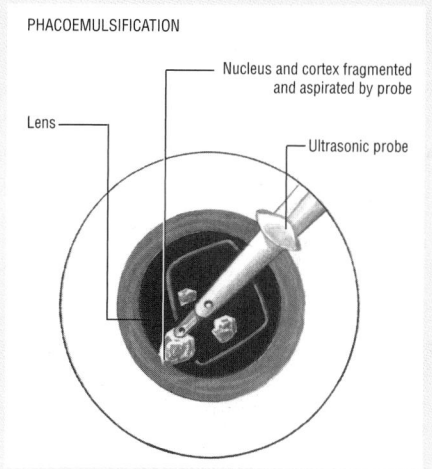

Nucleus and cortex fragmented and aspirated by probe
Lens — Ultrasonic probe

○ sustain no harm or injury
○ voice feelings and concerns
○ regain visual function.

Nursing interventions

○ Perform routine postoperative care.
○ Assist with early ambulation.
○ Apply an eye shield or eye patch postoperatively, as ordered.

Monitoring

○ Vital signs
○ Visual acuity
○ Complications of surgery

Patient teaching

Be sure to cover:
○ the need to avoid activities that increase intraocular pressure, such as straining with coughing, bowel movements, or lifting
○ the need to abstain from sexual intercourse until the patient receives physician's approval
○ proper instillation of ophthalmic ointment or drops.

Alert

If the patient has increased eye discharge, sharp eye pain that's unrelieved by analgesics, or deterioration in vision, instruct him to notify his physician immediately.

Cellulitis

Overview

Description

- Acute infection of the dermis and subcutaneous tissue causing inflammation of the cells
- May follow damage to the skin, such as a bite or wound
- Prognosis usually good with timely treatment
- With other comorbidities, such as diabetes, increased risk of developing or spreading cellulitis

Pathophysiology

- A break in skin integrity almost always precedes infection.
- As the offending organism invades the compromised area, it overwhelms the defensive cells, including the neutrophils, eosinophils, basophils, and mast cells, that normally contain and localize the inflammation.
- As cellulitis progresses, the organism invades tissue around the initial wound site.

Causes

- Bacterial infections, usually by *Staphylococcus aureus* and *group A beta-hemolytic streptococci*
- Fungal infections
- Extension of a skin wound or ulcer
- Furuncles or carbuncles

Risk factors

- Venous and lymphatic compromise
- Edema
- Diabetes mellitus
- Underlying skin lesion
- Prior trauma

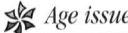 *Age issue*

Cellulitis of the lower extremity is more likely to develop into thrombophlebitis in an elderly patient.

Incidence

- Occurs most commonly in the lower extremities
- Affects males and females equally

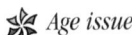 *Age issue*

Perianal cellulitis occurs more commonly in children, especially boys.

Common characteristics

- Tenderness
- Pain
- Erythema
- Warmth
- Edema

Complications

- Sepsis
- Deep vein thrombosis (DVT)
- Progression of cellulitis
- Local abscesses
- Thrombophlebitis
- Lymphangitis
- Amputation

Assessment

History

- Presence of one or more risk factors
- Tenderness
- Pain at the site and possibly surrounding area
- Erythema and warmth
- Edema
- Possible fever, chills, malaise

Physical findings

- Erythema with indistinct margins
- Fever
- Warmth and tenderness of the skin
- Regional lymph node enlargement and tenderness
- Red streaking visible in skin proximal to area of cellulitis

Test results

Laboratory
- White blood cell count showing mild leukocytosis
- Erythrocyte sedimentation rate showing mild elevation
- Culture and Gram stain possibly showing the causative organism

Treatment

General

- Immobilization and elevation of the affected extremity
- Moist heat
- Well-balanced diet
- Bed rest possibly necessary in severe infection

Medications

- Antibiotics
- Topical antifungals
- Analgesics

Surgery

- Tracheostomy possibly needed for severe cellulitis of head and neck
- Possible abscess drainage
- Amputation (with gas-forming cellulitis [gangrene])

Nursing considerations

Key outcomes

The patient will:
- avoid injury
- express feelings of increased comfort
- remain free from signs and symptoms of infection
- verbalize feelings and concerns.

Nursing interventions

- Give prescribed drugs.
- Elevate affected extremity.
- Apply moist heat, as ordered.
- Encourage a well-balanced diet.
- Encourage adequate fluid intake.
- Encourage verbalization of feelings and concerns.
- Institute safety precautions.

Monitoring

- Vital signs
- Pain control
- Edema
- Laboratory results
- Signs and symptoms of infection
- Complications
- Cellulitis progression

Patient teaching

Be sure to cover:
- the disorder, diagnosis, and treatment
- medications and possible adverse reactions
- when to notify the physician
- use of warm compresses
- signs and symptoms of infection
- prevention of injury and trauma
- infection control
- signs and symptoms of DVT.

Discharge planning

- Refer the patient for management of diabetes mellitus, as indicated.

Cerebral contusion

Overview

Description
○ Ecchymosis of brain tissue that results from injury to the head

Pathophysiology
○ Trauma to the head causes tearing or twisting of the structures and blood vessels of the brain.
○ Scattered hemorrhages form over the surface.
○ Functional disruption occurs and may be prolonged.

Causes
○ Acceleration-deceleration or coup-contrecoup injuries
○ Head trauma

Risk factors
○ Unsteady gait
○ Participation in contact sports
○ Receiving anticoagulant therapy

Incidence
○ Occurs at any age

Common characteristics
○ Change in level of consciousness
○ Hypotension
○ Dizziness
○ Headache
○ Nausea and vomiting
○ Pupil changes
○ Hemiparesis
○ Memory loss or forgetfulness
○ Seizure

Complications
○ Intracranial hemorrhage
○ Hematoma
○ Tentorial herniation
○ Increased intracranial pressure (see *What happens with increased ICP*)

Assessment

History
○ Head injury or motor vehicle accident
○ Loss of consciousness

Physical findings
○ Unconscious patient: pale and motionless; altered vital signs
○ Conscious patient: drowsy or easily disturbed
○ Scalp wound
○ Possible involuntary evacuation of bowel and bladder
○ Hemiparesis

Test results
Imaging
○ Computed tomography scan shows areas of damage.

Treatment

General
○ Establishment of a patent airway
○ Administration of I.V. fluids
○ Minimization of environmental stimuli
○ Nothing by mouth until fully conscious
○ Activity based on neurologic status
○ Initially, bed rest
○ Avoidance of contact sports

Medications
○ Nonopioid analgesics

Surgery
○ Craniotomy

Nursing considerations

Key outcomes
The patient will:
○ use support systems to assist with coping
○ maintain a stable neurologic state
○ express feelings of comfort and pain relief
○ maintain adequate fluid volume.

Nursing interventions
○ Perform neurologic examinations.
○ Maintain a patent airway.
○ Give prescribed drugs (no aspirin).
○ Protect from injury.

Monitoring
○ Vital signs
○ Neurologic status
○ Check for cerebrospinal fluid (CSF) leakage

Patient teaching

Be sure to cover:
○ the need to avoid coughing, sneezing, or blowing the nose until after recovery
○ observation for CSF drainage
○ how to detect and report mental status changes
○ signs and symptoms of infection.

Discharge planning
○ Refer the patient to a neurologist for follow-up, as indicated.

What happens with increased ICP

Intracranial pressure (ICP) is the pressure exerted within the intact skull by the intracranial volume — about 10% blood, 10% cerebrospinal fluid (CSF), and 80% brain tissue water. The rigid skull allows very little space for expansion of these substances. When ICP increases to pathologic levels, brain damage can result.

The brain compensates for increases in ICP by regulating the volumes of the three substances in the following ways:
- limiting blood flow to the head
- displacing CSF into the spinal canal
- increasing absorption or decreasing production of CSF — withdrawing water from brain tissue into the blood and excreting it through the kidneys.

When compensatory mechanisms become overworked, small changes in volume lead to large changes in pressure.

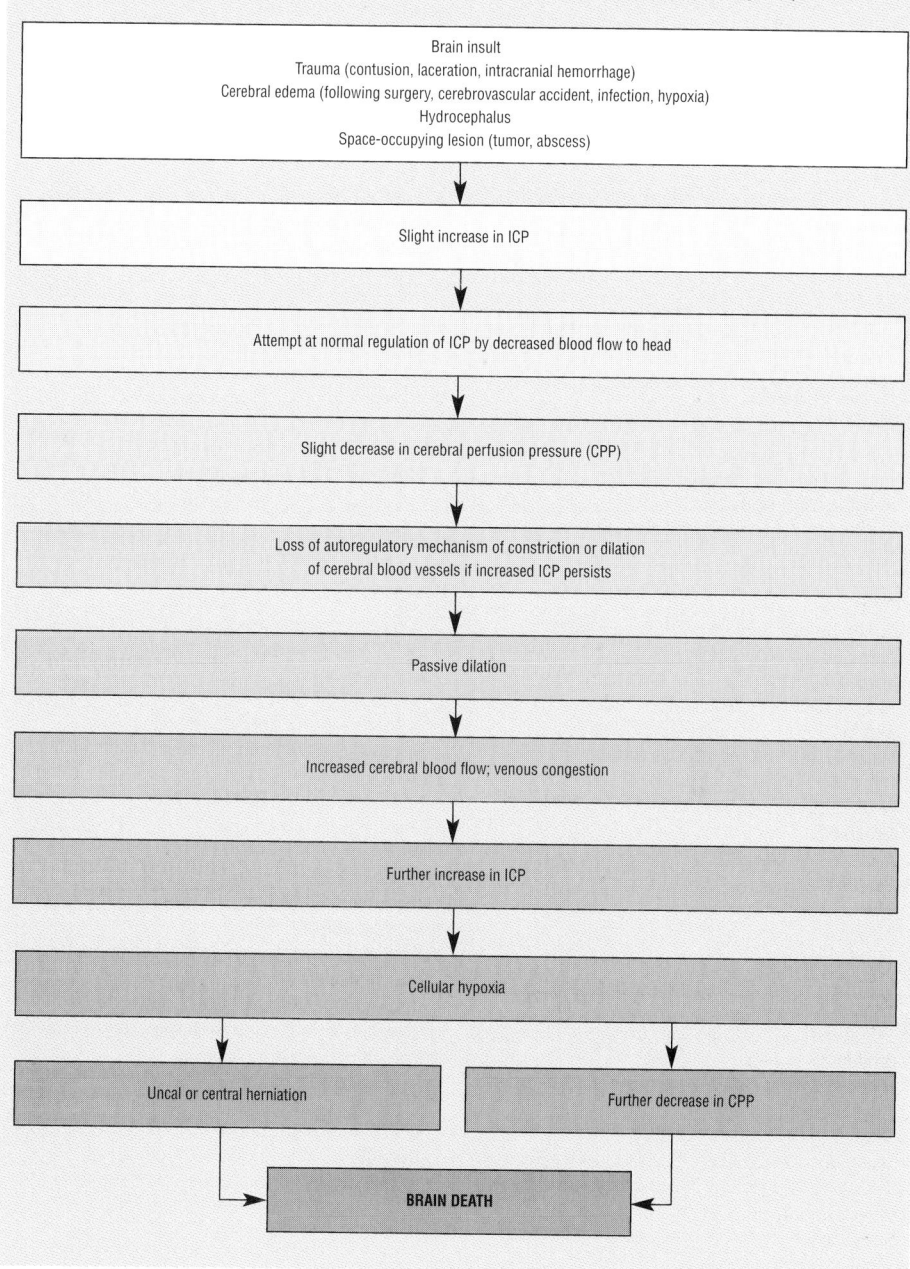

Cerebral palsy

Overview

Description

- Most common crippling neuromuscular disease in children
- Comprises several neuromuscular disorders
- Results from prenatal, perinatal, or postnatal central nervous system (CNS) damage
- Three types (sometimes occur in mixed forms):
  - spastic (affecting about 70% of children with cerebral palsy)
  - athetoid (affecting about 20%)
  - ataxic (affecting about 10%)
- Motor impairment may be minimal or severely disabling
- Associated defects:
  - seizures
  - speech disorders
  - mental retardation
- Prognosis varies

Pathophysiology

- A lesion or an abnormality occurs in the early stages of brain development.
- Structural and functional defects occur, impairing motor or cognitive function.
- Defects may not be distinguishable until months after birth.

Causes

- Conditions that result in cerebral anoxia, hemorrhage, or other CNS damage
- *Prenatal causes*
- Rh factor incompatibility
- ABO blood type incompatibility
- Maternal infection (especially rubella in the first trimester)
- Maternal diabetes
- Irradiation
- Anoxia
- Toxemia
- Malnutrition
- Abnormal placental attachment
- Isoimmunization
- *Parturition causes*
- Trauma during delivery
- Depressed maternal vital signs from general or spinal anesthesia
- Asphyxia from the cord wrapping around the neck
- Prematurity
- Prolonged or unusually rapid labor
- Multiple births (neonates born last in a multiple birth have an especially high rate of cerebral palsy)
- *Postnatal causes*
- Infections, such as meningitis and encephalitis
- Head trauma

- Poisoning
- Any condition resulting in cerebral thrombus or embolus

Incidence

- Highest in premature neonates and in those who are small for gestational age
- Slightly more common in boys than in girls
- More common in whites

Common characteristics

- Excessive lethargy or irritability
- High-pitched cry
- Poor head control
- Weak sucking reflex
- Delayed motor development
- Abnormal head circumference
- Abnormal postures
- Abnormal reflexes
- Abnormal muscle tone and performance

Complications

- Seizure disorders
- Speech, vision, and hearing problems
- Language and perceptual deficits
- Mental retardation (in up to 40% of patients)
- Dental problems
- Respiratory difficulties
- Poor swallowing and gag reflexes

Assessment

History

- Maternal or patient history reveals possible cause (see *When to suspect cerebral palsy*)

Physical findings

- Child with retarded growth and development
- Difficulty chewing and swallowing
- *Spastic cerebral palsy*
- Underdevelopment of affected limbs
- Characteristic scissors gait
- Walks on toes
- Crosses one foot in front of the other
- Hyperactive deep tendon reflexes
- Increased stretch reflexes
- Rapid alternating muscle contraction and relaxation
- Muscle weakness
- Impaired fine and gross motor skills
- Contractures in response to manipulation of muscles
- *Athetoid cerebral palsy*
- Involuntary movements
- Grimacing
- Wormlike writhing
- Dystonia
- Sharp jerks that impair voluntary movement
- Involuntary facial movements (speech difficult)
- Drooling

Ataxic cerebral palsy

- Lack of leg movement during infancy
- Wide gait when child begins to walk
- Disturbed balance
- Incoordination (especially of the arms)
- Hypoactive reflexes
- Nystagmus
- Muscle weakness
- Tremors

Test results

Imaging

- Computed tomography scan and magnetic resonance imaging of the brain may show structural abnormalities of the brain such as cerebral atrophy.
- EEG may show the source of seizure activity.

Treatment

General

- Braces or splints
- Special appliances, such as adapted eating utensils and low toilet seat with arms
- Range-of-motion (ROM) exercises
- Prescribed exercises to maintain muscle tone

Medications

- Anticonvulsants
- Muscle relaxants
- Antianxiety agents

Surgery

- Orthopedic surgery
- Neurosurgery

Nursing considerations

Key outcomes

The patient will:
- consume calorie requirements daily
- express positive feelings about self
- maintain joint mobility and ROM
- develop adequate coping mechanisms
- develop effective communication skills.

Nursing interventions

- Speak slowly and distinctly.
- Give all care in an unhurried manner.
- Allow participation in care decisions.
- Provide a diet with adequate calories. Stroking the throat may aid swallowing.
- Provide frequent mouth and dental care.
- Provide skin care.
- Perform prescribed exercises to maintain muscle tone.
- Care for associated hearing and vision disturbances, as necessary.
- Postoperatively, give analgesics, as ordered.
- Provide a safe physical environment.

When to suspect cerebral palsy

Early detection of cerebral palsy is essential for effective treatment and requires careful clinical observation during infancy and precise neurologic assessment. Suspect cerebral palsy whenever a neonate:

- has difficulty sucking or keeping the nipple or food in his mouth
- seldom moves voluntarily or has arm or leg tremors with voluntary movement
- crosses his legs when lifted from behind rather than pulling them up or bicycling like a normal neonate
- has legs that are hard to separate, making diaper changing difficult
- persistently uses only one hand or, as he gets older, uses his hands well but not his legs.

Monitoring

- Pain relief
- Seizure activity
- Speech
- Visual and auditory acuity
- Respiratory status
- Swallowing function
- Reflexes
- Nutritional status
- Skin integrity
- Motor development
- Muscle strength

Patient teaching

Be sure to cover:
- the prescribed medication regimen
- adverse drug reactions
- daily skin inspection and daily massage
- the need to place food far back in patient's mouth to facilitate swallowing
- the need to chew food thoroughly
- drinking through a straw
- sucking lollipops to develop muscle control
- proper nutrition
- opportunities for learning, such as summer camps or Special Olympics.
- correct use of assistive devices.

Discharge planning

- Refer family members to community support groups such as the local chapter of the United Cerebral Palsy Association.

Cervical cancer

Overview

Description
○ Proliferation of cancer cells in the cervix
○ Third most common cancer of the female reproductive system
○ Classified as either preinvasive (curable in 75% to 90% of patients with early detection and proper treatment) or invasive

Pathophysiology
Preinvasive cancer
○ Preinvasive cancer ranges from minimal cervical dysplasia, in which the lower third of the epithelium contains abnormal cells, to carcinoma in situ, in which the full thickness of epithelium contains abnormally proliferating cells.
Invasive cancer
○ Cancer cells penetrate the basement membrane and can spread directly to contiguous pelvic structures or disseminate to distant sites by way of lymphatic routes.
○ Most (95%) cases are squamous cell carcinoma; 5% of cases are adenocarcinomas.

Causes
○ Unknown

Risk factors
○ Frequent intercourse at a young age (under age 16)
○ Multiple sexual partners
○ Multiple pregnancies
○ Human papillomavirus (HPV)
○ Bacterial or viral venereal infections
○ Exposure to diethylstilbestrol in utero
○ Human immunodeficiency virus
○ Smoking

Incidence
○ Typically occurs between ages 30 and 45; rarely, under age 20

Common characteristics
○ Abnormal vaginal bleeding

Complications
○ Renal failure
○ Distant metastasis
○ Vaginal stenosis
○ Ureterovaginal or vesicovaginal fistula
○ Proctitis
○ Cystitis
○ Bowel obstruction

Assessment

History
○ One or more risk factors present
Preinvasive cancer
○ No symptoms or other clinical changes
Invasive cancer
○ Abnormal vaginal bleeding or discharge
○ Gradually increasing flank pain

Physical findings
○ Vaginal discharge
○ Postcoital bleeding
○ Irregular bleeding

Test results
Imaging
○ Lymphangiography can show metastasis.
○ Cystography can show metastasis.
○ Organ and bone scans can show metastasis.
Diagnostic procedures
○ Papanicolaou (Pap) test shows abnormal cells, and colposcopy shows the source of the abnormal cells seen on the Pap test. (See *Testing for cervical cancer.*)
○ Cone or punch biopsy is performed if endocervical curettage is positive.
○ Vira Pap test (investigational) permits examination of the specimen's deoxyribonucleic acid structure to detect HPV.

Treatment

General
○ Accurate clinical staging used to determine type of treatment
○ Well-balanced diet, as tolerated

Medications
○ Multidrug chemotherapy regimens

Surgery
Preinvasive lesions
○ Total excisional biopsy
○ Cryosurgery
○ Laser destruction
○ Conization, followed by frequent Pap test follow-ups
○ Hysterectomy (rare)
Invasive squamous cell carcinoma
○ Radical hysterectomy and radiation therapy (internal, external, or both)
○ Pelvic exenteration (rare; may be performed for recurrent cervical cancer)

To analyze cervical cells, the ThinPrep may be collected in the same manner as a Papanicolaou (Pap) test using a cytobrush and plastic spatula. The specimens are deposited in a bottle provided with a fixative and sent to the laboratory. A filter is then inserted into the bottle and excess mucus, blood, and inflammatory cells are filtered out by centrifuge. Remaining cells are then placed on a slide in a uniform, thin layer and read as a Pap test. This causes fewer slides to be classified as unreadable, significantly reducing the incidence of false negatives and the need for repeat tests.

When the ThinPrep test is used, screening can also be easily done for the human papillomavirus (HPV), of which certain strains have been identified as the primary cause of cervical cancer. The Digene hc2 HPV deoxyribonucleic acid (DNA) test has been approved by the Food and Drug Administration to determine if those identified as high risk for developing cervical cancer have been exposed to HPV. The specimen is collected as a Pap smear but is dispersed with ThinPrep solution. Separate aliquots are used for each test, from brushings of the endocervix. The brush is then inserted into the specialized tube and snapped off at the shaft, capping securely. The target solution in the tube disrupts the virus and releases target DNA, which combines with specific ribonucleic acid (RNA) probes creating RNA:DNA hybrids. The hybrids are captured, bound and able to be magnified and measured using a luminometer.

If a patient is positive for HPV, it means she had been infected with the virus. Depending on the type of HPV found through DNA testing, those harboring high-risk HPV strains have a high risk of developing cervical cancer. These patients should have a colposcopy in which the cervix is viewed under microscope and a biopsy taken from the tissue sample.

Nursing considerations

Key outcomes

The patient will:
○ express increased comfort and decreased pain
○ express feelings and perceptions about changes in sexual activity
○ maintain joint mobility and range of motion
○ experience no signs or symptoms of infection
○ use support systems and develop coping strategies.

Nursing interventions

○ Encourage verbalization and provide support.
○ Give prescribed drugs.

Monitoring

○ Vital signs
○ Complications
○ Pain control
○ Vaginal discharge
○ Renal status
○ Response to treatment

Patient teaching

Be sure to cover:
○ the disease process, diagnosis, and treatment
○ importance of follow-up care
○ how treatment won't radically alter the patient's lifestyle or prohibit sexual intimacy
○ drugs and their administration, dosage, and adverse effects.

Discharge planning

○ Refer the patient to resource and support services.

Chalazion

Overview

Description
○ Painless, slowly growing nodule on the eyelid
○ Common disorder of the sebaceous gland in the eyelid
○ May become large enough to press on the eyeball, producing astigmatism
○ May be chronic

Pathophysiology
○ Granulomatous inflammation in the upper or lower eyelid, the result of an obstruction of the meibomian (sebaceous) gland duct
○ Edema usually contained on the conjunctival portion of the eyelid

Causes
○ Rosacea
○ Chronic blepharitis
○ Seborrhea
○ Meibomian cancer

Incidence
○ Higher incidence in fair-skinned males than in other groups, possibly because of that group's higher incidence of rosacea and blepharitis
○ More common in adults ages 30 to 50

Common characteristics
○ Painless, hard lump that usually points toward the conjunctival side of the eyelid

Complications
○ Cosmetic deformity
○ Bleeding after surgery

Recognizing chalazion

A chalazion is a nontender granulomatous inflammation of a meibomian gland on the upper or lower eyelid.

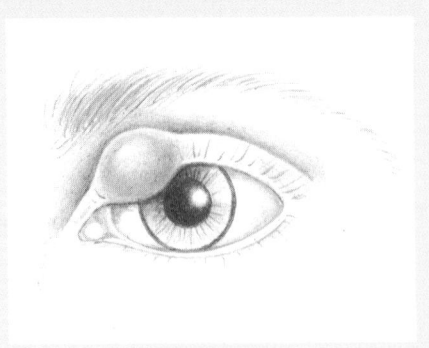

○ Infection
○ Vision disturbance

Assessment

History
○ Nodule on eyelid
○ Rosacea or blepharitis

Physical findings
○ Palpable small lump in the eyelid
○ Red, elevated area on the conjunctival surface (see *Recognizing chalazion*)

Test results
Other
○ Visual examination and palpation of the eyelid
○ Biopsy, to rule out meibomian cancer

Treatment

General
○ Warm compresses to the affected eyelid

Medications
○ Sulfonamide eyedrops
○ Steroid injection
○ Tetracycline
○ Antimicrobial eyedrops after surgical removal

Surgery
○ Incision and curettage of the chalazion under local anesthetic may be necessary.

Nursing considerations

Key outcomes
The patient will:
○ report improvement of condition of eyelid
○ maintain positive outlook regarding body image
○ remain free from signs of bleeding or infection.

Nursing interventions
○ Apply warm compress after surgery.
○ Apply eye patch to the affected eye for 24 hours. (See *Applying an eye patch.*)
○ Instill eyedrops, as ordered.

Monitoring
○ Bleeding (after surgery)

Patient teaching

Be sure to cover:
○ proper instillation of eyedrops
○ signs and symptoms of infection
○ reporting recurrence.

Applying an eye patch

You may apply an eye patch for various reasons: to protect the eye after injury or surgery, to prevent accidental damage to an anesthetized eye, to promote healing, to absorb secretions, to protect the eye from drying when the patient is comatose or unable to close the eye as in Bell's palsy, or to prevent the patient from touching or rubbing his eye.

A thicker patch, called a *pressure patch,* may be used to help corneal abrasions heal, compress postoperative edema, or control hemorrhage from traumatic injury. Application requires an ophthalmologist's prescription and supervision.

To apply a patch, choose a gauze pad of appropriate size for the patient's face, place it gently over the closed eye (as shown), and secure it with two or three strips of tape. Extend the tape from midforehead across the eye to below the earlobe.

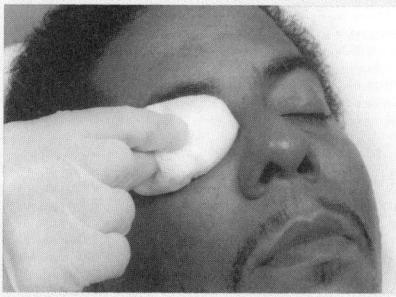

A pressure patch, which is markedly thicker than a single-thickness gauze patch, exerts extra tension against the closed eye. After placing the initial gauze pad, build it up with additional gauze pieces. Tape it firmly so that the patch exerts even pressure against the closed eye (as shown).

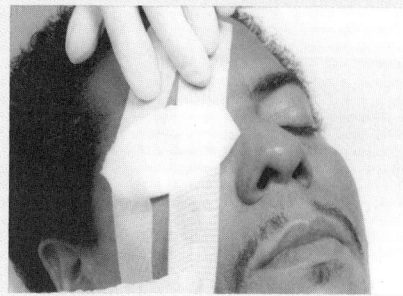

For increased protection of an injured eye, place a plastic or metal shield (as shown) on top of the gauze pads and apply tape over the shield.

Occasionally, you may use a head dressing to secure a pressure patch. The dressing applies additional pressure or, in burn patients, holds the patch in place without tape.

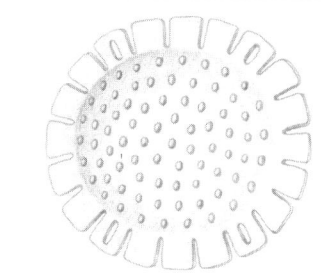

 Alert

Tell the patient to start applying warm compresses at the first sign of lid irritation to increase the blood supply and keep the lumen open.

Discharge planning

○ Encourage follow-up care, as ordered.

Chancroid

Overview

Description
- Sexually transmitted disease
- Characterized by painful genital ulcers and inguinal adenitis
- Common cause of genital ulcers in patients in developing countries

Pathophysiology
- Organisms are carried from the site of entry through the lymphatics to regional lymph nodes, resulting in node swelling.
- The initial lesion is a papule that ulcerates within 24 hours. (See *Chancroidal lesion.*)
- Untreated infections disseminate to other organs, causing systemic inflammation and specific organ dysfunction.

Causes
- *Haemophilus ducreyi*, a short, nonmotile, gram-negative bacillus

Risk factors
- Poor personal hygiene
- Unprotected sex
- Multiple sex partners
- Uncircumcised males

Incidence
- Increasing in the United States

Chancroidal lesion

Chancroid produces a soft, painful chancre, similar to that of syphilis. Without treatment, it may progress to inguinal adenitis and formation of buboes (enlarged, inflamed lymph nodes).

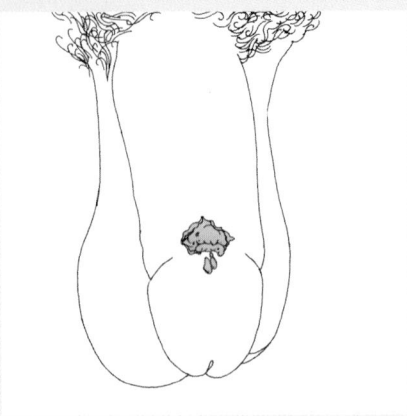

- More common in males than in females
- Occurs at any age but is most common among young, sexually active people

Common characteristics
- Multiple papules that ulcerate
- Lesions may heal spontaneously and usually respond well to treatment when no secondary infections present

Complications
- Phimosis and urethral fistulas in men
- Secondary infection
- Abscess formation
- Inguinal adenitis and formation of buboes

Assessment

History
- May report unprotected sexual contact with an infected person or with unknown or multiple partners
- Pain from ulcers and lymphadenopathy
- Headaches and malaise

Physical findings
- Genital area initially with single or multiple papules surrounded by redness that rapidly become pustular and then ulcerate
- Ulcers nonindurated with ragged edges, a base of granulation tissue, and bleed easily; range from 1 to 2 mm in diameter
- Lesions on the tongue, lip, or breast
- Suppuration with bubo formation in the untreated patient; rupture of abscess may follow
- Tender, fluctuant inguinal nodes

Test results
Laboratory
- Cultures from the lesion showing *H. ducreyi*

Treatment

General
- Aspiration of fluid-filled nodes
- Careful personal hygiene
- Abstinence from sexual activity until genital lesions are healed
- Evaluation of patient for syphilis, herpes simplex virus, and human immunodeficiency virus (HIV)

Medications
- Antibiotics

Surgery
- Surgical drainage for large abscess

Nursing considerations

Key outcomes

The patient will:
- communicate feelings about changes in body image
- regain skin integrity with decrease in size of chancroids
- state infection risk factors
- voice feelings about changes in sexual activity.

Nursing interventions

- Follow standard precautions.
- Give prescribed drugs.
- Wash the affected area with soap and water, followed by a bactericidal agent.
- Dry the affected area thoroughly.
- Report all cases of chancroid to the local board of health.

Monitoring

- Response to treatment
- Adverse effects of medications
- Compliance with treatment regimen
- Complications

Patient teaching

Be sure to cover:
- need to avoid applying creams, lotions, or oils on or near genitalia or on other lesion sites
- abstaining from sexual contact until follow-up shows that healing is complete
- proper washing techniques of the genitalia
- HIV infection and recommend testing
- following safe sex practices.

Discharge planning

- Refer the patient and affected sexual partners for treatment.

Chlamydial infections

Overview

Description

○ Infection that results in urethritis in men, cervicitis in women, and lymphogranuloma venereum in both sexes
○ Trachoma inclusion conjunctivitis: seldom occurs in United States, but is leading cause of blindness in developing countries
○ Most common sexually transmitted disease (STD) in the United States

Pathophysiology

○ Chlamydial infections are transmitted by direct contact (such as sexual).
○ Infection produces local inflammation.
○ Endometritis and salpingitis occur as the organism ascends the genitourinary tract.

Causes

○ Transmission of *Chlamydia trachomatis,* by sexual contact (oral, anal, or vaginal)
○ Neonate infection caused by transport through the infected mother's birth canal

Risk factors

○ Multiple sex partners or new sex partner
○ Unprotected sex
○ Coinfection with another STD

Incidence

○ Approximately 4 million cases reported annually
○ Affects primarily the Native American population of the southwest United States
○ Occurs more commonly among minorities and lower socioeconomic groups and people living in urban areas

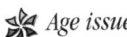 *Age issue*

Chlamydial infections have a 10% incidence among sexually active adolescent girls.

Common characteristics

○ Primarily follows vaginal or rectal intercourse or oral-genital contact with an infected person
○ Late appearance of signs and symptoms during the course of the disease
○ No symptoms in 75% of women, 50% of men
○ Sexual transmission of organism occurs unknowingly

Complications

○ Infertility
○ Pelvic inflammatory disease
○ Urethral and rectal strictures
○ Perihepatitis
○ Cervical cancer
○ Trachoma
○ Urethritis and epididymitis (in males)
○ Sterility
○ Stillbirth, neonatal death, premature labor (with infected pregnant females)

Assessment

History

○ Unprotected sexual contact with an infected person
○ Previous STD

Physical findings

○ Two-thirds of patients asymptomatic
Female
○ Pelvic or abdominal pain
○ Dyspareunia
○ Cervical erosion
○ Mucopurulent discharge
○ Dysuria
○ Urinary frequency
Male
○ Dysuria
○ Urinary frequency
○ Pruritus
○ Urethral discharge (copious and purulent)
○ Meatal erythema
○ Severe scrotal pain
Lymphogranuloma venereum
○ Painless vesicle or nonindurated ulcer, 2 to 3 mm in diameter, on the glans or shaft of the penis; on the labia, vagina, or cervix; or in the rectum
○ Enlarged inguinal lymph nodes
○ Regional nodes appear as series of bilateral buboes
○ Untreated buboes may rupture and form sinus tracts that discharge thick, yellow, granular secretion

Test results

Laboratory
○ Swab culture of the infection site showing *C. trachomatis* (see Chlamydia trachomatis)
○ Culture of aspirated blood, pus, or cerebrospinal fluid establishing epididymitis, prostatitis, and lymphogranuloma venereum
○ Serologic studies revealing previous exposure
○ Enzyme-linked immunosorbent assay showing *C. trachomatis* antibody

Treatment

General

○ Symptomatic treatment (sex partners also treated)
○ Abstinence from sexual activity until infection resolved

Medications

○ Antibiotics

Nursing considerations

Key outcomes

The patient will:
○ voice feelings about changes in sexuality
○ express concern about self-concept, self-esteem, and body image
○ exhibit improved or healed lesions or wounds
○ express relief from pain.

Nursing interventions

○ Follow standard precautions.
○ Check the neonate of an infected mother for signs of infection.
○ Give prescribed drugs.
○ Provide appropriate skin care.
○ If required in your state, report cases of chlamydial infection to the local board of health for follow-up on sexual contacts.

Monitoring

○ Response to treatment
○ Adverse effects of medication
○ Complications

Patient teaching

Be sure to cover:
○ the disorder, signs and symptoms, and treatment
○ proper hand-washing technique
○ abstinence from intercourse or use of condoms
○ importance of getting tested for the human immuno-deficiency virus
○ dealing with long-term risks and complications from infection
○ transmission of infection
○ prevention of STDs by following safe sex practices
○ follow-up care
○ complications.

Discharge planning

○ Refer the patient to support services.
○ Advise rescreenings at 3 to 4 months and annual screenings for sexually active teens and females ages 20 to 25.

Chlamydia trachomatis

In chlamydial infections, microscopic examination reveals *Chlamydia trachomatis*, a unicellular parasite with a rigid cell wall.

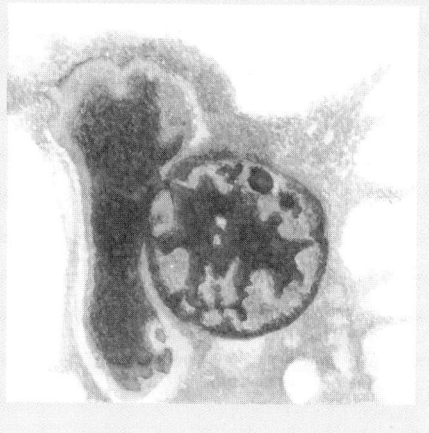

Cholelithiasis, cholecystitis, and related disorders

Overview

Description

Cholelithiasis
- Leading biliary tract disease
- Formation of calculi (gallstones) in the gallbladder
- Prognosis usually good with treatment, unless infection occurs

Cholecystitis
- Related disorder that arises from formation of gallstones
- Acute or chronic inflammation of gallbladder
- Usually caused by a gallstone lodged in the cystic duct
- Acute form most common during middle age
- Chronic form most common among elderly persons
- Prognosis good with treatment

Choledocholithiasis
- Related disorder that arises from formation of gallstones
- Partial or complete biliary obstruction due to gallstones lodged in the common bile duct
- Prognosis good unless infection occurs

Cholangitis
- Related disorder that arises from formation of gallstones
- Infected bile duct
- Commonly linked to choledocholithiasis
- Rapid response of nonsuppurative type to antibiotic treatment
- Poor prognosis of suppurative type unless surgery to correct obstruction and drain infected bile performed promptly

Gallstone ileus
- Related disorder that arises from formation of gallstones
- Obstruction of the small bowel by a gallstone
- Most common in elderly persons
- Prognosis good with surgery

Pathophysiology

- Calculi formation in the biliary system causes obstruction.
- Obstruction of hepatic duct leads to intrahepatic retention of bile; increased release of bilirubin into the bloodstream occurs.
- Obstruction of cystic duct leads to inflammation of the gallbladder; increased gallbladder contraction and peristalsis occurs.
- Obstruction of bile causes impairment of digestion and absorption of lipids.

Causes
- Calculi formation; type of disorder that develops depends on where in the gallbladder or biliary tract the calculi collect
- Acute cholecystitis also a result of conditions that alter gallbladder's ability to fill or empty (trauma, reduced blood supply to the gallbladder, prolonged immobility, chronic dieting, adhesions, prolonged anesthesia, and opioid abuse)

Risk factors
- High-calorie, high-cholesterol diet
- Linked to obesity
- Elevated estrogen levels from hormonal contraceptive use, postmenopausal hormone-replacement therapy, or pregnancy
- Diabetes mellitus, ileal disease, hemolytic disorders, hepatic disease (cirrhosis), or pancreatitis
- Rapid weight loss

Incidence
- Six times more common in women between ages 20 and 50
- Men and women equal after age 50; increases with each succeeding decade

Common characteristics
- Epigastric or right upper quadrant abdominal pain
- Nausea, vomiting
- Low-grade fever
- Abdominal distention

Complications

Cholelithiasis
- Cholangitis
- Cholecystitis
- Choledocholithiasis
- Gallstone ileus

Cholecystitis
- Gallbladder complications, such as empyema, hydrops or mucocele, and gangrene
- Chronic cholecystitis and cholangitis

Choledocholithiasis
- Cholangitis
- Obstructive jaundice
- Pancreatitis
- Secondary biliary cirrhosis

Cholangitis
- Septic shock
- Death

Gallstone ileus
- Bowel obstruction

Assessment

History
- Gallbladder disease may produce no symptoms (even when X-rays reveal gallstones).

Gallbladder attack

- ❍ Sudden onset of severe steady or aching pain in the midepigastric region or the right upper abdominal quadrant
- ❍ Pain radiating to the back, between the shoulder blades or over the right shoulder blade, or just to the shoulder area
- ❍ Attack occurring after eating a fatty meal or a large meal after fasting for an extended time
- ❍ Attack occurring in the middle of the night
- ❍ Nausea, vomiting, and chills
- ❍ Low-grade fever
- ❍ History of milder GI symptoms that preceded the acute attack; indigestion, vague abdominal discomfort, belching, and flatulence after eating meals or snacks rich in fats

Physical findings

- ❍ Severe pain
- ❍ Pallor
- ❍ Diaphoresis
- ❍ Low-grade fever (high in cholangitis)
- ❍ Exhaustion
- ❍ Jaundice (chronic)
- ❍ Dark-colored urine and clay-colored stools
- ❍ Tachycardia
- ❍ Tenderness over the gallbladder, which increases on inspiration (Murphy's sign)
- ❍ Palpable, painless, sausagelike mass (calculus-filled gallbladder without ductal obstruction)
- ❍ Hypoactive bowel sounds

Test results

Laboratory

- ❍ Blood studies possibly revealing elevated levels of serum alkaline phosphatase, lactate dehydrogenase, aspartate aminotransferase, icteric index, and total bilirubin; white blood cell count slightly elevated during cholecystitis attack

Imaging

- ❍ Plain abdominal X-rays show gallstones if they contain enough calcium to be radiopaque. X-rays are also helpful in identifying porcelain gallbladder, limy bile, and gallstone ileus.
- ❍ Ultrasonography of the gallbladder confirms cholelithiasis in most patients and distinguishes between obstructive and nonobstructive jaundice; calculi as small as 2 mm can be detected.
- ❍ Oral cholecystography confirms the presence of gallstones, although this test is gradually being replaced by ultrasonography.
- ❍ Technetium-labeled iminodiacetic acid scan of the gallbladder indicates cystic duct obstruction and acute or chronic cholecystitis if the gallbladder can't be seen.

Diagnostic procedures

- ❍ Percutaneous transhepatic cholangiography, imaging performed under fluoroscopic guidance, supports the diagnosis of obstructive jaundice and is used to visualize calculi in the ducts.

Treatment

General

- ❍ Endoscopic retrograde cholangiopancreatography to visualize and remove calculi
- ❍ Lithotripsy
- ❍ Low-fat diet
- ❍ Nothing by mouth if surgery required
- ❍ Activity, as tolerated

Medications

- ❍ Gallstone dissolution therapy
- ❍ Bile salts
- ❍ Analgesics
- ❍ Antispasmodics
- ❍ Anticholinergics
- ❍ Antiemetics
- ❍ Antibiotics

Surgery

- ❍ Cholecystectomy (laparoscopic or abdominal), cholecystectomy with operative cholangiography, choledochostomy, or exploration of the common bile duct

Nursing considerations

Key outcomes

The patient will:
- ❍ express feelings of increased comfort
- ❍ show no signs of infection
- ❍ have laboratory values that return to within normal parameters
- ❍ avoid complications.

Nursing interventions

- ❍ Give prescribed drugs.

Monitoring

- ❍ Vital signs
- ❍ Intake and output
- ❍ Pain control

After surgery

- ❍ Signs and symptoms of bleeding, infection, or atelectasis
- ❍ Wound site
- ❍ T tube patency and drainage

Patient teaching

Be sure to cover:
- ❍ the disease, diagnosis, and treatment
- ❍ how to breathe deeply, cough, expectorate, and perform leg exercises that are necessary after surgery
- ❍ dietary modifications
- ❍ medication administration, dosage, and possible adverse effects
- ❍ wound care.

Cholera

Overview

Description

○ Acute enterotoxin-mediated GI infection
○ Transmitted through food and water contaminated with fecal material from carriers or people with active infections.
○ Food poisoning caused by *Vibrio parahaemolyticus,* a similar bacterium (see Vibrio parahaemolyticus *food poisoning*)
○ Also known as *Asiatic cholera* or *epidemic cholera*

Pathophysiology

○ Humans are the only hosts and victims of *V. cholerae,* a motile, aerobic organism.

Causes

○ The gram-negative bacillus *V. cholerae*

Risk factors

○ Deficiency or absence of hydrochloric acid

Incidence

○ Most common in Africa, Southern and Southeast Asia, and the Middle East, although outbreaks have occurred in Japan, Australia, and Europe
○ Occurs during the warmer months and is most prevalent among lower socioeconomic groups
○ Common among children ages 1 to 5 in India, but equally distributed among all age-groups in other endemic areas

---

Vibrio parahaemolyticus food poisoning

Vibrio parahaemolyticus is a common cause of gastroenteritis in Japan. Outbreaks also occur on American cruise ships and in the eastern and southeastern coastal areas of the United States, especially during the summer.

V. parahaemolyticus, which thrives in a salty environment, is transmitted through the ingestion of uncooked or undercooked contaminated shellfish, particularly crab and shrimp. After an incubation period of 2 to 48 hours, *V. parahaemolyticus* causes watery diarrhea, moderately severe cramps, nausea, vomiting, headache, weakness, chills, and fever. Food poisoning is usually self-limiting and subsides spontaneously within 2 days. Occasionally, however, it's more severe, and may even be fatal in debilitated or elderly persons.

Diagnosis requires bacteriologic examination of vomitus, blood, stool smears, or fecal specimens collected by rectal swab. Diagnosis must rule out not only other causes of food poisoning but also other acute GI disorders.

Treatment is supportive, consisting primarily of bed rest and oral fluid replacement. I.V. replacement therapy is seldom necessary, but oral tetracycline may be prescribed. Thorough cooking of seafood prevents this infection.

Common characteristics

○ Acute, painless, profuse, watery diarrhea
○ Effortless vomiting (without preceding nausea)

Complications

○ Dehydration
○ Hypovolemic shock
○ Metabolic acidosis
○ Uremia
○ Coma and death

Assessment

History

○ Profuse, watery diarrhea
○ Vomiting
○ Intense thirst
○ Weakness
○ Muscle cramps (especially in the extremities)

Physical findings

○ Stools containing white flecks of mucus (rice-water stools)
○ Loss of skin turgor, wrinkled skin, sunken eyes
○ Pinched facial expression
○ Cyanosis
○ Tachycardia, tachypnea
○ Thready or absent peripheral pulses
○ Decreased blood pressure
○ Fever
○ Inaudible, hypoactive bowel sounds

Test results

Laboratory
○ A culture of *V. cholerae* from feces or vomitus indicates cholera.
○ Microscopic examination of fresh feces shows rapidly moving bacilli (like shooting stars).
○ Agglutination reveals reactions to group- and type-specific antisera.

Others
○ In endemic areas or during epidemics, typical clinical features strongly suggest cholera.

Treatment

General

○ Enteric precautions
○ Supportive care
○ Increased fluid intake

Medications

○ Rapid I.V. infusion of large amounts (50 to 100 ml/minute) of isotonic saline solution, alternating with isotonic sodium bicarbonate or sodium lactate
○ Tetracycline

Nursing considerations

Key outcomes

The patient will:
○ regain and maintain adequate fluid and electrolyte balance
○ have normal elimination patterns
○ have stable vital signs
○ produce adequate urine volume.

Nursing interventions

○ Wear a gown and gloves when handling feces-contaminated articles.
○ Carefully observe neck veins.
○ Auscultate the lungs frequently.

Monitoring

○ Vital signs
○ Intake and output
○ Laboratory values
○ I.V. infusion
○ Neck veins

Patient teaching

Be sure to cover:
○ administration of cholera vaccine to travelers in endemic areas
○ proper hand-washing technique
○ need for increased fluid intake.

Discharge planning

○ Explain the use of oral tetracycline to family members.
○ If the physician orders a cholera vaccine, tell the patient that he'll need a booster 3 to 6 months later for continuing protection.

Chronic fatigue and immune dysfunction syndrome

Overview

Description

- Characterized by prolonged overwhelming fatigue
- Also called *chronic fatigue syndrome, chronic Epstein-Barr virus, myalgic encephalomyelitis,* and *Yuppie flu*

Pathophysiology

- Infectious agents or environmental factors trigger an abnormal immune response and hormonal alterations.

Causes

- Exact cause unknown
- Possibly cytomegalovirus, herpes simplex virus types 1 and 2, human herpesvirus 6, Inoue-Melnick virus, human adenovirus 2, enteroviruses, measles virus, or a retrovirus that resembles human T-cell lymphotropic virus type II
- May result from overactive immune system

Risk factors

- Genetic predisposition
- Hormonal balance
- Neuropsychiatric factors
- Sex
- Previous illness
- Stressful environment

Diagnosing chronic fatigue syndrome

Chronic fatigue and immune dysfunction syndrome is defined by:
- New or relapsing fatigue that isn't the result of ongoing exertion or alleviated by rest and reduces occupational, educational, social, or personal activities or efforts.
- Four or more of the following symptoms, occurring for 6 months or more:
  - self-reported impairment in short-term memory or concentration
  - sore throat
  - tender cervical or axillary nodes
  - muscle pain
  - multiple joint pain without redness or swelling
  - headaches of a new pattern or severity
  - nonrefreshing sleep
  - postexertional malaise lasting 24 hours or longer.

Incidence

- Chronic fatigue and immune dysfunction syndrome affects people of all ages, occupations, and income levels.
- It's more common in women than in men or children, especially women younger than age 45.
- Sporadic incidence and epidemic clusters have been observed.
- Estimated to affect approximately 200 out of every 100,000 persons in the United States

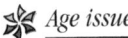 *Age issue*

Chronic fatigue and immune dysfunction syndrome is most prevalent among professionals in their 20s and 30s.

Common characteristics

- Suggests viral illness in some cases
- Characterized by incapacitating fatigue
- Waxing and waning symptoms
- Severely debilitating and can last for months or years
- Depression and anxiety after the syndrome's onset
- Fever
- Pharyngitis
- Lymphadenopathy

Complications

- Social and occupational impairment

Assessment

History

- Characteristic complaints of prolonged, overwhelming fatigue (see *Diagnosing chronic fatigue syndrome*)

Physical findings

- Myalgia
- Cognitive dysfunction

Test results

Laboratory
- Lymphocyte differential revealing reduced natural killer cell cytotoxicity, abnormal CD4+:CD8+ T-cell ratios, and mild lymphocytosis
- Immunoglobulin profile showing decreased immunoglobulin subclasses
- Immune complex profile revealing circulating immune complexes
- Antimicrosomal antibody testing revealing increased levels of antimicrosomal antibodies

---

Treatment

General

- Focus on supportive care
- Psychiatric evaluation
- Behavioral therapy
- Well-balanced diet high in vitamins and minerals
- Physical therapy
- Frequent rest periods, as needed
- Avoidance of strenuous activities

Medications

- Nonsteroidal anti-inflammatory drugs
- Antidepressants
- Antihistamines

Nursing considerations

Key outcomes

The patient will:
- verbally report having an increased energy level
- express feelings about diminished capacity to perform usual roles
- recognize limitations imposed by illness
- make decisions regarding the course of treatment and management of the illness
- voice feelings related to self-esteem.

Nursing interventions

- Provide emotional support.
- Begin a graded exercise program.

Monitoring

- Response to treatment
- Adverse effects of medication
- Complications

Patient teaching

Be sure to cover:
- the need to decrease activities when fatigue is greatest
- the need to avoid bed rest, which has no proven therapeutic value
- medication administration, dosage, and possible adverse effects
- appropriate activity planning.

Discharge planning

- Refer the patient to support services.

Cirrhosis

Overview

Description
- Chronic hepatic disease
- Several types

Pathophysiology
- Diffuse destruction and fibrotic regeneration of hepatic cells occurs.
- Necrotic tissue yields to fibrosis.
- Liver structure and normal vasculature are altered.
- Blood and lymph flow are impaired.
- Hepatic insufficiency occurs.

Causes
Laënnec's or micronodular cirrhosis (alcoholic or portal cirrhosis)
- Chronic alcoholism
- Malnutrition

Postnecrotic or macronodular cirrhosis
- Complication of viral hepatitis
- Possible after exposure to such liver toxins as arsenic, carbon tetrachloride, and phosphorus

Biliary cirrhosis
- Prolonged biliary tract obstruction or inflammation

Idiopathic cirrhosis (cryptogenic)
- No known cause
- Sarcoidosis
- Chronic inflammatory bowel disease

Risk factors
- Alcoholism
- Toxins
- Biliary obstruction
- Hepatitis
- Metabolic disorders

Incidence
- Tenth most common cause of death in the United States
- Most common among those ages 45 to 75
- Occurs in two times as many men as women

Common characteristics
- Abdominal pain
- Pruritus
- Jaundice
- Ascites
- Indigestion
- Anemia

Complications (advanced cirrhosis)
- Portal hypertension
- Bleeding esophageal varices
- Hepatic encephalopathy
- Hepatorenal syndrome
- Death

Ascites / Hepatitis

Assessment

History
- Chronic alcoholism
- Malnutrition
- Viral hepatitis
- Exposure to liver toxins such as arsenic and certain medications
- Prolonged biliary tract obstruction or inflammation

Early stage
- Vague signs and symptoms
- Abdominal pain
- Diarrhea, constipation
- Fatigue
- Nausea, vomiting
- Muscle cramps

Later stage
- Chronic dyspepsia
- Constipation
- Pruritus
- Weight loss
- Bleeding tendency, such as frequent nosebleeds, easy bruising, and bleeding gums

Physical findings
- Telangiectasis on the cheeks
- Spider angiomas on the face, neck, arms, and trunk
- Gynecomastia
- Umbilical hernia
- Distended abdominal blood vessels
- Ascites
- Testicular atrophy
- Menstrual irregularities
- Palmar erythema
- Clubbed fingers
- Thigh and leg edema
- Ecchymosis
- Anemia
- Jaundice
- Palpable, large, firm liver with a sharp edge (early finding)
- Enlarged spleen
- Asterixis
- Slurred speech, paranoia, hallucinations

Test results
Laboratory
- Elevated levels of liver enzymes, such as alanine aminotransferase, aspartate aminotransferase, total serum bilirubin, and indirect bilirubin; decreased total serum albumin and protein levels; prolonged prothrombin time; decreased hemoglobin, hematocrit, and serum electrolyte levels; deficient vitamins A, C, and K
- Increased urine levels of bilirubin and urobilinogen; decreased fecal urobilinogen levels

Imaging
- Abdominal X-rays show liver and spleen size and cysts or gas in the biliary tract or liver; liver calcification; and massive ascites.

○ Computed tomography and liver scans determine liver size, identify liver masses, and visualize hepatic blood flow and obstruction.
○ Radioisotope liver scans show liver size, blood flow, or obstruction.

Diagnostic procedures
○ Liver biopsy is the definitive test for cirrhosis, revealing hepatic tissue destruction and fibrosis.
○ Esophagogastroduodenoscopy reveals bleeding esophageal varices, stomach irritation or ulceration, and duodenal bleeding and irritation.

Treatment

General
○ Removal or alleviation of underlying cause
○ Paracentesis
○ Esophageal balloon tamponade
○ Sclerotherapy
○ I.V. fluids
○ Blood transfusion
○ Restricted sodium consumption
○ Restricted fluid intake
○ No alcohol intake
○ High-calorie diet
○ Frequent rest periods, as needed

Medications
○ Vitamin and nutritional supplements
○ Antacids
○ Potassium-sparing diuretics
○ Beta-adrenergic blockers and vasopressin
○ Ammonia detoxicant
○ Antiemetics

Surgery
○ May be required to divert ascites into venous circulation; if so, peritoneovenous shunt is used
○ Portal-systemic shunts

Nursing considerations

Key outcomes
The patient will:
○ maintain caloric intake, as required
○ maintain normal fluid volume
○ incur no injuries
○ exhibit no bleeding.

Nursing interventions
○ Give prescribed I.V. fluids and blood products.
○ Give prescribed drugs.
○ Encourage verbalization and provide support.
○ Provide appropriate skin care.

Monitoring
○ Vital signs
○ Laboratory values
○ Hydration and nutritional status

○ Abdominal girth
○ Weight
○ Bleeding tendencies
○ Skin integrity
○ Changes in mentation, behavior
○ Ammonia level

Patient teaching

Be sure to cover:
○ the disorder, diagnosis, and treatment
○ over-the-counter medications that may increase bleeding tendencies
○ dietary modifications
○ the need to avoid infections and abstain from alcohol
○ the need to avoid sedatives and acetaminophen (hepatotoxic)
○ high-calorie diet and small, frequent meals.

Discharge planning
○ Refer the patient to Alcoholics Anonymous, if appropriate.
○ Refer the patient for psychological counseling, if needed.

Cleft lip and cleft palate

Overview

Description

○ Front and sides of the face and the palatine shelves fuse imperfectly during pregnancy
○ May occur separately or in combination
○ Can occur unilaterally, bilaterally or, rarely, in the midline.
○ May affect just the lip or extend into the upper jaw or nasal cavity (see *Types of cleft deformities*)

Pathophysiology

○ Chromosomal abnormality, exposure to teratogens, genetic abnormality, or environmental factors cause the lip or palate to fuse imperfectly during the second month of pregnancy.
○ A complete cleft includes the soft palate, the bones of the maxilla, and the alveolus on one or both sides of the premaxilla.
○ A double cleft runs from the soft palate forward to either side of the nose, separating the maxilla and premaxilla into freely moving segments. The tongue and other muscles can displace the segments, enlarging the cleft.

 Alert

Isolated cleft palate occurs more commonly with congenital defects other than isolated cleft lip. The constellation of U-shaped cleft palate, mandibular hypoplasia, and glossoptosis known as Robin sequence, *can occur as an isolated defect or one feature of many different syndromes. These infants should have comprehensive genetic evaluation. Because of their mandibular hypoplasia and glossoptosis, the airway in infants with Robin sequence must be carefully evaluated and managed.*

Causes

○ Chromosomal or Mendelian syndrome (cleft defects caused by more than 300 syndromes)
○ Exposure to teratogens during fetal development
○ Combined genetic and environmental factors

Incidence

○ Twice as common in males than in females
○ More common in children with a family history of cleft defects
○ Cleft lip with or without cleft palate occurs in about 1 in 1,000 births among Whites; incidence is higher in Asians (1.7 in 1,000) and Native Americans (more than 3.6 in 1,000), but lower in Blacks (1 in 2,500)

Common characteristics

○ Obvious cleft lip or cleft palate
○ Feeding difficulties from incomplete fusion of the palate

Complications

○ Malnutrition
○ Hearing impairment
○ Permanent speech impediment

Assessment

History

○ Family history of cleft defects
○ Maternal exposure to teratogens during pregnancy

Physical findings

○ Cleft that runs from the soft palate forward to either side of the nose

Test results

Imaging
○ Prenatal targeted ultrasound reveals abnormality.
Others
○ Clinical presentation, obvious at birth

Treatment

General

○ Orthodontic prosthesis to improve sucking
○ Use of a contoured speech bulb attached to the posterior of a denture to occlude the nasopharynx when a wide horseshoe defect makes surgery impossible (to help the child develop intelligible speech)
○ Use of a large, soft nipple with large holes, such as a lamb's nipple, to improve feeding patterns and promote adequate nutrition

Medications

 Alert

Daily use of folic acid before conception decreases the risk for isolated (not associated with another genetic or congenital malformation) cleft lip or palate by up to 25%. Women of childbearing age should be encouraged to take a daily multivitamin containing folic acid until menopause or until they're no longer fertile.

Surgery

○ Surgical correction of cleft lip in the first few days of life and again at 12 to 18 months, after the infant gains weight and is infection-free

Nursing considerations

Key outcomes

The patient will:
○ exhibit normal growth and development patterns within the confines of the disorder
○ not aspirate feedings.

The family will:
○ express an understanding of the condition and treatment
○ seek appropriate resources to assist with coping.

Nursing interventions

○ Encourage the mother of an infant with cleft lip to breast-feed if the cleft doesn't prevent effective sucking.
○ Suction, as necessary.
○ Help the parents deal with their feelings about the child's deformity.

 Alert

Never place a child with Robin sequence on his back because his tongue could fall back and obstruct his airway. Place the infant on his side for sleeping. Most other infants with a cleft palate can sleep on their backs without difficulty.

Monitoring

○ Swallowing ability
○ Weight gain
○ Intake and output

Patient teaching

Be sure to cover:
○ treatment plan
○ how to best feed the infant
○ burping the infant frequently
○ gently cleaning the palatal cleft with a cotton-tipped applicator dipped in half-strength hydrogen peroxide or water after each feeding.

Discharge planning

○ Refer the patient to speech therapy to correct speech patterns.
○ Refer the parents to a social worker who can guide them to community resources, if needed, and to a genetic counselor to determine the recurrence risk.

Types of cleft deformities

These illustrations show variations of cleft lip and cleft palate.

NOTCH IN THE VERMILLION BORDER
(JUNCTION OF THE LIP AND SURROUNDING SKIN)

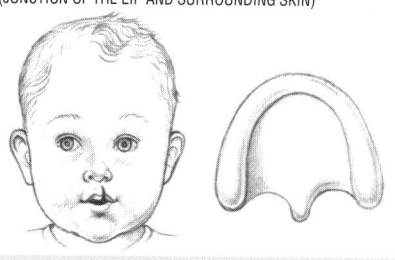

UNILATERAL CLEFT LIP AND PALATE

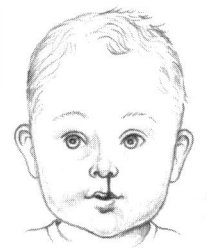
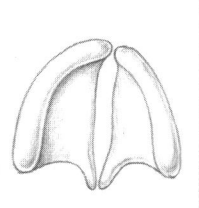

BILATERAL CLEFT LIP AND PALATE

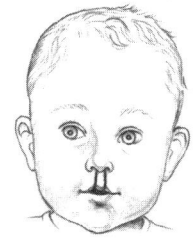
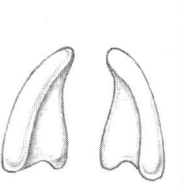

CLEFT PALATE

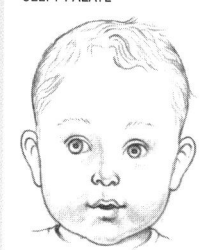
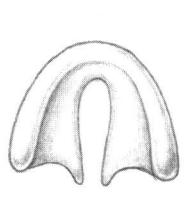

Clostridium difficile infection

Overview

Description

- A gram-positive anaerobic bacterium often resulting in antibiotic-associated diarrhea
- Symptoms ranging from asymptomatic carrier states to severe pseudomembranous colitis caused by exotoxins (Toxin A is an enterotoxin and toxin B is a cytotoxin.)
- Within 14 to 30 days of treatment, recurrence with the same organism possible in 10% to 20% of patients

Pathophysiology

- Antibiotics may trigger toxin production.
- Toxin A mediates alteration in fluid secretion, enhances inflammation, and causes leakage of albumin from the postcapillary venules.
- Toxin B causes damage and exfoliation to the superficial epithelial cells and inhibits adenosine diphosphate ribosylation of Rho proteins.
- Both toxins cause electrophysiologic alterations of colonic tissue.

Causes

- Antibiotics that disrupt the bowel flora
- Enemas and intestinal stimulants
- Transmission from infected person
- Some antifungal and antiviral agents

Risk factors

- Contaminated equipment and surfaces
- Antibiotics
- Abdominal surgery
- Antineoplastic agents that have an antibiotic activity
- Immunocompromised state

Incidence

- More common in people in nursing homes and daycare facilities
- One of the most common nosocomial infections (Approximately 20% of hospitalized patients taking antibiotics contract C. difficile infection.)

Common characteristics

- Watery, foul-smelling diarrhea

Complications

- Electrolyte abnormalities
- Hypovolemic shock
- Toxic megacolon
- Colonic perforation
- Peritonitis
- Sepsis
- Hemorrhage
- Pseudomembranous colitis

Assessment

History

- Recent antibiotic therapy
- Abdominal pain
- Cramping

Physical findings

- Soft, unformed, or watery diarrhea (more than three stools in a 24-hour period) that may be foul smelling or grossly bloody
- Abdominal tenderness
- Fever

Test results

Laboratory

- Cell cytotoxin test showing toxins A and B
- Enzyme immunoassay identifying *C. difficile;* slightly less sensitive than cell cytotoxin test but has turnaround time of only a few hours
- Stool culture identifying *C. difficile*

Treatment

General

- Withdrawal of causative antibiotic
- Avoidance of antimotility agents
- Good skin care
- Well-balanced diet
- Increased fluid intake, if appropriate
- Rest periods, if fatigued

Medications

- Metronidazole
- Vancomycin
- If relapse and previous treatment was metronidazole, low-dose vancomycin may be effective
- Combination of vancomycin and rifampin
- Experimental treatments involve the administration of yeast *Saccharomyces boulardii* with metronidazole or vancomycin and biologic vaccines to restore the normal GI flora
- Lactobacillus
- Cholestyramine

Nursing considerations

Key outcomes

The patient will:
- maintain stable vital signs
- maintain normal electrolyte levels
- maintain adequate fluid volume
- maintain skin integrity.

Nursing interventions

○ Give prescribed drugs.
○ Institute enteric precautions for those with active diarrhea.
○ Wash your hands with an antiseptic soap after direct contact with the patient or his immediate environment.
○ Make sure reusable equipment is disinfected before it's used on another patient.

Monitoring

○ Vital signs
○ Intake and output
○ Complications
○ Serum electrolytes
○ Adverse effects of medication
○ Response to treatment
○ Amount and characteristics of stools
○ Skin integrity

Patient teaching

Be sure to cover:
○ the disorder, diagnosis, and treatment
○ proper hand-washing technique
○ proper disinfection of contaminated clothing or household items
○ adequate fluid intake
○ signs and symptoms of dehydration
○ medications and potential adverse reactions
○ complications and when to notify the physician
○ perirectal skin care.

Clubfoot

Overview

Description

- A deformed talus and shortened Achilles tendon give the foot a characteristic clublike appearance. In talipes equinovarus, the foot points downward (equinus) and turns inward (varus), and the front of the foot curls toward the heel (forefoot adduction).
- Clubfoot, also known as talipes, is the most common congenital disorder of the lower extremities

Pathophysiology

- Unknown
- Possible contributing factors:
  - defective cartilage with ligamentous laxity
  - muscle imbalance
  - abnormal intrauterine position
  - central nervous system anomaly
  - persistence of a normal fetal relationship

Causes

- Combination of genetic and environmental factors in utero
- Heredity
- Idiopathic
- Suspected muscle abnormalities, leading to variations in length and tendon insertions

Incidence

- 1 per 1,000 live births
- Usually occurs bilaterally
- Twice as common in boys as it is in girls
- May be linked to other birth defects, such as myelomeningocele, spina bifida, and arthrogryposis

Common characteristics

- Inward deformity of the foot (see *Recognizing clubfoot*)

Complications

- Abnormal gait
- Stress changes on lateral side of the foot
- Residual deformity

Assessment

History

- Family history
- Muscular atrophy or dystrophy

Recognizing clubfoot

Clubfoot (talipes) may have various names, depending on the orientation of the deformity, as shown in the illustrations at right.

TALIPES EQUINUS
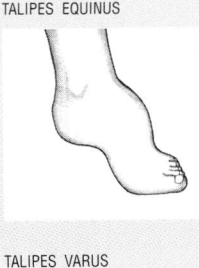

TALIPES CALCANEUS
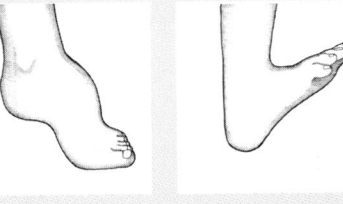

TALIPES CAVUS
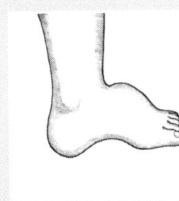

TALIPES VARUS
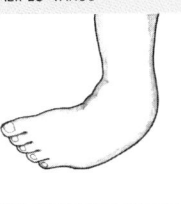

TALIPES EQUINOVARUS
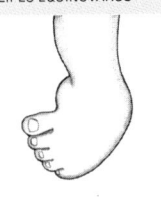

TALIPES CALCANEOVARUS
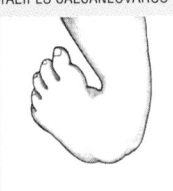

TALIPES VALGUS
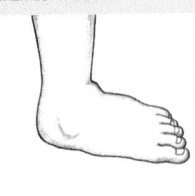

TALIPES CALCANEOVALGUS
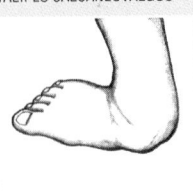

TALIPES EQUINOVALGUS
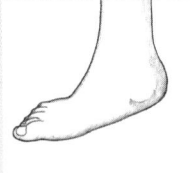

Physical findings

○ Deformed talus with a shortened Achilles tendon, the calcaneus somewhat shortened and flattened
○ Shortened, underdeveloped calf muscles, with soft tissue contractures at the site of the deformity
○ Foot tight in its deformed position and resistant of manual efforts to push it back into normal position

Test results

Imaging

○ X-rays show superimposition of the talus and the calcaneus and a ladderlike appearance of the metatarsals.

Others

○ Physical examination reveals clubfoot.

Treatment

General

○ Correction of the deformity
○ Activity according to ability
○ Maintaining the correction until the foot regains normal muscle balance
○ Close observation to prevent the deformity from recurring

Sequential correction

○ Forefoot adduction; uncurling the front of the foot away from the heel (forefoot abduction)
○ Varus deformity; turning the foot so the sole faces outward (eversion)
○ Equinus; casting the foot with the toes pointing up (dorsiflexion).

Surgery

○ Subcutaneous tenotomy of the Achilles tendon and posterior capsulotomy of the ankle joint may need to be done with the equinus stage of correction.
○ In severe cases, bone surgery (wedge resections, osteotomy, or astragalectomy) may be appropriate. After surgery, a cast is applied to preserve the correction.

Nursing considerations

Key outcomes

The patient will:
○ maintain joint mobility and range of motion
○ maintain muscle strength
○ show no evidence of complications.

Nursing interventions

○ After casting, elevate the child's feet with pillows.
○ Perform proper skin and cast care.

Monitoring

○ Neurovascular status of affected extremity after casting or surgery

○ Proper foot alignment
○ Pain control

Patient teaching

Be sure to cover:
○ the need for prompt treatment
○ signs of circulatory impairment
○ proper skin care
○ use of exercise, night splints, and orthopedic shoes to maintain alignment.

Coarctation of the aorta

Overview

Description

- A narrowing of the aorta, usually just below the left subclavian artery, near the site where the ligamentum arteriosum (the remnant of the ductus arteriosus, a fetal blood vessel) joins the pulmonary artery to the aorta
- May occur with aortic valve stenosis (usually of a bicuspid aortic valve) and with severe cases of hypoplasia of the aortic arch, patent ductus arteriosus (PDA), and ventricular septal defect
- Ineffective pumping of the heart and increased risk from heart failure due to the obstruction of blood flow

Pathophysiology

- Coarctation of the aorta may develop as a result of spasm and constriction of the smooth muscle in the ductus arteriosus as it closes.
- This contractile tissue extends into the aortic wall, causing narrowing.
- The obstructive process causes hypertension in the aortic branches above the constriction (arteries that supply the arms, neck, and head) and diminished pressure in the vessel below the constriction.
- Restricted blood flow through the narrowed aorta increases the pressure load on the left ventricle and causes dilation of the proximal aorta and ventricular hypertrophy.
- As oxygenated blood leaves the left ventricle, a portion travels through the arteries that branch off the aorta proximal to the coarctation.
- If PDA is present, the rest of the blood travels through the coarctation, mixes with deoxygenated blood from the PDA, and travels to the legs.
- If PDA is closed, the legs and lower portion of the body must rely solely on the blood that gets through the coarctation.

Causes

- Unknown
- Turner's syndrome

Incidence

- Accounts for about 7% of all congenital heart defects in children
- Twice as common in males as it is in females
- In females, commonly linked to Turner's syndrome, a chromosomal disorder that causes ovarian dysgenesis

Common characteristics

- Resting systolic hypertension in the upper body
- Absent or diminished femoral pulses
- Wide pulse pressure
- Signs and symptoms of heart failure

Complications

- Heart failure
- Severe hypertension
- Cerebral aneurysms and hemorrhage
- Rupture of the aorta
- Aortic aneurysm
- Infective endocarditis

Assessment

History

- Tachypnea
- Dyspnea
- Failure to thrive
- Headache
- Vertigo
- Epistaxis
- Claudication

Physical findings

- Pallor
- Hypertension
- Crackles
- Edema
- Tachycardia
- Cardiomegaly
- Hepatomegaly
- Hypertension
- Pink upper arms and cyanotic legs
- Absent or diminished femoral pulses
- Arm blood pressure greater than leg blood pressure
- Chest and arms more developed than legs

Test results

Imaging
- Chest X-rays may show left ventricular hypertrophy, heart failure, a wide ascending and descending aorta, and notching of the ribs' undersurfaces due to erosion by collateral circulation. (See *Recognizing coarctation of the aorta.*)
- Echocardiography may show increased left ventricular muscle thickness, coexisting aortic valve abnormalities, and the coarctation site.

Diagnostic procedures
- Electrocardiography may reveal left ventricular hypertrophy.
- Cardiac catheterization evaluates collateral circulation and measures pressure in the right and left ventricles and in the ascending and descending aortas (on both sides of the obstruction).
- Aortography locates the site and extent of coarctation.

Treatment

General

- Low-sodium diet
- Fluid restrictions
- Limited activity

Medications

○ Digoxin
○ Diuretics
○ Oxygen
○ Sedatives
○ Prostaglandin infusion to keep the ductus open
○ Antibiotic prophylaxis
○ Antihypertensive therapy

Surgery

○ A flap of the left subclavian artery may be used to reconstruct the aorta.
○ Balloon angioplasty or resection with end-to-end anastomosis or use of a tubular graft may also be performed.

Nursing considerations

Key outcomes

The patient will:
○ carry out activities of daily living without weakness or fatigue
○ maintain hemodynamic stability
○ remain free from signs and symptoms of infection.

Nursing interventions

○ Offer emotional support.
○ Regulate environmental temperature.
○ Give prescribed drugs.

Monitoring

○ Vital signs
○ Intake and output
○ Oxygenation
○ Blood glucose levels
○ Postoperative pain
○ Signs of infection

Patient teaching

Be sure to cover:
○ the disorder, diagnosis, and treatment
○ exercise restrictions
○ endocarditis prophylaxis.

Discharge planning

○ Stress the need for follow-up care, as ordered.

Recognizing coarctation of the aorta

Collateral circulation develops to bypass the occluded aortic lumen, and can be seen on X-ray as notching of the ribs. By adolescence, palpable, visible pulsations may be evident.

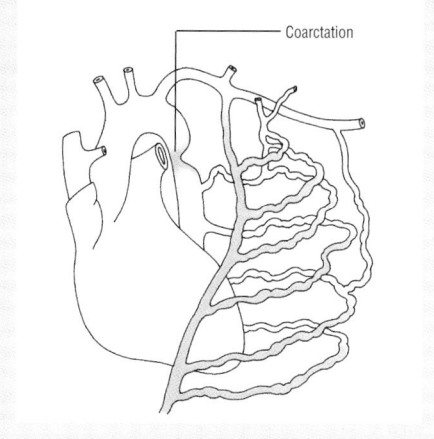

Coarctation

Coccidioidomycosis

Overview

Description
○ Fungal infection that occurs primarily as a respiratory tract infection, although generalized dissemination may occur
○ Also known as *valley fever* or *San Joaquin Valley fever*

Pathophysiology
○ After spores are inhaled, cell activation and cytokine formation stimulate inflammatory cells and facilitate killing of the organism.
○ Immunosuppression may delay resolution of the infection.

Causes
○ Inhaled spores of *Coccidioides immitis* found in the soil
○ Dressings or plaster casts of infected persons

Incidence
○ Disseminated illness more common in dark-skinned men, pregnant women, and patients receiving an immunosuppressant
○ Endemic to the southwestern United States, especially between the San Joaquin Valley in California and southwestern Texas; also found in Mexico, Guatemala, Honduras, Venezuela, Colombia, Argentina, and Paraguay
○ Generally affects Filipino Americans, Mexican Americans, Native Americans, and Blacks because of population distribution and an occupational link (common in migrant farm laborers)

Common characteristics
Primary coccidioidomycosis
○ Acute or subacute respiratory signs and symptoms
○ Fever that persists for weeks
Disseminated coccidioidomycosis
○ Fever
○ Abscesses throughout the body, especially in skeletal, central nervous system, splenic, hepatic, renal, and subcutaneous tissues

Complications
○ Meningitis
○ Bronchiectasis
○ Osteomyelitis
○ Hepatosplenomegaly
○ Liver failure

Assessment

History
○ Living or traveling to an endemic area
○ Fever
○ Dry cough
○ Pleuritic chest pain
○ Sore throat
○ Chills
○ Malaise
○ Headache
○ Joint pain

Physical findings
○ Fever
○ Itchy macular rash
○ Hemoptysis
○ Local swelling and redness in involved sites (with musculoskeletal involvement)
○ Bronchial breath sounds

Test results
Laboratory
○ Complement fixation for immunoglobulin G antibodies
○ Positive serum precipitins (immunoglobulins)
○ *C. immitis* spores detected through immunodiffusion testing of sputum, pus from lesions, and tissue biopsy
○ Presence of antibodies in pleural and joint fluid and a rising serum or body fluid antibody titer (indicate dissemination)
○ Increased white blood cell count
○ Increased eosinophil count
○ Increased erythrocyte sedimentation rate
Imaging
○ Chest X-ray shows bilateral diffuse infiltrates.
Others
○ Abnormal coccidioidin skin test result

Treatment

General
○ Bed rest
○ Symptomatic measures

Medications
○ I.V. fluids
○ Amphotericin B
○ Analgesics

Surgery
○ Excision or drainage of lesions
○ Lobectomy for severe pulmonary lesions

Nursing considerations

Key outcomes

The patient will:
○ be free from pain
○ maintain a patent airway
○ cough effectively.

Nursing interventions

○ Encourage bed rest.
○ Encourage adequate fluid intake.
○ Provide measures to relieve pain and increase comfort.

Monitoring

○ Intake and output
○ Vital signs
○ Sputum color, consistency, and amount
○ Respiratory status

Patient teaching

Be sure to cover:
○ the disorder, diagnosis, and treatment
○ proper hand-washing technique
○ wound care.

Cold injuries

Overview

Description

- Injury caused by overexposure to cold air or water
- Includes localized injuries (frostbite) and systemic injuries (hypothermia)
- Frostbite: superficial or deep; can lead to gangrene
- Hypothermia: core body temperature below 95° F (35° C)

Pathophysiology

- Cold temperature causes ice crystals to form within and around tissue cells.
- Cell membranes rupture and enzymatic activities are interrupted.
- Histamine is released.
- Aggregation of red blood cells results.

Causes

- Prolonged exposure to freezing temperatures
- Prolonged exposure to cold, wet environments
- Administration of large amounts of cold blood

Risk factors

- Lack of insulating body fat
- Substance abuse
- Cardiac disease
- Poverty, homelessness
- Immersion in cold water
- Altered mental state

Incidence

- More common in men than women

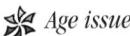 *Age issue*

Patients who are very young or elderly have an increased risk of hypothermia.

Common characteristics

Frostbite
- Initial coldness
- Stinging, burning, throbbing
- Numbness, followed by complete loss of sensation
- Loss of fine-muscle dexterity
- Loss of large-muscle dexterity
- Severe joint pain

Hypothermia
- Severe shivering, slurred speech, and amnesia
- Confusion
- Apathy
- Unresponsiveness, with peripheral cyanosis and muscle rigidity
- Shock
- Cardiopulmonary arrest

Complications

- Renal failure
- Rhabdomyolysis
- Avascular necrosis
- Gangrene
- Severe infection
- Aspiration pneumonia
- Cardiac arrhythmias
- Hypoglycemia or hyperglycemia
- Metabolic acidosis
- Pancreatitis

Assessment

History

- Burning, numbness, tingling, and itching of affected area
- Paresthesia and stiffness while the part is still frozen
- Burning pain when the part thaws

Physical findings

Frostbite
- Superficial — swollen, with a mottled, blue-gray skin color
- Deep — white or yellow until thawed; then turns purplish blue
- Edema, skin blisters, and necrosis
- Skin immobility
- Presence or absence of associated peripheral pulses

Hypothermia
- Mild — severe shivering, slurred speech, and amnesia
- Moderate — unresponsive, with peripheral cyanosis and muscle rigidity
- Severe — appears dead, with no palpable pulse and no audible heart sounds

Test results

Laboratory
- Complete blood count and coagulation profile possibly showing blood loss related to clotting abnormalities
- Elevated serum amylase
- Serum glucose possibly showing hypoglycemia or hyperglycemia
- Liver function studies possibly showing hepatic failure
- Elevated serum corticotropin
- Elevated serum thyroid-stimulating hormone
- Elevated white blood cell count
- Arterial blood gas levels showing acid-base derangements; hypoxia
- Serum electrolytes showing electrolyte derangements

Imaging
- Technetium pertechnetate scanning shows perfusion defects, deep tissue damage, and nonviable bone.
- Doppler and plethysmographic studies locate pulses and show extent of frostbite.

Treatment

General

Frostbite injuries
○ Rapid rewarming of injured part
○ Whirlpool treatments
○ Active range-of-motion exercises
○ Elevation of extremity after rewarming

 Alert

Never rub the injured area because this can aggravate tissue damage. Don't rupture any blebs.

Hypothermia
○ Remove wet clothing
○ Supportive measures
○ Cardiopulmonary resuscitation
○ Administration of oxygen
○ Endotracheal intubation with controlled ventilation
○ Warmed I.V. fluids
○ Treat metabolic acidosis
○ Nothing by mouth until fully alert
○ Warm fluids to drink
○ Rest until rewarmed

Medications

Frostbite injuries
○ Tetanus toxoid
○ Antibiotics
Hypothermia
○ Antiarrhythmics, as needed

Surgery

○ Fasciotomy or amputation for extensive tissue damage

Nursing considerations

Key outcomes
The patient will:
○ maintain adequate ventilation
○ regain skin integrity
○ express feelings of increased comfort
○ maintain a normal body temperature
○ prevent recurrent episodes of hypothermia.

Nursing interventions

Frostbite
○ Remove constrictive clothing and jewelry.
○ Perform rewarming measures.
○ Give prescribed drugs.
○ Never rub the injured area; this aggravates tissue damage.

Hypothermia
○ Remove wet clothing.
○ Maintain airway, breathing, and circulation.
○ Perform rewarming measures.
○ Perform supportive measures, as needed.

Monitoring
○ Core body temperature
○ Vital signs
○ Cardiac status
○ Peripheral vascular circulation

Patient teaching

Be sure to cover:
○ the disorder, diagnosis, and treatment
○ measures to avoid hypothermia
○ complications and when to notify the physician.

Discharge planning
○ Refer the patient to resource and support services.

Colorectal cancer

Overview

Description

- Malignant tumors of colon or rectum almost always adenocarcinomas (about half are sessile lesions of rectosigmoid area; all others are polypoid lesions)
- Slow progression
- Five-year survival rate 50%; potentially curable in 75% of patients if early diagnosis allows resection before nodal involvement
- Second most common visceral neoplasm in United States and Europe

Pathophysiology

- Most lesions of the large bowel are moderately differentiated adenocarcinomas.
- Tumors tend to grow slowly and remain asymptomatic for long periods.
- Tumors in the sigmoid and descending colon undergo circumferential growth and constrict the intestinal lumen.
- Tumors in the ascending colon are usually large at diagnosis and are palpable on physical examination.

Causes

- Unknown

Risk factors

- Excessive intake of saturated animal fat
- Digestive tract diseases
- Over age 40
- History of ulcerative colitis
- Familial polyposis
- Family history of colon cancer
- High-protein, low-fiber diet

Incidence

- Equally distributed among men and women
- Greater in areas of higher economic development

Common characteristics

- Changes in bowel habits
- Symptoms of direct extension to bladder, prostate, ureters, vagina, or sacrum
- Symptoms of local obstruction

Complications

- Abdominal distention and intestinal obstruction as tumor growth encroaches on abdominal organs
- Anemia

Assessment

History

- Right colon tumors: no signs and symptoms in early stages because stool is liquid in that part of colon
- Black, tarry stools
- Abdominal aching, pressure, or dull cramps
- Weakness
- Diarrhea, anorexia, obstipation, weight loss, and vomiting
- Rectal bleeding
- Intermittent abdominal fullness
- Rectal pressure
- Urgent need to defecate on arising

Physical findings

- Abdominal distention or visible masses
- Enlarged abdominal veins
- Enlarged inguinal and supraclavicular nodes
- Abnormal bowel sounds
- Abdominal masses (right-side tumors that usually feel bulky; tumors of transverse portion more easily detected)
- Generalized abdominal tenderness

Test results

Laboratory
- Fecal occult blood test possibly showing blood in stools, a warning sign of rectal cancer
- Carcinoembryonic antigen permitting patient monitoring before and after treatment to detect metastasis or recurrence

Imaging
- Excretory urography verifies bilateral renal function and allows inspection for displacement of the kidneys, ureters, or bladder by a tumor pressing against these structures.
- Barium enema studies use a dual contrast of barium and air and reveal the location of lesions that aren't detectable manually or visually. Barium examination shouldn't precede colonoscopy or excretory urography because barium sulfate interferes with these tests.
- Computed tomography scan allows better visualization if a barium enema yields inconclusive results or if metastasis to the pelvic lymph nodes is suspected.

Diagnostic procedures
- Proctoscopy or sigmoidoscopy permits visualization of the lower GI tract. It can detect up to 66% of colorectal cancers.
- Colonoscopy permits visual inspection and photography of the colon up to the ileocecal valve and provides access for polypectomies and biopsies of suspected lesions.

Other
- Digital rectal examination can be used to detect almost 15% of colorectal cancers; specifically, it can be used to detect suspicious rectal and perianal lesions.

Treatment

General

○ Radiation preoperatively and postoperatively to induce tumor regression
○ High-fiber diet
○ After surgery, avoidance of heavy lifting and contact sports

Medications

○ Chemotherapy for metastasis, residual disease, or recurrent inoperable tumor
○ Analgesics

Surgery

○ Resection or right hemicolectomy for advanced disease; surgery may include resection of the terminal segment of the ileum, cecum, ascending colon, and right half of the transverse colon with corresponding mesentery
○ Right colectomy that includes the transverse colon and mesentery corresponding to midcolic vessels, or segmental resection of the transverse colon and associated midcolic vessels
○ Resection surgery usually limited to the sigmoid colon and mesentery
○ Anterior or low anterior resection (newer method, using a stapler, allows for much lower resections than previously possible)
○ Abdominoperineal resection and permanent sigmoid colostomy required

Nursing considerations

Key outcomes

The patient will:
○ maintain normal fluid volume
○ maintain intact mucous membranes
○ report feeling less pain
○ express increased sense of well-being
○ use support systems and employ coping strategies.

Nursing interventions

○ Provide support and encourage verbalization.
○ Give prescribed drugs.

Monitoring

○ Stools
○ Diet
Postoperative
○ Vital signs
○ Intake and output
○ Hydration and nutritional status
○ Electrolyte levels
○ Wound site
○ Postoperative complications
○ Bowel function
○ Pain control
○ Psychological status

Patient teaching

Be sure to cover:
○ the disease process, treatment, and postoperative course
○ stoma care
○ avoidance of heavy lifting
○ the need for keeping follow-up appointments
○ risk factors and signs of reoccurrence.

Discharge planning

○ Refer the patient to resource and support services.

Common cold

Overview

Description

- Acute, usually afebrile viral infection that causes inflammation of the upper respiratory tract
- Transmission through airborne respiratory droplets or through contact with contaminated objects, including hands
- Accounts for 30% to 50% of time lost from work by adults and 60% to 80% of time lost from school by children, more than any other illness
- Communicable for 2 to 3 days after onset of symptoms
- Usually benign and self-limiting

Pathophysiology

- Rhinoviruses have been found to infect cells by attaching to specific receptors.
- Infiltration with neutrophils, lymphocytes, plasma cells, and eosinophils occurs.
- Mucus-secreting glands become hyperactive and nasal turbinates become engorged. (See *What happens in the common cold.*)

Causes

- Viral infection of the upper respiratory tract passages and consequent mucous membrane inflammation responsible for 90% of cases
- More than 200 viruses, including rhinoviruses, coronaviruses, myxoviruses, adenoviruses, coxsackieviruses, and echoviruses
- Mycoplasma

Incidence

- Most common infectious disease
- More prevalent in children, adolescent boys, and women
- In temperate climates, occurs more often in the colder months
- In the tropics, occurs more often during the rainy season

Common characteristics

- Initial complaints of nasal congestion, headache, and burning, watery eyes, chills, myalgia, arthralgia, malaise, lethargy, sore throat, and a hacking, nonproductive or nocturnal cough
- Most patients afebrile, although fever may occur, especially in children

Complications

- Secondary bacterial infection causing sinusitis, otitis media, pharyngitis, or lower respiratory tract infection

Assessment

History

- Exposure to persons with the common cold
- Sore throat
- Fatigue
- Malaise
- Myalgia
- Fever

Physical findings

- Copious nasal discharge that often irritates the nose
- Increased erythema of nasal and pharyngeal mucous membranes
- Nasal quality to voice
- Excoriated skin around nose

Test results

- There isn't an explicit diagnostic test.

Laboratory

- White blood cell count and differential are within normal limits.

Treatment

General

- Use of humidified inspired air
- Prevention of chilling
- Increased fluid intake
- Rest periods, as needed

Medications

- Acetylsalicylate acid
- Ibuprofen
- Acetaminophen
- Throat lozenges
- Antitussives
- In infants, saline nose drops and mucus aspiration with a bulb syringe
- Vitamin therapy, interferon administration, and experimental vaccines (under investigation)

Nursing considerations

Key outcomes

The patient will:
- express feeling of increased comfort
- cope effectively with illness
- reestablish normal temperature
- have respiratory secretions that remain clear and odorless
- maintain adequate air exchange.

Nursing interventions

- Give prescribed drugs.
- A lubricant on nostrils can decrease irritation.

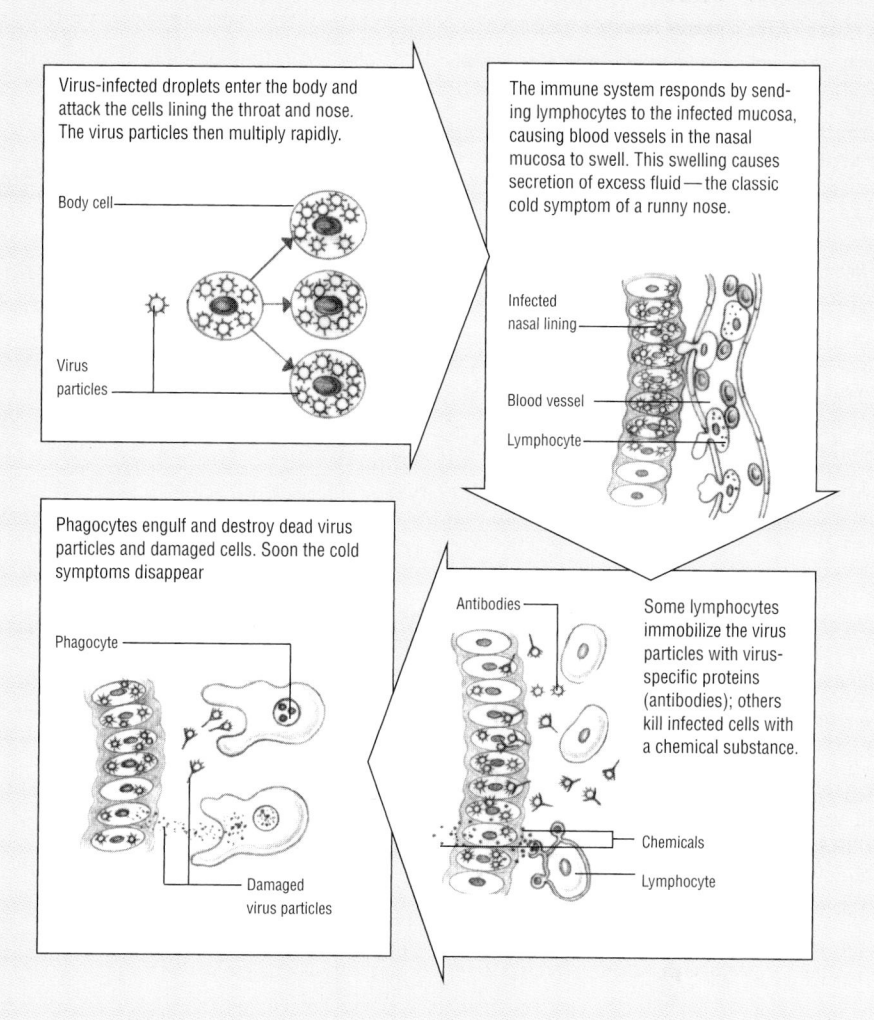

Virus-infected droplets enter the body and attack the cells lining the throat and nose. The virus particles then multiply rapidly.

Body cell

Virus particles

The immune system responds by sending lymphocytes to the infected mucosa, causing blood vessels in the nasal mucosa to swell. This swelling causes secretion of excess fluid — the classic cold symptom of a runny nose.

Infected nasal lining

Blood vessel

Lymphocyte

Phagocytes engulf and destroy dead virus particles and damaged cells. Soon the cold symptoms disappear

Phagocyte

Damaged virus particles

Some lymphocytes immobilize the virus particles with virus-specific proteins (antibodies); others kill infected cells with a chemical substance.

Antibodies

Chemicals

Lymphocyte

○ Relieve throat irritation with sugarless hard candy or cough drops.
○ A warm bath or heating pad can reduce aches and pains.
○ Suggest a hot or cold steam vaporizer to relieve nasal congestion.

Monitoring

○ Body temperature
○ Respiratory status
○ Response to treatment
○ Adverse effects of medication
○ Complications

Patient teaching

Be sure to cover:
○ advice against overuse of nose drops or sprays
○ how to avoid spreading colds
○ proper hand-washing technique.

Discharge planning

○ Refer the patient for medical care if a high fever persists, level of consciousness changes, or significant respiratory symptoms develop.

Complex regional pain syndrome

Overview

Description

- A chronic pain disorder that results from abnormal healing after minor or major injury to a bone, muscle, or nerve
- Also known as *reflex sympathetic dystrophy (RSD/CRPS1)* or *causalgia (CRPS2)*

Pathophysiology

- Abnormal functioning of the sympathetic nervous system that causes development of symptoms commonly disproportionate to the injury's severity
- Interference with normal signals for sensations, temperature, and blood flow possibly caused by impaired communication between the damaged nerves of the sympathetic nervous system and the brain

Causes

- Exact cause unknown

Precipitating factors

- Trauma
- Neurologic disorder
- Herpes zoster infection
- Myocardial infarction
- Musculoskeletal disorder (shoulder rotator cuff injury)
- Malignancy

Incidence

- Can occur at any age but is less common in children
- Reported more commonly in women

Common characteristics

- Severe, constant pain

Complications

- Impaired mobility
- Depression

Assessment

History

- Injury
- Severe pain that worsens after activity

Physical findings

- Altered blood flow, feeling either warm or cool to the touch, with discoloration, sweating, or swelling to the affected extremity
- Skin, hair, and nail changes
- Impaired mobility and weakness
- Muscle wasting (see *Stages of complex regional pain syndrome*)

Test results

Imaging

- Bone X-rays to rule out other conditions

Treatment

General

- Physical therapy
- Activity, as tolerated

Medications

- Anti-inflammatories
- Antidepressants
- Vasodilators
- Analgesics

Surgery

- Nerve or regional blocks

Nursing considerations

Key outcomes

The patient will:

- express increased comfort
- use support systems and develop coping techniques
- demonstrate effective relaxation techniques.

Nursing interventions

- Offer emotional support.
- Apply antiembolism stockings.
- Apply heat or cold therapy.

Monitoring

- Pain control
- Effects of medications
- Blood glucose level

Patient teaching

Be sure to cover:

- the disease and treatment
- relaxation techniques
- medication administration, dosage, and adverse effects.

Discharge planning

- Refer the patient for home therapy.
- Refer the patient to a pain care specialist.
- Refer the patient for psychological counseling and support groups, as indicated.

Stages of complex regional pain syndrome

Complex regional pain syndrome is divided into three stages. The stages aren't always distinct and not all of the signs may be present.

Stage	Duration	Pain, swelling, and immobility	Skin	Hair and nails	Osteoporosis
I (ACUTE)					
	• Symptoms begin within hours, days, or weeks of the injury; this stage lasts several weeks	• Gradual or abrupt onset of severe aching, throbbing, and burning pain at site of injury • Pain may be accompanied by sensitivity to touch, swelling, muscle spasm, stiffness, and limited mobility	• Warm, red, dry skin at onset; changes to bluish and becomes cold and sweaty	• Accelerated hair and nail growth	• Early osteoporosis symptoms
II (SUBACUTE OR DYSTROPHIC)					
	• Lasts 3 to 6 months	• Continuous burning, aching, or throbbing pain that's more severe than stage I • Swelling spreads and changes from soft to brawny and firm • Loss of range of motion, muscle wasting	• Cool, pale, bluish, sweaty	• Altered hair growth; cracked, grooved, or ridged nails	• More apparent osteoporosis
III (CHRONIC OR ATROPHIC)					
	• Lasts more than 6 months	• Pain spreads proximately and may be intractable, but sometimes lessens and stabilizes • More distinct dystrophic changes and irreversible tissue damage • Muscle atrophy and contractures	• Thin, shiny	• Increasingly brittle and ridged nails	• Marked diffuse osteoporosis

Concussion

Overview

Description

- Blow to the head forceful enough to jostle the brain and make it strike the skull
- Acceleration-deceleration injury
- Causes temporary (less than 48 hours) neural dysfunction

Pathophysiology

- Concussion causes diffuse soft tissue damage.
- Inflammation occurs.
- Structural damage is usually minimal.

Causes

- Trauma to the head

Incidence

- More than 2 million instances of concussion per year in the United States
- May occur in up to 20% of football players
- More common in males than in females
- Most commonly affects those ages 15 to 24

Common characteristics

- Short-term loss of consciousness
- Nausea and vomiting
- Dizziness
- Retrograde amnesia
- Erratic behavior
- Headache
- Blurred vision

Complications

- Seizures
- Persistent vomiting
- Intracranial hemorrhage (rare)

What to look for after a concussion

Before the patient's discharge, follow these teaching guidelines: Instruct the caregiver to awaken the patient every 2 hours through the night and to ask his name and whether he can identify the caregiver.

Advise the caregiver to return the patient to the facility immediately if he is difficult to arouse, is disoriented, has seizures, or experiences a persistent or worsening headache, forceful or constant vomiting, blurred vision, changes in personality, abnormal eye movements, a staggering gait, or twitching. If the patient is a child, explain to the parents that some children have no apparent ill effects immediately after a concussion but may grow lethargic or somnolent a few hours later. Teach the patient the signs of postconcussion syndrome — headache, vertigo, anxiety, personality changes, memory loss, and fatigue. Explain that these signs may persist for several weeks.

Assessment

History

- Trauma to head
- Short-term loss of consciousness
- Vomiting
- Antegrade and retrograde amnesia
- Change in level of consciousness (LOC)
- Dizziness
- Nausea
- Severe headache

Physical findings

- Tenderness or hematomas on skull palpation

Test results

Imaging
- Computed tomography scan and magnetic resonance imaging help to rule out fractures and more serious injuries.

Treatment

General

- Observation for changes in mental status
- Clear liquids if vomiting occurs
- Bed rest initially
- Avoidance of contact sports until fully recovered

Medications

- Nonopioid analgesics

Nursing considerations

Key outcomes

The patient will:
- state appropriate interactions for pain relief
- maintain stable vital signs
- identify factors that increase the potential for injury
- recover or be rehabilitated from physical injuries to the extent possible.

Nursing interventions

- Give prescribed drugs, and avoid opioids that may decrease LOC.
- Reorient to time and place, if necessary.

Monitoring

- Vital signs
- Neurologic status
- Pain

Patient teaching

Be sure to cover:
○ the injury, diagnosis, and treatment
○ nonopioid analgesics for a headache and avoidance of products containing aspirin
○ change in LOC or projectile vomiting, which requires a return to the hospital
○ signs and symptoms of increased intracranial pressure.

Discharge planning

○ Arrange for continued observation at home. (See *What to look for after a concussion.*)

Conjunctivitis

Overview

Description

○ Inflammation of palpebral or bulbar conjunctiva
○ Characterized by hyperemia of the conjunctiva
○ Usually spreads rapidly from one eye to the other
○ Usually benign and self-limiting
○ Seldom affects vision
○ If chronic, may signal degenerative changes or damage from repeated acute attacks
○ Acute bacterial conjunctivitis (pink eye) usually lasting about 2 weeks
○ Other viral conjunctival infections lasting 2 to 3 weeks; chronic and may produce severe disability

Pathophysiology

○ Conjunctivitis is an inflammatory response of the conjunctiva that usually begins in one eye and may rapidly spread to the other eye.
○ Vernal conjunctivitis is linked to a severe form of immunoglobulin E-mediated mast cell hypersensitivity reaction.

Causes

○ Allergens
○ Bacteria
○ Viruses
○ Chemical irritations

Recognizing conjunctival papillae

If you see papillae in the conjunctiva of the upper eyelid, your patient may have vernal (allergic) conjunctivitis. These cobblestone bumps are the telltale sign. They result from swollen lymph tissue within the conjunctival membrane.

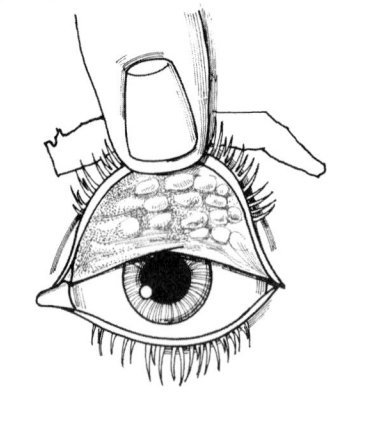

○ Transmission by contaminated towels, washcloths, or one's own hand
○ Systemic diseases, such as erythema multiforme and thyroid disease
○ Candidal infection

Incidence

○ Most common eye disorder in the Western hemisphere
○ Responsible for about 30% of all eye complaints

Common characteristics

○ Reddened conjunctiva
○ Edema of eyelid
○ Pain in the eye
○ Increased lacrimation
○ Burning in eyes

Complications

○ Tic
○ Corneal infiltrates
○ Corneal ulcers
○ Eye loss

Assessment

History

○ Eye pain
○ Photophobia
○ Burning, itching, and sensation of a foreign body in the eye
○ Sore throat and fever, in children

Physical findings

○ Conjunctival hyperemia
○ Discharge
○ Tearing
○ Crust of sticky, mucopurulent discharge (in bacterial conjunctivitis)
○ Profuse, purulent discharge (in gonococcal conjunctivitis)
○ Copious tearing and minimal discharge (in viral conjunctivitis)
○ Conjunctival papillae (in vernal conjunctivitis) (see *Recognizing conjunctival papillae*)
○ Ipsilateral preauricular lymph node enlargement (in viral conjunctivitis)

Test results

Laboratory
○ Culture and sensitivity tests possibly identifying the bacterial pathogen
○ Stained smears of conjunctival scrapings possibly showing mostly monocytes with viral conjunctivitis; polymorphonuclear cells (neutrophils) predominating with bacterial conjunctivitis; and eosinophils predominating with allergic conjunctivitis

Treatment

General

○ Warm compresses
○ Depends on cause

Medications

○ Antibiotics
○ Antivirals
○ Corticosteroids
○ Histamine-1 receptor antagonists
○ Oral antihistamines

Nursing considerations

Key outcomes

The patient will:
○ maintain current health status
○ sustain no harm or injury
○ exhibit no signs of infection
○ regain visual function.

Nursing interventions

○ Apply warm compresses.
○ Apply therapeutic ointment or eyedrops, as ordered.
○ Avoid irrigating the eye to prevent the spread of infection.
○ Notify public health officials if culture results identify *Neisseria gonorrhoeae.*
○ Obtain culture specimens before antibiotic therapy.

Monitoring

○ Response to treatment
○ Signs and symptoms of complications
○ Adverse reactions
○ Visual acuity

Patient teaching

Be sure to cover:
○ proper hand-washing technique
○ instillation of eyedrops and ointments
○ completing the prescribed antibiotics
○ methods for preventing disease transmission
○ importance of avoiding chemical irritants
○ avoiding eye makeup and contact lens use until the infection has cleared.

 Alert

Caution the patient to avoid rubbing the infected eye so that he can prevent the spread of infection to the other eye or to other people.

Corneal abrasion

Overview

Description
○ Scratch on the epithelial surface of the cornea
○ Prognosis usually good with appropriate treatment

Pathophysiology
○ Epithelial layers of cornea are lost due to trauma.
○ Superficial abrasions don't involve the Bowman's membrane.
○ Deep abrasions penetrate the Bowman's membrane.

Causes
○ Eye trauma
○ Foreign bodies embedded under eyelid
○ Contact lenses
○ Chemicals
○ Fingernails
○ Hair brushes
○ Tree branches
○ Dust

Incidence
○ Affects males and females equally

Common characteristics
○ Difficulty opening the eye
○ Eye pain
○ Erythema
○ Feeling of foreign body in eye
○ Increased lacrimation

Complications
○ Corneal erosion
○ Corneal ulceration
○ Permanent vision loss
○ Secondary infection

Assessment

History
○ Eye trauma
○ Prolonged contact lens wear
○ Sensation of foreign body in eye
○ Sensitivity to light
○ Decreased visual acuity
○ Eye pain

Physical findings
○ Redness in eye
○ Increased tearing
○ Possibly a foreign object embedded under the eyelid, uncovered by eyelid eversion
○ Disruption of corneal surface

Test results
Diagnostic procedures
○ Fluorescein staining of the injured area of the cornea appears green when illuminated.
○ Slit-lamp examination discloses the depth of the abrasion.

Treatment

General
○ Eye irrigation (see *Performing eye irrigation*)
○ Removal of foreign body
○ Warm compresses
○ Eye patch for 24 hours
○ Eye protection with potentially dangerous activities

Medications
○ Antibiotic eyedrops or ointment

Surgery
○ Surgical repair of corneal lacerations by an ophthalmologist

Nursing considerations

Key outcomes
The patient will:
○ regain visual function
○ sustain no harm or injury
○ express feelings of increased comfort
○ verbalize feelings and concerns

Nursing interventions
○ Use a flashlight to inspect the cornea.
○ Check visual acuity before treatment begins.
○ If a foreign body is present, irrigate the eye with 0.9% sodium chloride solution.
○ Give prescribed antibiotics and cycloplegics.
○ Instill prescribed topical anesthetics.

 Alert

Never give the patient topical anesthetic drops for self-administration. Abuse of this medication can delay healing, especially if the patient rubs the numb eye and further injures it.

Monitoring
○ Visual acuity
○ Response to treatment

 Alert

Pulse oximeter probes should be applied to the middle, ring, or preferably little finger, but never the index finger, in order to minimize the likeli-

SQUEEZE BOTTLE

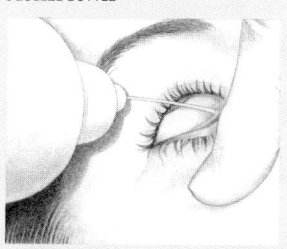

I.V. TUBE

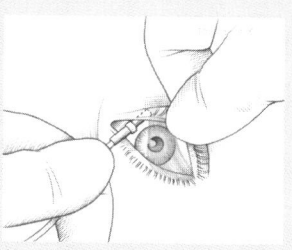

MORGAN LENS

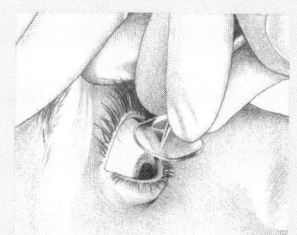

For moderate-volume irrigation — to remove eye secretions, for example — apply sterile ophthalmic irrigant to the eye directly from the squeeze bottle container. Direct the stream at the inner canthus and position the patient so that the stream washes across the cornea and exits at the outer canthus.

For copious irrigation — to treat chemical burns, for example — set up an I.V. bag and tubing without a needle. Use the procedure described for moderate irrigation to flush the eye for at least 15 minutes. Alkali burns may require irrigation for several hours.

Connected to irrigation tubing, a Morgan lens permits continuous lavage and delivers medication to the eye. Use an adapter to connect the lens to the I.V. tubing and the solution container. Begin the irrigation at the prescribed flow rate. To insert the device, ask the patient to look down as you insert the lens under the upper eyelid. Then have her look up as you retract and release the lower eyelid over the lens.

hood of corneal abrasion, especially as patients emerge from anesthesia.

Patient teaching

Be sure to cover:
○ healing process
○ proper instillation of antibiotic eyedrops or ointment
○ effects of untreated corneal infection
○ need to wear safety glasses in the workplace, if appropriate
○ contact lens care and instructions for wear.

Coronary artery disease

Overview

Description

- Heart disease that results from narrowing of coronary arteries over time due to atherosclerosis
- Primary effect: loss of oxygen and nutrients to myocardial tissue because of diminished coronary blood flow

Pathophysiology

- Increased blood levels of low-density lipoprotein (LDL) irritate or damage the inner layer of coronary vessels.
- LDL enters the vessel after damaging the protective barrier, accumulates, and forms a fatty streak.
- Smooth muscle cells move to the inner layer to engulf the fatty substance, produce fibrous tissue, and stimulate calcium deposition.
- Cycle continues, resulting in transformation of the fatty streak into fibrous plaque and, eventually, a coronary artery disease (CAD) lesion evolves.
- Oxygen deprivation forces the myocardium to shift from aerobic to anaerobic metabolism, leading to accumulation of lactic acid and reduction of cellular pH.
- The combination of hypoxia, reduced energy availability, and acidosis rapidly impairs left ventricular function.
- The strength of contractions in the affected myocardial region is reduced as the fibers shorten inadequately, resulting in less force and velocity.
- Wall motion is abnormal in the ischemic area, resulting in less blood being ejected from the heart with each contraction.

Causes

- Atherosclerosis
- Dissecting aneurysm
- Infectious vasculitis
- Syphilis
- Congenital defects
- Coronary artery spasm

Risk factors

- Family history
- High cholesterol level
- Smoking
- Diabetes
- Hormonal contraceptives
- Obesity
- Sedentary lifestyle
- Stress
- Increased homocystine levels

Incidence

- Occurs after age 40
- Men eight times more susceptible than pre-menopausal women
- Risk increased by positive family history
- White men more susceptible than nonwhite men; nonwhite women more susceptible than white women
- Occurs in approximately 11 million Americans

Common characteristics

- Angina

Complications

- Arrhythmias
- Myocardial infarction (MI)
- Heart failure

Assessment

History

- Angina that may radiate to the left arm, neck, jaw, or shoulder blade
- Commonly occurs after physical exertion but may also follow emotional excitement, exposure to cold, or a large meal
- May develop during sleep; symptoms wake the patient
- Nausea
- Vomiting
- Fainting
- Sweating
- Stable angina (predictable and relieved by rest or nitrates)
- Unstable angina (increases in frequency and duration and is more easily induced and generally indicates extensive or worsening disease and, untreated, may progress to MI)
- Crescendo angina (an effort-induced pain that occurs with increasing frequency and with decreasing provocation)
- Prinzmetal's or variant angina pectoris (severe non-effort-produced pain occurs at rest without provocation)

Physical findings

- Cool extremities
- Xanthoma
- Arteriovenous nicking of the eye
- Obesity
- Hypertension
- Positive Levine sign (holding fist to chest)
- Decreased or absent peripheral pulses

Test results

Imaging
- Myocardial perfusion imaging with thallium 201 during treadmill exercise shows ischemic areas of the myocardium, visualized as "cold spots."
- Pharmacologic myocardial perfusion imaging in arteries with stenosis shows decrease in blood flow proportional to the percentage of occlusion.

- Multiple-gated acquisition scanning demonstrates cardiac wall motion and reflects injury to cardiac tissue.

Diagnostic procedures
- Electrocardiography may be normal between anginal episodes. During angina, it may show ischemic changes.
- Exercise testing may be performed to detect ST-segment changes during exercise, indicating ischemia, and to determine a safe exercise prescription.
- Coronary angiography reveals the location and degree of coronary artery stenosis or obstruction, collateral circulation, and the condition of the artery beyond the narrowing.
- Stress echocardiography may show abnormal wall motion.

Treatment

General
- Stress reduction techniques essential, especially if known stressors precipitate pain
- Lifestyle modifications, such as smoking cessation and maintaining ideal body weight (see *Preventing coronary artery disease*)
- Low-fat, low-sodium diet
- Activity restrictions possible
- Regular exercise

Medications
- Aspirin
- Nitrates
- Beta-adrenergic blockers
- Calcium channel blockers
- Antiplatelets
- Antilipemics
- Antihypertensives
- Estrogen replacement therapy

Surgery
- Coronary artery bypass graft
- "Keyhole" or minimally invasive surgery
- Angioplasty
- Endovascular stent placement
- Laser angioplasty
- Atherectomy

Nursing considerations

Key outcomes
The patient will:
- maintain hemodynamic stability
- plan menus appropriate to prescribed diet
- demonstrate understanding of the disease process
- express concern about self-concept, self-esteem, and body image
- express feelings of increased comfort and decreased pain.

Preventing coronary artery disease

Because coronary artery disease is so widespread, prevention is important. Dietary restrictions aimed at reducing the intake of calories (in obesity) and of salt, fats, and cholesterol minimize the risk, especially when supplemented with regular exercise. Abstention from smoking and reduction of stress are also essential.

Other preventive actions include control of hypertension (with diuretics or sympathetic beta-adrenergic blockers), control of elevated serum cholesterol or triglyceride levels (with antilipemics such as HMG-CoA reductase inhibitors, including atorvastatin, pravastatin, or simvastatin), and measures to minimize platelet aggregation and the danger of blood clots (with aspirin, for example).

Nursing interventions
- Ask the patient to grade the severity of his pain on a scale of 1 to 10.
- Keep nitroglycerin available for immediate use. Instruct the patient to call immediately whenever he feels pain and before taking nitroglycerin.
- Observe for signs and symptoms that may signify worsening of condition.
- Perform vigorous chest physiotherapy and guide the patient in pulmonary self-care.

Monitoring
- Vital signs
- Intake and output
- Effectiveness of pain medication during anginal episodes
- Abnormal bleeding and distal pulses following intervention procedures
- Breath sounds
- Chest tube drainage, after surgery
- Cardiac rate and rhythm

Patient teaching

Be sure to cover:
- risk factors for CAD
- avoidance of activities that precipitate episodes of pain
- effective coping mechanisms to deal with stress
- the need to follow the prescribed drug regimen
- low-sodium and low-calorie diet
- the importance of regular, moderate exercise.

Discharge planning
- Refer the patient to a weight-loss program, if needed.
- Refer the patient to a smoking-cessation program, if needed.
- Refer the patient to a cardiac-rehabilitation program, if indicated.

Cor pulmonale

Overview

Description
- Hypertrophy and dilation of the right ventricle secondary to disease affecting the structure or function of the lungs or their vasculature
- Can occur at the end stage of various chronic disorders of the lungs, pulmonary vessels, chest wall, or respiratory control center
- Also called *right-sided heart failure*

Pathophysiology
- An occluded vessel impairs the heart's ability to generate enough pressure.
- Increased blood flow creates pulmonary hypertension.
- Pulmonary hypertension increases the heart's workload.
- To compensate, the right ventricle hypertrophies to force blood through the lungs.

Cor pulmonale: An overview

Although pulmonary restrictive disorders (such as fibrosis or obesity), obstructive disorders (such as bronchitis), or primary vascular disorders (such as recurrent pulmonary emboli) may cause cor pulmonale, these disorders share this common pathway.

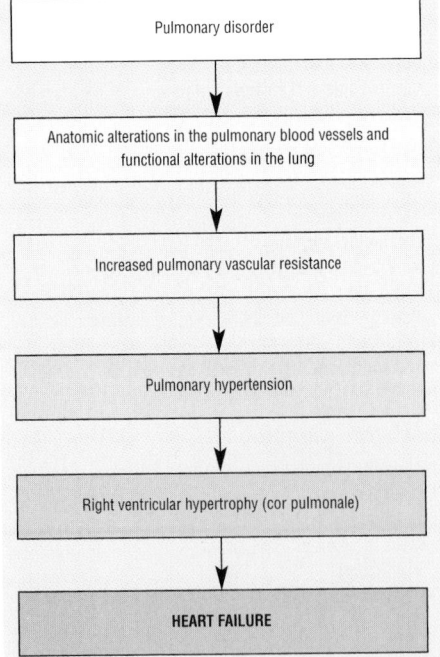

- In response to hypoxia, the bone marrow produces more red blood cells, causing polycythemia.
- The blood's viscosity increases, further aggravating pulmonary hypertension. This increases the right ventricle's workload, causing heart failure. (See *Cor pulmonale: An overview.*)

Causes
- Disorders affecting the pulmonary parenchyma
- Chronic obstructive pulmonary disease
- Bronchial asthma
- Primary pulmonary hypertension
- Vasculitis
- Pulmonary emboli
- External vascular obstruction resulting from a tumor or aneurysm
- Kyphoscoliosis
- Pectus excavatum (funnel chest)
- Muscular dystrophy
- Poliomyelitis
- Obesity
- High altitude

Incidence
- Accounts for 6% to 7% of all types of adult heart disease in the United States
- Affects males and females equally

Common characteristics
- Dyspnea
- Tachypnea
- Signs of heart failure

Complications
- Right- and left-sided heart failure
- Hepatomegaly
- Edema
- Ascites
- Pleural effusions
- Thromboembolism due to polycythemia

Assessment

History
- Dyspnea
- Chronic productive cough
- Fatigue
- Weakness

Physical findings
- Wheezing respirations
- Tachypnea
- Dependent edema
- Distended neck veins
- Enlarged, tender liver
- Hepatojugular reflux
- Tachycardia
- Pansystolic murmur at the lower left sternal border

Test results

Laboratory

○ Arterial blood gas analysis detects decreased partial pressure of arterial oxygen (usually less than 70 mm Hg and rarely more than 90 mm Hg).
○ Hematocrit level is typically over 50%.
○ Serum hepatic tests may show an elevated level of aspartate aminotransferase levels.

Imaging

○ Echocardiography demonstrates right ventricular enlargement.
○ Angiography shows right ventricular enlargement.
○ Chest X-rays reveal large central pulmonary arteries and right ventricular enlargement.
○ Magnetic resonance imaging measures the right ventricular mass, wall thickness, and ejection fraction.
○ Cardiac catheterization measures pulmonary vascular pressures.

Diagnostic procedures

○ Electrocardiography shows arrhythmias, such as premature atrial and ventricular contractions and atrial fibrillation during severe hypoxia, and also right bundle branch block, right axis deviation, prominent P waves, and an inverted T wave in right precordial leads.
○ Pulmonary function studies reflect underlying pulmonary disease.

Other

○ Pulmonary artery catheterization shows increased right ventricular and pulmonary artery pressures.

Treatment

General

○ Low-sodium diet
○ Fluid restrictions
○ Limited activity or bed rest
○ Phlebotomy, if necessary

Medications

○ Digoxin
○ Antibiotics
○ Vasodilators
○ Oxygen

Nursing considerations

Key outcomes

The patient will:
○ maintain adequate cardiac output
○ maintain adequate ventilation
○ use support services and develop coping mechanisms.

Nursing interventions

○ Reposition the patient often.
○ Give prescribed drugs.

Monitoring

○ Vital signs
○ Oxygenation
○ Intake and output
○ Laboratory values
○ Respiratory status

Patient teaching

Be sure to cover:
○ the disorder, diagnosis, and treatment
○ dietary restrictions
○ medication administration and potential adverse reactions.

Discharge planning

○ Refer the patient for home services, as indicated.

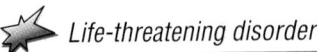 *Life-threatening disorder*

Creutzfeldt-Jakob disease

Overview

Description

○ Rapidly progressive prion disease that attacks the central nervous system (CNS)
○ Manifested by progressive dementia, tremors, and muscle wasting
○ Always fatal
○ Not transmitted by normal casual contact (although iatrogenic transmission can occur)
○ Has a 15- to 20-month incubation period
○ Typical duration is 6 months
○ New variant of Creutzfeldt-Jakob disease emerged in Europe in 1996 (see *Understanding new-variant Creutzfeldt-Jakob disease*)
○ No cure and progress can't be slowed
○ Also known as *CJD*

Pathophysiology

○ CJD is caused by the abnormal accumulation or metabolism of prion proteins.
○ These modified proteins are resistant to proteolytic digestion and aggregate in the brain to produce rod-like particles.
○ The accumulation of these modified cellular proteins results in neuronal degeneration and spongiform changes in brain tissue.

Understanding new-variant Creutzfeldt-Jakob disease

Like conventional Creutzfeldt-Jakob disease (CJD), new-variant CJD (nvCJD) is a rare, fatal neurodegenerative disease. Most cases have been reported in the United Kingdom, and it's most likely caused by exposure to bovine spongiform encephalopathy (BSE), a fatal brain disease in cattle also known as *mad cow disease*. Ingestion of beef products from cattle with BSE is the most probable route of exposure.

NvCJD affects patients at a much younger age than CJD, and the duration of the illness is much longer (14 months versus 6 months).

Regulations have been established in Europe to control outbreaks of BSE in cattle and to prevent contaminated meat from entering the food supply. NvCJD and its relationship with BSE are still being explored by the Centers for Disease Control and Prevention and World Health Organization.

A European commission report released in 2000 placed Canada in the second rank of risk for mad cow disease.

Causes

○ Familial or genetically inherited form
○ Sporadic form of unknown etiology
○ Iatrogenic or acquired form due to inadvertent exposure to CJD-contaminated equipment or material as a result of brain surgery, corneal grafts, or use of human pituitary-derived growth hormones or gonadotropin

Incidence

○ About one case in 1 million people worldwide annually
○ Most cases sporadic, accounting for approximately 85% of all cases
○ Approximately 5% to 15% of cases familial, with an autosomal dominant pattern of inheritance
○ Usually patients over age 55; median age of death in the United States is 68
○ Affects men and women of diverse ethnic backgrounds
○ Most cases in Libya, North Africa, and Slovakia

Common characteristics

○ Rapidly progressive dementia
○ Prominent myoclonus

Complications

○ Severe, progressive dementia
○ CNS abnormalities
○ Death

Assessment

History

○ Mood changes
○ Emotional lability
○ Poor concentration
○ Lethargy
○ Impaired judgment
○ Memory loss
○ Involuntary muscle movements
○ Vision disturbances or other types of hallucinations
○ Gait disturbances

Physical findings

○ Dementia
○ Myoclonus
○ Spasticity
○ Agitation
○ Tremor
○ Clumsiness
○ Ataxia
○ Hypokinesis and rigidity
○ Hyperreflexia

Test results

Laboratory
○ Cerebral spinal fluid (CSF) immunoassay may show abnormal protein species.
○ CSF analysis may show mildly elevated protein level.

Imaging

○ Computed tomography scan and magnetic resonance imaging of the brain may show evidence of generalized cortical atrophy.

Diagnostic procedures

○ EEG may show burst suppression changes in brain wave activity
○ Brain biopsy may show spongiform changes.

Other

○ Autopsy of brain tissue allows definitive diagnosis.

Treatment

General

○ Palliative care to make the patient comfortable and to ease symptoms
○ Well-balanced diet
○ Adequate fluid intake
○ Activity, as tolerated

Medications

○ Amantadine
○ Pramental

Surgery

○ Possible brain biopsy for diagnosis

Nursing considerations

Key outcomes

The patient will:
○ verbalize feelings of anxiety and fear
○ demonstrate effective coping techniques
○ remain free from injury
○ maintain social interaction to the extent possible
○ utilize support systems.

Nursing interventions

○ Assist the patient and his family through the grieving process.
○ Follow standard precautions.
○ Encourage verbalization of concerns and fears.
○ Encourage involvement of the patient and his family in care decisions.

Monitoring

○ Vital signs
○ Intake and output
○ Neurologic status
○ Mental status

Patient teaching

Be sure to cover:
○ the disorder, diagnosis, and supportive treatment
○ prevention of disease transmission
○ effective coping strategies
○ safety precautions.

Discharge planning

○ Refer the patient and his family to CJD support groups.
○ Refer the patient for hospice care, as appropriate.

Crohn's disease

Overview

Description

- ◯ Inflammatory bowel disease that may affect any part of the GI tract but commonly involves the terminal ileum
- ◯ Fifty percent of cases involve colon and small bowel; 33% involve terminal ileum; 10% to 20% involve only colon
- ◯ Extends through all layers of the intestinal wall; may involve regional lymph nodes and mesentery

Pathophysiology

- ◯ Crohn's disease involves slow, progressive inflammation of the bowel.
- ◯ Lymphatic obstruction is caused by enlarged lymph nodes.
- ◯ Edema, mucosal ulceration, fissures, and abscesses occur.
- ◯ Elevated patches of closely packed lymph follicles (Peyer's patches) develop in the small intestinal lining.
- ◯ Fibrosis occurs, thickening the bowel wall and causing stenosis.
- ◯ Inflamed bowel loops adhere to other diseased or normal loops.
- ◯ The diseased bowel becomes thicker, shorter, and narrower.

Causes

- ◯ Exact cause unknown
- ◯ Lymphatic obstruction and infection among contributing factors

Risk factors

- ◯ History of allergies
- ◯ Immune disorders
- ◯ Genetic predisposition — 10% to 20% of patients with the disease have one or more affected relatives; sometimes occurs in monozygotic twins

Incidence

- ◯ Occurs equally in males and females
- ◯ More common in Jewish people
- ◯ Onset usually before age 30

Common characteristics

- ◯ Diarrhea
- ◯ Abdominal pain
- ◯ Weight loss

Complications

- ◯ Anal fistula
- ◯ Perineal abscess
- ◯ Fistulas of the bladder or vagina or to the skin in an old scar area
- ◯ Intestinal obstruction
- ◯ Perforation
- ◯ Nutritional deficiencies caused by malabsorption and maldigestion

Assessment

History

- ◯ Gradual onset of signs and symptoms, marked by periods of remission and exacerbation
- ◯ Fatigue and weakness
- ◯ Fever, flatulence, nausea
- ◯ Steady, colicky, or cramping abdominal pain that usually occurs in the right lower abdominal quadrant
- ◯ Diarrhea that may worsen after emotional upset or ingestion of poorly tolerated foods, such as milk, fatty foods, and spices
- ◯ Weight loss

Physical findings

- ◯ Possible soft or semiliquid stool, usually without gross blood
- ◯ Right lower abdominal quadrant tenderness or distention
- ◯ Possible abdominal mass, indicating adherent loops of bowel
- ◯ Hyperactive bowel sounds
- ◯ Bloody diarrhea
- ◯ Perianal and rectal abscesses

Test results

Laboratory
- ◯ Occult blood in stools
- ◯ Decreased hemoglobin and hematocrit levels
- ◯ Increased white blood cell count and erythrocyte sedimentation rate
- ◯ Decreased serum potassium, calcium, magnesium, and hemoglobin (Hb)
- ◯ Hypoglobulinemia from intestinal protein loss
- ◯ Vitamin B_{12} and folate deficiency

Imaging
- ◯ Small bowel X-rays may show irregular mucosa, ulceration, and stiffening.
- ◯ Barium enema reveals the string sign (segments of stricture separated by normal bowel) and may also show fissures and narrowing of the lumen.

Diagnostic procedures
- ◯ Sigmoidoscopy and colonoscopy show patchy areas of inflammation and may also reveal the characteristic coarse irregularity (cobblestone appearance) of the mucosal surface.
- ◯ Biopsy reveals granulomas in up to half of all specimens.

Treatment

General

- ◯ Stress reduction
- ◯ Avoidance of foods that worsen diarrhea

- Avoidance of raw fruits and vegetables if blockage occurs
- Adequate caloric, protein, and vitamin intake
- Parenteral nutrition, if necessary
- Reduced physical activity

Medications

- Corticosteroids
- Immunosuppressant agents
- Sulfonamides
- Anti-inflammatory agents
- Antibacterial and antiprotozoal agents
- Antidiarrheals
- Opioids
- Vitamin supplements
- Antispasmodics

Surgery

- Indicated for acute intestinal obstruction
- Colectomy with ileostomy

Nursing considerations

Key outcomes

The patient will:
- maintain adequate caloric intake
- maintain normal fluid volume
- regain normal bowel movements
- verbalize understanding of the disease process and treatment regimen
- exhibit adequate coping mechanisms and seek appropriate sources of support.

Nursing interventions

- Provide emotional support to the patient and his family.
- Provide meticulous skin care after each bowel movement.
- Schedule patient care to include rest periods throughout the day.
- Assist with dietary modification.
- Give prescribed iron supplements and blood transfusions.
- Give prescribed analgesics.

Monitoring

- Abdominal pain and distention
- Vital signs
- Intake and output, including amount of stool
- Daily weight
- Serum electrolytes and glucose, Hb, and stools for occult blood
- Signs of infection or obstruction
- Bleeding, especially with steroid use

Patient teaching

Be sure to cover:
- information about the disease, symptoms, and complications
- ordered diagnostic tests and pretest guidelines
- the importance of adequate rest
- how the patient can identify and reduce sources of stress
- prescribed dietary changes
- prescribed medications, administration, and possible adverse reactions.

Discharge planning

- Refer the patient to a smoking-cessation program, if appropriate.
- Refer the patient to enterostomal therapist, if indicated.

Croup

Overview

Description

- Viral infection causing severe inflammation and obstruction of the upper airway
- Childhood disease manifested by acute laryngotracheobronchitis (most commonly), laryngitis, acute spasmodic laryngitis, and febrile rhinitis
- Incubation period about 3 to 6 days; contagious while febrile
- Recovery usually complete

Pathophysiology

- Viral invasion of the laryngeal mucosa leads to inflammation, hyperemia, edema, epithelial necrosis, and shedding.
- This leads to irritation and cough, reactive paralysis and continuous stridor, or collapsible supraglottic or inspiratory stridor and respiratory distress.
- A thin, fibrinous membrane covers the mucosa of the epiglottis, larynx, and trachea. (See *How croup affects the upper airways.*)

Causes

- Parainfluenza viruses
- Adenoviruses
- Respiratory syncytial virus
- Influenza viruses
- Measles viruses
- Bacteria (pertussis and diphtheria)

Incidence

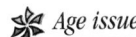 *Age issue*

Occurs mainly in children ages 3 months to 5 years

- Affects boys more commonly than girls
- Usually occurs in late autumn and early winter

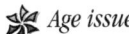 *Age issue*

Acute spasmodic laryngitis affects children between ages 1 and 3, particularly those with allergies

Common characteristics

- Sharp, barklike, or brassy cough that progresses to stridor
- Hoarse or muffled vocal sounds

Complications

- Airway obstruction
- Respiratory failure
- Dehydration
- Ear infection
- Pneumonia
- Hypoxia
- Hypercapnia

Assessment

History

- Recent upper respiratory infection

Laryngotracheobronchitis
- Fever and breathing problems that usually occur at night
- Difficulty exhaling

Laryngitis in children
- Mild sore throat
- Cough
- Marked hoarseness (rare)
- No respiratory distress

Laryngitis in infants
- Respiratory distress

Acute spasmodic laryngitis
- Mild to moderate hoarseness
- Nasal discharge
- Characteristic cough and noisy inspiration
- Anxiety
- Increased dyspnea
- Transient cyanosis

Physical findings

- Rhinorrhea
- Use of accessory muscles
- Nasal flaring
- Barklike cough
- Hoarse, muffled vocal sounds
- Inspiratory stridor
- Diminished breath sounds

Laryngotracheobronchitis
- Edema of bronchi and bronchioles
- Decreased breath sounds
- Expiratory rhonchi
- Scattered crackles

Laryngitis
- Suprasternal and intercostal retractions
- Inspiratory stridor
- Dyspnea, tachypnea
- Diminished breath sounds
- Severe dyspnea and exhaustion in later stages

Acute spasmodic laryngitis
- Labored breathing with retractions
- Clammy skin
- Rapid pulse rate

Test results

Laboratory
- Throat cultures show bacteria and sensitivity to antibiotics.

Imaging
- ○ Neck X-ray may show upper airway narrowing and edema in subglottic folds; helps to differentiate croup from bacterial epiglottitis.
- ○ Computed tomography scan helps differentiate between croup, epiglottitis, and noninfection.

Diagnostic procedures
- ○ Laryngoscopy may reveal inflammation and obstruction in epiglottal and laryngeal areas.

Treatment

General
- ○ Home or hospitalized care
- ○ Humidification during sleep
- ○ Intubation if other means of preventing respiratory failure are unsuccessful
- ○ Diet, as tolerated
- ○ Parenteral fluids, if required
- ○ Rest periods

Medications
- ○ Oxygen therapy, as needed
- ○ Antipyretics
- ○ Antibiotics if cause is bacterial
- ○ Aerosolized racemic epinephrine for moderately severe croup
- ○ Corticosteroids for acute laryngotracheobronchitis (controversial)

Surgery
- ○ Tracheostomy (rare)

Nursing considerations

Key outcomes
The patient will:
- ○ maintain adequate ventilation
- ○ maintain normal temperature
- ○ maintain a patent airway
- ○ use effective coping strategies
- ○ verbalize understanding of the disorder.

Nursing interventions
- ○ Give prescribed drugs.
- ○ Provide quiet diversional activities.
- ○ Engage parents in the care of the infant or child.
- ○ Position an infant in an infant seat or prop him up with a pillow.
- ○ Position an older child in Fowler's position.
- ○ Provide humidification.
- ○ Avoid mild-based fluids if the patient has thick mucus or swallowing difficulties.
- ○ Provide frequent mouth care.
- ○ Isolate patients for respiratory syncytial virus and parainfluenza infections.
- ○ Use sponge baths and hypothermia blanket, as ordered, for temperatures above 102° F (38.9° C).

How croup affects the upper airways

In croup, inflammatory swelling and spasms constrict the larynx, thereby reducing airflow. This cross-sectional drawing (from chin to chest) shows the upper airway changes caused by croup. Inflammatory changes almost completely obstruct the larynx (which includes the epiglottis) and significantly narrow the trachea.

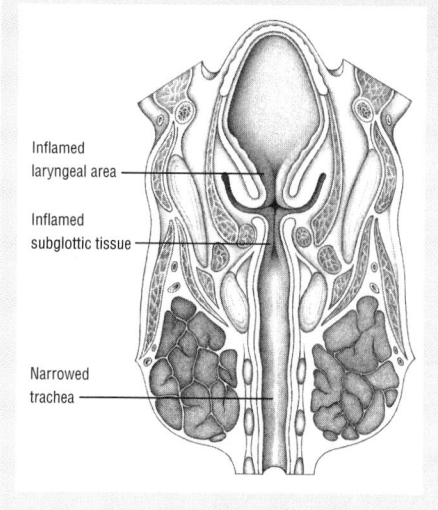

Inflamed laryngeal area

Inflamed subglottic tissue

Narrowed trachea

Monitoring
- ○ Vital signs
- ○ Intake and output
- ○ Respiratory status
- ○ Signs and symptoms of dehydration

Patient teaching

Be sure to cover:
- ○ the disorder, diagnosis, and treatment
- ○ medications and possible adverse reactions
- ○ when to notify the physician
- ○ humidification
- ○ hydration
- ○ signs and symptoms of ear infection
- ○ signs and symptoms of pneumonia.

Cryptococcosis

Overview

Description

○ Yeast infection that usually begins as asymptomatic pulmonary infection in patient who presents with meningoencephalitis on diagnosis
○ Fungal infection also known as *torulosis* and *European blastomycosis*

Pathophysiology

○ Small granulomas and cysts in the cerebral cortex and, later, in deep cerebral tissues produce a minimal inflammatory response.
○ In chronic cases, dense basilar arachnoiditis occurs.
○ Lung lesions with intense granulomatous inflammation occur.

Causes

○ Airborne fungus *Cryptococcus neoformans* found in dust particles contaminated by pigeon stool
○ Transmission by inhalation of cryptococci

Incidence

○ Prevalent in immunocompromised patients and those taking immunosuppressant drugs
○ Increasing, especially in patients with acquired immunodeficiency syndrome

Common characteristics

○ Disseminates to extrapulmonary sites, including the central nervous system (CNS), skin, bones, prostate gland, liver, and kidneys
○ Without treatment, leads to CNS infection and death
○ Mortality dramatically reduced with treatment; neurologic deficits, such as paralysis and hydrocephalus, not necessarily reduced with treatment

Complications

○ Optic atrophy
○ Ataxia
○ Hydrocephalus
○ Deafness
○ Paralysis
○ Organic mental syndrome
○ Personality changes
○ Coma
○ Death

Assessment

History

○ Human immunodeficiency virus infection or another immunosuppressive disorder
○ Usually asymptomatic but patient may complain of dull chest pain and cough producing slight amount of white, blood-streaked sputum

Physical findings

○ Progressively severe frontal and temporal headache
○ Diplopia, blurred vision, papilledema
○ Tinnitus, dizziness, ataxia, and aphasia
○ Vomiting
○ Memory changes, inappropriate behavior, irritability, and psychosis
○ Facial weakness
○ Hyperactive reflexes and seizures in the late stage
○ Pain in the long bones, skull, spine, and joints
○ Red facial papules and other skin abscesses, with or without ulceration
○ Rarely, pleural friction rub or crackles
○ Photophobia

Test results

Imaging
○ Chest X-ray or computed tomography scan of the chest reveals lesions in pulmonary cryptococcosis.
Laboratory
○ Analysis or cultures of the sputum, urine, prostatic secretions, or bone marrow aspirate shows *C. neoformans*
○ Tissue or neural biopsy shows myriad cryptococci
○ India ink preparation of cerebrospinal fluid (CSF) diagnosing CNS infection when *C. neoformans* is detected
○ Positive blood cultures only in severe infection
○ Elevated antigen titer in serum and CSF in disseminated infection
○ Elevated protein levels and white blood cell count in CNS infection
○ Moderately decreased CSF glucose levels decreased in about 50% of patients
Other
○ Lumbar puncture shows increased CSF pressure

Treatment

General

○ Early treatment for cryptococcal disease

Medications

○ Combination of antifungal antibiotics amphotericin B and flucytosine, or amphotericin B alone

Nursing considerations

Key outcomes

The patient will:
○ be free from pain
○ be free from injury
○ maintain patent airway
○ increase activity, as tolerated.

Nursing interventions

○ Give prescribed drugs.
○ Before therapy, draw serum for testing to determine electrolyte levels and baseline renal status.

- Observe for adverse effects such as diarrhea.
- Evaluate the need for long-term venous access for administering amphotericin B.
- Provide psychological support to help the patient cope with long-term treatment.
- If vision loss occurs, provide a safe environment.
- Encourage verbalization and provide support.

Monitoring

- Vital signs
- Neurologic checks
- Headache, vomiting, and nuchal rigidity
- Urine output
- Blood urea nitrogen, creatinine levels, and complete blood count results
- Urinalysis results
- Magnesium and potassium levels and hepatic function test results
- Blood levels of flucytosine

Patient teaching

Be sure to cover:
- the disorder and treatment
- medication therapy, including dosage, desired drug actions, adverse effects, and need for long-term treatment.

Discharge planning

- Urge the patient to return for follow-up care and evaluation every few months for 1 year.
- Refer the patient for resource and support services, as needed.

Cryptorchidism

Overview

Description

- Congenital disorder in which one or both testes fail to descend into the scrotum, remaining in the abdomen or inguinal canal or at the external ring
- May be bilateral, but more commonly affects the right testis (see *Varieties of cryptorchidism*)

Pathophysiology

- In the male fetus, testosterone normally stimulates the formation of the gubernaculum. A fibromuscular band connects the testes to the scrotal floor.
- This band probably helps pull the testes into the scrotum by shortening as the fetus grows.
- Thus, cryptorchidism may result from inadequate testosterone levels or a defect in the testes or the gubernaculum.
- Because the testis is maintained at a higher temperature, spermatogenesis is impaired, leading to reduced fertility.

- True undescended testes remain along the path of normal descent, while ectopic testis deviate from that path.

Causes

- Hormonal factors
- Testosterone deficiency
- Structural factors
- Genetic predisposition

Incidence

- Occurs in 30% of premature male neonates, but in only 3% of those born at term
- In about 80% of affected infants, the testes descend spontaneously during the first year; in the rest, the testes may descend later

Common characteristics

- Testis on the affected side not palpable in the scrotum; underdeveloped scrotum (unilateral cryptorchidism)
- Scrotum enlarged on the unaffected side
- Infertility

Varieties of cryptorchidism

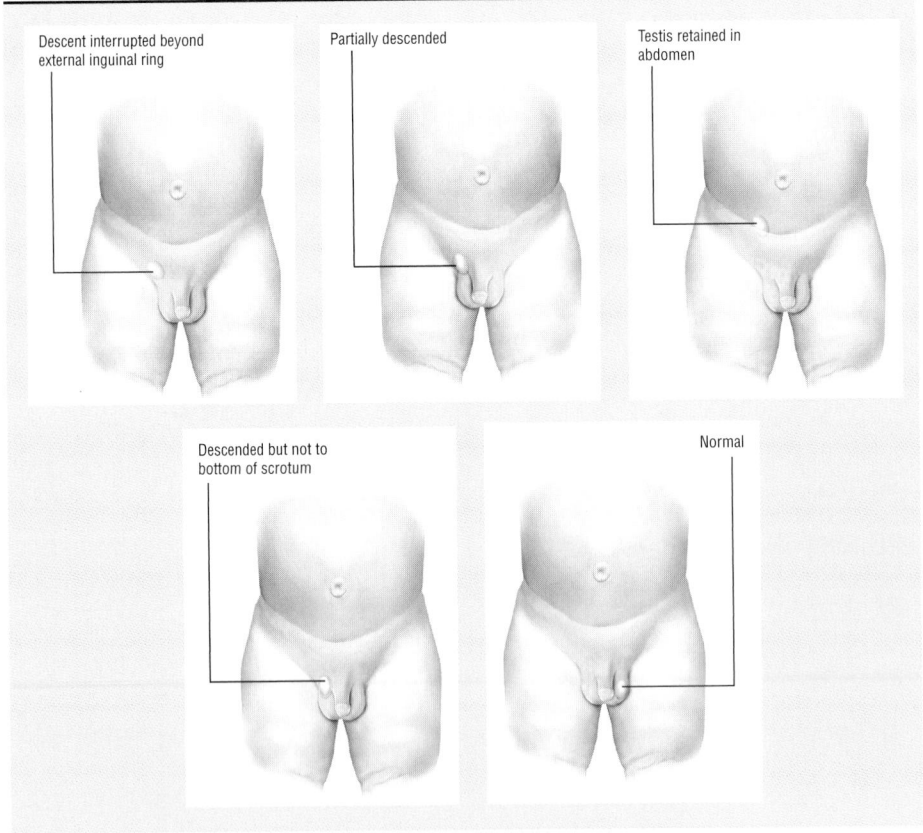

Descent interrupted beyond external inguinal ring

Partially descended

Testis retained in abdomen

Descended but not to bottom of scrotum

Normal

Complications

○ Sterility
○ Increased risk for testicular cancer
○ Increased vulnerability of the testes to trauma

Assessment

Physical findings

○ Nonpalpable testes
○ Underdeveloped scrotum

Test results

Laboratory
○ Buccal smear (cells from oral mucosa) determines genetic sex (a male sex chromatin pattern).
○ Serum gonadotropin confirms the presence of testes by showing presence of circulating hormone.
Other
○ Physical examination

Treatment

Medications

○ Human chorionic gonadotropin

Surgery

○ Orchiopexy

Nursing considerations

Key outcomes

The patient will:
○ express or demonstrate feelings of increased comfort
○ be free from complications.

Nursing interventions

○ Encourage the parents of the child with undescended testes to express their concern about his condition.
○ Tell the parents that a rubber band may be taped to the patient's thigh for about 1 week after surgery to keep the testis in place. Explain that his scrotum may swell but shouldn't be painful.

Monitoring

After surgery
○ Vital signs
○ Intake and output
○ Operative site

Patient teaching

Be sure to cover:
○ the disorder, treatment, and effect on reproduction
○ surgery or medications prescribed.

Cushing's syndrome

Overview

Description

- Clinical manifestations of glucocorticoid excess, particularly cortisol
- May also reflect excess secretion of mineralocorticoids and androgens
- Classified as primary, secondary, or iatrogenic, depending on etiology
- Prognosis dependent on early diagnosis, identification of underlying cause, and effective treatment

Pathophysiology

- A loss of normal feedback inhibition by cortisol occurs.
- Elevated levels of cortisol don't suppress hypothalamic and anterior pituitary secretion of corticotropin-releasing hormone and adrenocorticotropic hormone (ACTH).
- The result is excessive levels of circulating cortisol.

Causes

- Pituitary microadenoma
- Excess production of corticotropin
- Corticotropin-producing tumor in another organ
- Chronic use of synthetic glucocorticoids or corticotropin
- Cortisol-secreting adrenal tumor

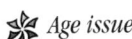 *Age issue*

In neonates, the usual cause of Cushing's syndrome is adrenal carcinoma.

Incidence

- More common in females than in males
- Can affect a person at any age

Common characteristics

- Adiposity of the face, neck, and trunk
- Purple striae on the skin
- Truncal weight gain
- Glucose intolerance

Complications

- Osteoporosis and pathologic fractures
- Peptic ulcer
- Dyslipidemia
- Impaired glucose tolerance
- Diabetes mellitus
- Frequent infections
- Slow wound healing
- Suppressed inflammatory response
- Hypertension
- Ischemic heart disease; heart failure
- Menstrual disturbances
- Sexual dysfunction
- Psychiatric problems, ranging from mood swings to frank psychosis

Assessment

History

- Use of synthetic steroids
- Fatigue
- Muscle weakness
- Sleep disturbances
- Polyuria
- Thirst
- Frequent infections
- Water retention
- Amenorrhea
- Decreased libido
- Irritability; emotional instability
- Symptoms resembling those of hyperglycemia
- Impotence
- Headache

Physical findings

- Thin hair
- Moon-shaped face
- Hirsutism
- A buffalo-humplike back
- Thin extremities
- Muscle wasting and weakness
- Petechiae, ecchymoses, and purplish striae
- Delayed wound healing
- Swollen ankles
- Hypertension
- Central obesity
- Acne

Test results

Laboratory
- Elevated salivary free cortisol
- Decreased ACTH in adrenal disease and increase in excess pituitary or ectopic secretion of ACTH
- Blood chemistry may show hypernatremia, hypokalemia, hypocalcemia, and elevated blood glucose
- Elevated urinary free cortisol
- Elevated serum cortisol in the morning
- Glycosuria

Imaging
- Ultrasonography, computed tomography scan, and magnetic resonance imaging may show the location of a pituitary or adrenal tumor.

Diagnostic procedures
- A low-dose dexamethasone suppression test shows failure of plasma cortisol levels to be suppressed.

Treatment

General

○ Management to restore hormone balance and reverse Cushing's syndrome, including radiation, drug therapy, or surgery
○ High-protein, high-potassium, low-calorie, low-sodium diet
○ Activity, as tolerated

Medications

○ Aminoglutethimide
○ Antifungal agents
○ Antihypertensives
○ Diuretics
○ Glucocorticoids
○ Potassium supplements
○ Antineoplastic, antihormone agents

 Alert

Glucocorticoid administration on the morning of surgery can help prevent acute adrenal insufficiency during surgery. Cortisol therapy is essential during and after surgery to help the patient tolerate the physiologic stress caused by removal of the pituitary or adrenal glands.

Surgery

○ Possible hypophysectomy or pituitary irradiation
○ Bilateral adrenalectomy
○ Excision of nonendocrine, corticotropin-producing tumor, followed by drug therapy

Nursing considerations

Key outcomes

The patient will:
○ maintain skin integrity
○ remain free from infection
○ perform activities of daily living as tolerated within the confines of the disorder
○ express positive feelings about self
○ express understanding of disorder.

Nursing interventions

○ Give prescribed drugs.
○ Consult a dietitian.
○ Use protective measures to reduce the risk of infection.
○ Use meticulous hand-washing technique.
○ Schedule adequate rest periods.
○ Institute safety precautions.
○ Provide meticulous skin care.
○ Encourage verbalization of feelings.
○ Offer emotional support.
○ Help to develop effective coping strategies.

With transsphenoidal approach to hypophysectomy

○ Keep the head of the bed elevated at least 30 degrees.
○ Maintain nasal packing.
○ Provide frequent mouth care.
○ Avoid activities that increase intracranial pressure (ICP).

Monitoring

○ Vital signs
○ Intake and output
○ Daily weights
○ Serum electrolyte results

After bilateral adrenalectomy and hypophysectomy

○ Neurologic and behavioral status
○ Severe nausea, vomiting, and diarrhea
○ Bowel sounds
○ Adrenal hypofunction
○ Increased ICP
○ Hypopituitarism
○ Transient diabetes insipidus
○ Hemorrhage and shock

After transsphenoidal approach to hypophysectomy

○ Cerebrospinal fluid leak

Patient teaching

Be sure to cover:
○ the disorder, diagnosis, and treatment
○ medications and potential adverse reactions
○ when to notify the physician
○ lifelong steroid replacement
○ signs and symptoms of adrenal crisis
○ medical identification bracelet
○ prevention of infection
○ stress reduction strategies.

Discharge planning

○ Refer the patient to a mental health professional for additional counseling, if necessary.

Cystic fibrosis

Overview

Description

- Chronic, progressive, inherited, incurable disease affecting exocrine (mucus-secreting) glands
- Transmitted as an autosomal recessive trait
- Genetic mutation that involves chloride transport across epithelial membranes (more than 100 specific mutations of the gene identified)
- Characterized by major aberrations in sweat gland, respiratory, and GI functions
- Accounts for almost all cases of pancreatic enzyme deficiency in children
- Clinical effects apparent soon after birth or take years to develop
- Death typically from pneumonia, emphysema, or atelectasis

Pathophysiology

- The viscosity of bronchial, pancreatic, and other mucous gland secretions increases, obstructing glandular ducts.
- The accumulation of thick, tenacious secretions in the bronchioles and alveoli causes respiratory changes, eventually leading to severe atelectasis and emphysema.
- The disease also causes characteristic GI effects in the intestines, pancreas, and liver.
- Obstruction of the pancreatic ducts results in a deficiency of trypsin, amylase, and lipase. This prevents the conversion and absorption of fat and protein in the intestinal tract and interferes with the digestion of food and absorption of fat-soluble vitamins.
- In the pancreas, fibrotic tissue, multiple cysts, thick mucus, and fat replace the acini, producing signs of pancreatic insufficiency.

Causes

- Autosomal recessive mutation of gene on chromosome 7
- Causes of symptoms: increased viscosity of bronchial, pancreatic, and other mucous gland secretions and consequent destruction of glandular ducts

Incidence

- Most common fatal genetic disease of white children
- Twenty-five percent chance of transmission with each pregnancy when both parents are carriers of the recessive gene
- Highest in people of northern European ancestry
- Less common in Blacks, Native Americans, and people of Asian ancestry
- Equally common in both sexes

Common characteristics

- Wheezy respirations
- Dry, nonproductive, paroxysmal cough

- Dyspnea
- Poor weight gain

Complications

- Bronchiectasis
- Pneumonia
- Atelectasis
- Dehydration
- Distal intestinal obstructive syndrome
- Malnutrition
- Gastroesophageal reflux
- Cor pulmonale
- Hepatic disease
- Diabetes
- Arthritis
- Biliary disease
- Clotting problems
- Retarded bone growth
- Delayed sexual development
- Azoospermia in males
- Secondary amenorrhea in females
- Electrolyte imbalances
- Cardiac arrhythmias
- Potentially fatal shock
- Death

Assessment

History

- Recurring bronchitis and pneumonia
- Nasal polyps and sinusitis
- Wheezing
- Dry, nonproductive cough
- Shortness of breath
- Abdominal distention, vomiting, constipation
- Frequent, bulky, foul-smelling, and pale stool with a high fat content
- Poor weight gain
- Poor growth
- Ravenous appetite
- Hematemesis

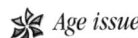 *Age issue*

Neonates may exhibit meconium ileus and develop symptoms of intestinal obstruction: abdominal distention, vomiting, constipation, dehydration, and electrolyte imbalance.

Physical findings

- Wheezy respirations
- Dry, nonproductive, paroxysmal cough
- Dyspnea
- Tachypnea
- Bibasilar crackles and hyperresonance
- Barrel chest
- Cyanosis, and clubbing of the fingers and toes
- Distended abdomen
- Thin extremities

- Sallow skin with poor turgor
- Delayed sexual development
- Neonatal jaundice
- Hepatomegaly
- Rectal prolapse
- Failure to thrive

Test results

Laboratory
- Sweat test reveals sodium and chloride values
- Stool specimen analysis shows absence of trypsin
- Deoxyribonucleic acid testing shows presence of the delta F 508 deletion
- Liver enzyme tests may show hepatic insufficiency
- Sputum culture may show such organisms as *Pseudomonas* and *Staphylococcus*
- Decreased serum albumin level
- Serum electrolytes may show hypochloremia and hyponatremia
- Arterial blood gas shows hypoxemia

Imaging
- Chest X-rays may show early signs of lung obstruction.
- High-resolution chest computed tomography scan shows bronchial wall thickening, cystic lesions, and bronchiectasis.

Diagnostic procedures
- Sweat tests using pilocarpine solution show positive results.
- Pulmonary function tests show decreased vital capacity, elevated residual volume, and decreased forced expiratory volume in 1 second.

Treatment

General
- Based on organ systems involved
- Chest physiotherapy, nebulization, and breathing exercises several times per day
- Postural drainage
- Gene therapy (experimental)
- Annual influenza vaccination
- Salt supplements
- High-fat, high-protein, high-calorie diet
- Activity, as tolerated

Medications
- Dornase alfa, a pulmonary enzyme given by aerosol nebulizer
- Antibiotics
- Oxygen therapy, as needed
- Oral pancreatic enzymes
- Bronchodilators
- Prednisone
- Vitamin A, D, E, and K supplements

Surgery
- Heart-lung transplantation

Nursing considerations

Key outcomes
The patient will:
- maintain a patent airway and adequate ventilation
- consume adequate calories daily
- use a support system to assist with coping
- express an understanding of the illness.

Nursing interventions
- Give prescribed drugs.
- Administer pancreatic enzymes with meals and snacks.
- Perform chest physiotherapy and postural drainage.
- Administer oxygen therapy, as needed.
- Provide a well-balanced, high-calorie, high-protein diet; include adequate fats.
- Provide vitamin A, D, E, and K supplements, if indicated.
- Ensure adequate oral fluid intake.
- Provide exercise and activity periods.
- Encourage breathing exercises.
- Provide the young child with play periods.
- Enlist the help of the physical therapy department and play therapists, if available.
- Provide emotional support.
- Include family members in all phases of the child's care.

Monitoring
- Vital signs
- Intake and output
- Daily weight
- Hydration
- Pulse oximetry
- Respiratory status

Patient teaching

Be sure to cover:
- the disorder, diagnosis, and treatment
- medications and potential adverse reactions
- when to notify the physician
- aerosol therapy
- chest physiotherapy
- signs and symptoms of infection
- complications.

Discharge planning
- Refer family members for genetic counseling, as appropriate.
- Refer the patient and his family to a local support group such as the Cystic Fibrosis Foundation.

Cytomegalovirus infection

Overview

Description
- A member of the herpesvirus group
- Also called *generalized salivary gland disease* and *cytomegalic inclusion disease*

Pathophysiology
- Cytomegalovirus (CMV) is found in the saliva, urine, semen, breast milk, feces, blood, and vaginal and cervical secretions of infected people. It can be detected in body fluids for weeks or months after infection.
- CMV usually remains latent, but reactivation occurs when T-lymphocyte-mediated immunity is compromised, as in organ transplantation, lymphoid neoplasms, and certain acquired immunodeficiencies.
- CMV spreads through the body in lymphocytes or mononuclear cells to the lungs, liver, GI tract, eyes, and central nervous system (CNS), typically producing inflammatory reactions.

Causes
- Results from a deoxyribonucleic acid virus belonging to the herpes family
- Transmitted by human contact; once infected, a person carries CMV for life
- Transmission through direct contact with secretions and excretions, through blood transfusions, transplacentally, and through transplanted organs
- May be transmitted in semen during homosexual activity (such transmission not yet proved in heterosexual men)

Incidence
- Occurs worldwide
- Occurs in approximately 30% to 50% of acquired immunodeficiency syndrome patients
- One of the most opportunistic pathogens in patients infected with human immunodeficiency virus

Common characteristics
- Mild fatigue, myalgia, and headache or no clinical symptoms

Complications
- Pneumonia
- Hepatitis
- Ulceration of the GI tract and esophagus
- Retinitis
- Encephalopathy

Neonatal complications
- Stillbirth
- Neonatal retinitis
- Microcephaly
- Mental retardation
- Seizures
- Hearing loss
- Thrombocytopenia
- Hemolytic anemia

Assessment

History
- Immunosuppressive condition

Physical findings
- Fever common
- Lethargy
- In immunocompetent patient with CMV mononucleosis, 3 or more weeks of irregular high fever may be the only finding
- Tachypnea
- Dyspnea
- Cyanosis
- Cough
- Jaundice
- Spider angiomas
- Hepatomegaly
- Splenomegaly
- In infants, CNS damage (mental retardation, hearing loss, seizures), jaundice, petechial rash, respiratory distress

Test results
Laboratory
- Isolating the virus or demonstrating increasing serologic titers by complement fixation studies, hemagglutination inhibition antibody tests and, in congenital infections, indirect immunofluorescent tests for CMV immunoglobulin M antibody allowing diagnosis

Imaging
- Chest X-ray reveals bilateral, diffuse, white infiltrates.
- Computed tomography scan or magnetic resonance imaging shows CNS involvement.

Diagnostic procedures
- Endoscopy shows GI involvement.
- Fundoscopy may show retinitis.

Treatment

General
- Currently no treatment for CMV infection in the healthy individual
- Antiviral therapy that's now being evaluated in neonates
- Vaccines that are still in the research and development stage
- Rest, as needed

Medications
- Antiviral agents
- Immune serums

Nursing considerations

Key outcomes

The patient will:
- maintain normal temperature
- maintain adequate caloric intake
- demonstrate skill in conserving energy while carrying out daily activities to tolerance level
- verbally report having an increased energy level
- articulate factors that intensify pain and modify behavior accordingly
- maintain respiratory rate within 5 breaths of baseline
- express feeling of comfort while maintaining air exchange.

Nursing interventions

- Institute standard precautions.
- Give prescribed drugs.
- If vision impairment occurs, provide a safe environment and encourage optimal independence.

Monitoring

- Intake and output
- Ventilation and oxygenation if the respiratory system is involved

Patient teaching

Be sure to cover:
- proper hand-washing technique
- need for parents to wear gloves when in contact with secretions or changing diapers and to dispose of diapers or soiled articles properly and wash hands thoroughly
- need for female health care workers trying to get pregnant to have CMV titers drawn to identify their risk of contracting the infection
- need for an immunosuppressed or pregnant patient to avoid contact with any person who has confirmed or suspected CMV infection
- need for an immunosuppressed patient who's CMV-seronegative to carry this information with him so he won't be given CMV-positive blood.

Discharge planning

- Provide emotional support and counseling to the parents of a child with severe CMV infection. Help them find support systems, and coordinate referrals to other health care professionals.
- For information and support, refer the patient and his family to a local chapter of the National Center for Infectious Diseases.

Dacryocystitis

Overview

Description
○ Infection of the lacrimal sac resulting from obstruction of the nasolacrimal duct
○ Acute or chronic

Pathophysiology
○ The lacrimal excretory system is a mucus membrane-lined tract that's contiguous with conjuctival and nasal mucosa
○ Conjuctival and nasal mucosa are normally colonized with bacteria
○ Inability to drain tears due to a blocked lacrimal drainage system results in infection (see *A close look at tears*)

Causes
Acute form
○ *Staphylococcus aureus*
○ Beta-hemolytic streptococci
○ Nasal disease
Chronic form
○ *Streptococcus pneumonia*
○ Fungus, such as *Actinomyces* or *Candida albicans*
○ Chronic mucosal degeneration

Incidence
○ More common in adults older than age 40
○ Occurs more commonly on the left side than the right side
○ Rare in blacks
○ Affects females more commonly than males

Common characteristics
Acute form
○ Sudden onset of pain
○ Redness in the medial canthal region
Chronic form
○ Incidious onset of watery eyes

Complications
○ Hemorrhage
○ Infection
○ Cerebrospinal fluid leakage

Assessment

History
○ Eye pain
○ Fever

Physical findings
○ Severe erythematous swelling around nasal aspect of lower eyelid
○ Tenderness of eyelid

A close look at tears

Tears begin in the lacrimal gland and drain through the nasolacrimal duct into the nose.

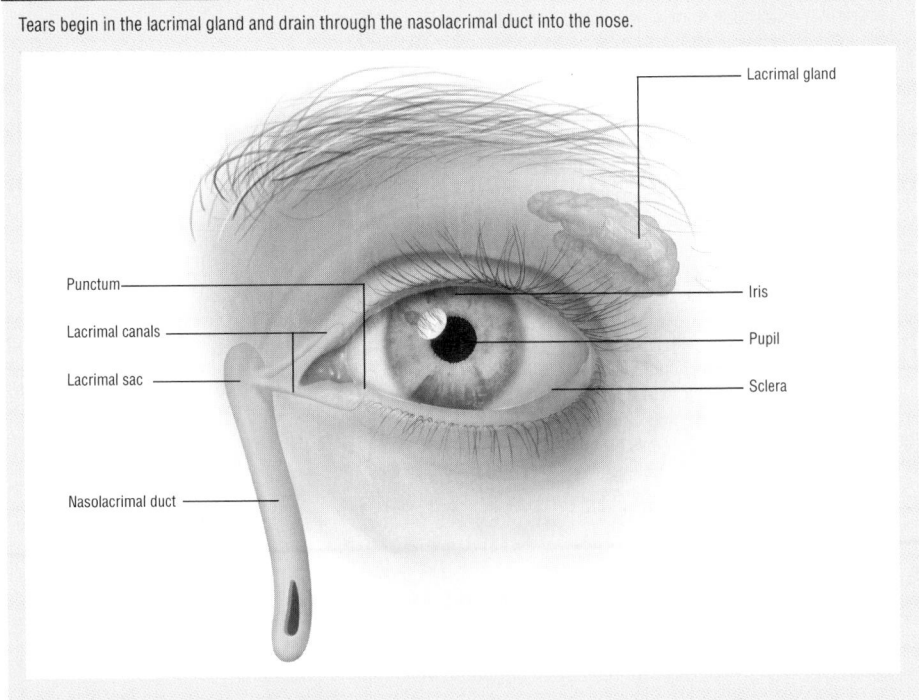

Punctum

Lacrimal canals

Lacrimal sac

Nasolacrimal duct

Lacrimal gland

Iris

Pupil

Sclera

- Tearing
- Conjunctival injection
- Palpable mass inferior to the medial canthal tendon
- Decreased visual acuity
- Orbital cellulitis

Test results

Laboratory
- Culture of discharge demonstrates organism
- Elevated white blood cell count

Imaging
- X-ray after injection of radiopaque medium locates atresia
- Dacryocystography and dacryoscintigraphy identify anatomical abnormalities of the nasolacrimal drainage system

Other
- Physical examination

Treatment

General
- Warm compresses
- Activity, as tolerated

Medication
- Topical polymyxin/trimethoprim eyedrops
- Systemic amoxicillin
- I.V. antibiotics

Surgery
- Incision and drainage
- Dacryocystorhinostomy (chronic cases)

Nursing considerations

Key outcomes
The patient will:
- express feelings of increased comfort
- remain free from signs of infection.

Nursing interventions
- Give prescribed antibiotics.
- Apply compresses.

Monitoring
- Bleeding
- Pain

Patient teaching

Be sure to cover:
- the disorder, diagnosis, and treatment
- applying warm compresses and eyedrops
- reporting signs of worsening infection.

Dermatitis

Overview

Description

- Skin condition characterized by inflammation
- Can be acute or chronic
- Occurs in several forms, including contact, seborrheic, nummular, exfoliative, and stasis dermatitis (see *Types of dermatitis*, pages 228 and 229)
- Typically associated with other atopic diseases

Pathophysiology

- The allergic mechanism of hypersensitivity results in a release of inflammatory mediators through sensitized antibodies of immunoglobulin (Ig) E.
- Histamine and other cytokines induce an inflammatory response resulting in edema, skin breakdown, and pruritus.

Causes

- Exact cause unknown
- Possible underlying metabolic or biochemical causes
- Possible genetic link to elevated serum IgE levels
- Possible defective T-cell function
- Precipitating factors:
  - Infections
  - Allergens
  - Temperature extremes
  - Humidity
  - Sweating
  - Stress

Incidence

- Common in infants and toddlers between ages 6 months and 2 years
- Common in those with strong family histories of atopic disease
- Affects about 9 of every 1,000 persons

Common characteristics

- Pruritus
- Skin lesions

Complications

- Permanent skin damage
- Lichenification
- Altered pigmentation
- Scarring
- Bacterial, fungal, and viral infections
- Kaposi's varicelliform eruption

Assessment

History

- Depends on type of dermatitis
- Family history of atopic dermatitis
- Exposure to an allergen or irritant
- Intense itching

Physical findings

- Depend on type of dermatitis
- Erythematous patches in excessively dry areas

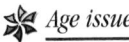 *Age issue*

In children, look for lesions on the forehead, cheeks, and extensor surfaces of the arms and legs.

- Lesions usually at flexion points in adults
- During a flare-up: edema, scaling, and vesiculation; pus-filled vesicles
- In chronic disease: multiple areas of dry, scaly skin, with white dermatographism, blanching, and lichenification

Test results

- Depend on type of dermatitis

Laboratory
- Serum analysis showing elevated IgE levels
- Tissue cultures possibly ruling out bacterial, viral, or fungal superinfections
- Allergy testing possibly disclosing allergic rhinitis or asthma

Diagnostic procedures
- Patch testing and distribution of lesions are used to pinpoint the provoking allergen.

Other
- Firm stroking of the patient's skin with a blunt instrument causes a white — not reddened — hive to appear on the skin of 70% of patients with atopic dermatitis.
- Food elimination diet may help to identify at least one allergen.

Treatment

General

- Depends on type of dermatitis
- Elimination of allergens
- Avoidance of precipitating factors
- Ultraviolet B light therapy to increase the thickness of the stratum corneum
- Avoid food allergens
- Avoid overheating

Medication

- Antihistamines
- Corticosteroids
- Bland emollients
- Antibiotics
- Antifungals
- Antivirals

Surgery

○ Vein stripping, sclerotherapy, or skin grafts in stasis dermatitis

Nursing considerations

Key outcomes

The patient will:
○ exhibit improved or healed lesions or wounds
○ avoid complications
○ demonstrate understanding of skin care regimen
○ verbalize feelings about altered body image.

Nursing interventions

○ Nursing interventions are guided by the type of dermatitis.
○ Assist with daily skin care.
○ Apply intermittent occlusive dressings to lichenified skin.
○ Apply cool, moist compresses.
○ Encourage verbalization of feelings.
○ Offer emotional support and reassurance.

Monitoring

○ Adverse reactions
○ Response to treatment
○ Complications

Patient teaching

Be sure to cover:
○ the disorder, diagnosis, and treatment
○ skin care
○ prescribed drugs and potential adverse reactions
○ signs and symptoms of corticosteroid overdose and notifying the physician immediately if they occur
○ control of pruritus
○ meticulous hand washing and good personal hygiene
○ use of plain, tepid water (96° F [35.6° C]) and non-fatty, nonperfumed soaps
○ application of occlusive dressings
○ application of wet-to-dry dressings
○ identification and avoidance of aggravating factors.

Discharge planning

○ Refer the patient to the American Academy of Dermatology.

Types of dermatitis

Type	Causes	Assessment findings	Diagnosis	Treatment and intervention
CHRONIC DERMATITIS				
Characterized by inflammatory eruptions of the hands and feet	• Usually unknown but may result from progressive contact dermatitis • Secondary factors: trauma, infections, redistribution of normal flora, photosensitivity, and food sensitivity, which may perpetuate this condition	• Thick, lichenified, single or multiple lesions on any part of the body (commonly on the hands) • Inflammation and scaling • Recurrence after long remissions	• No characteristic pattern or course; diagnosis based on detailed history and physical findings	• Elimination of known allergens and decreased exposure to irritants, wearing protective clothing such as gloves, and washing immediately after contact with irritants or allergens • Antibiotics for secondary infection • Avoidance of excessive washing and drying of hands and of accumulation of soaps and detergents under rings • Use of emollients with topical steroids
CONTACT DERMATITIS				
Commonly, sharply demarcated skin inflammation and irritation due to contact with concentrated substances to which the skin is sensitive, such as perfumes or chemicals	• Mild irritants: chronic exposure to detergents or solvents • Strong irritants: damage on contact with acids or alkalis • Allergens: sensitization after repeated exposure	• Mild irritants and allergens: erythema and small vesicles that ooze, scale, and itch • Strong irritants: blisters and ulcerations • Classic allergic response: clearly defined lesions, with straight lines following points of contact • Severe allergic reaction: marked edema of affected areas	• Patient history • Patch testing to identify allergens • Shape and distribution of lesions	• Same as for chronic dermatitis • Topical anti-inflammatory agents (such as steroids), systemic steroids for edema and bullae, antihistamines, and local applications of Burow's solution (for blisters) • Other nursing interventions similar to those for atopic dermatitis
EXFOLIATIVE DERMATITIS				
Severe, chronic skin inflammation characterized by redness and widespread erythema and scaling	• Progression of preexisting skin lesions to exfoliative stage, as in contact dermatitis, drug reaction, lymphoma, or leukemia	• Generalized dermatitis, with acute loss of stratum corneum, and erythema and scaling • Sensation of tight skin • Hair loss • Possibly fever, sensitivity to cold, shivering, gynecomastia, and lymphadenopathy	• Identification of the underlying cause	• Hospitalization, with protective isolation and hygienic measures to prevent secondary bacterial infection • Open wet dressings, with colloidal baths • Bland lotions over topical steroids • Maintenance of constant environmental temperature to prevent chilling or overheating • Careful monitoring of renal and cardiac status • Systemic antibiotics and steroids • Other nursing interventions similar to those for atopic dermatitis
LOCALIZED NEURODERMATITIS (LICHEN SIMPLEX CHRONICUS, ESSENTIAL PRURITUS)				
Superficial skin inflammation characterized by itching and papular eruptions that appear on thickened, hyperpigmented skin	• Chronic scratching or rubbing of a primary lesion or insect bite, or other skin irritation	• Intense, sometimes continual scratching • Thick, sharp-bordered, possibly dry, scaly lesions, with raised papules • Usually affects easily reached areas, such as ankles, lower legs, anogenital area, back of neck, and ears	• Physical findings	• Scratching must stop; then erosions will disappear in 2 weeks • Fixed dressing or Unna's boot to cover affected area • Topical steroids (occlusive dressings or intralesional injections) • Antihistamines and open wet dressings • Emollients

Type	Causes	Assessment findings	Diagnosis	Treatment and intervention
NUMMULAR DERMATITIS				
Chronic form of dermatitis characterized by coin-shaped, vesicular, crusted scales and, possibly, pruritic lesions	• Possibly precipitated by stress; or dryness, irritants, or scratching	• Round, nummular (coin-shaped) lesions, usually on arms and legs, with distinct borders of crusts and scales • Possibly oozing and severe itching • Summertime remissions common, with wintertime recurrence	• Physical findings and patient history; history of atopic dermatitis in middle-aged or older patient • Exclusion of fungal infections, atopic or contact dermatitis, and psoriasis	• Elimination of known irritants • Measures to relieve dry skin: increased humidification, limited frequency of baths and use of bland soap and bath oils, and application of emollients • Wet dressings in acute phase • Topical steroids (occlusive dressings or intralesional injections) for persistent lesions • Tar preparations and antihistamines for itching and antibiotics for secondary infection • Other interventions similar to those for atopic dermatitis
SEBORRHEIC DERMATITIS				
An acute or subacute disease that affects the scalp, face and, occasionally, other areas and is characterized by lesions covered with yellow or brownish gray scales	• Unknown; stress and neurologic conditions may be predisposing factors	• Eruptions in areas with many sebaceous glands (usually scalp, face, and trunk) and in skin folds • Itching, redness, and inflammation of affected areas; lesions that may appear greasy; possibly fissures • Indistinct, occasionally yellowish scaly patches from excess stratum corneum (dandruff may be mild seborrheic dermatitis)	• Patient history and physical findings, especially distribution of lesions in sebaceous gland areas • Exclusion of psoriasis	• Removal of scales by frequent washing and shampooing with selenium sulfide suspension, zinc pyrithione, tar and salicylic acid shampoo or ketoconazole shampoo • Application of topical steroids and antifungal agents to nonhairy areas • For infants, baby shampoo
STASIS DERMATITIS				
Condition usually caused by impaired circulation and characterized by eczema of the legs with edema, hyperpigmentation, and persistent inflammation	• Secondary to peripheral vascular diseases affecting legs, such as recurrent thrombophlebitis and resultant chronic venous insufficiency	• Varicosities and edema common, but obvious vascular insufficiency not always present • Usually affects the lower leg, just above internal malleolus, or sites of trauma or irritation • Early signs: dusky red deposits of hemosiderin in skin, with itching and dimpling of subcutaneous tissue; later signs: edema, redness, and scaling of large area of legs • Possibly fissures, crusts, and ulcers	• Positive history of venous insufficiency and physical findings such as varicosities	• Measures to prevent venous stasis: avoidance of prolonged sitting or standing, use of support stockings, and weight reduction for obese patients • Corrective surgery for underlying cause • After ulcer develops, rest periods with legs elevated; open wet dressings; Unna's boot (provides continuous pressure to areas); and antibiotics for secondary infection after wound culture

Developmental dysplasia of the hip

Overview

Description

- An abnormality of the hip joint present at birth
- The most common disorder affecting the hip joints in children younger than 3 years

Degrees of hip dysplasia

Normally, the head of the femur fits snugly into the acetabulum, allowing the hip to move properly. In congenital hip dysplasia, flattening of the acetabulum prevents the head of the femur from rotating adequately. The child's hip may be unstable, subluxated (partially dislocated), or completely dislocated, with the femoral head lying totally outside the acetabulum. The degree of dysplasia and the child's age are considered in determining the treatment choice.

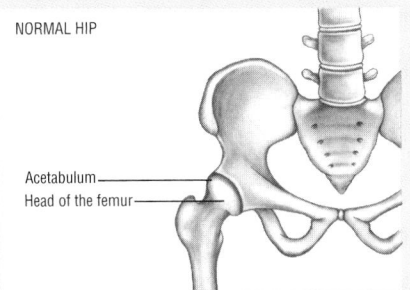

NORMAL HIP

Acetabulum
Head of the femur

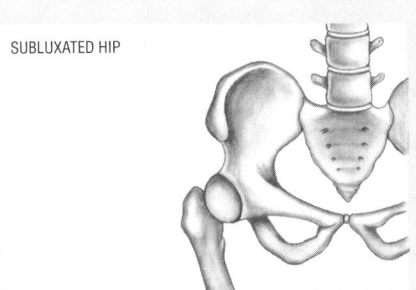

SUBLUXATED HIP

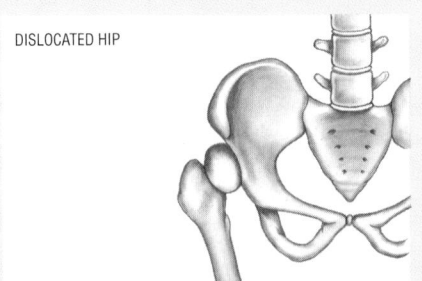

DISLOCATED HIP

- Can be unilateral or bilateral
- Occurs in three forms of varying severity (see *Degrees of hip dysplasia*)

Causes

- Precise cause unknown

Risk factors

- Breech delivery
- Elevated maternal relaxin (hormone secreted by the corpus luteum during pregnancy that causes relaxation of pubic symphysis and cervical dilation)
- Large neonates and twins

Pathophysiology

- Excessive or abnormal movement of the joint during a traumatic birth may cause dislocation.
- Displacement of bones within the joint may damage joint structures, including articulating surfaces, blood vessels, tendons, ligaments, and nerves.
- Disruption of blood flow to the joint may lead to ischemic necrosis.

Incidence

- About 85% of affected infants are females.

Common characteristics

- Level of knees uneven
- Limited abduction on the dislocated side
- Buttock fold on the affected side higher with the child lying prone (also restricted abduction of the affected hip) (see *Ortolani's and Trendelenburg's signs of DDH*)

Complications

- Degenerative hip changes
- Abnormal acetabular development
- Lordosis (abnormally increased concave curvature of the lumbar and cervical spine)
- Joint malformation
- Sciatic nerve injury (paralysis)
- Avascular necrosis of femoral head
- Soft tissue damage
- Permanent disability

Assessment

History

- Traumatic birth
- Large birth size
- Twin

Physical findings

- Extra fold on the thigh of the affected side
- Limited abduction on the dislocated side
- Level of knees uneven
- Swaying from side to side ("duck waddle") because of uncorrected bilateral dysplasia
- Limp due to uncorrected unilateral dysplasia

Test results

Imaging
- X-rays show the location of the femur head and a shallow acetabulum.
- Sonography and magnetic resonance imaging assess reduction.

Other
- Physical examination

Treatment

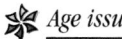 *Age issue*

Treatment of developmental dysplasia of the hip varies with the patient's age.

Younger than age 3 months:

- *Gentle manipulation to reduce the dislocation, followed by splint-brace or harness*
- *Splint-brace or harness worn continuously for 2 to 3 months, then a night splint for another month*

Older than age 3 months:

- *Bilateral skin traction (in infants) or skeletal traction (in children who have started walking)*
- *Bryant's traction or divarication traction (both extremities placed in traction, even if only one is affected, to help maintain immobilization) for children younger than 3 years and weighing less than 35 lb (15.9 kg) for 2 to 3 weeks*
- *Immobilization in a spica cast for approximately 3 months for children ages 6 to 12 months*

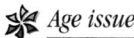 *Age issue*

Treatment begun after age 5 rarely restores satisfactory hip function.

General
- Activity, as tolerated
- No dietary restriction

Surgery
- Gentle closed reduction under general anesthesia to further abduct the hips, followed by a spica cast for 3 months (if traction fails)
- In children older than age 18 months, open reduction and pelvic or femoral osteotomy to correct bony deformity followed by immobilization in a spica cast for 6 to 8 weeks
- In children ages 2 to 5 years, skeletal traction and subcutaneous adductor tenotomy (surgical cutting of the tendon)

Ortolani's and Trendelenburg's signs of DDH

A positive Ortolani's or Trendelenburg's sign confirms developmental dysplasia of the hip (DDH).

Ortolani's sign
- Place the infant on his back, with hip flexed and in abduction. Adduct the hip while pressing the femur downward. This will dislocate the hip.
- Next, abduct the hip while moving the femur upward. A click or a jerk (produced by the femoral head moving over the acetabular rim) indicates subluxation in an infant younger than 1 month. The sign indicates subluxation or complete dislocation in an older infant.

Trendelenburg's sign
- When the child rests his weight on the side of the dislocation and lifts his other knee, the pelvis drops on the normal side because abductor muscles in the affected hip are weak.
- However, when the child stands with his weight on the normal side and lifts the other knee, the pelvis remains horizontal.

Nursing considerations

Key outcomes
The patient will:
- maintain joint mobility and range of motion
- maintain muscle strength
- achieve the highest level of mobility possible within the confines of the disease.

Nursing interventions
- Provide reassurance to the parents.
- Turn the child every 2 hours.
- Provide appropriate cast care.

Monitoring
- Parental care of cast or equipment
- Skin integrity
- Color, sensation, and motion of the infant's legs and feet
- Comfort

Patient teaching

Be sure to cover:
- how to correctly splint or brace the hips, as ordered
- good hygiene
- signs and symptoms of cast compression (cyanosis, cool extremities, or pain).

Discharge planning
- Stress the need for frequent checkups.
- Refer the child and parents to a child life specialist to ensure continued developmental progress.

Diabetes insipidus

Overview

Description

- Disorder of water balance regulation characterized by excessive fluid intake and hypotonic polyuria
- Two types: primary and secondary
- May occur transiently during pregnancy, usually after the 5th or 6th month of gestation
- Impaired or absent thirst mechanism increases risk of complications
- If uncomplicated, prognosis is good
- If complicated by underlying disorder, such as cancer, prognosis varies
- Also referred to as *DI*

Pathophysiology

- Vasopressin (antidiuretic hormone) is synthesized in the hypothalamus and stored by the posterior pituitary gland.
- Once released into the general circulation, vasopressin acts on the distal and collecting tubules of the kidneys.
- Vasopressin increases the water permeability of the tubules and causes water reabsorption.
- The absence of vasopressin allows filtered water to be excreted in the urine instead of being reabsorbed.

Causes

- Failure of vasopressin secretion in response to normal physiologic stimuli
- Failure of the kidneys to respond to vasopressin, called nephrogenic DI
- Familial
- Idiopathic
- Congenital malformation of the central nervous system (CNS)
- Infection
- Trauma
- Tumors
- Neurosurgery, skull fracture, or head trauma
- Granulomatous disease
- Vascular lesions
- Psychogenic
- Pregnancy (gestational DI)
- Damage to hypothalamus or pituitary gland
- Certain medications such as lithium

Incidence

- Affects men and women equally
- Primary DI in 50% of patients

Common characteristics

- Polyuria with low specific gravity and osmolality
- Nocturia
- Dehydration
- Polydipsia

- Weight loss
- Fatigue

Complications

- Hypovolemia
- Hyperosmolality
- Circulatory collapse
- Loss of consciousness
- CNS changes
- Bladder distention
- Hydroureter
- Hydronephrosis

Assessment

History

- Abrupt onset of extreme polyuria
- Extreme thirst
- Extraordinarily large oral fluid intake
- Weight loss
- Dizziness; weakness; fatigue
- Constipation
- Nocturia

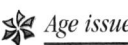 *Age issue*

In children, reports of enuresis, sleep disturbances, irritability, anorexia, thirst, and decreased weight gain and linear growth are common.

Physical findings

- Signs of dehydration
- Fever
- Dyspnea
- Pale, voluminous urine
- Poor skin turgor
- Tachycardia
- Decreased muscle strength
- Hypotension

Test results

Laboratory
- Urinalysis showing colorless urine with low osmolality and specific gravity
- Increased serum sodium
- Increased serum osmolality
- Decreased serum vasopressin
- 24-hour urine showing decreased specific gravity and increased volume
- Elevated blood urea nitrogen (BUN) and creatinine levels

Diagnostic procedures
- Dehydration test or water deprivation test shows an increase in urine osmolality after vasopressin administration exceeding 9%.

Treatment

General

- ○ Identification and treatment of underlying cause
- ○ Control of fluid balance
- ○ Dehydration prevention
- ○ Free access to oral fluids
- ○ With nephrogenic DI, low-sodium diet

Medication

- ○ Vasopressin
- ○ Synthetic vasopressin analogue
- ○ Vasopressin stimulant
- ○ Thiazide diuretics in nephrogenic DI
- ○ I.V. fluids:
  - − If serum sodium >150: 5% dextrose in water
  - − If serum sodium < 150: normal saline solution

Surgery

- ○ Not indicated, unless required to treat underlying cause such as a tumor

Nursing considerations

Key outcomes

The patient will:
- ○ demonstrate balanced fluid volume
- ○ display adaptive coping behaviors
- ○ avoid complications
- ○ demonstrate normal laboratory values.

Nursing interventions

- ○ Administer medications, as ordered.
- ○ Provide meticulous skin and mouth care.

 Alert

Use caution when administering vasopressin to a patient with coronary artery disease because it can cause coronary artery constriction.

- ○ Encourage verbalization of feelings.
- ○ Offer encouragement while providing a realistic assessment of the situation.
- ○ Help the patient develop effective coping strategies.

Monitoring

- ○ Intake and output
- ○ Vital signs
- ○ Daily weight
- ○ Urine specific gravity
- ○ Serum electrolytes and BUN
- ○ Signs and symptoms of hypovolemic shock
- ○ Changes in mental or neurologic status
- ○ Cardiac rhythm

Patient teaching

Be sure to cover:
- ○ the disorder, diagnosis, and treatment
- ○ medication and potential adverse reactions
- ○ when to notify the physician
- ○ signs and symptoms of dehydration
- ○ daily weight
- ○ intake and output
- ○ use of a hydrometer to measure urine specific gravity
- ○ need for medical identification jewelry
- ○ need for ongoing medical care.

Discharge planning

- ○ Refer the patient to a mental health professional for additional counseling as indicated.

Diabetes mellitus

Overview

Description
○ Chronic disease of absolute or relative insulin deficiency or resistance
○ Characterized by disturbances in carbohydrate, protein, and fat metabolism
○ Two primary forms:
  – Type 1, characterized by absolute insufficiency
  – Type 2, characterized by insulin resistance with varying degrees of insulin secretory defects

Pathophysiology
○ The effects of diabetes mellitus (DM) result from insulin deficiency or resistance to endogenous insulin.
○ Insulin allows glucose transport into the cells for use as energy or storage as glycogen.
○ Insulin also stimulates protein synthesis and free fatty acid storage in the adipose tissues.
○ Insulin deficiency compromises the body tissues' access to essential nutrients for fuel and storage.

Causes
○ Genetic factors
○ Autoimmune disease (type 1)

Risk factors
○ Viral infections (type 1)
○ Obesity (type 2)
○ Physiologic or emotional stress
○ Sedentary lifestyle (type 2)
○ Pregnancy
○ Medication, such as thiazide diuretics, adrenal corticosteroids, and hormonal contraceptives

Incidence
○ Type 1 — usually occurs before age 30, although it may occur at any age
○ More common in men
○ Type 2 — usually occurs in obese adults after age 30, although it may be seen in obese North American youths of African-American, Native American, or Hispanic descent
○ Affects about 8% of the population of the United States
○ About one-third of patients undiagnosed
○ Increases with age (type 2)

Common characteristics
○ Polyuria
○ Polydipsia
○ Polyphagia
○ Weight loss
○ Fatigue

Complications
○ Ketoacidosis
○ Hyperosmolar, hyperglycemic syndrome
○ Cardiovascular disease
○ Peripheral vascular disease
○ Retinopathy, blindness
○ Nephropathy
○ Diabetic dermopathy
○ Impaired resistance to infection
○ Cognitive depression

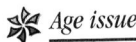 *Age issue*

Neonates of diabetic mothers have a two to three times greater incidence of congenital malformations and fetal distress unless the mothers' blood glucose levels are well-controlled prior to conception and during pregnancy.

Assessment

History
○ Polyuria, nocturia
○ Dehydration
○ Polydipsia
○ Dry mucous membranes
○ Poor skin turgor
○ Weight loss and hunger
○ Weakness; fatigue
○ Vision changes
○ Frequent skin and urinary tract infections
○ Dry, itchy skin
○ Sexual problems
○ Numbness or pain in the hands or feet
○ Postprandial feeling of nausea or fullness
○ Nocturnal diarrhea
Type 1
○ Rapidly developing symptoms
Type 2
○ Vague, long-standing symptoms that develop gradually
○ Family history of DM
○ Pregnancy
○ Severe viral infection
○ Other endocrine diseases
○ Recent stress or trauma
○ Use of drugs that increase blood glucose levels

Physical findings
○ Retinopathy or cataract formation
○ Skin changes, especially on the legs and feet
○ Muscle wasting and loss of subcutaneous fat (type 1)
○ Obesity, particularly in the abdominal area (type 2)
○ Poor skin turgor
○ Dry mucous membranes
○ Decreased peripheral pulses
○ Cool skin temperature
○ Diminished deep tendon reflexes

- ○ Orthostatic hypotension
- ○ Characteristic "fruity" breath odor in ketoacidosis
- ○ Possible hypovolemia and shock in ketoacidosis and hyperosmolar hyperglycemic state

Test results

Laboratory

- ○ Fasting plasma glucose level greater than or equal to 126 mg/dl on at least two occasions
- ○ Random blood glucose level greater than or equal to 200 mg/dl
- ○ Two-hour postprandial blood glucose level greater than or equal to 200 mg/dl
- ○ Glycosylated hemoglobin (Hb) increased
- ○ Urinalysis possibly showing acetone or glucose

Diagnostic procedures

- ○ Ophthalmologic examination may show diabetic retinopathy.

Treatment

General

- ○ Exercise and diet control
- ○ Tight glycemic control for prevention of complications
- ○ Modest caloric restriction for weight loss or maintenance
- ○ American Diabetes Association recommendations to reach target glucose, Hb A_{1c} lipid, and blood pressure levels
- ○ Regular aerobic exercise

Medication

- ○ Exogenous insulin (type 1 or possibly type 2)
- ○ Oral antihyperglycemic drugs (type 2)

Surgery

- ○ Pancreas transplantation

Nursing considerations

Key outcomes

The patient will:
- ○ maintain optimal body weight
- ○ remain free from infection
- ○ avoid complications
- ○ verbalize understanding of the disorder and treatment
- ○ demonstrate adaptive coping behaviors.

Nursing interventions

- ○ Give prescribed drugs.
- ○ Give rapidly absorbed carbohydrates for hypoglycemia or, if the patient is unconscious, glucagon or I.V. dextrose, as ordered.
- ○ Administer I.V. fluids and insulin replacement for hyperglycemic crisis, as ordered.
- ○ Provide meticulous skin care, especially to the feet and legs.

- ○ Treat all injuries, cuts, and blisters immediately.
- ○ Avoid constricting hose, slippers, or bed linens.
- ○ Encourage adequate fluid intake.
- ○ Encourage verbalization of feelings.
- ○ Offer emotional support.
- ○ Help to develop effective coping strategies.

Monitoring

- ○ Vital signs
- ○ Intake and output
- ○ Daily weight
- ○ Serum glucose
- ○ Urine acetone
- ○ Renal status
- ○ Cardiovascular status
- ○ Signs and symptoms of:
  - – Hypoglycemia
  - – Hyperglycemia
  - – Hyperosmolar coma
  - – Urinary tract and vaginal infections
  - – Diabetic neuropathy

Patient teaching

Be sure to cover:
- ○ the disorder, diagnosis, and treatment
- ○ medication and potential adverse reactions
- ○ when to notify the physician
- ○ prescribed meal plan
- ○ prescribed exercise program
- ○ signs and symptoms of:
  - – infection
  - – hypoglycemia
  - – hyperglycemia
  - – diabetic neuropathy
- ○ self-monitoring of blood glucose
- ○ complications of hyperglycemia
- ○ foot care
- ○ annual regular ophthalmologic examinations
- ○ safety precautions
- ○ management of diabetes during illness.

Discharge planning

- ○ Refer the patient to a dietitian.
- ○ Refer the patient to a podiatrist if indicated.
- ○ Refer the patient to an ophthalmologist.
- ○ Refer adult diabetic patients who are planning families for preconception counseling.
- ○ Refer the patient to the Juvenile Diabetes Research Foundation, the American Association of Diabetes Educators, and the American Diabetes Association to obtain additional information.

Diphtheria

Overview

Description
- Acute, highly contagious, toxin-mediated infection that usually infects the respiratory tract — primarily the tonsils, nasopharynx, and larynx
- GI and urinary tracts, conjunctivae, and ears rarely involved

Pathophysiology
- Proliferation of organism at site of implantation
- Endotoxin: produced, absorbed by the blood, and transported to the heart and central nervous system

Causes
- *Corynebacterium diphtheriae,* a gram-positive rod
- Transmission usually through intimate contact, airborne respiratory droplets, or a break in the skin

Incidence
- More prevalent during the colder months
- Rare in many parts of the world, including the United States
- Incidence of cutaneous diphtheria on the increase since 1972, especially in the Pacific Northwest and the Southwest
- More prevalent in children younger than age 15

Common characteristics
- Thick, patchy, grayish green membrane over the mucous membranes of the pharynx, larynx, tonsils, soft palate, and nose
- Symptoms similar to croup
- Bleeding when attempting to remove membrane
- In cutaneous diphtheria, yellow spots or skin lesions (resembles impetigo)

Complications
- Thrombocytopenia
- Myocarditis
- Neurologic involvement (primarily affecting motor fibers but possibly also sensory neurons)
- Renal involvement
- Pulmonary involvement (bronchopneumonia)

Assessment

History
- Fever
- Sore throat
- Rasping cough
- Malaise
- Vomiting
- Dysphagia

Physical findings
- Hoarseness or stridor
- Thick, patchy, grayish green membrane over the mucous membranes of the pharynx, larynx, tonsils, soft palate, and nose
- Swelling of the palate
- Yellow spots or lesions (cutaneous)

Test results
Laboratory
- Throat culture or culture of other suspect lesions grows *C. diphtheriae.*

Treatment

General
- Symptomatic
- Droplet precautions (see *Droplet precautions*)
- Activity, as tolerated
- Diet, as tolerated

Medication
- Diphtheria antitoxin
- Antibiotics

Surgery
- Tracheotomy if airway obstruction occurs.

Nursing considerations

Key outcomes
The patient will:
- maintain patent airway
- have adequate ventilation
- remain free from signs and symptoms of infection.

Nursing interventions
- Enforce strict isolation techniques.
- Give prescribed drugs.
- Obtain cultures, as ordered.
- Report all cases to local public health authorities.

Droplet precautions

Droplet precautions prevent the spread of infectious diseases transmitted by contact with nasal or oral secretions (droplets arising from coughing or sneezing) from the infected patient with the mucous membranes of the susceptible host.

Effective droplet precautions require a single room (not necessarily a negative-pressure room), and the door doesn't need to be closed. Persons having direct contact with, or who will be within 3 feet of, the patient should wear a surgical mask covering the nose and mouth.

When handling infants or young children who require droplet precautions, you may also need to wear gloves and a gown to prevent soiling of clothing with nasal and oral secretions.

Monitoring
○ Pulse oximetry
○ Airway
○ Signs of shock
○ Cardiac rhythm

Patient teaching

Be sure to cover:
○ proper disposal of nasopharyngeal secretions
○ maintaining infection precautions until after two consecutive negative nasopharyngeal cultures — at least 1 week after drug therapy stops.

Discharge planning
○ Stress the need for childhood immunizations to all parents.

Dislocations and subluxations

Overview

Description

- Dislocation — displacement of joint bones so that articulating surfaces totally lose contact (see *Common dislocation*)
- Subluxation — partial displacement of articulating surfaces
- May accompany fractures of joints

Pathophysiology

- Trauma causes displacement of the joint.
- Joint structures (blood vessels, ligaments, tendons, and nerves) are damaged.

Common dislocation

The elbow is a common site of dislocation.

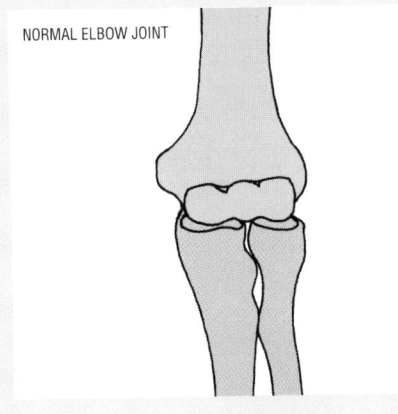

NORMAL ELBOW JOINT

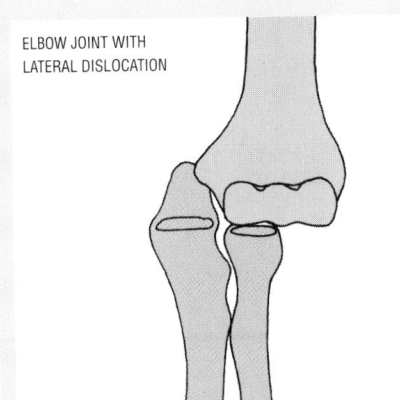

ELBOW JOINT WITH LATERAL DISLOCATION

- Injuries may result in deposition of fracture fragments between joint surfaces, damaging surrounding structures.
- Joint function is impaired.

Causes

- Congenital
- Trauma
- Paget's disease of surrounding joint tissues

Risk factors

- Participation in contact sports

Incidence

- Shoulder dislocations — account for more than half of dislocations seen in emergency rooms
- Hip dislocations — from trauma are more common in those younger than age 35; from falls are more common in those older than age 65

Common characteristics

- Visible deformity of affected extremity
- Shortening of affected extremity
- Local pain
- Swelling
- Limitation of function
- Numbness of affected extremity

Complications

- Avascular necrosis
- Bone necrosis

Assessment

History

- Trauma or fall
- Extreme pain at injury site
- Participation in contact sports

Physical findings

- Joint surface fractures
- Deformity around the joint
- Change in the length of the involved extremity
- Impaired joint mobility
- Point tenderness

Test results

Imaging
- X-rays confirm the diagnosis and show any associated fractures.

Treatment

General

- Immediate reduction and immobilization
- Nothing by mouth if surgery scheduled
- Activity limitations based on injury

○ Active range-of-motion (ROM) exercises for adjacent joints that aren't immobilized

Medication

○ Sedation
○ Analgesics
○ Muscle relaxants

Surgery

○ Open reduction
○ Skeletal traction
○ Ligament repair

Nursing considerations

Key outcomes

The patient will:
○ identify factors that intensify pain
○ identify factors that increase the potential for injury
○ maintain muscle strength and tone
○ maintain joint ROM.

Nursing interventions

○ Give prescribed drugs.
○ Provide proper positioning of the affected area.
○ Apply ice, as ordered.
○ Encourage ROM exercises, as ordered, for adjacent nonmobilized joints.
○ Provide meticulous skin care.

 Alert

Immediately report signs and symptoms of severe vascular compromise, such as pallor, pain, loss of pulse, paralysis, and paresthesia; the patient needs an immediate orthopedic examination and emergency reduction.

Monitoring

○ Respiratory status when I.V. sedatives used
○ Neurovascular status of involved extremity
○ Integrity of skin

Patient teaching

Be sure to cover:
○ the need to report numbness, pain, cyanosis, and coldness of the extremity below the cast or splint
○ how to evaluate skin integrity
○ how to assess neurovascular status
○ the use of assistive devices
○ the importance of follow-up visits
○ drug administration, dosage, and possible adverse effects.

Discharge planning

○ Refer the patient to a rehabilitation program if appropriate.
○ Refer the patient for home health care if appropriate.

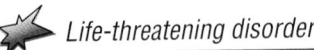 *Life-threatening disorder*

Disseminated intravascular coagulation

Overview

Description

- Syndrome of activated coagulation characterized by bleeding or thrombosis
- Complicates diseases and conditions that accelerate clotting, causing occlusion of small blood vessels, organ necrosis, depletion of circulating clotting factors and platelets, and activation of the fibrinolytic system
- Also known as *DIC, consumption coagulopathy,* and *defibrination syndrome*

Pathophysiology

- Typical accelerated clotting results in generalized activation of prothrombin and a consequent excess of thrombin.
- Excess thrombin converts fibrinogen to fibrin, producing fibrin clots in the microcirculation.
- This process consumes exorbitant amounts of coagulation factors (especially platelets, factor V, prothrombin, fibrinogen, and factor VIII), causing thrombocytopenia, deficiencies in factors V and VIII, hypoprothrombinemia, and hypofibrinogenemia.
- Circulating thrombin activates the fibrinolytic system, which lyses fibrin clots into fibrinogen degradation products (FDPs).
- The hemorrhage that occurs may be due largely to the anticoagulant activity of FDPs and depletion of plasma coagulation factors.

Causes

- Infection, sepsis
- Obstetric complications
- Neoplastic disease
- Disorders that produce necrosis, such as extensive burns and trauma
- Other disorders, such as heatstroke, shock, incompatible blood transfusion, drug reactions, cardiac arrest, surgery necessitating cardiopulmonary bypass, acute respiratory distress syndrome, diabetic ketoacidosis, pulmonary embolism, and sickle cell anemia

Incidence

- Depends on the cause

Common characteristics

- Abnormal bleeding
- Hemorrhage

Complications

- Renal failure
- Hepatic damage
- Stroke
- Ischemic bowel
- Respiratory distress
- Death (mortality is greater than 50%)

Assessment

History

- Abnormal bleeding *without* a history of a serious hemorrhagic disorder; bleeding may occur at all bodily orifices
- Possible presence of one of the causes of DIC
- Possible signs of bleeding into the skin, such as cutaneous oozing, petechiae, ecchymoses, and hematomas
- Possible bleeding from surgical or invasive procedure sites, such as incisions or venipuncture sites
- Possible nausea and vomiting; severe muscle, back, and abdominal pain; chest pain; hemoptysis; epistaxis; seizures; and oliguria
- Possible GI bleeding, hematuria

Physical findings

- Petechiae
- Acrocyanosis
- Dyspnea, tachypnea
- Mental status changes, including confusion

Test results

Laboratory

- Decreased serum platelet count (less than 150,000/mm^3)
- Decreased serum fibrinogen level (less than 170 mg/dl)
- Prolonged prothrombin time (more than 19 seconds)
- Prolonged partial thromboplastin time (more than 40 seconds)
- Increased FDPs (commonly greater than 45 mcg/ml, or positive at less than 1:100 dilution)
- Positive D-dimer test (specific fibrinogen test for DIC) at less than 1:8 dilution
- Prolonged thrombin time
- Diminished blood clotting factors V and VIII
- Complete blood count showing decreased hemoglobin levels (less than 10 g/dl)
- Elevated blood urea nitrogen (greater than 25 mg/dl) and elevated serum creatinine levels (greater than 1.3 mg/dl)

Treatment

General

- ○ Treat underlying condition
- ○ Possibly supportive care alone if the patient isn't actively bleeding
- ○ Activity, as tolerated

Medication

If the patient is actively bleeding

- ○ Administration of blood, fresh frozen plasma, platelets, or packed red blood cells
- ○ Cryoprecipitate
- ○ Antithrombin III and gabexate
- ○ Fluid replacement

Nursing considerations

Key outcomes

The patient will:
- ○ maintain balanced intake and output
- ○ maintain adequate ventilation
- ○ express feelings of increased comfort and decreased pain
- ○ have laboratory values return to normal
- ○ use available support systems to assist in coping with fears.

Nursing interventions

 Alert

Focus on early recognition of signs of abnormal bleeding, prompt treatment of the underlying disorders, and prevention of further bleeding.

- ○ Provide emotional support.
- ○ Provide adequate rest periods.
- ○ Give prescribed analgesics as necessary.
- ○ Reposition the patient every 2 hours and provide meticulous skin care.
- ○ Give prescribed oxygen therapy.

 Alert

To prevent clots from dislodging and causing fresh bleeding, don't vigorously rub the affected areas when bathing.

- ○ Protect the patient from injury.
- ○ If bleeding occurs, use pressure and topical hemostatic agents to control bleeding.
- ○ Limit venipunctures whenever possible.
- ○ Watch for transfusion reactions and signs of fluid overload.
- ○ Measure the amount of blood lost, weigh dressings and linen and record drainage.
- ○ Weigh the patient daily, particularly in renal involvement.

Monitoring

- ○ Vital signs
- ○ Results of serial blood studies
- ○ Signs of shock
- ○ Intake and output, especially when administering blood products

Patient teaching

Be sure to cover (for the patient and his family):
- ○ an explanation of the disorder
- ○ the signs and symptoms of the problem, diagnostic procedures required, and treatment that the patient is to receive.

Diverticular disease

Overview

Description
- Bulging pouches (diverticula) in GI wall pushing the mucosal lining through surrounding muscle
- Sigmoid colon is most common site, but may develop anywhere, from proximal end of the pharynx to the anus
- Other typical sites:
  - The duodenum, near the pancreatic border or the ampulla of Vater
  - The jejunum
- Diverticular disease of the ileum (Meckel's diverticulum) — most common congenital anomaly of the GI tract
- Two clinical forms:
  - Diverticulosis: diverticula are present but don't cause symptoms
  - Diverticulitis: diverticula become inflamed and may cause complications

Pathophysiology
- Pressure in the intestinal lumen is exerted on weak areas, such as points where blood vessels enter the intestine, causing a break in the muscular continuity of the GI wall, creating a diverticulum.
- Diverticulitis occurs when retained undigested food mixed with bacteria accumulates in the diverticulum, forming a hard mass (fecalith). This substance cuts off the blood supply to the diverticulum's thin walls, increasing its susceptibility to attack by colonic bacteria.
- Inflammation follows bacterial infection, causing abdominal pain.

Causes
- Diminished colonic motility and increased intraluminal pressure
- Defects in colon wall strength

Risk factors
- Age
- Low-fiber diet

Incidence
- Most common in adults ages 45 and older
- Affects 30% of adults older than age 60
- More common in women than men

Common characteristics
- Left lower quadrant abdominal pain
- Abdominal pain
- Diarrhea or constipation
- Palpable mass
- Nausea, vomiting

Complications
- Ruptured diverticula that cause abdominal abscesses or peritonitis
- Intestinal obstruction
- Rectal hemorrhage
- Portal pyemia
- Fistula

Assessment

History
Diverticulosis
- May be symptom-free
- Occasional intermittent pain in the left lower abdominal quadrant, which may be relieved by defecation or the passage of flatus
- Alternating bouts of constipation and diarrhea

Diverticulitis
- History of diverticulosis
- Low fiber consumption
- Recent consumption of foods containing seeds or kernels or indigestible roughage, such as celery and corn
- Complaints of moderate dull or steady pain in the left lower abdominal quadrant, aggravated by straining, lifting, or coughing
- Mild nausea, gas, diarrhea, or intermittent bouts of constipation, sometimes accompanied by rectal bleeding

Physical findings
Diverticulitis
- Distressed appearance
- Left lower quadrant abdominal tenderness
- Low-grade fever
- Palpable mass

Acute diverticulitis
- Muscle spasms
- Signs of peritoneal irritation
- Guarding and rebound tenderness

Test results
Laboratory
- Complete blood count revealing leukocytosis
- Erythrocyte sedimentation rate elevated in diverticulitis
- Stool test positive for occult blood in 25% of patients with diverticulitis

Imaging
- Barium studies reveal barium-filled diverticula or outlines, but barium doesn't fill diverticula blocked by impacted stools. This procedure isn't performed for acute diverticulitis due to potential rupture.
- Radiography may reveal colonic spasm if irritable bowel syndrome accompanies diverticular disease.
- Abdominal X-rays rule out perforation.

Diagnostic procedures
- Colonoscopy or flexible sigmoidoscopy shows diverticula or inflamed mucosa. It isn't usually performed in the acute phase.

- Biopsy results may rule out cancer.
- Computed tomography scan of the abdomen evaluates the presence of abscess.

Treatment

General

- No treatment for asymptomatic diverticulosis required
- Nasogastric (NG) decompression for severe diverticulitis
- Bed rest

For diverticulosis

- Liquid or low-residue diet (if experiencing pain)
- Increased water consumption if appropriate
- High-residue diet

For severe diverticulitis

- Nothing by mouth

Medication

For diverticulosis

- Stool softeners
- Bulk medication

For diverticulitis

- Antibiotics
- Analgesics
- Antispasmodics
- I.V. therapy for severe diverticulitis

Surgery

- Colon resection
- May require temporary colostomy to drain abscesses or to rest the colon for 6 to 8 weeks
- Needed for rupture or to correct cases refractory to medical treatment

Nursing considerations

Key outcomes

The patient will:

- express feelings of increased comfort
- maintain normal fluid volume
- have bowel movements that return to normal
- verbalize understanding of the disease process and treatment regimen.

Nursing interventions

 Alert

Remember that diverticulitis produces more serious signs and symptoms, as well as complications, and requires more interventions than diverticulosis.

- If the patient is anxious, provide psychological support.
- Give prescribed drugs.
- Maintain bed rest for acute diverticulitis.

- Maintain the prescribed diet.
- If surgery is scheduled, provide routine preoperative care.

After colon resection

- Provide meticulous wound care.
- Encourage coughing and deep breathing to prevent atelectasis.
- Give I.V. fluids and prescribed drugs.
- Provide colostomy care if appropriate.

Monitoring

- Pain control
- Stools for color, consistency, and frequency
- NG drainage if appropriate
- Signs and symptoms of complications

After colon resection

- Signs of infection and postoperative bleeding
- Intake and output
- Vital signs

Patient teaching

Be sure to cover:

- bowel and dietary habits (in uncomplicated diverticulosis)
- the disorder, diagnosis, and treatment
- preoperative teaching (for a patient needing surgery)
- postoperative teaching (for a patient who must care for his colostomy as needed)
- the desired actions and possible adverse effects of prescribed medications.

Discharge planning

- Refer the patient to an enterostomal therapist if appropriate.
- Refer the patient to a dietitian if needed.

Down syndrome

Overview

Description

- A chromosomal aberration that results in mental retardation, abnormal facial features, and other distinctive physical abnormalities
- Commonly associated with heart defects and other congenital disorders
- Average IQ between 30 and 50 (some higher)
- Also known as *mongolism* and *trisomy 21 syndrome*

Pathophysiology

- Down syndrome is an aberration in which chromosome 21 has three copies instead of the normal two because of faulty meiosis (nondisjunction) of the ovum or, sometimes, the sperm.
- There's unbalanced translocation, in which the long arm of chromosome 21 breaks and attaches to another chromosome.
- The result is a karyotype of 47 chromosomes instead of the normal 46.

Causes

- Trisomy 21
- Deterioration of the oocyte resulting from age or cumulative effects of radiation and viruses

Risk factors

- Maternal age, especially if the mother is older than age 35

Incidence

- Occurs in 1 per 800 to 1,000 live births
- Increases with maternal age, especially after age 35

Common characteristics

- Characteristic craniofacial appearance

Complications

- Death
- Congenital heart defects
- Premature senile dementia
- Leukemia
- Acute and chronic infections
- Diabetes mellitus
- Thyroid disorders

Assessment

History

- Neonate lethargic and a poor feeder

Physical findings

- Slanting, almond-shaped eyes
- Small, open mouth, protruding tongue
- Single transverse palmar crease
- Brushfield's spots on the iris
- Small skull
- Flat bridge across the nose
- Flattened face
- Small external ears
- Short neck with excess skin
- Dry, sensitive skin with decreased elasticity
- Umbilical hernia
- Short stature
- Short extremities with broad, flat, and squarish hands and feet
- Dysplastic middle phalanx of the fifth finger
- Wide space between the first and second toes
- Abnormal fingerprints and footprints
- Impaired reflex development
- Absent Moro's reflex and hyperextensible joints
- Impaired posture, coordination, and balance
- Clubfoot
- Imperforate anus
- Cleft lip and palate
- Pelvic bone abnormalities

Test results

Laboratory
- Karyotype analysis or chromosome mapping showing the chromosomal abnormality and confirming the diagnosis of Down syndrome
- Serum alpha-fetoprotein revealing reduced levels of alpha-fetoprotein prenatally

Imaging
- Prenatal ultrasonography can suggest Down syndrome if a duodenal obstruction or an atrioventricular canal defect is present.
- Amniocentesis allows prenatal diagnosis.

Other
- Developmental screening tests show severity and progress of retardation.

Treatment

General

- Early intervention
- Special education programs
- Special athletic programs
- Maximal environmental simulation for infants
- Safety precautions for children and adults in a controlled environment

Medication

- Antibiotic therapy for recurrent infections
- Thyroid hormone replacement for hypothyroidism

Surgery

- Open-heart surgery to correct cardiac defects, such as ventricular septal defects or atrial septal defects
- Plastic surgery to correct congenital abnormalities, such as protruding tongue, cleft lip, and cleft palate

Nursing considerations

Key outcomes

The patient will:
○ demonstrate age-appropriate skills and behaviors to the extent possible
○ perform health maintenance activities according to level of ability
○ participate in developmental stimulation programs to increase skill levels.

Nursing interventions

○ Establish a trusting relationship with the child's parents.
○ Encourage verbalization and provide support.
○ Encourage the parents to hold and nurture their child.

Monitoring

○ Response to treatment
○ Signs and symptoms of infection
○ Complications
○ Nutritional status
○ Growth and development
○ Thyroid function test results
○ Heart sounds

Patient teaching

Be sure to cover:
○ the need for adequate exercise and maximal environmental stimulation
○ realistic goals for the parents and child
○ information about a balanced diet
○ the importance of remembering the emotional needs of other children in the family.

Discharge planning

○ Refer the parents to infant stimulation classes.
○ Refer the parents and older siblings for genetic and psychological counseling, as appropriate.
○ Refer the patient and his parents to support services.

Dysmenorrhea

Overview

Description

○ Painful menstruation associated with ovulation that isn't related to pelvic disease
○ Most common gynecologic complaint
○ Leading cause of absenteeism from school and work
○ A primary disorder or secondary to an underlying disease

Causes

Primary
○ Unrelated to an identifiable cause
Secondary
○ Endometriosis
○ Cervical stenosis
○ Uterine leiomyomas (benign fibroid tumors)
○ Pelvic inflammatory disease
○ Pelvic tumors (see *Causes of pelvic pain*)

Risk factors

Primary
○ Hormonal imbalance
○ Psychogenic factors

Pathophysiology

○ Pain may result from increased prostaglandin secretion in menstrual blood, which intensifies normal uterine contractions.
○ Prostaglandins intensify myometrial smooth muscle contraction and uterine blood vessel constriction, thereby worsening the uterine hypoxia normally associated with menstruation.
○ Intense muscle contractions and hypoxia cause the intense pain of dysmenorrhea.

Causes of pelvic pain

The characteristic pelvic pain of dysmenorrhea must be distinguished from the acute pain caused by many other disorders, such as:
○ *GI disorders*: appendicitis, acute diverticulitis, acute or chronic cholecystitis, chronic cholelithiasis, acute pancreatitis, peptic ulcer perforation, intestinal obstruction
○ *urinary tract disorders:* cystitis, renal calculi
○ *reproductive disorders:* acute salpingitis, chronic inflammation, degenerative fibroid, ovarian cyst torsion
○ *pregnancy disorders:* impending abortion (pain and bleeding early in pregnancy), ectopic pregnancy, abruptio placentae, uterine rupture, leiomyoma degeneration, toxemia
○ *emotional conflicts:* psychogenic (functional) pain.
Other conditions that may mimic dysmenorrhea include ovulation and normal uterine contractions experienced in pregnancy.

Incidence

○ Affects 10% of high school girls each month
○ Incidence usually peaks in the early 20s, then slowly decreases
○ Generally secondary after age 20

Common characteristics

○ Sharp, intermittent, cramping, lower abdominal pain, usually radiating to the back, thighs, groin, and vulva
○ Pain typically starting with or immediately before menstrual flow and peaking within 24 hours

Complications

○ Dehydration

Assessment

History

○ Pelvic disease
○ Urinary frequency
○ Nausea
○ Vomiting
○ Diarrhea
○ Headache
○ Backache
○ Chills
○ Depression
○ Irritability

Physical findings

○ Abdominal bloating
○ Painful breasts

Test results

Imaging
○ Laparoscopy, hysteroscopy, and pelvic ultrasound help in diagnosing underlying disorders in secondary dysmenorrhea.
Other
○ Pelvic examination and a detailed patient history help to identify causation.

Treatment

General

○ Heat applied locally to the lower abdomen
○ Increased fluid intake
○ Activity, as tolerated

Medication

○ Analgesics
○ Prostaglandin inhibitors
○ Sex steroids (primary)

Surgery

○ Surgical treatment of underlying disorders, such as endometriosis or uterine leiomyomas (secondary)

Nursing considerations

Key outcomes

The patient will:
○ remain free from pain
○ express understanding of disorder.

Nursing interventions

○ Provide emotional support.
○ Give prescribed analgesics.

Monitoring

○ Depression
○ Hydration
○ Pain control

Patient teaching

Be sure to cover:
○ explanation of normal female anatomy and physiology as well as the nature of dysmenorrhea
○ information on pregnancy and contraception
○ keeping a detailed record of her menstrual cycle and symptoms
○ seeking medical care if symptoms persist.

Discharge planning

○ Refer the patient for psychological counseling, if appropriate.

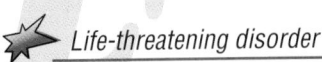
Life-threatening disorder

Ebola virus infection

Overview

Description
○ An unclassified ribonucleic acid virus that results in bleeding
○ Four known strains: Ebola Zaire, Ebola Sudan, Ebola Tai, and Ebola Reston (affects only monkeys)
○ Poor prognosis

Pathophysiology
○ Transmitted by direct contact with infected blood, body secretions, or organs
○ Nosocomial and community-acquired transmission
○ Viral replication (causes focal tissue necrosis, most severely in the liver)
○ Microvasculature damage (causes increased vascular permeability and bleeding)
○ Remains contagious even after the patient has died

Causes
○ Infection with one of three of the four presently known subtypes of Ebola: EBO-Z, EBO-S, and EBO-C

Incidence
○ Not endemic to the United States
○ Affects men and women of all ages

Preventing the spread of Ebola virus

The Centers for Disease Control and Prevention recommends the following guidelines to help prevent the spread of this deadly disease:
○ Keep the patient in isolation throughout the course of the disease.
○ If possible, place the patient in a negative-pressure room at the beginning of hospitalization to avoid the need for transfer as the disease progresses.
○ Restrict nonessential staff members from entering the patient's room.
○ Make sure that anyone who enters the patient's room wears gloves and a gown to prevent contact with any surface in the room that may have been soiled.
○ Use barrier precautions to prevent skin and mucous membrane exposure to blood or other body fluids, secretions, or excretions when caring for the patient.
○ If you must come within 3' (1 m) of the patient, also wear a face shield or a surgical mask and goggles or eyeglasses with side shields.
○ Don't reuse gloves or gowns unless they have been completely disinfected.
○ Make sure any patient who dies of the disease is promptly buried or cremated. Precautions to avoid contact with the patient's body fluids and secretions should continue even after the patient's death.

Common characteristics
○ Flulike symptoms
○ Severe diarrhea
○ Vomiting
○ Internal and external hemorrhage

Complications
○ Liver and kidney dysfunction
○ Dehydration
○ Hemorrhage
○ Abortion

Assessment

History
○ Contact with an infected person
○ Headache
○ Malaise
○ Myalgia
○ Fever
○ Cough
○ Sore throat

Physical findings
○ Conjunctival injection
○ Bruising
○ Maculopapular eruptions
○ Melena
○ Hematemesis
○ Bleeding gums

Test results
Laboratory
○ Blood studies reveal specific antigens or antibodies and may show the isolated virus.
○ Blood studies reveal neutrophil leukocytosis, hypofibrinogenemia, thrombocytopenia, and microangiopathic hemolytic anemia.

Treatment

General
○ Supportive care
○ Strict isolation (see *Preventing the spread of Ebola virus*)
○ Diet as tolerated or total parental nutrition
○ Bed rest or limited activity

Medication
○ I.V. fluids
○ Blood transfusions

Nursing considerations

Key outcomes
The patient will:
○ maintain adequate fluid balance

○ remain hemodynamically stable
○ understand the implications of his illness.

Nursing interventions

○ Enforce strict isolation.
○ Provide emotional support.
○ Give prescribed I.V. solutions and blood products.
○ Provide safety precautions.

Monitoring

○ Vital signs
○ Signs of bleeding
○ Intake and output
○ Laboratory studies

Patient teaching

Be sure to cover:
○ the disorder, diagnosis, and treatment
○ signs of bleeding
○ isolation precautions.

Discharge planning

○ Refer the patient for home care if appropriate.
○ Stress to the patient the need for continued follow-up care.

Ectopic pregnancy

Overview

Description

- Implantation of a fertilized ovum outside the uterine cavity, most commonly in the fallopian tube (see *Implantation sites of ectopic pregnancy*)
- Prognosis good with prompt diagnosis, appropriate surgical intervention, and control of bleeding
- Very few fetuses carried to term; rarely, with abdominal implantation, fetus survives to term
- About one in three chance of giving birth to live neonate in subsequent pregnancy

Pathophysiology

- Transport of a blastocyst to the uterus is delayed.
- The blastocyst implants at another available vascularized site, usually the fallopian tube lining.
- Normal signs of pregnancy are initially present.
- Uterine enlargement occurs in about 25% of cases.
- Human chorionic gonadotropin (HCG) hormonal levels are lower than in uterine pregnancies.
- If not interrupted, internal hemorrhage occurs with rupture of the fallopian tube.

Causes

- Endosalpingitis
- Diverticula
- Tumors pressing against the tube
- Previous surgery, such as tubal ligation or resection
- Transmigration of the ovum
- Congenital defects in reproductive tract
- Ectopic endometrial implants in the tubal mucosa
- Sexually transmitted tubal infection
- Intrauterine device

Implantation sites of ectopic pregnancy

In about 95% of patients with ectopic pregnancy, the ovum implants in part of the fallopian tube: the fimbria, ampulla, or isthmus. Other possible abnormal sites of implantation include the interstitium, ovarian ligament, ovary, abdominal viscera, and internal cervical os.

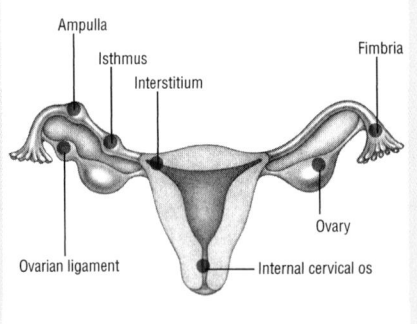

Incidence

- In whites, about 1 of 200 pregnancies
- In nonwhites, about 1 of 120 pregnancies

Common characteristics

- Abdominal tenderness
- Abdominal discomfort
- Minimal vaginal bleeding
- Amenorrhea

Complications

- Rupture of fallopian tube
- Hemorrhage
- Shock
- Peritonitis
- Infertility
- Disseminated intravascular coagulation
- Death

Assessment

History

- Amenorrhea
- Abnormal menses (after fallopian tube implantation)
- Slight vaginal bleeding
- Unilateral pelvic pain over the mass
- If fallopian tube ruptures, sharp lower abdominal pain, possibly radiating to the shoulders and neck

 Alert

Ectopic pregnancy sometimes produces symptoms of normal pregnancy or no symptoms other than mild abdominal pain (especially in abdominal pregnancy), making diagnosis difficult.

Physical findings

- Possible extreme pain when cervix is moved and adnexa palpated
- Boggy and tender uterus
- Adnexa may be enlarged

Test results

Laboratory
- Serum HCG abnormally low; when repeated in 48 hours, level remaining lower than levels found in a normal intrauterine pregnancy

Imaging
- Real-time ultrasonography shows intrauterine pregnancy or ovarian cyst.

Diagnostic procedures
- Culdocentesis shows free blood in the peritoneum.
- Laparoscopy may reveal pregnancy outside the uterus.

Treatment

General

- Initially, in the event of pelvic-organ rupture, management of shock
- Diet determined by clinical status
- Activity determined by clinical status

Medication

- Transfusion with whole blood or packed red blood cells
- Broad-spectrum I.V. antibiotics
- Supplemental iron
- Methotrexate

Surgery

- Laparotomy and salpingectomy if culdocentesis shows blood in the peritoneum; possibly after laparoscopy to remove affected fallopian tube and control bleeding
- Microsurgical repair of the fallopian tube for patients who wish to have children
- Oophorectomy for ovarian pregnancy
- Hysterectomy for interstitial pregnancy
- Laparotomy to remove the fetus for abdominal pregnancy

Nursing considerations

Key outcomes

The patient will:
- have stable vital signs
- express feelings about the current situation
- use available support systems to aid in coping.

Nursing interventions

- Prepare the patient with excessive blood loss for emergency surgery.
- Give prescribed blood transfusions.
- Provide emotional support.
- Give prescribed analgesics.
- Administer $Rh_o(D)$ immune globulin (RhoGAM), as ordered, if the patient is Rh-negative.
- Determine the date and description of her last menstrual period.
- Provide a quiet, relaxing environment.
- Encourage the patient to express her feelings of fear, loss, and grief.
- Help the patient to develop effective coping strategies.

Monitoring

- Vital signs
- Vaginal bleeding
- Pain
- Intake and output
- Signs of hypovolemia
- Signs of impending shock

Patient teaching

Be sure to cover:
- the disorder, diagnosis, and treatment
- postoperative care
- prevention of recurrent ectopic pregnancy
- prompt treatment of pelvic infections
- risk factors for ectopic pregnancy, including surgery involving the fallopian tubes and pelvic inflammatory disease.

Discharge planning

- Refer the patient to a mental health professional for additional counseling, if necessary.

Electric shock

Overview

Description

○ Electric current passing through body
○ Physical damage depends on intensity of current, resistance of the tissues it passes through, type of current, and frequency and duration of current flow
○ Classified as lightning, low voltage (less than 600 V), and high voltage (greater than 600 V)

Pathophysiology

○ Electrical energy results in altered cell membrane resting potential, causing depolarization in muscles and nerves.
○ Electric shock alters normal electrical activity of the heart and brain.
○ Electric shock resulting from a high-frequency current generates more heat in tissues than a low-frequency current, resulting in burns and local tissue coagulation and necrosis.
○ Muscle tetany is elicited.
○ Tissue destruction and coagulative necrosis occurs.

Causes

○ Accidental contact with an exposed part of an electrical appliance or wiring
○ Lightning
○ Flash of electric arcs from high-voltage power lines or machines

Incidence

○ Causes more than 500 deaths annually
○ More common in men ages 20 to 40

Common characteristics

○ Cutaneous burn
○ Variable deep tissue damage

Complications

○ Sepsis
○ Neurologic dysfunction
○ Cardiac dysfunction
○ Psychiatric dysfunction
○ Renal failure
○ Electrolyte abnormalities
○ Peripheral nerve injuries
○ Vascular disruption
○ Thrombi
○ Death

Assessment

History

○ Exposure to electricity or lightning
○ Loss of consciousness
○ Muscle pain
○ Fatigue
○ Headache
○ Nervous irritability

Physical findings

○ Determined by voltage exposure
○ Burns
○ Local tissue coagulation
○ Entrance and exit injuries
○ Cyanosis
○ Apnea
○ Markedly decreased blood pressure
○ Cold skin
○ Unconsciousness
○ Numbness or tingling or sensorimotor deficits

Test results

Laboratory
○ Laboratory test results evaluate internal damage and guide treatment:
  – Arterial blood gas analysis
  – Urine analysis, urine myoglobin tests
  – Complete blood count
  – Electrolytes
  – Blood urea nitrogen, creatinine

Imaging
○ Chest X-rays, if chest injury or shortness of breath occurred, evaluate internal damage and guide treatment.

Other
○ Electrocardiogram (ECG) evaluates internal damage and guide treatment.

Treatment

General

○ Separation of victim from current source
○ Stabilization of cervical spine
○ Emergency measures
○ Treatment of acid-base imbalance
○ Vigorous fluid replacement
○ No dietary restrictions if swallowing ability intact
○ Activity based on outcome of interventions

Medication

○ Osmotic diuretic
○ Tetanus prophylaxis

Nursing considerations

Key outcomes

The patient will:
○ maintain stable cardiac rhythm
○ maintain cardiac output
○ regain skin integrity
○ have wounds and incisions that appear clean, pink, and free from purulent drainage.

Nursing interventions

○ Separate the victim from the current source.
○ Provide emergency treatment.
○ Give rapid I.V. fluid infusion.
○ Obtain a 12-lead ECG.
○ Give prescribed drugs.

Monitoring

○ Cardiac rhythm (continuously)
○ Intake and output (hourly)
○ Neurologic status
○ Sensorimotor deficits
○ Peripheral neurovascular status

Patient teaching

Be sure to cover:
○ information about the injury, diagnosis, and treatment
○ how to avoid electrical hazards at home and at work
○ electrical safety regarding children.

Emphysema

Overview

Description

- Chronic lung disease characterized by permanent enlargement of air spaces distal to the terminal bronchioles and by exertional dyspnea
- One of several diseases usually labeled collectively as chronic obstructive pulmonary disease or chronic obstructive lung disease

Pathophysiology

- Recurrent inflammation associated with the release of proteolytic enzymes from lung cells causes abnormal, irreversible enlargement of the air spaces distal to the terminal bronchioles.
- This enlargement leads to the destruction of alveolar walls, which results in a breakdown of elasticity. (See *What happens in emphysema.*)

Causes

- Genetic deficiency of alpha$_1$-antitrypsin
- Cigarette smoking

Incidence

- Most common cause of death from respiratory disease in the United States
- More prevalent in men than in women
- Approximately 2 million Americans affected
- Affects 1 in 3,000 neonates

Common characteristics

- Exertional dyspnea
- Chronic cough
- Shortness of breath
- Anorexia and weight loss
- Malaise

Complications

- Recurrent respiratory tract infections
- Cor pulmonale
- Respiratory failure
- Peptic ulcer disease
- Spontaneous pneumothorax
- Pneumomediastinum

Assessment

History

- Smoking
- Shortness of breath
- Chronic cough
- Anorexia and weight loss
- Malaise

Physical findings

- Barrel chest
- Pursed-lip breathing
- Use of accessory muscles
- Cyanosis
- Clubbed fingers and toes
- Tachypnea
- Decreased tactile fremitus
- Decreased chest expansion
- Hyperresonance
- Decreased breath sounds
- Crackles
- Inspiratory wheeze
- Prolonged expiratory phase with grunting respirations
- Distant heart sounds

Test results

Laboratory

- Arterial blood gas analysis showing decreased partial pressure of oxygen; partial pressure of carbon dioxide normal until late in the disease
- Red blood cell count showing an increased hemoglobin level late in the disease

Imaging

- Chest X-ray may show:
  - a flattened diaphragm
  - reduced vascular markings at the lung periphery
  - overaeration of the lungs
  - a vertical heart
  - enlarged anteroposterior chest diameter
  - large retrosternal air space.

Diagnostic procedures

- Pulmonary function tests typically show:
  - increased residual volume and total lung capacity
  - reduced diffusing capacity
  - increased inspiratory flow.
- Electrocardiography may show tall, symmetrical P waves in leads II, III, and aV$_F$; a vertical QRS axis; and signs of right ventricular hypertrophy late in the disease.

Treatment

General

- Chest physiotherapy
- Possible transtracheal catheterization and home oxygen therapy
- Adequate hydration
- High-protein, high-calorie diet
- Activity, as tolerated

Medication

- Bronchodilators
- Anticholinergics
- Mucolytics
- Corticosteroids
- Antibiotics
- Oxygen

Surgery

- Chest tube insertion for pneumothorax

Nursing considerations

Key outcomes

The patient will:
- maintain a patent airway and adequate ventilation
- demonstrate energy conservation techniques
- express understanding of the illness
- demonstrate effective coping strategies.

Nursing interventions

- Give prescribed drugs.
- Provide supportive care.
- Help the patient adjust to lifestyle changes necessitated by a chronic illness.
- Encourage the patient to express his fears and concerns.
- Perform chest physiotherapy.
- Provide a high-calorie, protein-rich diet.
- Give small, frequent meals.
- Encourage daily activity and diversional activities.
- Provide frequent rest periods.

Monitoring

- Vital signs
- Intake and output
- Daily weight
- Complications
- Respiratory status
- Activity tolerance

Patient teaching

Be sure to cover:
- the disorder, diagnosis, and treatment
- medication and potential adverse reactions
- when to notify the physician
- avoidance of smoking and areas where smoking is permitted
- avoidance of crowds and people with known infections
- home oxygen therapy, if indicated
- transtracheal catheter care, if needed
- coughing and deep-breathing exercises
- the proper use of handheld inhalers
- high-calorie, protein-rich diet
- adequate oral fluid intake
- avoidance of respiratory irritants
- signs and symptoms of pneumothorax.

 Alert

Urge the patient to notify the physician if he experiences a sudden onset of worsening dyspnea or sharp pleuritic chest pain exacerbated by chest movement, breathing, or coughing.

What happens in emphysema

In normal, healthy breathing, air moves in and out of the lungs to meet metabolic needs. A change in airway size compromises the lungs' ability to circulate sufficient air.

In a patient with emphysema, recurrent pulmonary inflammation damages and eventually destroys the alveolar walls, creating large air spaces. This breakdown leaves the alveoli unable to recoil normally after expanding and results in bronchiolar collapse on expiration. This traps air within the lungs.

Associated pulmonary capillary destruction usually allows a patient with severe emphysema to match ventilation to perfusion and thus avoid cyanosis.

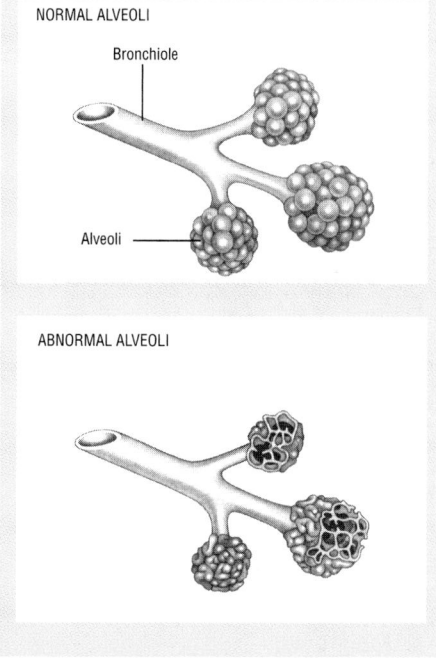

NORMAL ALVEOLI

Bronchiole

Alveoli

ABNORMAL ALVEOLI

Discharge planning

- Refer the patient to a smoking-cessation program if indicated.
- Refer the patient for influenza and pneumococcal pneumonia immunizations as needed.
- Refer the family of patients with familial emphysema for alpha$_1$-antitrypsin deficiency screening.

Encephalitis

Overview

Description
○ Severe inflammation of the brain

Pathophysiology
○ Intense lymphocytic infiltration of brain tissues and the leptomeninges results in:
  – cerebral edema
  – degeneration of the brain's ganglion cells
  – diffuse nerve cell destruction (gray matter more than white).

Causes
○ Mosquito- or tick-borne arboviruses specific to rural areas
○ Enteroviruses in urban areas (coxsackievirus, poliovirus, and echovirus)
○ Herpesvirus
○ Mumps virus
○ Adenoviruses
○ Demyelinating diseases after measles, varicella, rubella, or vaccination
○ Human immunodeficiency virus

Incidence
○ Determining true incidence nearly impossible because reporting policies differ

Common characteristics
○ Dysuria; pyuria
○ Fever
○ Nausea and vomiting
○ Myalgia
○ Photophobia
○ Stiff neck; headache
○ Localized seizures
○ Acute confusion or amnesic state

Complications
○ Bronchial pneumonia
○ Urinary retention and urinary tract infection
○ Pressure ulcers
○ Coma
○ Epilepsy
○ Parkinsonism
○ Mental deterioration

Assessment

History
○ Systemic symptoms include:
  – headache
  – muscle stiffness and malaise
  – sore throat and upper respiratory tract symptoms
  – sudden onset of altered levels of consciousness
  – seizures.

Physical findings
○ Confusion, disorientation, or hallucinations
○ Tremors
○ Cranial nerve palsies
○ Exaggerated deep tendon reflexes and absent superficial reflexes
○ Paresis or paralysis of the extremities
○ Stiff neck when the head is bent forward
○ Fever
○ Nausea and vomiting
○ Cerebral hemispheres
○ Aphasia
○ Involuntary movements
○ Ataxia
○ Sensory defects

Test results
Laboratory
○ Blood analysis identifying the virus
○ Serologic studies in herpes encephalitis showing rising titers of complement-fixing antibodies
Imaging
○ Computed tomography scan to rule out cerebral hematoma
Diagnostic procedures
○ Cerebrospinal fluid (CSF) analysis identifies the virus.
○ Lumbar puncture discloses CSF pressure.
Other
○ EEG shows slowing of waveforms.
○ Diagnosis is readily made from the clinical findings and patient history.

Treatment

General
○ Supportive measures
○ Airway maintenance
○ Oxygen administration
○ Adequate fluid and electrolyte intake
○ Diet as tolerated
○ Activity as tolerated

Medication
○ Osmotic diuretics
○ Corticosteroids
○ Anticonvulsants
○ Aspirin or acetaminophen
○ Antibiotics
○ Antiviral agent vidarabine

Nursing considerations

Key outcomes

The patient will:
○ maintain adequate ventilation
○ exhibit fluid balance within normal limits
○ exhibit temperature within normal limits
○ consume adequate calorie requirements daily
○ verbalize feelings of increased comfort and relief from pain.

Nursing interventions

○ Assure adequate fluid intake.
○ Give prescribed drugs.
○ Position and turn the patient often.
○ Assist with range-of-motion exercises.
○ Maintain adequate nutrition.
○ Administer laxatives or stool softeners.
○ Administer mouth care.
○ Maintain a quiet environment.
○ Start seizure precautions if necessary.
○ Reorient the patient often if necessary.

Monitoring

○ Neurologic function (continuous) for cranial nerve involvement
○ Intake and output
○ Response to medications
○ Intracranial pressure (severe cases)

Patient teaching

Be sure to cover:
○ the disorder, diagnosis, and treatment
○ transient behavior changes
○ the medication regimen
○ adverse effects of medication
○ follow-up care.

Discharge planning

○ Refer the patient to an outpatient rehabilitation program as indicated.

Endocarditis

Overview

Description

- Infection of the endocardium, heart valves, or cardiac prosthesis

Pathophysiology

- Fibrin and platelets cluster on valve tissue and engulf circulating bacteria or fungi. (See *Degenerative changes in endocarditis*.)
- This produces vegetation, which in turn may cover the valve surfaces, causing deformities and destruction of valvular tissue and may extend to the chordae tendineae, causing them to rupture, leading to valvular insufficiency.
- Vegetative growth on the heart valves, endocardial lining of a heart chamber, or the endothelium of a blood vessel may embolize to the spleen, kidneys, central nervous system, and lungs.

Causes

- Cardiac valvular disease
- I.V. drug use
- Rheumatic heart disease
- Prosthetic heart valves
- Congenital heart disease
- Mitral valve prolapse
- Degenerative heart disease
- Calcific aortic stenosis (in elderly patients)
- Asymmetrical septal hypertrophy
- Marfan syndrome
- Syphilitic aortic valve
- Long-term hemodialysis

Incidence

- Up to 40% of affected patients have no underlying heart disease.

Native valve endocarditis
- More common in males than in females
- Most patients are older than age 50
- Uncommon in children
- Rheumatic valvular disease in about 25% of all cases
- Mitral valve most commonly involved valve
- Drug abusers with endocarditis (frequently males)

Common characteristics

- Heart murmur

Complications

- Left-sided heart failure
- Valve stenosis or regurgitation
- Myocardial erosion
- Embolic debris lodged in the small vasculature of the visceral tissue

Assessment

History

- Patient may report predisposing condition and complain of nonspecific symptoms, such as weakness, fatigue, weight loss, anorexia, arthralgia, night sweats, and intermittent fever that may recur for weeks.

Physical findings

- Petechiae on the skin (especially common on the upper anterior trunk) and on the buccal, pharyngeal, or conjunctival mucosa
- Splinter hemorrhages under the nails
- Clubbing of the fingers in patients with long-standing disease
- Heart murmur in all patients except those with early acute endocarditis and I.V. drug users with tricuspid valve infection
- Osler's nodes
- Roth's spots
- Janeway lesions
- A murmur that changes suddenly or a new murmur that develops in the presence of fever (classic physical sign)
- Splenomegaly in long-standing disease
- Dyspnea, tachycardia, and bibasilar crackles possible with left-sided heart failure
- Splenic infarction causing pain in the upper left quadrant, radiating to the left shoulder, and abdominal rigidity
- Renal infarction causing hematuria, pyuria, flank pain, and decreased urine output
- Cerebral infarction causing hemiparesis, aphasia, and other neurologic deficits
- Pulmonary infarction causing cough, pleuritic pain, pleural friction rub, dyspnea, and hemoptysis
- Peripheral vascular occlusion causing numbness and tingling in arm, leg, finger, or toe or signs of impending peripheral gangrene

Test results

Laboratory
- Three or more blood cultures during a 24- to 48-hour period identifying the causative organism (in up to 90% of patients)
- White blood cell count and differential normal or elevated
- Complete blood count and anemia panel showing normocytic, normochromic anemia in subacute infective endocarditis
- Erythrocyte sedimentation rate and serum creatinine levels elevated
- Serum rheumatoid factor positive in about half of all patients with endocarditis after the disease is present for 6 weeks
- Urinalysis showing proteinuria and microscopic hematuria

Imaging
○ Echocardiography may identify valvular damage in up to 80% of patients with native valve disease.
Diagnostic procedures
○ An electrocardiogram reading may show atrial fibrillation and other arrhythmias that accompany valvular disease.

Treatment

General
○ Prompt therapy that continues for several weeks
○ Selection of anti-infective drug based on type of infecting organism and sensitivity studies
○ If blood cultures negative (10% to 20% of subacute cases), possible I.V. antibiotic therapy (usually for 4 to 6 weeks) against probable infecting organism
○ Sufficient fluid intake
○ Bed rest

Medication
○ Aspirin
○ Antibiotics

Surgery
○ With severe valvular damage, especially aortic insufficiency or infection of a cardiac prosthesis, possible corrective surgery if refractory heart failure develops or if an infected prosthetic valve must be replaced

Nursing considerations

Key outcomes
The patient will:
○ carry out activities of daily living without weakness or fatigue
○ maintain hemodynamic stability with adequate cardiac output
○ exhibit no arrhythmias
○ maintain adequate ventilation
○ express feelings about diminished capacity to perform usual roles.

Nursing interventions
○ Stress the importance of bed rest.
○ Provide a bedside commode.
○ Allow the patient to express his concerns.
○ Obtain a history of allergies.
○ Administer antibiotics on time.
○ Administer oxygen.

Monitoring

 Alert

Watch for signs of embolization, a common occurrence during the first 3 months of treatment. Tell the patient to watch for and report these signs.

Degenerative changes in endocarditis

This illustration shows typical vegetations on the endocardium produced by fibrin and platelet deposits on infection sites.

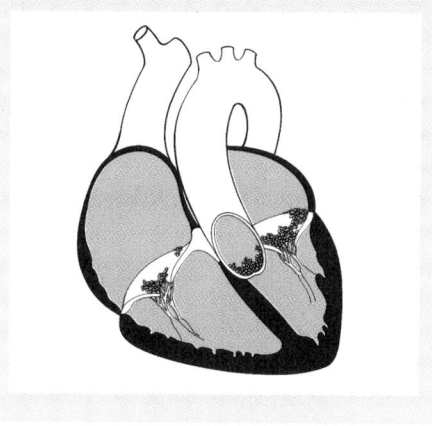

○ Renal status
○ Frequent cardiovascular status assessment
○ Arterial blood gas analysis as needed

Patient teaching

Be sure to cover:
○ the disorder, diagnosis, and treatment
○ anti-infectives the patient needs to continue taking
○ the need to watch closely for fever, anorexia, and other signs of relapse about 2 weeks after treatment stops
○ the need for prophylactic antibiotics before dental work and some surgical procedures
○ proper dental hygiene and avoiding flossing the teeth
○ how to recognize symptoms of endocarditis and to notify the physician immediately if such symptoms occur.

Discharge planning
○ Encourage follow-up care with cardiologist.

Endometriosis

Overview

Description

- Poorly understood gynecologic condition characterized by pain that occurs with menstruation
- Endometrial tissue — appears outside uterine cavity lining
- Ectopic tissue — generally confined to the pelvic area, but can appear anywhere in the body

Pathophysiology

- Endometrial cells respond to estrogen and progesterone with proliferation and secretion.
- During menstruation, ectopic tissue bleeds and causes inflammation of the surrounding tissues.
- Inflammation leads to fibrosis.
- Fibrosis leads to adhesions that produce pain and infertility.

Causes

- Direct cause unknown
- Familial susceptibility
- Direct implantation
- Transportation (retrograde menstruation)
- Formation in situ
- Induction
- Immune system defects
- Lymphatic spread theory
- Inflammatory influence
- Environmental contaminants

Incidence

- Usually occurs between ages 20 and 40
- More common in women who postpone childbearing
- Uncommon before age 20

Common characteristics

- Early menarche
- Menstrual flow lasting more than 7 days
- Cycles lasting more than 27 days
- Family history of endometriosis
- Multiparity
- Cyclic pelvic pain
- Severe dysmenorrhea

Complications

- Infertility
- Spontaneous abortion
- Anemia secondary to excessive bleeding
- Emotional problems secondary to infertility
- Pelvic adhesions
- Severe dysmenorrhea
- Ovarian cyst

Assessment

History

- Cyclic pelvic pain that peaks 5 to 7 days before menses and lasts 2 to 3 days
- Infertility
- Acquired dysmenorrhea
- Pain in lower abdomen, vagina, posterior pelvis and back; often radiates down legs
- Additional symptoms depending on site of involvement:
  - Hypermenorrhea (oviducts and ovaries)
  - Deep-thrust dyspareunia (ovaries and cul-de-sac)
  - Suprapubic pain, dysuria, and hematuria (bladder)
  - Dyschezia, rectal bleeding with menses, and pain in the coccyx or sacrum (rectovaginal septum and colon)
  - Nausea and vomiting that worsen before menses (small bowel and appendix)
  - Abdominal cramps (small bowel and appendix)

Physical findings

- Multiple tender nodules on uterosacral ligaments or rectovaginal septum
- Enlarged nodules (tender during menses)
- Ovarian enlargement with endometrial cysts on the ovaries
- Thickened, nodular adnexa

Test results

Diagnostic procedures

- A scoring and staging system created by the American Fertility Society quantifies endometrial implants according to size, character, and location:
  - Stage I indicates minimal disease (1 to 5 points).
  - Stage II indicates mild disease (6 to 15 points).
  - Stage III indicates moderate disease (16 to 40 points).
  - Stage IV indicates severe disease (more than 40 points).
- Laparoscopy results confirm the diagnosis and identify the disease stage.

Treatment

General

- Stage of disease, patient's age, and desire to have children determine course of treatment
- Pregnancy, if possible, is temporary treatment
- Activity, as tolerated

Medication

- Progestins
- Hormonal contraceptives
- Gonadotropin-releasing analogues
- Androgens
- Analgesics

Surgery

○ Laparoscopy to lyse adhesions, remove small implants, and cauterize implants; for laser vaporization of implants; usually followed by hormonal therapy to suppress return of endometrial implants
○ Total abdominal hysterectomy with bilateral salpingo-oophorectomy in stages III and IV

Nursing considerations

Key outcomes

The patient will:
○ express feelings of increased comfort
○ exhibit no signs of infection
○ express understanding of the disorder and treatment
○ develop adequate coping behaviors.

Nursing interventions

○ Encourage the patient to express her feelings about the disorder.
○ Offer the patient emotional support.
○ Encourage using open communication before and during intercourse.
○ Help the patient to develop effective coping strategies.

Monitoring

○ Effect of treatment
○ Complications
○ Adverse drug reactions
○ Coping ability

Patient teaching

Be sure to cover:
○ the disorder, diagnosis, and treatment
○ associated complications
○ avoiding minor gynecologic procedures immediately before and during menstruation
○ not postponing childbearing due to potential for infertility
○ annual pelvic examination and Papanicolaou test.

Discharge planning

○ Refer the patient and her partner to a mental health professional for additional counseling if necessary.
○ Refer the patient to a support group such as the Endometriosis Association.

Enterobacteriaceae infections

Overview

Description

○ Variety of infections caused by a family of mostly aerobic, gram-negative bacilli
○ Cause local and systemic infections, including invasive diarrhea resembling shigellosis and noninvasive, toxin-mediated diarrhea resembling cholera
○ *Escherichia coli* is the cause of most nosocomial infections

Pathophysiology

○ When infected, incubation takes 12 to 72 hours.
○ Noninvasive diarrhea results from two toxins produced by enterotoxigenic or enteropathogenic strains of *E. coli.*
○ Toxins interact with intestinal juices and promote excessive loss of chloride and water.
○ The invasive form directly attacks the intestinal mucosa without producing enterotoxins, causing local irritation, inflammation, and diarrhea. This form produces sporadic and outbreak-associated bloody diarrhea due to hemorrhagic colitis, which can be life-threatening at age extremes.

Causes

○ Some strains of *E. coli* that are part of normal GI flora but cause infection in immunocompromised patients
○ Infection usually from nonindigenous strains
○ Transmission directly from an infected person
○ Ingestion of contaminated food or water or contact with contaminated utensils
○ Enterotoxigenic *E. coli* (major cause of diarrhea among those who travel from industrialized to developing regions)
○ Most common food source is chopped beef

Incidence

○ May be major cause of diarrheal illness in children in United States
○ Incidence highest among travelers returning from abroad, especially Mexico (noninvasive form), Southeast Asia (noninvasive form), and South America (invasive form)

Common characteristics

○ Diarrhea (cardinal symptom)

Complications

○ Bacteremia
○ Severe dehydration and life-threatening electrolyte disturbances
○ Acidosis
○ Shock

Assessment

History

○ Recent travel to another country
○ Ingestion of contaminated food or water
○ Recent close contact with a person who has diarrhea
○ Abrupt onset of watery diarrhea

Physical findings

○ Cramping abdominal pain with hyperactive bowel sounds
○ Blood and pus in infected stools
○ Vomiting and anorexia
○ Low-grade fever
○ Signs of dehydration, especially in children
○ Signs and symptoms of hyponatremia, hypokalemia, hypomagnesemia, and hypocalcemia from electrolyte losses
○ Orthostatic hypotension
○ Rapid, thready pulse
○ Initially in infants, loose, watery stools that change from yellow to green and contain little mucus or blood
○ Listlessness and irritability in infants

Test results

Laboratory

○ Cultures — growth of *E. coli* in a normally sterile location, including the bloodstream, cerebrospinal fluid, biliary tract, pleural fluid, or peritoneal cavity — suggesting *E. coli* infection at that site

Treatment

General

○ Enteric precautions
○ Correction of fluid and electrolyte imbalances
○ Initially, nothing by mouth
○ Increased fluid intake (if appropriate)
○ Avoidance of foods that cause diarrhea
○ Small frequent meals until bowel function returns to normal
○ Activity, as tolerated.

Medication

○ I.V. antibiotics
○ Bismuth subsalicylate or tincture of opium

Nursing considerations

Key outcomes

The patient will:
○ regain or maintain normal fluid and electrolyte balance
○ have an elimination pattern that returns to normal
○ show no further evidence of weight loss
○ maintain normal cardiac output.

Nursing interventions

○ Institute contact precautions and use proper hand-washing technique.
○ Replace fluids and electrolytes as needed.
○ Clean the perianal area and lubricate it after each episode of diarrhea.
○ Give prescribed antibiotics.
○ During epidemics, screen all facility personnel and visitors for diarrhea, and prevent people with the disorder from having direct patient contact.

Monitoring

○ Intake and output
○ Stool volume measurement and presence of blood and pus
○ Serum electrolyte results
○ Signs and symptoms of gram-negative septic shock
○ Signs and symptoms of dehydration
○ Vital signs

Patient teaching

Be sure to cover:
○ the disorder, diagnosis, and treatment
○ proper hand-washing technique
○ the need to avoid unbottled water, ice, unpeeled fruit, and uncooked vegetables in other countries
○ signs of dehydration and seeking prompt medical attention if these occur (if the patient is to be cared for at home).

Epididymitis

Overview

Description

○ Infection of the epididymis (cordlike excretory duct of the testis)
○ One of most common infections of the male reproductive tract

Pathophysiology

○ Organisms enter the epididymis by the vas deferens or lymphatics.
○ Inflammation occurs.
○ Other organs, such as the testes and prostate, may be affected.

Causes

○ Pyogenic organisms, such as staphylococci, *Escherichia coli*, streptococci, chlamydia, *Neisseria gonorrhoeae*, and *Treponema pallidum*
○ Tuberculosis
○ Sarcoidosis
○ Brucellosis
○ Leprosy
○ Trauma
○ Certain drus (such as amiodarone)
○ Obstruction

Risk factors

○ Urinary tract infection
○ Unprotected sex
○ Prostatitis
○ Trauma

Understanding orchitis

Orchitis, an infection of the testes, is a serious complication of epididymitis. It may also result from mumps, which can lead to sterility or, less commonly, another systemic infection.
Signs and symptoms
Typical effects of orchitis include unilateral or bilateral tenderness and redness, sudden onset of pain, and swelling of the scrotum and testes. Nausea and vomiting also occur. Sudden cessation of pain indicates testicular ischemia, which can cause permanent damage to one or both testes. Hydrocele may also be present.
Treatment
Appropriate treatment consists of immediate antibiotic therapy in bacterial infection or, in mumps orchitis, injection of 20 ml of lidocaine near the spermatic cord of the affected testis, which may relieve swelling and pain. Severe orchitis may require surgery to incise and drain the hydrocele and to improve testicular circulation. Other treatments are similar to those for epididymitis.
   To prevent mumps orchitis, suggest that prepubertal males receive the mumps vaccine (or gamma globulin injection after contracting mumps).

Incidence

○ Usually affects boys and men ages 15 to 30 or older than 60
○ Affects 1 in 1,000 men anually
○ Rare before puberty

Common characteristics

○ Dull, aching groin pain
○ Fever

Complications

○ Orchitis (see *Understanding orchitis*)
○ Infertility
○ Abscess
○ Atrophy
○ Pyocele
○ Infarction

Assessment

History

○ Unilateral, dull, aching pain
○ Pain radiates to spermatic cord, lower abdomen, and flank
○ Extremely heavy feeling in scrotum
○ Dysuria
○ Mild scrotal cellulitis

Physical findings

○ Erythema
○ High fever
○ Characteristic waddle (attempt to protect groin and scrotum while walking)
○ Urethral discharge
○ Prehn sign: elevation of hemiscrotum relieves pain

Test results

Laboratory
○ Urinalysis showing an increased white blood cell (WBC) count, indicating infection
○ Urine culture and sensitivity tests possibly showing the causative organism
○ Serum WBC count greater than 10,000/µl, indicating infection
Imaging
○ Ultrasonography shows enlarged epididymis (larger than 17 mm); can rule out testicular torsion

Treatment

General

○ Scrotal elevation
○ Ice bag to groin
○ Increased oral fluids
○ Bed rest until condition improves
○ Use of an athletic supporter until recovered

Medication

- Broad-spectrum antibiotics
- Analgesics
- Antipyretics

Surgery

- Scrotal exploration for complications of acute epididymitis
- Epididymectomy under local anesthesia when disease is refractory to antibiotic therapy

Nursing considerations

Key outcomes

The patient will:
- avoid or have minimal complications
- express feelings of increased comfort
- express concern about self-concept and body image
- express feelings about potential or actual changes in sexual activity.

Nursing interventions

- Give prescribed drugs.
- Apply ice packs for comfort.

Monitoring

- Signs of abscess formation
- Vital signs
- Pain control
- Intake and output

Patient teaching

Be sure to cover:
- the disorder, diagnosis, and treatment
- drug administration, dosage, and possible adverse effects
- the use of a scrotal support while sitting, standing, or walking
- safe sex practices.

Epidural hematoma

Overview

Description

○ Acceleration-deceleration or coup-contrecoup injuries that disrupt normal nerve functions in bruised area and cause intracranial bleeding

Pathophysiology

○ Injury is directly beneath the site of impact when the brain rebounds against the skull from the force of a blow (a beating with a blunt instrument, for example), when the force of the blow drives the brain against the opposite side of the skull, or when the head is hurled forward and stopped abruptly (as in an automobile accident when a driver's head strikes the windshield).
○ Brain continues moving and slaps against the skull (acceleration), then rebounds (deceleration). Brain may strike bony prominences inside the skull (especially the sphenoidal ridges), causing intracranial hemorrhage or hematoma that may result in tentorial herniation.

Causes

○ Trauma
○ Anticoagulation
○ Thrombolysis
○ Lumbar puncture
○ Epidural anesthesia
○ Coagulopathy or bleeding diathesis
○ Hepatic disease with portal hypertension
○ Vascular malformation
○ Disk herniation
○ Paget disease of bone
○ Valsalva's maneuver
○ Hypertension

Incidence

○ Rare in children younger than age 2 and patients older than age 60
○ Four times more common in men than in women

Common characteristics

○ Brief loss of consciousness
○ Headache
○ Deteriorating mental status

Complications

○ Increased intracranial pressure (ICP)
○ Seizures
○ Respiratory depression and failure

Assessment

History

○ Injury to head
○ Headache
○ Nausea, vomiting
○ Change in mental status

Physical findings

○ Head wound
○ Neurologic signs based on the extent of bleeding—dilated pupils, weakness, sensory deficits, alterations in reflexes, alterations in bladder or anal sphincter tone
○ Bradycardia and hypertension (with increased ICP)

Test results

Laboratory
○ Coagulation studies show clotting abnormalities (if cause is anticoagulation).
Imaging
○ Computed tomography scan or magnetic resonance imaging identifies abnormal masses or structural shifts within the cranium.

Treatment

General

○ Supportive: airway, breathing, circulation
○ Wound care
○ Head of the bed elevated 30 degrees with intracerebral injury
○ Diet based on extent of injury
○ Nothing by mouth if surgery is necessary
○ Bed rest initially, then activity, as tolerated

Medication

○ Vitamin K, fresh frozen plasma, platelets, or clotting products (if coagulation studies are abnormal)
○ Analgesics (after extent of injury is determined)
○ Osmotic diuretics
○ Anticonvulsants
○ Prophylactic antibiotics
○ Corticosteroids

Surgery

○ Placement of burr holes
○ Evacuation of the hematoma
○ Craniotomy

Nursing considerations

Key outcomes

The patient will:
○ be hemodynamically stable

- recover or be rehabilitated from physical injuries to the greatest extent possible
- use support systems to assist with coping
- express a feeling of increased comfort and pain relief.

Nursing interventions

- Provide appropriate wound care.
- Give prescribed drugs.
- Provide emotional support.
- Institute seizure precautions.

Monitoring

- Vital signs
- Neurologic status
- Wound healing
- Seizure activity
- Respiratory status

Patient teaching

Be sure to cover:
- reporting changes in neurologic status
- avoiding aspirin as a pain treatment
- observing for cerebrospinal fluid drainage and signs of infection.

Discharge planning

- Refer the patient to physical, occupational, and speech therapy, as appropriate.
- Refer the patient to social service for extended services, as appropriate.

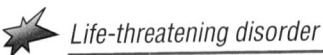

Epiglottiditis

Overview

Description

- ○ Acute inflammation of the epiglottis and surrounding area
- ○ Life-threatening emergency that rapidly causes edema and induration
- ○ If untreated, results in complete airway obstruction
- ○ Mortality 8% to 12%, typically in children ages 2 to 8

Pathophysiology

- ○ An infection of the epiglottis and surrounding area leads to intense inflammation of the supraglottic region.
- ○ Swelling of the epiglottis, aryepiglottic folds, arytenoid cartilage, and ventricular bands leads to acute airway obstruction.

Causes

- ○ Bacterial infection, usually *Haemophilus influenzae* type B
- ○ Pneumococci or group A streptococci

Incidence

- ○ Occurs from infancy to adulthood
- ○ Occurs in any season

Common characteristics

- ○ Sore throat
- ○ Dysphagia
- ○ Apprehension
- ○ Irritability

Airway crisis

Epiglottiditis can progress to complete airway obstruction within minutes. To prepare for this medical emergency, keep these tips in mind:
- ○ Watch for the inability to speak; weak, ineffective cough; high-pitched sounds or no sounds while inhaling; increased difficulty breathing; and possible cyanosis. These are warning signs of total airway obstruction and the need for an emergency tracheotomy.
- ○ Keep the following equipment available at the patient's bedside in case of sudden, complete airway obstruction: a tracheotomy tray, endotracheal tubes, a hand-held resuscitation bag, oxygen equipment, and a laryngoscope with blades of various sizes.
- ○ Remember that using a tongue blade or throat culture swab can initiate sudden, complete airway obstruction.
- ○ Before examining the patient's throat, request trained personnel, such as an anesthesiologist, to stand by if emergency airway insertion is needed.

Complications

- ○ Airway obstruction
- ○ Death

Assessment

History

- ○ Recent upper respiratory tract infection
- ○ Sore throat
- ○ Dysphagia
- ○ Sudden onset of high fever

Physical findings

- ○ Red and inflamed throat
- ○ Fever
- ○ Drooling
- ○ Pale or cyanotic skin
- ○ Restlessness and irritability
- ○ Nasal flaring
- ○ Patient may sit in tripod position
- ○ Thick and muffled voice sounds

Test results

Laboratory
- ○ Arterial blood gas (ABG) analysis possibly showing hypoxia

Imaging
- ○ Lateral neck X-rays show an enlarged epiglottis and distended hypopharynx.

Diagnostic procedures
- ○ Direct laryngoscopy shows swollen, beefy-red epiglottis.

Other
- ○ Pulse oximetry may show decreased oxygen saturation.

Treatment

General

- ○ Emergency hospitalization
- ○ Humidification of airway
- ○ Parenteral fluids
- ○ Activity, as tolerated

Medication

- ○ Parenteral antibiotics
- ○ Corticosteroids
- ○ Oxygen therapy

Surgery

- ○ Possible tracheotomy

Nursing considerations

Key outcomes

The patient will:
- ○ maintain adequate ventilation
- ○ maintain adequate fluid volume

○ maintain a patent airway (see *Airway crisis*)
○ use alternate means of communication.

Nursing interventions

○ Give prescribed drugs.
○ Place the patient in a sitting position.
○ Place the patient in a cool-mist tent.
○ Encourage the parents to remain with their child.
○ Offer reassurance and support.
○ Ensure adequate fluid intake.
○ Minimize external stimuli.

Monitoring

○ Vital signs
○ Intake and output
○ Respiratory status
○ ABG results
○ Pulse oximetry
○ Signs and symptoms of secondary infection
○ Signs and symptoms of dehydration

Patient teaching

Be sure to cover:
○ the disorder, diagnosis, and treatment
○ prescribed drugs and potential adverse effects
○ when to call the physician
○ humidification
○ signs and symptoms of respiratory distress
○ signs and symptoms of dehydration.

Discharge planning

○ Refer the patient for *H. influenzae* b conjugate vaccine, preferably at age 2 months, if indicated.

Epilepsy

Overview

Description

○ Neurologic condition characterized by recurrent seizures
○ Doesn't affect intelligence
○ About 80% of patients have good seizure control with strict adherence to prescribed treatment
○ Also known as *seizure disorder*

Pathophysiology

○ Seizures are paroxysmal events involving abnormal electrical discharges of neurons in the brain and cell membrane potential.
○ On stimulation, the neuron fires, the discharge spreads to surrounding cells, and stimulation continues to one side or both sides of the brain, resulting in seizure activity.

Causes

○ Half of cases are idiopathic
Nonidiopathic epilepsy
○ Birth trauma
○ Anoxia
○ Perinatal infection
○ Genetic abnormalities (tuberous sclerosis and phenylketonuria)
○ Perinatal injuries
○ Metabolic abnormalities (hypoglycemia, pyridoxine deficiency, hypoparathyroidism)
○ Brain tumors or other space-occupying lesions
○ Meningitis, encephalitis, or brain abscess
○ Traumatic injury
○ Ingestion of toxins, such as mercury, lead, or carbon monoxide
○ Cerebrovascular accident
○ Apparent familial incidence in some seizure disorders

Incidence

○ Usually occurs in patients younger than age 20
○ Affects both sexes
○ First seizure usually experienced during childhood or after age 50

Common characteristics

○ Recurring seizures

Complications

○ Anoxia
○ Traumatic injury

Assessment

History

○ Seizure occurrence unpredictable and unrelated to activities
○ Precipitating factors or events possibly reported
○ Headache
○ Mood changes
○ Lethargy
○ Myoclonic jerking
○ Description of an aura
○ Pungent smell
○ GI distress
○ Rising or sinking feeling in the stomach
○ Dreamy feeling
○ Unusual taste in the mouth
○ Visual disturbance

Physical findings

○ Findings possibly normal while patient isn't having a seizure and when the cause is idiopathic
○ Findings related to underlying cause of the seizure

Test results

Laboratory
○ Serum glucose and calcium study results ruling out other diagnoses
Imaging
○ Computed tomography scan and magnetic resonance imaging may indicate abnormalities in internal structures.
○ Skull radiography may show certain neoplasms within the brain substance or skull fractures.
○ Brain scan may show malignant lesions when X-ray findings are normal or questionable.
○ Cerebral angiography may show cerebrovascular abnormalities, such as aneurysm or tumor.
Other
○ EEG shows paroxysmal abnormalities. (A negative EEG doesn't rule out epilepsy because paroxysmal abnormalities occur intermittently.)

Treatment

General

○ Airway protection during seizure
○ Vagal nerve stimulation by pacemaker (see *Vagal nerve stimulation*)
○ A detailed presurgical evaluation to characterize seizure type, frequency, site of onset, psychological functioning, and degree of disability to select candidates for surgery in medically intractable patients
○ No dietary restrictions
○ Safety measures
○ Activity as tolerated

Medication

○ Anticonvulsants

Vagal nerve stimulation

The vagal nerve stimulator is a Food and Drug Administration–approved method to treat medically refractory epilepsy. The stimulator device is about the size of a pacemaker and is surgically placed in a pocket under the skin in the upper chest. Leadwires from the stimulator are tunneled under the skin to a neck incision where the vagal nerve has been exposed. The electrode coils are then placed around the nerve. The treating physician has a computer, which can be used to alter the stimulation parameters, thereby optimizing the treatment of seizures.

The device stimulates the vagus nerve for 30 seconds every 5 minutes to prevent seizure occurrence. A magnet over the area can activate the device to give extra, on-demand stimulation if the patient feels a seizure coming on. Adverse effects are voice change, throat discomfort, shortness of breath, and coughing and are usually experienced only when the device is "on."

○ the importance of carrying a medical identification card or wearing medical identification jewelry.

Discharge planning

○ Refer the patient to the Epilepsy Foundation of America.
○ Refer the patient to his state's motor vehicle department for information about a driver's license.

Surgery

○ Removal of a demonstrated focal lesion
○ Correction of the underlying problem

Nursing considerations

Key outcomes

The patient will:
○ remain free from injury
○ communicate understanding of the condition and treatment regimen
○ use support systems and develop adequate coping
○ maintain usual participation in social situations and activities.

Nursing interventions

○ Institute seizure precautions.
○ Prepare the patient for surgery if indicated.
○ Give prescribed anticonvulsants.

Monitoring

○ Response to anticonvulsants
○ Vital signs
○ Seizure activity
○ Respiratory status
○ Adverse drug reactions
○ Associated injuries

Patient teaching

Be sure to cover:
○ the disorder, diagnosis, and treatment
○ maintaining a normal lifestyle
○ compliance with the prescribed drug schedule
○ adverse drug effects
○ care during a seizure
○ the importance of regular meals and checking with the physician before dieting

Erectile dysfunction

Overview

Description

○ Inability to attain or maintain penile erection long enough to complete intercourse
○ Classified as primary or secondary:
  – Primary impotence — never achieving sufficient erection
  – Secondary impotence — patient has achieved erection and completed intercourse in the past
○ Also called *impotence*

Pathophysiology

○ A lack of autonomic signal or impairment of perfusion may interfere with arteriolar dilation due to inappropriate adrenergic stimulation
○ Premature collapse of the sacs of the corpus cavernosum occurs.
○ Pelvic steal syndrome can cause loss of erection before ejaculation due to increased blood flow to pelvic muscles.

Causes

○ 80% of cases believed to have an organic cause, such as vascular insufficiency and veno-occlusive dysfunction
○ 20% of cases believed to be psychogenic in origin

Risk factors

○ Medication
○ Pelvic injury or surgery
○ Alcohol use
○ Increasing age
○ Smoking
○ Obesity
○ Hypertension
○ Diabetes mellitus
○ Scleroderma
○ Renal failure
○ Cancer treatment
○ Stroke
○ Multiple sclerosis
○ Alzheimer's disease
○ Depression

Incidence

○ Affects men of all age-groups but incidence increases with age

Common characteristics

○ Depression
○ Inability to obtain or maintain an erection

Complications

○ Serious disruption of marital or other sexual relationships

Assessment

History

○ Long-standing inability to achieve erection
○ Sudden loss of erectile function
○ Gradual decline in sexual function
○ Medical disorders, drug therapy, or psychological trauma
○ Achievement of erection through masturbation but not with a partner

Physical findings

○ Anxious appearance
○ Signs of depression

DSM-IV-TR criteria

○ Diagnosis confirmed when patient meets either of two criteria:
  – Persistent or recurrent partial or complete failure to attain or maintain erection until completion of sexual activity
  – Marked distress or interpersonal difficulty occurs as a result of erectile dysfunction
○ Disorder doesn't occur only during course of other Axis I disorder such as major depression

Test results

Laboratory
○ Hormone levels may be decreased
○ Tests to evaluate cause such as HbA_{1c}, serum chemistries, lipid profile, and prostate-specific antigen
Imaging
○ Ultrasonography evaluates vascular function
Diagnostic procedures
○ Angiography evaluates vaso-occlusive disease
Other
○ Direct injection of PGE_1 (alprostadil) into the corpora evaluates the quality of erection
○ Nocturnal penile tumescence testing helps distinguish psychogenic impotence from organic impotence

Treatment

General

○ Sex therapy for psychogenic impotence
○ Treatment of cause for organic impotence
○ Psychological counseling
○ Avoidance of alcohol
○ External vacuum device

Medication

○ Intracavernosal injection therapy
○ Mediaction Urethral System for Erections (MUSE) intraurethral suppository
○ Sildenafil
○ Vardenafil

Surgery
○ Surgically inserted inflatable or semirigid penile prosthesis

Nursing considerations

Key outcomes
The patient will:
○ acknowledge a problem in sexual function
○ discuss feelings and perceptions about changes in sexual performance
○ develop and maintain a positive attitude toward sexuality and sexual performance.

Nursing interventions
○ Encourage verbalization and provide support.
○ As needed, refer the patient to a physician, nurse, psychologist, social worker, or counselor trained in sex therapy.

After penile prosthesis surgery
○ Apply ice packs to the penis for 24 hours.
○ Empty the drainage device when it's full.
○ If the patient has an inflatable prosthesis, provide instructions for use.

Monitoring
○ Response to treatment
○ Adverse effects of medication
○ Complications
○ Postoperative bleeding
○ Postoperative infection

Patient teaching

Be sure to cover:
○ the disorder, diagnosis, and treatment
○ the anatomy and physiology of the reproductive system and the human sexual response cycle
○ the need to avoid intercourse until the incision heals, usually 6 weeks after penile implant surgery
○ signs of infection.

Discharge planning
○ Refer the patient to support services.

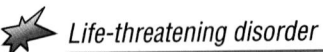
Erythroblastosis fetalis

Overview

Description

- Hemolytic disease of the fetus and neonate
- Stems from an incompatibility of fetal and maternal blood
- Also known as *hemolytic disease of the newborn*

Pathophysiology

ABO incompatibility

- Each blood group has specific antigens on red blood cells (RBCs) and specific antibodies in the serum.
- The maternal immune system forms antibodies against fetal cells when blood groups differ.

What happens in RH isoimmunization

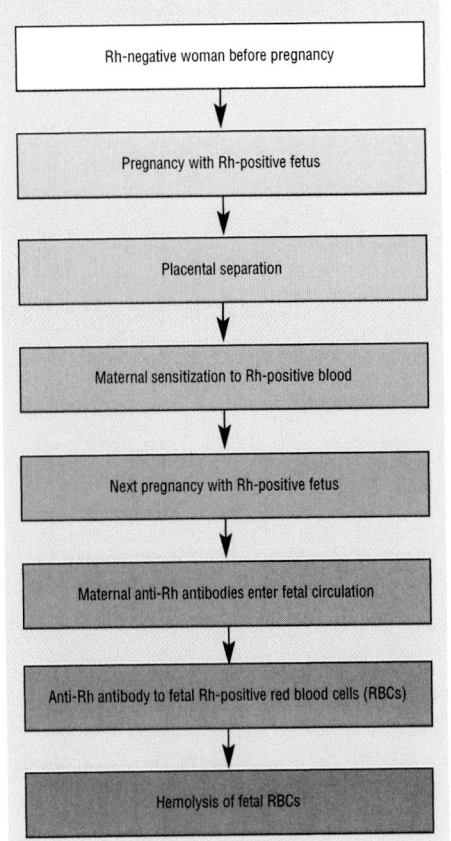

- This can cause hemolytic disease even if fetal erythrocytes don't escape into the maternal circulation during pregnancy.

Rh incompatibility

- During her first pregnancy, an Rh-negative female becomes sensitized (during delivery or abortion) by exposure to Rh-positive fetal blood antigens inherited from the father.
- A female may also become sensitized from receiving blood transfusions with alien Rh antigens; from inadequate doses of $Rh_O(D)$ (Rh_OGAM); or from failure to receive $Rh_O(D)$ after significant fetal-maternal leakage during abruptio placentae (premature detachment of the placenta).
- A subsequent pregnancy with an Rh-positive fetus provokes maternal production of agglutinating antibodies, which cross the placental barrier, attach to Rh-positive cells in the fetus, and cause hemolysis and anemia.
- To compensate, the fetal blood forming organs step up the production of RBCs, and erythroblasts (immature RBCs) appear in the fetal circulation.
- Extensive hemolysis releases more unconjugated bilirubin than the liver can conjugate and excrete, causing hyperbilirubinemia and hemolytic anemia.

Causes

- ABO incompatibility
- Rh isoimmunization (see *What happens in Rh isoimmunization*)
- Rh negativity — more common in Whites than Blacks and rare in Asians
- Rh sensitization — 11 cases per 10,000 births
- ABO incompatibility — frequently occurs during first pregnancy; present in approximately 12% of pregnancies

Common characteristics

- Jaundice
- Anemia
- Hepatosplenomegaly

Complications

- Fetal death in utero
- Severe anemia
- Heart failure
- Kernicterus

Assessment

History

- Mother Rh-positive; father Rh-negative
- Antigen-antibody response developed during previous pregnancy
- Blood transfusion
- Maternal history (for erythroblastotic stillbirths, abortions, previously affected children, previous anti-Rh titers)

Physical findings

- Pallor
- Edema
- Petechiae
- Bile-stained umbilical cord
- Yellow- or meconium-stained amniotic fluid
- Mild to moderate hepatosplenomegaly
- Pulmonary crackles
- Heart murmur
- Jaundice

Test results

Laboratory

- Paternal blood typing for ABO and Rh
- Amniotic fluid analysis showing increased bilirubin and anti-Rh titers
- Direct Coombs' test of umbilical cord blood to measure RBC (Rh-positive) antibodies in the neonate (positive only when the mother is Rh negative and the fetus is Rh positive)
- Cord hemoglobin level in neonate less than 10 g, indicating severe disease
- Many nucleated peripheral RBCs

Imaging

- Radiologic studies showing edema and, in hydrops fetalis, the halo sign (edematous, elevated, subcutaneous fat layers) and the Buddha position (fetus's legs are crossed)

Treatment

General

- Phototherapy (exposure to ultraviolet light to reduce bilirubin levels)
- Intubation of neonate
- Removal of excess fluid
- Maintenance of body temperature

Medication

- Intrauterine-intraperitoneal transfusion (if amniotic fluid analysis suggests the fetus is severely affected and isn't mature enough to deliver)
- Exchange transfusion
- Albumin infusion
- Gamma globulin containing anti-Rh antibody ($Rh_o[D]$)

Surgery

- Planned delivery (usually 2 to 4 weeks before term date, depending on maternal history, serologic test results, and amniocentesis)

Nursing considerations

Key outcomes

The patient will:
- exhibit adequate ventilation
- remain hemodynamically stable
- maintain fluid balance within normal limits
- maintain normal temperature.

Nursing interventions

- Encourage expression of fears by parents concerning possible complications of treatment.
- Promote normal parental bonding.
- Administer $Rh_o(D)$ I.M., as ordered.

Monitoring

- Cardiac rhythm and rate
- Temperature
- Airway and ventilation
- Transfusion complications
- Intake and output

Patient teaching

Be sure to cover:
- the disorder, diagnosis, and treatment
- medications, drug routes, and administration
- preventive measures for reoccurrence.

Discharge planning

- Encourage follow-up appointments.

Esophageal cancer

Overview

Description

- Esophageal tumors usually fungating and infiltrating and nearly always fatal
- Common sites of metastasis are liver and lungs
- Includes two types of malignant tumors: squamous cell carcinoma and adenocarcinoma
- Grim prognosis (5-year survival rates occur in less than 5% of cases; most patients die within 6 months of diagnosis)

Pathophysiology

- Most esophageal cancers are poorly differentiated squamous cell carcinomas, with 50% occurring in the lower portion of the esophagus, 40% in the middle portion, and 10% in the upper or cervical esophagus.
- Adenocarcinomas occur less frequently and are contained to the lower third of the esophagus.
- The tumor partially constricts the lumen of the esophagus.
- Regional metastasis occurs early by way of submucosal lymphatics, often fatally invading adjacent vital intrathoracic organs. (If the patient survives primary extension, the liver and lungs are the usual sites of distant metastases; unusual metastasis sites include the bone, kidneys, and adrenal glands.)

Causes

- Unknown

Risk factors

- Chronic irritation from heavy smoking
- Excessive use of alcohol
- Stasis-induced inflammation, as in achalasia or stricture
- Previous head and neck tumors
- Nutritional deficiency, such as in untreated sprue and Plummer-Vinson syndrome

Incidence

- Most common in men older than age 60
- Occurs worldwide, but most common in Japan, Russia, China, the Middle East, and the Transkei region of South Africa

Common characteristics

- Dysphagia
- Weight loss
- Esophageal obstruction
- Acute pain
- Hoarseness, coughing
- Cachexia

Complications

- Direct invasion of adjoining structures
- Inability to control secretions
- Obstruction of the esophagus
- Loss of lower esophageal sphincter control (may result in aspiration pneumonia)

Assessment

History

- Feeling of fullness, pressure, indigestion, or substernal burning
- Dysphagia and weight loss; the degree of dysphagia varies, depending on the extent of disease
- Hoarseness
- Pain on swallowing or pain that radiates to the back
- Anorexia, vomiting, and regurgitation of food

Physical findings

- Chronic cough (possibly from aspiration)
- Cachexia and dehydration

Test results

Imaging
- X-rays of the esophagus, with barium swallow and motility studies, are used to delineate structural and filling defects and reduced peristalsis.
- Computed tomography scan may help to diagnose and monitor esophageal lesions.
- Magnetic resonance imaging permits evaluation of the esophagus and adjacent structures.

Diagnostic procedures
- Esophagoscopy, punch and brush biopsies, and exfoliative cytologic tests confirm esophageal tumors.
- Bronchoscopy (usually performed after an esophagoscopy) may reveal tumor growth in the tracheobronchial tree.
- Endoscopic ultrasonography of the esophagus combines endoscopy and ultrasound technology to measure the depth of penetration of the tumor.

Treatment

General

- Surgery and other treatments to relieve disease effects
- Palliative therapy used to keep esophagus open:
  - Dilatation of the esophagus
  - Laser therapy
  - Radiation therapy
  - Installation of prosthetic tubes (such as Celestin's tube)
- Liquid to soft diet, as tolerated
- High-calorie supplements

Medication

- Chemotherapy and radiation therapy
- Analgesics

Surgery

○ Radical surgery to excise tumor and resect esophagus or stomach and esophagus
○ Gastrostomy or jejunostomy

Other

○ Endoscopic laser treatment and bipolar electrocoagulation

Nursing considerations

Key outcomes

The patient will:
○ maintain weight
○ maintain fluid volumes within the normal range
○ not aspirate
○ express feelings of increased comfort and decreased pain.

Nursing interventions

○ Provide support and encourage verbalization.
○ Position the patient properly to prevent food aspiration.
○ Provide tube feedings, as ordered.
○ Give prescribed drugs.

Monitoring

○ Vital signs
○ Hydration and nutritional status
○ Electrolyte levels
○ Intake and output
○ Postoperative complications
○ Swallowing ability
○ Pain control

Patient teaching

Be sure to cover:
○ the disease process, treatment, and postoperative course
○ dietary needs
○ the need for rest between activities.

Discharge planning

○ Arrange for home care follow-up after discharge.
○ Refer the patient to the American Cancer Society.

Exophthalmos

Overview

Description

- Unilateral or bilateral bulging or protrusion of the eyeballs or their apparent forward displacement (with lid retraction)
- Also called *proptosis*

Pathophysiology

- Increase in volume within the fixed bony orbital confines displaces the globular orbit anteriorly.

Causes

- Ophthalmic Graves' disease
- Trauma
- Hemorrhage
- Varicosities
- Thrombosis
- Edema
- Infection
- Orbital cellulitis
- Panophthalmitis
- Tumors and neoplastic diseases

Incidence

- Occurs more often in women than in men
- Can occur at any age, but more common between ages 30 and 50

Common characteristics

- Bulging eyeball (see *Recognizing exophthalmos*)
- Diplopia

Complications

- Vision changes

Assessment

History

- Vision changes

Recognizing exophthalmos

This photo shows the characteristic forward protrusion of the eyes from the orbit associated with exophthalmos.

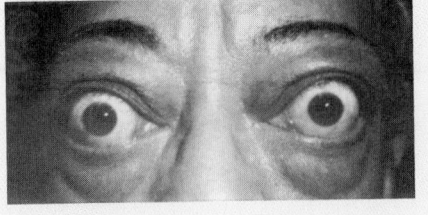

- Eye trauma

Physical findings

- Eye protrusion (see *Detecting unilateral exophthalmos*)
- Visible rim of the sclera
- Infrequent blinking
- Limited ocular movement
- Ocular tenderness

Test results

Laboratory
- Culture of discharge determines the infecting organism
- Sensitivity testing indicates appropriate antibiotic therapy.

Imaging
- Computed tomography scan detects swollen extraocular muscles or lesions within the orbit.

Diagnostic procedures
- Exophthalmometer readings confirm diagnosis by showing the degree of anterior projection and asymmetry between the eyes. (Normal bar readings range from 12 to 20 mm.)

Other
- Physical examination

Treatment

General

- Cold and warm compresses (trauma)
- Activity, as tolerated

Medication

- Antibiotics (infection)
- Antithyroid therapy (Graves' disease)
- Corticosteroids (optic neuropathy)
- Eye lubricants

Surgery

- Orbital decompression (removal of the superior and lateral orbital walls) if vision is threatened, followed by lid (blepharoplasty) and muscle surgery
- Surgical exploration of the orbit and excision of the tumor

Nursing considerations

Key outcomes

The patient will:
- maintain functional eyesight
- understand cause and treatment of exopthalmus
- experience normal eye movement.

Nursing interventions

- Give prescribed drugs.
- Apply cold and warm compresses, as ordered, for fracture or other trauma.
- Provide postoperative care.

If one of the patient's eyes seems more prominent than the other, examine both eyes from above the patient's head. Look down across his face, gently draw his lids up, and compare the relationship of the corneas to the lower lids. Abnormal protrusion of one eye suggests unilateral exophthalmos.

Don't perform this test if you suspect eye trauma.

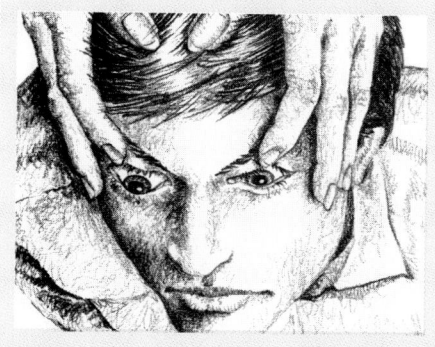

○ Provide emotional support.
○ Protect the exposed cornea with lubricants to prevent corneal drying.

Monitoring

○ Response to therapy
○ Visual acuity

Patient teaching

Be sure to cover:
○ the disorder, diagnosis, and treatment.

Discharge planning

○ Encourage follow-up care.

Fibromyalgia syndrome

Overview

Description

○ A diffuse pain syndrome
○ Referred to as *FMS*
○ Previously called fibrositis

Pathophysiology

○ Several theories describe FMS:
  – Blood flow to the muscle is decreased (due to poor muscle aerobic conditioning, rather than other physiologic abnormalities).
  – Blood flow in the thalamus and caudate nucleus is decreased, leading to a lowered pain threshold.
  – Endocrine dysfunction—such as abnormal pituitary-adrenal axis responses or abnormal levels of the neurotransmitter serotonin in brain centers—affects pain and sleep.
  – The functioning of other pain-processing pathways is abnormal.

Causes

○ Unknown
○ May be primary disorder or associated with underlying disease
○ Possible association with infection
○ May be multifactorial and influenced by stress, physical conditioning, abnormal-quality sleep, neuroendocrine factors, psychiatric factors and, possibly, hormonal factors (due to predominance in women)

Incidence

○ Observed in up to 15% of patients seen in general rheumatology practice and 5% of general medicine clinic patients
○ More common in women than in men
○ May occur at almost any age; peak incidence among those ages 20 to 60

Common characteristics

○ Widespread pain and fatigue

Complications

○ Pain
○ Depression
○ Sleep deprivation

Assessment

History

○ Diffuse, dull, aching pain across neck and shoulders and in lower back and proximal limbs
○ Pain typically worse in morning, sometimes with stiffness; can be exacerbated by stress, lack of sleep, weather changes, and inactivity
○ Sleep disturbances with frequent arousal and fragmented sleep or frequent waking throughout night (patient unaware of arousals)
○ Possible report of irritable bowel syndrome, tension headaches, puffy hands, and paresthesia

Physical findings

○ Tender points are elicited by applying a moderate amount of pressure to a specific location. (See *Tender points of fibromyalgia.*)

Test results

○ Diagnostic testing in FMS not associated with an underlying disease is generally negative for significant abnormalities.

Treatment

General

○ Massage therapy
○ Ultrasound treatments
○ Regular, low-impact aerobic exercise program such as water aerobics
○ Preexercise and postexercise stretching to minimize injury

Medication

○ Amitriptyline, nortriptyline, or cyclobenzaprine
○ Tricyclic antidepressant and serotonin uptake inhibitor
○ Nonsteroidal anti-inflammatory drugs
○ Magnesium supplements
○ Steroid or lidocaine injections

Nursing considerations

Key outcomes

The patient will:
○ express feelings of increased comfort and decreased pain
○ attain the highest degree of mobility possible within the confines of the disease
○ express feelings about limitations
○ express an increased sense of well-being.

Nursing interventions

○ Give prescribed drugs.
○ Provide emotional support.
○ Encourage the patient to perform regular stretching exercises safely and effectively.
○ Provide reassurance that FMS can be treated.

Monitoring

○ Sensory disturbances
○ Level of pain
○ Response to treatment
○ Fatigue
○ Depression

Tender points of fibromyalgia

The patient with fibromyalgia syndrome may complain of specific areas of tenderness, which are shown in the illustrations below.

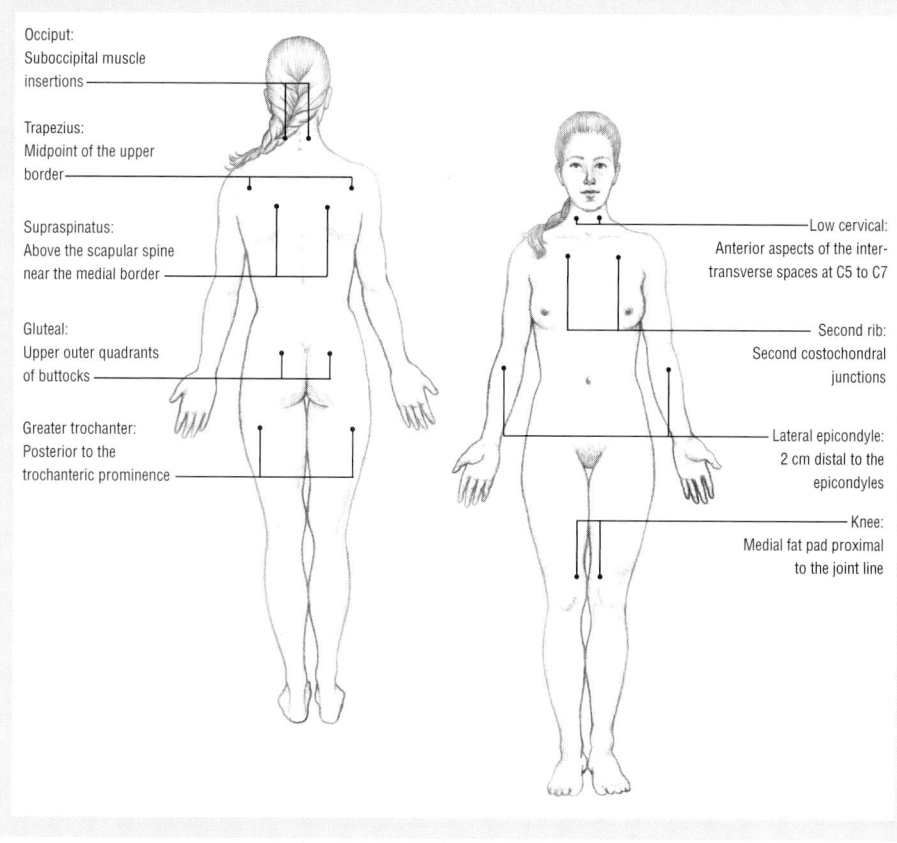

Occiput:
Suboccipital muscle insertions

Trapezius:
Midpoint of the upper border

Supraspinatus:
Above the scapular spine near the medial border

Gluteal:
Upper outer quadrants of buttocks

Greater trochanter:
Posterior to the trochanteric prominence

Low cervical:
Anterior aspects of the inter-transverse spaces at C5 to C7

Second rib:
Second costochondral junctions

Lateral epicondyle:
2 cm distal to the epicondyles

Knee:
Medial fat pad proximal to the joint line

Patient teaching

Be sure to cover:
- the disorder, diagnosis, and treatment
- the importance of exercise in maintaining muscle conditioning, improving energy and, possibly, improving sleep quality
- the importance of taking the tricyclic antidepressant dose 1 to 2 hours before bedtime, which can improve sleep benefits while reducing the morning-after effect
- the avoidance of decongestants and caffeine before bedtime
- the need for a low-fat diet, high in complex carbohydrates, to decrease symptoms.

Discharge planning

- Refer the patient to appropriate counseling as needed.

Folliculitis, furunculosis, and carbunculosis

Overview

Description

Folliculitis
- Superficial bacterial infection of hair follicles that usually heals without scarring
- Characterized by the formation of pustules
- Typically a localized eruption
- Predilection for perifollicular (hairy) areas and flexural surfaces
- May occur in the beard region (sycosis barbae)
- May occur in the scalp or on extremities (follicular impetigo)
- May lead to the development of furuncles (furunculosis) or carbuncles
- Prognosis depends on severity, the patient's physical condition, and ability to resist infection

Furunculosis
- Deeper infections characterized by deeper, more tender, and erythematous nodules or "boils"
- Exacerbated by irritation, friction, or perspiration

Hair follicles and bacterial infection

The degree of hair follicle involvement in bacterial skin infection ranges from superficial folliculitis (erythema and a pustule in a single follicle) to deep folliculitis (extensive follicle involvement), to furunculosis (red, tender nodules that surround follicles with a single draining point) and, finally, to carbunculosis (deep abscesses that involve several follicles with multiple draining points).

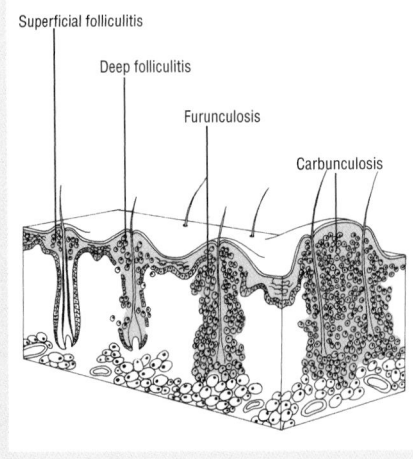

Superficial folliculitis

Deep folliculitis

Furunculosis

Carbunculosis

Carbunculosis
- Abscess of adjacent furuncles
- Develops more slowly

Pathophysiology
- The infecting organism invades the hair follicle.
- An inflammatory reaction within the hair follicle results. (See *Hair follicles and bacterial infection.*)

Causes
- Bacterial infection, typically coagulase-positive *Staphylococcus aureus*
- Contamination from an infected wound elsewhere on the body

Risk factors
- Poor personal hygiene
- Debilitation
- Immunosuppression
- Diabetes mellitus
- Occlusive agents or chemicals such as cosmetics
- Tight-fitting clothing
- Improper shaving technique
- Occlusive therapy, using steroids
- Obesity
- Chronic colonization of *S. aureus* in nares or perineum

Incidence

Folliculitis
- Common infection
- Affects all ages
- Affects males more commonly than females

Furunculosis
- Uncommon in children unless immunocompromised
- Increased frequency after puberty
- More common in adolescents and young adults
- Affects males and females equally

Carbunculosis
- Affects males more commonly than females
- Not uncommon for several family members to be affected at the same time
- More common in patients with diabetes and in patients who are immunocompromised

Common characteristics
- Pustules
- Pain
- Erythema

Complications
- Cellulitis
- Septicemia
- Hematogenous seeding to heart valves, joints, and other organs
- Residual scarring

Assessment

History
- Presence of risk factors
- Pain and erythema for several days or more
- Malaise

Physical findings

Folliculitis
- Localized pustules, usually on the scalp or extremities
- Pustules possibly also in beard area or on eyelids (styes)

Furunculosis
- Hard, painful, or fluctuant nodules usually on neck, face, axillae, or buttocks
- If nodules enlarge and rupture, pus and necrotic material on the skin surface
- Erythema that may persist for days or weeks after nodule rupture

Carbunculosis
- Fever
- Extremely painful, deep abscesses
- Abscesses drain through multiple openings onto the skin surface
- Pain, tenderness, and edema around pustule sites
- Hard or fluctuant nodules under skin surface
- Localized lymphadenopathy

Test results

Laboratory
- Wound culture and sensitivity results showing the infecting organism
- Complete blood count possibly revealing leukocytosis

Treatment

General
- Thorough cleaning of infected area with soap and water
- Avoidance of occlusive agents
- Application of warm, moist compresses

Medication
- Topical or systemic antibiotics

Surgery
- Possible incision and drainage in patients with furunculosis or carbunculosis

Nursing considerations

Key outcomes
The patient will:
- avoid or minimize complications
- exhibit improved or healed wounds or lesions
- report feelings of increased comfort

- demonstrate understanding of proper skin care regimen.

Nursing interventions
- Perform wound care.
- Properly dispose of contaminated dressings.
- Follow standard precautions.
- Apply warm, moist compresses.
- Assist with general hygiene and comfort measures as needed.
- Give prescribed pain medications and antibiotics.

Monitoring
- Adverse drug reactions
- Response to treatment
- Level of comfort
- Complications

Patient teaching

Be sure to cover:
- the disorder, diagnosis, and treatment
- meticulous hand-washing technique
- good personal hygiene
- how to prevent the spread of the infection
- lesion care
- the prescribed medication and potential adverse reactions.

Discharge planning
- Refer patients with recurrent furunculosis for a physical examination to assess for underlying diseases.

Fragile X syndrome

Overview

Description

- Fragile X syndrome is the most common inherited cause of mental retardation.
- Approximately 85% of males and 50% of females who inherit the fragile X mental retardation-1 (FMR1) gene will demonstrate clinical features of the syndrome.
- Postpubescent males with fragile X syndrome often have distinct physical features, behavioral difficulties, and cognitive impairment.
- Females with fragile X syndrome tend to have more subtle symptoms.

Pathophysiology

- This X-linked condition doesn't follow a simple X-linked inheritance pattern.
- Full mutation typically causes abnormal methylation (methyl groups attach to components of the gene) of FMR1.
- Methylation inhibits gene transcription and, thus, protein production.
- The reduced or absent protein production leads to the clinical features of fragile X syndrome.

Causes

- Genetic defect of the X-chromosome
- Well-defined mutation at a specific location on the FMR1 gene

Incidence

- Estimated to occur in about 1 in 1,500 males and 1 in 2,500 females
- Occurs in almost all races and ethnic populations

Common characteristics

Males
- Prominent jaw and forehead
- Head circumference exceeding the 90th percentile
- Long, narrow face with long or large ears that may be posteriorly rotated
- Connective tissue abnormalities, including hyperextension of the fingers, a floppy mitral valve (in 80% of adults), and mild to severe pectus excavatum
- Unusually large testes, found in most affected males after puberty
- Average IQ between 30 and 70
- Hyperactivity, speech difficulties, language delay, and autistic-like behaviors

Females
- Some degree of cognitive impairment, most commonly learning disabilities (math difficulties, language deficits, and attentional problems)
- IQ scores in the mental retardation range
- Autistic-like features (rare)
- Excessive shyness or social anxiety

- Prominent ears and connective tissue manifestations (possibly as significant as in males)

Complications

- Behavioral or learning difficulties
- Cognitive impairment
- Connective tissue abnormalities

Assessment

History

- Average IQ between 30 and 70
- Hyperactivity, speech difficulties, language delay, and autistic-like behaviors
- Excessive shyness or social anxiety

Physical findings

- A prominent jaw and forehead
- Head circumference exceeding the 90th percentile
- Long, narrow face with long or large ears that may be posteriorly rotated
- Hyperextension of the fingers
- Unusually large testes

Test results

Laboratory
- Positive genetic test, preferably deoxyribonucleic acid analysis of blood or buccal samples to detect the size of the cytosine-guanine-guanine repeat and the methylation status of FMR1

Other
- Identification of clinical symptoms

Treatment

General

- Controlling individual symptoms
- Activity, as tolerated

Medication

- Anticonvulsants
- Antidepressants
- Sedatives

Surgery

- Mitral valve repair

Nursing considerations

Key outcomes

The patient will:
- function at the highest level possible
- be free from signs and symptoms of infection
- demonstrate effective learning related to potential.

Nursing interventions

- Give prescribed drugs.

- Provide emotional support to the patient and his family.
- Encourage appropriate activities for the patient's ability.

Monitoring

- Language development
- Seizures
- Hyperactivity

Patient teaching

Be sure to cover:
- drug administration and adverse effects.

Discharge planning

- Refer the patient and family for genetic counseling.
- Refer the family to a support group.
- Advocate for special education services and individualized speech, language, and occupational therapy services during the patient's schooling.

Gas gangrene

Overview

Description

○ Rare condition caused by local infection with an anaerobic, spore-forming, gram-positive, rod-shaped bacillus *Clostridium perfringens* or another clostridial species
○ Occurs in devitalized tissues and results from compromised arterial circulation

Pathophysiology

○ Incubation is 1 to 4 days but can vary from 3 hours to 6 weeks or longer.
○ *C. perfringens* invades soft tissues, producing thrombosis of regional blood vessels, tissue necrosis, and localized edema. (See *Effects of* Clostridium perfringens.)
○ Necrosis releases carbon dioxide and hydrogen subcutaneously, producing interstitial gas bubbles.

Causes

○ *C. perfringens*
○ Transmission occurs when the organism enters the body during trauma or surgery

Risk factor

○ Diabetes mellitus

Incidence

○ Rare, although more than 30% of deep wounds infected with clostridia
○ Most common in deep wounds, especially when tissue necrosis further reduces oxygen supply

---

Effects of *Clostridium perfringens*

As *C. perfringens* grows in a closed wound, it destroys cell walls and causes hemolysis, local tissue death, and increasing edema.

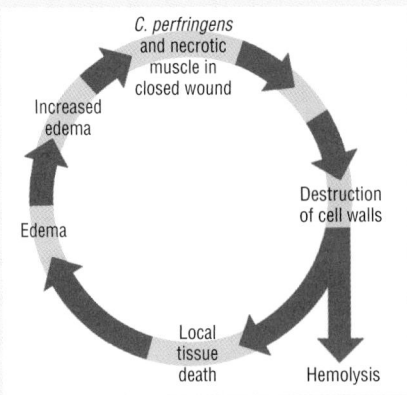

○ Most common in extremities and abdominal wounds; less common in uterus

Common characteristics

○ Sudden, severe pain at wound site

Complications

○ Renal failure
○ Hypotension and shock
○ Hemolytic anemia
○ Tissue death requiring amputation of the affected body part

Assessment

History

○ Recent surgery (within 72 hours)
○ Traumatic injury
○ Septic abortion
○ Delivery

Physical findings

○ Normothermia, followed by a moderate increase, usually not above 101° F (38.3° C)
○ Toxemia (hypotension, tachycardia, tachypnea)
○ Localized swelling and discoloration (often dusky brown or reddish)
○ Bullae and tissue necrosis
○ Dark red or black necrotic muscle
○ Foul-smelling, watery or frothy discharge
○ Subcutaneous emphysema (hallmark of gas gangrene)
○ In later stages, altered level of consciousness that may deteriorate to delirium and coma

Test results

Laboratory
○ Anaerobic cultures of wound drainage showing *C. perfringens*
○ Gram stain of wound drainage showing large, gram-positive, rod-shaped bacteria
○ Blood studies showing leukocytosis and, later, hemolysis
Imaging
○ X-rays reveal gas in tissues.

Treatment

General

○ Hyperbaric oxygenation
○ Adequate hydration
○ Nothing by mouth if surgery is planned
○ Bed rest until recovery begins

Medication

○ I.V. antibiotics
○ Analgesics

Surgery

○ Immediate wide surgical excision of all affected tissues and necrotic muscle in myositis
○ Amputation of the affected part

Nursing considerations

Key outcomes

The patient will:
○ maintain hemodynamic stability
○ have skin that remains warm, dry, and intact
○ maintain collateral circulation
○ express feelings of increased comfort and relief from pain.

Nursing interventions

○ Give prescribed analgesics.
○ Prepare for surgery, if indicated.
○ Provide adequate fluid replacement.
○ Maintain the airway and ventilation.
○ Provide appropriate skin care and meticulous wound care; place the patient on an air mattress or an air-fluidized bed.
○ Encourage verbalization and provide support.

Monitoring

○ Vital signs
○ Intake and output
○ Pulmonary and cardiac function
○ Wound site

Patient teaching

Be sure to cover:
○ the disorder, diagnosis, and treatment
○ the need to report severe pain at the wound site immediately
○ the need to report foul odor or drainage from the wound site.

Discharge planning

○ After recovery, refer the patient for physical rehabilitation as necessary.
○ After extensive surgery, such as amputation, refer the patient for psychological support as necessary.

Gastric cancer

Overview

Description

- Cancer of the GI tract classified according to gross appearance (polypoid, ulcerating, ulcerating and infiltrating, or diffuse)
- Prognosis depends on stage of disease at time of diagnosis (5-year survival rate about 15%)

Pathophysiology

- The most commonly affected areas of the stomach are the pylorus and antrum.
- The remaining areas affected in order of descending frequency are the lesser curvature of the stomach, the cardia, the body of the stomach, and the greater curvature of the stomach.
- Rapid metastasis occurs to the regional lymph nodes, omentum, liver, and lungs.

Causes

- Unknown

Risk factors

- Gastritis with gastric atrophy
- Type A blood (10% increased risk)
- Family history of gastric cancer
- Smoked foods, pickled vegetables, and salted fish and meat
- High alcohol consumption
- Smoking

Incidence

- Common worldwide in all races
- Incidence greater in men older than age 40
- Mortality high in Japan, Iceland, Chile, and Austria
- Incidence decreased 50% over the past 25 years, with the resulting death rate now one-third of the death rate 30 years ago

Common characteristics

- Feeling of fullness
- Abdominal distention
- Back, epigastric, or retrosternal pain

Complications

- Malnutrition
- GI obstruction
- Iron deficiency anemia
- Metastasis

Assessment

History

- Back, epigastric, or retrosternal pain not relieved with nonprescription medications
- Vague feeling of fullness, heaviness, and moderate abdominal distention after meals
- Weight loss, nausea, vomiting
- Weakness and fatigue
- Dysphagia

Physical findings

- Abdominal distention
- Palpable mass
- Palpable lymph nodes, especially the supraclavicular and axillary nodes
- Other assessment findings that depend on extent of disease and location of metastasis

Test results

Laboratory

- Complete blood count possibly showing iron deficiency anemia
- Liver function studies possibly elevated with metastatic spread of tumor to liver
- Carcinoembryonic antigen radioimmunoassay possibly elevated

Imaging

- Barium X-rays of the GI tract with fluoroscopy show changes that suggest gastric cancer, including a tumor or filling defect in the outline of the stomach, loss of flexibility and distensibility, and abnormal gastric mucosa with or without ulceration.

Diagnostic procedures

- Gastroscopy with fiber-optic endoscope helps rule out other diffuse gastric mucosal abnormalities by allowing direct visualization.
- Gastroscopic biopsy permits evaluation of gastric mucosal lesions.

Other

- Gastric acid stimulation test discloses whether the stomach secretes acid properly.

Treatment

General

- Radiation therapy combined with chemotherapy (not indicated preoperatively because it may damage viscera and impede healing)
- Diet based on the extent of the disorder and clinical condition
- Parenteral feeding with an inability to consume adequate calories

Medication

- Chemotherapy
- Antiemetics
- Sedatives and tranquilizers
- Opioid analgesics

Surgery

- Excision of lesion with appropriate margins (in more than one-third of patients)
- Gastroduodenostomy
- Gastrojejunostomy

- Partial gastric resection
- Total gastrectomy (If metastasis has occurred, omentum and spleen may have to be removed)

Nursing considerations

Key outcomes

The patient will:
- not lose more weight
- express feelings of increased energy
- report feeling less tension and pain
- maintain skin integrity.

Nursing interventions

- Provide a high-protein, high-calorie diet with dietary supplements.
- Give prescribed drugs.
- Provide parenteral nutrition as appropriate.
- After surgery, provide supportive care.

Monitoring

- Pain control
- Vital signs
- Hydration and nutritional status
- Nasogastric tube function and drainage
- Wound site
- Postoperative complications
- Effects of medication

Patient teaching

Be sure to cover (with the patient or his family):
- the disorder, diagnosis, and treatment
- the dietary plan
- effective pulmonary toileting
- avoidance of crowds and people with known infection
- relaxation techniques
- all drugs, including administration, dosage, and possible adverse effects

Discharge planning

- Direct the patient and his family to support services.
- Refer the patient for home services as necessary.
- Refer the patient for physical or occupational therapy as necessary.

Gastritis

Overview

Description

- ○ Inflammation of the gastric mucosa
- ○ May be acute or chronic
- ○ Most common stomach disorder (acute)

Pathophysiology

Acute gastritis
- ○ The protective mucosal layer is altered.
- ○ Acid secretion produces mucosal reddening, edema, and superficial surface erosion.

Chronic gastritis
- ○ Progressive thinning and degeneration of gastric mucosa occur.

Causes

Acute gastritis
- ○ Chronic ingestion of irritating foods and alcohol
- ○ Such drugs as aspirin and other nonsteroidal anti-inflammatory agents (in large doses), cytotoxic agents, caffeine, corticosteroids, antimetabolites, phenylbutazone, and indomethacin
- ○ Ingested poisons, especially dichloro-diphenyl-trichloroethane (DDT), ammonia, mercury, carbon tetrachloride, or corrosive substances
- ○ Endotoxins released from infecting bacteria, such as staphylococci, *Escherichia coli,* and salmonella
- ○ Complication of acute illness

Chronic gastritis
- ○ Recurring exposure to irritating substances, such as drugs, alcohol, cigarette smoke, and environmental agents
- ○ Pernicious anemia, renal disease, or diabetes mellitus
- ○ *Helicobacter pylori* infection (common cause of nonerosive gastritis)

Risk factors

- ○ Older than age 60
- ○ Exposure to toxic substances
- ○ Hemodynamic disorder

Incidence

- ○ May occur at any age; increased incidence of *H. pylori* in people older than age 60
- ○ Occurs equally in men and women
- ○ Acute gastritis in 8 of 1,000 people; chronic gastritis in 2 of 10,000 people

Common characteristics

- ○ Abdominal pain
- ○ Indigestion

Complications

- ○ Hemorrhage
- ○ Obstruction
- ○ Perforation
- ○ Peritonitis
- ○ Gastric cancer

Assessment

History

- ○ Patient reveals one or more causative agents
- ○ Rapid onset of symptoms (acute gastritis)
- ○ Epigastric discomfort
- ○ Indigestion
- ○ Cramping
- ○ Anorexia
- ○ Nausea, hematemesis, and vomiting
- ○ Coffee-ground emesis or melena if GI bleeding is present

Physical findings

- ○ Possible normal appearance
- ○ Grimacing
- ○ Restlessness
- ○ Pallor
- ○ Tachycardia
- ○ Hypotension
- ○ Abdominal distention, tenderness, and guarding
- ○ Normoactive to hyperactive bowel sounds

Test results

Laboratory
- ○ Occult blood in vomitus or stools (or both) if the patient has gastric bleeding
- ○ Decreased hemoglobin (Hb) level and hematocrit
- ○ Urea breath test showing *H. pylori*

Diagnostic procedures
- ○ Upper GI endoscopy reveals gastritis when it's performed within 24 hours of bleeding.
- ○ Biopsy reveals inflammatory process.

Treatment

General

- ○ Elimination of cause
- ○ For massive bleeding:
  - – Blood transfusion
  - – Iced saline lavage
  - – Angiography with vasopressin
- ○ Nothing by mouth if bleeding occurs
- ○ Elimination of irritating foods
- ○ Activity, as tolerated (encourage mobilization)

Medication

- ○ Histamine antagonists
- ○ Antacids
- ○ Proton pump inhibitors
- ○ Prostaglandins
- ○ Vitamin B_{12}
- ○ Triple therapy — two antibiotics and bismuth subsalicylate
- ○ Dual therapy — antibiotic and proton pump inhibitor

Surgery

○ When conservative treatment fails
○ Vagotomy, pyloroplasty
○Partial or total gastrectomy (rarely)

Nursing considerations

Key outcomes

The patient will:
○ express feelings of increased comfort
○ maintain normal fluid volume
○ maintain weight
○ express concerns about current condition
○ verbalize understanding of the disorder and treatment regimen.

Nursing interventions

○ Provide physical and emotional support.
○ Give prescribed drugs and I.V. fluids.
○ Assist the patient with diet modification.
○ If surgery is necessary, prepare the patient preoperatively and provide appropriate postoperative care.
○ Consult a dietitian as necessary.

Monitoring

○ Vital signs
○ Fluid intake and output
○ Electrolyte and Hb levels
○ Returning symptoms as food is reintroduced
○ Response to medication
○ Pain control

Patient teaching

Be sure to cover:
○ the disorder, diagnosis, and treatment
○ lifestyle and diet modifications
○ preoperative teaching if surgery is necessary
○ stress-reduction techniques
○ drug administration and possible adverse effects.

Discharge planning

○ Refer the patient to a smoking-cessation program if indicated.

Gastroenteritis

Overview

Description

- Self-limiting inflammation of the stomach and small intestine
- Intestinal flu, traveler's diarrhea, viral enteritis, and food poisoning

Pathophysiology

- The bowel reacts to the various causes of gastroenteritis with increased luminal fluid that can't be absorbed.
- This results in abdominal pain, vomiting, severe diarrhea (primarily), and secondary depletion of intracellular fluid.
- Dehydration and electrolyte loss occur.

Causes

- Bacteria, such as *Staphylococcus aureus, Salmonella, Shigella, Clostridium botulinum, Clostridium perfringens, and Escherichia coli*
- Amoebae, especially *Entamoeba histolytica*
- Parasites, such as *Ascaris, Enterobius,* and *Trichinella spiralis*

Preventing traveler's diarrhea

If the patient travels, especially to developing nations, discuss precautions that he can take to reduce his chances of getting traveler's diarrhea. Explain that traveler's diarrhea is caused by inadequate sanitation and occurs after bacteria-contaminated food or water is ingested. These organisms attach to the lining of the small intestine, where they release a toxin that causes diarrhea and cramps. To minimize this risk, advise him to:

- drink water (or brush his teeth with water) only if it's chlorinated or bottled (Chlorination protects the water supply from bacterial contaminants such as *Escherichia coli.*)
- avoid beverages in glasses that may have been washed in contaminated water
- refuse ice cubes that may have been made from contaminated water
- drink only beverages made with boiled water, such as coffee and tea, or those in bottles or cans
- sanitize impure water by adding 2% tincture of iodine (5 drops/L of clear water, 10 drops/L of cloudy water) or by adding liquid laundry bleach (about 2 drops/L of clear water; 4 drops/L of cloudy water)
- avoid uncooked vegetables, unpeeled fresh fruits, salads, unpasteurized milk, and other dairy products
- beware of foods offered by street vendors.

If traveler's diarrhea occurs despite precautions, bismuth subsalicylate, diphenoxylate with atropine, or loperamide can be used to relieve symptoms.

- Viruses, such as adenoviruses, echoviruses, and coxsackieviruses
- Ingestion of toxins, such as poisonous plants and toadstools
- Drug reactions from antibiotics
- Food allergens
- Enzyme deficiencies

Incidence

- Occurs at any age
- Major cause of morbidity and mortality in underdeveloped nations
- Ranks second to common cold as cause of lost work time in the United States
- Fifth most common cause of death among young children
- Can be life-threatening in elderly and debilitated patients

Common characteristics

- Diarrhea
- Nausea and vomiting

Complications

- Severe dehydration
- Electrolyte imbalance

Assessment

History

- Acute onset of diarrhea
- Abdominal pain and discomfort
- Nausea, vomiting
- Malaise and fatigue
- Exposure to contaminated food
- Recent travel (see *Preventing traveler's diarrhea*)

Physical findings

- Slight abdominal distention
- Poor skin turgor (with dehydration)
- Hyperactive bowel sounds
- Decreased blood pressure

Test results

Laboratory
- Gram stain, stool culture (by direct rectal swab), or blood culture showing the causative bacteria

Treatment

General

- Supportive treatment for nausea, vomiting, and diarrhea
- Rehydration
- Initially, clear liquids as tolerated
- Electrolyte solutions
- Avoidance of milk products
- Activity, as tolerated (encourage mobilization)

Medication

○ Antidiarrheal therapy
○ Antiemetics
○ Antibiotics
○ I.V. fluids

Nursing considerations

Key outcomes

The patient will:
○ maintain weight without further loss
○ express feelings of increased comfort
○ maintain adequate fluid volume
○ maintain normal vital signs.

Nursing interventions

○ Allow uninterrupted rest periods.
○ Replace lost fluids and electrolytes through diet or
  I.V. fluids.
○ Give prescribed drugs.

Monitoring

○ Intake and output
○ Vital signs
○ Signs of dehydration
○ Electrolytes

Patient teaching

Be sure to cover:
○ the disorder, diagnosis, and treatment
○ dietary modifications
○ all prescribed drugs, including administration and
  possible adverse effects
○ preventive measures
○ how to perform warm sitz baths three times per day
  to relieve anal irritation.

Gastroesophageal reflux disease

Overview

Description

○ Backflow of gastric or duodenal contents, or both, into the esophagus and past the lower esophageal sphincter (LES), without associated belching or vomiting
○ Reflux of gastric acid, causing acute epigastric pain, usually after a meal
○ Popularly called *heartburn*
○ Also called *GERD*

Pathophysiology

○ Reflux occurs when LES pressure is deficient or pressure in the stomach exceeds LES pressure. The LES relaxes, and gastric contents regurgitate into the esophagus.
○ The degree of mucosal injury is based on the amount and concentration of refluxed gastric acid, proteolytic enzymes, and bile acids.

Causes

○ Pyloric surgery (alteration or removal of the pylorus), which allows reflux of bile or pancreatic juice
○ Hiatal hernia with incompetent sphincter
○ Any condition or position that increases intra-abdominal pressure

Risk factors

○ Any agent that lowers LES pressure: acidic and fatty food, alcohol, cigarettes, anticholinergics (atropine, belladonna, propantheline) or other drugs (morphine, diazepam, calcium channel blockers, meperidine)
○ Nasogastric (NG) intubation for more than 4 days

Incidence

○ Affects approximately 7 million Americans
○ Affects all ethnic groups and socioeconomic classes
○ Most common in people ages 45 to 64

Common characteristics

○ Epigastric pain, usually after a meal or when lying down

Complications

○ Reflux esophagitis
○ Esophageal stricture
○ Esophageal ulcer
○ Barrett's esophagus (metaplasia and possible increased risk of neoplasm)
○ Anemia from esophageal bleeding
○ Reflux aspiration leading to chronic pulmonary disease

Assessment

History

○ Minimal or no symptoms in one-third of patients
○ Heartburn that typically occurs 1½ to 2 hours after eating
○ Heartburn that worsens with vigorous exercise, bending, lying down, wearing tight clothing, coughing, constipation, and obesity
○ Reported relief by using antacids or sitting upright
○ Regurgitation without associated nausea or belching
○ Feeling of fluid accumulation in the throat without a sour or bitter taste
○ Chronic pain radiating to the neck, jaws, and arms that may mimic angina pectoris
○ Nocturnal hypersalivation and wheezing

Physical findings

○ Odynophagia (sharp substernal pain on swallowing), possibly followed by a dull substernal ache
○ Bright red or dark brown blood in vomitus
○ Laryngitis and morning hoarseness
○ Chronic cough

Test results

Imaging
○ Barium swallow with fluoroscopy shows evidence of recurrent reflux.
Diagnostic procedures
○ Esophageal acidity test reveals degree of gastroesophageal reflux.
○ Gastroesophageal scintillation testing shows reflux.
○ Esophageal manometry reveals abnormal LES pressure and sphincter incompetence.
○ Acid perfusion (Bernstein) test result confirms esophagitis.
○ Esophagoscopy and biopsy results confirm pathologic changes in the mucosa.

Treatment

General

○ Modification of lifestyle
○ Positional therapy
○ Removal of cause
○ Weight reduction, if appropriate
○ Avoidance of dietary causes
○ Avoidance of eating 2 hours before sleep (see *Factors affecting LES pressure*)
○ Parenteral nutrition or tube feedings
○ No activity restrictions for medical treatment
○ Lifting restrictions for surgical treatment

Medication

○ Antacids
○ Cholinergics
○ Histamine-2 receptor antagonists
○ Proton pump inhibitors

Factors affecting LES pressure

Various dietary and lifestyle elements can increase or decrease lower esophageal sphincter (LES) pressure. Take these into account as you plan the patient's treatment program.

What increases LES pressure
- Protein
- Carbohydrates
- Nonfat milk
- Low-dose ethanol

What decreases LES pressure
- Fat
- Whole milk
- Orange juice
- Tomatoes
- Antiflatulent (simethicone)
- Chocolate
- High-dose ethanol
- Cigarette smoking
- Lying on right or left side
- Sitting

Surgery

- Hiatal hernia repair
- Vagotomy or pyloroplasty
- Esophagectomy

Nursing considerations

Key outcomes

The patient will:
- state and demonstrate understanding of the disorder and its treatment
- express feelings of increased comfort
- show no signs of aspiration
- have minimal or no complications.

Nursing interventions

- Offer emotional and psychological support.
- Assist with diet modification.
- Perform chest physiotherapy.
- Use semi-Fowler's position for the patient with an NG tube.

Monitoring

After surgery
- Respiratory status
- Pain control
- Intake and output
- Vital signs
- Chest tube drainage
- Bowel function

Patient teaching

Be sure to cover:
- the disorder, diagnosis, and treatment
- causes of gastroesophageal reflux
- prescribed antireflux regimen of medication, diet, and positional therapy
- developing a dietary plan
- the need to identify situations or activities that increase intra-abdominal pressure
- the need to refrain from using substances that reduce sphincter control
- signs and symptoms to watch for and report.

Generalized anxiety disorder

Overview

Description

- Feeling of apprehension sometimes described as an exaggerated feeling of impending doom, dread, or uneasiness
- Reaction to an internal threat
- Uncontrollable, unreasonable worry that persists for at least 6 months and narrows perceptions or interferes with normal functioning

Pathophysiology

- Little physiologic data
- Aberration in benzodiazepine receptor regulation occurs

Causes

- Conflict

Incidence

- Can begin at any age but typically begins between ages 20 and 40
- Equally common in men and women

Common characteristics

Mild anxiety
- Psychological symptoms
- Unusually self-aware and alert to surroundings

Moderate anxiety
- Selective inattention, but can concentrate on a single task

Severe anxiety
- Inability to concentrate on more than scattered details of a task
- Panic state with acute anxiety causing complete loss of concentration, typically with unintelligible speech

Complications

- Impaired social or occupational functioning
- Substance abuse

Assessment

History

- Muscle aches and spasms
- Headaches
- Inability to relax
- Apprehension
- Fear
- Anger
- Difficulty concentrating, eating, and sleeping

Physical findings

- Trembling

- Shortness of breath
- Tachycardia
- Sweating

DSM-IV-TR criteria

A diagnosis is confirmed when the patient's symptoms match the following criteria:
- Excessive anxiety and worry about a number of events or activities occur more days than not for at least 6 months.
- The person finds it difficult to control the worry.
- The anxiety and worry are associated with at least three of the following six symptoms:
  - restlessness or feeling keyed up or on edge
  - being easily fatigued
  - difficulty concentrating or mind going blank
  - irritability
  - muscle tension
  - sleep disturbances (difficulty falling or staying asleep, or restless, unsatisfying sleep).
- The focus of the anxiety and worry isn't confined to features of an axis disorder.
- The anxiety, worry, or physical symptoms cause clinically significant distress or impairment in social, occupational, or other important areas of functioning.
- The disturbance isn't due to the direct physiologic effects of a substance or a general medical condition and doesn't occur exclusively during a mood disorder, a psychotic disorder, or a pervasive, developmental disorder.

Test results

Laboratory
- Tests, such as cardiac enzymes, troponin level, and thyroid studies, rule out organic causes of symptoms.

Diagnostic procedures
- Electrocardiogram excludes myocardial ischemia.

Other
- Psychiatric evaluation

Treatment

General

- Psychotherapy
- Relaxation techniques

Medication

- Benzodiazepines
- Tricyclic antidepressants

Nursing considerations

Key outcomes

The patient will:
- develop effective coping strategies
- identify anxiety triggers
- experience reduced anxiety.

Nursing interventions

○ Give prescribed drugs.
○ Reduce environmental stimuli.
○ Help identify triggers to anxiety.
○ Provide emotional support.

Monitoring

○ Response to therapy

Patient teaching

Be sure to cover:
○ prescribed drugs
○ relaxation techniques
○ effective coping strategies.

Discharge planning

○ Refer the patient for psychological counseling.

Genital herpes

Overview

Description

○ Acute inflammatory disease of the genitalia
○ Usually self-limiting but may cause painful local or systemic disease (see *Understanding the genital herpes cycle*)

Pathophysiology

○ Virus invades and replicates in neurons and epidermal and dermal cells.
○ Birions travel to sensory dorsal root ganglion.
○ Replication in the sensory ganglia leads to recurrent clinical outbreaks.

Causes

○ Herpes simplex virus (HSV), type 1 or type 2
○ Typically transmitted through sexual intercourse, orogenital sexual activity, kissing, hand-to-body contact, and vaginal delivery

Incidence

○ One in five adults is serologically positive for HSV in the United States.

Understanding the genital herpes cycle

After a patient is infected with genital herpes, a latency period follows. The virus takes up permanent residence in the nerve cells surrounding the lesions, and intermittent viral shedding may take place.

Repeated outbreaks may develop at any time, again followed by a latent stage during which the lesions heal completely. Outbreaks may recur as often as three to eight times yearly.

Although the cycle continues indefinitely, some people remain symptom-free for years.

```
┌─────────────────────────────────────────┐
│              INITIAL INFECTION           │
│ Highly infectious period marked by fever,│
│   aches, adenopathy, pain, and ulcerated │
│        skin and mucous membranes         │
└─────────────────────────────────────────┘
```

```
┌─────────────────────────────────────────┐
│                  LATENCY                 │
│  Intermittently infectious period marked │
│  by viral dormancy or viral shedding and │
│         no disease symptoms              │
└─────────────────────────────────────────┘
```

```
    ┌─────────────────────────────────────┐
    │          RECURRENT INFECTION        │
    │  Highly infectious period similar to │
    │  initial infection with milder      │
    │  symptoms that resolve faster        │
    └─────────────────────────────────────┘
```

Common characteristics

○ Fluid-filled vesicles that develop into shallow, painful ulcers with yellow, oozing centers
○ Fever
○ Malaise
○ Dysuria

Complications

○ Herpetic keratitis, which may lead to blindness
○ Herpetic encephalitis

Assessment

History

○ Intimate contact with an infected person
○ Fever
○ Malaise
○ Dysuria
○ Leukorrhea (females)

Physical findings

○ Shallow, reddened, painful ulcers with yellow, oozing centers usually on the cervix (the primary infection site) and possibly on the labia, perianal skin, vulva, or vagina of the female and on the glans penis, foreskin, or penile shaft of the male
○ Extragenital lesions, possibly on the mouth or anus
○ Marked edema
○ Tender inguinal lymph nodes

Test results

Laboratory
○ Vesicular fluid reveals HSV.
○ Antigen testing identifies specific antigens.
Other
○ Physical examination and patient history

Treatment

General

○ Standard precautions
○ Adequate rest periods

Medication

○ Acyclovir
○ Famciclovir
○ Valacyclovir

Nursing considerations

Key outcomes

The patient will:
○ express an understanding of the disorder and its treatment
○ practice safe sex
○ report feelings of increased comfort
○ demonstrate improved skin integrity.

Nursing interventions

○ Encourage expression of feelings and concerns.
○ Keep lesions dry.
○ Follow standard precautions.

Monitoring

○ Response to treatment
○ Skin integrity
○ Wound healing

Patient teaching

Be sure to cover:
○ avoiding sexual intercourse during the active stage of this disease (while lesions are present)
○ using condoms during all sexual encounters
○ urging sexual partners to seek medical examination
○ having a Papanicolaou test every 6 months (females).

Discharge planning

○ Refer the patient to the Herpes Resource Center for support.

Genital warts

Overview

Description

- Papillomas that consist of fibrous tissue overgrowth from the dermis and thickened epithelial coverings
- Also known as venereal warts and condylomata acuminata

Pathophysiology

- Infection is transmitted by sexual contact and incubates for 1 to 6 months (2 months, average) before warts erupt.
- Infection of the basal cells occurs, with proliferation of all epidermal layers, producing acanthosis, parakeratosis, and hyperkeratosis.

Causes

- Infection with one of more than 60 known strains of human papillomavirus
- Possibly receptive anal intercourse

Incidence

- One of the most common sexually transmitted diseases (STDs) in the United States

Common characteristics

- Appearance of small, pink to red, moist warts with irregular surfaces (see *Recognizing genital warts*)
- Usually located around the external genitalia and possibly inside the urethra or vagina or on the cervix
- No symptoms in most patients

Complications

- During pregnancy, genital warts in the vaginal and cervical walls that grow large enough to impede vaginal delivery
- Genital tract dysplasia

Recognizing genital warts

Genital warts are marked by clusters of flesh-colored papillary growths that may be barely visible or several inches in diameter.

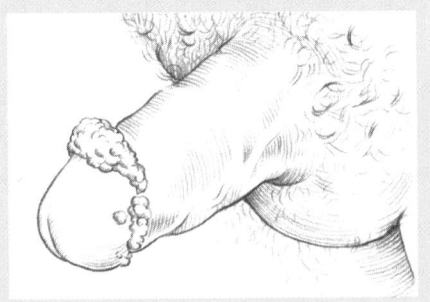

- Cervical and vulvar cancer in women, penile cancer in men, and some rectal carcinomas in both genders

Assessment

History

- Unprotected sexual contact with a partner with a known infection, a new partner, or many partners

Physical findings

- Warts on moist genital surfaces (subpreputial sac, urethral meatus, penile shaft, scrotum, vulva, vaginal and cervical walls)
- Tiny red or pink swellings that may grow as large as 10 cm and that may be pedunculated
- Infected lesions that become malodorous

Test results

Laboratory
- Dark-field microscopy of wart-cell scrapings showing marked epidermal cell vascularization
- Application of 5% acetic acid (white vinegar) turning warts white if they're papillomas

Treatment

General

- Circumcision may prevent recurrence

Medication

- Topical antimetabolites
- Topical podophyllum resin
- Topical interferon
- Vaccine preparations

Surgery

- Cryosurgery
- Electrodesiccation
- Surgical excision
- Laser ablation

Nursing considerations

Key outcomes

The patient will:
- remain free from all signs and symptoms of infection
- exhibit improved or healed lesions or wounds
- acknowledge the change in body image
- voice feelings about potential or actual changes in sexuality
- express feelings of increased comfort and decreased pain.

Nursing interventions

- Use standard precautions.
- Provide a nonthreatening, nonjudgmental atmosphere that encourages verbalization, and provide support.

○ Remove podophyllum resin with soap and water 4 to 6 hours after applying it to warts.

Monitoring

○ Response to treatment
○ Adverse effects of medication
○ Signs and symptoms of infection (postoperative)
○ Concomitant STDs or infections
○ Papanicolaou (Pap) test results

Patient teaching

Be sure to cover:
○ the disorder, diagnosis, and treatment
○ the need for sexual abstinence or condom use during intercourse until healing is complete
○ evaluation of the patient's sexual partners
○ the importance of testing for human immunodeficiency virus infection and other STDs
○ the emphasis that genital warts can recur and that the virus can mutate, causing infection with warts of a different strain
○ recommendation that female patients have a Pap test every 6 months.

Giardiasis

Overview

Description

- Infection of the small bowel by *Giardia lamblia,* a symmetrical flagellate protozoan
- Reinfection possible because infection doesn't confer immunity
- Also called G. enteritis and *lambliasis*

Pathophysiology

- Cysts enter the small bowel and release trophozoites, which attach to the bowel's epithelial surface.
- Attachment causes superficial mucosal invasion and destruction, inflammation, and irritation.
- Trophozoites become encysted again, travel down the colon, and are excreted. (Unformed stool may contain trophozoites as well as cysts.)

Causes

- Ingestion of *G. lamblia* cysts in stool-contaminated water
- Fecal-oral transfer of cysts from an infected person

Incidence

- Occurs worldwide but is most common in developing countries and other areas where sanitation and hygiene are poor (*G. lamblia* has been found in municipal water sources, nursing homes, and day-care centers.)
- Children are generally more likely to develop giardiasis than adults
- In the United States, most common in travelers recently returned from endemic areas, campers who drink water from contaminated streams, male homosexuals, patients with congenital immunoglobulin A deficiency, and children in day-care centers

Common characteristics

- Diarrhea
- Abdominal pain
- Bloating
- Belching
- Flatus
- Nausea and vomiting

Complications

- Malabsorption
- Dehydration
- Lactose intolerance
- Possible death, in hypogammaglobulinemia

Assessment

History

- Recent travel to an area with poor sanitation
- Sexual practices that involve oral-anal contact
- Drinking of suspect water
- Institutionalization

Physical findings

- Possibly, no intestinal symptoms in mild infection
- Abdominal cramps, bloating
- Belching, flatus
- Nausea, vomiting
- Explosive pale, loose, greasy, malodorous, frequent stools (occurring 2 to 10 times daily)
- Fatigue, weight loss
- Hyperactive bowel sounds in the right upper and left lower quadrants just before bowel movements
- General upper and right lower quadrant discomfort and guarding

Test results

Laboratory
- Examination of a fresh stool specimen showing cysts or examination of duodenal aspirate or biopsy showing trophozoites

Treatment

General

- Examination for possible testing and treatment for people living with an infected person or those who have had sexual contact with an infected person
- Parenteral fluid replacement to prevent dehydration

Medication

- Metronidazole
- Furazolidone

Nursing considerations

Key outcomes

The patient will:
- avoid skin breakdown or infection
- maintain stable vital signs
- maintain normal electrolyte levels
- have an elimination pattern that returns to normal
- express feelings of increased comfort and relief from pain.

Nursing interventions

- Institute enteric precautions, and quickly dispose of all fecal material.
- Place a child or an incontinent adult in a private room.
- Keep the perianal area clean, especially after each bowel movement.
- Administer I.V. fluid therapy, as needed.
- Provide nutritionally adequate foods.
- Give prescribed drugs.
- Report epidemic situations to public health authorities.

Monitoring

○ Frequency and characteristics of bowel movements
○ Nutritional intake (to prevent malnutrition)
○ Adverse drug effects
○ Skin integrity
○ Signs and symptoms of dehydration

Patient teaching

Be sure to cover:
○ prescribed drugs, including precautions and adverse effects
○ need for the patient who's taking metronidazole or furazolidone to avoid alcohol while taking the drug and for 3 days after completing treatment
○ need for the family and others in contact with the patient to have their stools tested for *G. lamblia* cysts
○ need for good personal hygiene, especially proper hand washing as well as correct handling of infectious material by the patient and his family
○ importance of safe sex practices
○ need for campers to purify all stream and lake water before drinking it
○ need for travelers to endemic areas to avoid drinking tap or suspect water and to avoid eating uncooked and unpeeled fruits or vegetables.

Discharge planning

○ Encourage the patient to return for follow-up appointments because relapses can occur.

Glaucoma

Overview

Description

- Eye disorder characterized by high intraocular pressure (IOP) and optic nerve damage
- Two forms:
  - Open-angle (also known as *chronic, simple,* or *wide-angle*) glaucoma, which begins insidiously and progresses slowly
  - Angle-closure (also known as *acute* or *narrow-angle*) glaucoma, which occurs suddenly and can cause permanent vision loss in 48 to 72 hours

Pathophysiology

Open-angle glaucoma
- Degenerative changes in the trabecular meshwork block the flow of aqueous humor from the eye, increasing IOP and resulting in optic nerve damage.

Angle-closure glaucoma
- Obstruction to the outflow of aqueous humor is caused by an anatomically narrow angle between the iris and the cornea.
- IOP increases suddenly.

Causes

Open-angle glaucoma
- Degenerative changes

Angle-closure glaucoma
- Anatomically narrow angle between the iris and the cornea
- Attacks triggered by trauma, pupillary dilation, stress, or ocular changes that push the iris forward

Optic disk changes

Ophthalmoscopy and slit-lamp examination show cupping of the optic disk, which is characteristic of glaucoma.

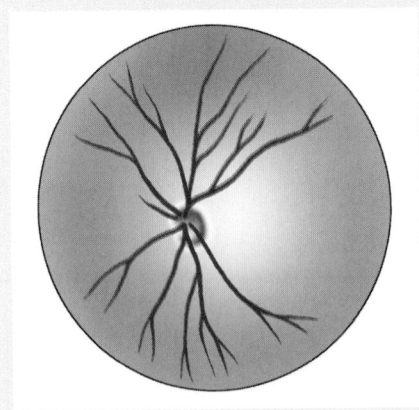

Risk factors

Open-angle glaucoma
- Family history
- Myopia
- Ethnic origin

Angle-closure glaucoma
- Family history
- Cataracts
- Hyperopia

Incidence

- A leading cause of blindness; accounts for about 12% of newly diagnosed blindness in the United States
- Affects about 2% of Americans older than age 40
- Highest incidence among males and Black and Asian populations
- Open-angle glaucoma commonly familial

Common characteristics

- Decreased visual acuity
- Nausea and vomiting
- Eye pain

Complications

- Varying degrees of vision loss
- Total blindness

Assessment

History

Open-angle glaucoma
- Possibly no symptoms
- Dull, morning headache
- Mild aching in the eyes
- Loss of peripheral vision
- Halos around lights
- Reduced visual acuity (especially at night) not corrected by glasses

Angle-closure glaucoma
- Pain and pressure over the eye
- Blurred vision
- Decreased visual acuity
- Halos around lights
- Nausea and vomiting (from increased IOP)

Physical findings

- Unilateral eye inflammation
- Cloudy cornea
- Moderately dilated pupil, nonreactive to light
- With gentle fingertip pressure to the closed eyelids, one eye feels harder than the other (in angle-closure glaucoma)

Test results

Diagnostic procedures
- Tonometry measurement shows increased IOP.
- Slit-lamp examination shows effects of glaucoma on the anterior eye structures.
- Gonioscopy shows angle of the eye's anterior chamber.

- Ophthalmoscopy aids visualization of the fundus. (See *Optic disk changes.*)
- Perimetry or visual field tests show extent of peripheral vision loss.
- Fundus photography shows optic disk changes.

Treatment

 Alert

Angle-closure glaucoma typically has a rapid onset and is an emergency.

General

- Reduction of IOP by decreasing aqueous humor production with medications
- Bed rest (with acute angle-closure glaucoma)

Medication

- Topical adrenergic agonists
- Cholinergic agonists
- Beta-adrenergic blockers
- Topical or oral carbonic anhydrase inhibitors

 Alert

Occasionally, systemic absorption of a beta-adrenergic blocker from eyedrops can be sufficient to cause bradycardia, hypotension, heart block, bronchospasm, impotence, or depression.

Surgery

- For patients who don't respond to drug therapy:
  - Argon laser trabeculoplasty
  - Trabeculectomy

Angle-closure glaucoma
- Laser iridectomy
- Surgical peripheral iridectomy
- In end-stage glaucoma, tube shunt or valve

Nursing considerations

Key outcomes

The patient will:
- express feelings of increased comfort
- express feelings and concerns
- sustain no harm or injury
- maintain present vision.

Nursing interventions

- Give prescribed drugs.
- Prepare for surgery, if indicated.
- After surgery, protect the affected eye.
- Encourage ambulation immediately after surgery.
- Encourage the patient to express his concerns related to the chronic condition.

Monitoring

- Vital signs
- Response to treatment
- Visual acuity

Patient teaching

Be sure to cover:
- the disorder, diagnosis, and treatment
- need for meticulous compliance with prescribed drug therapy
- all procedures and treatments, especially surgery
- fact that lost vision can't be restored but treatment can usually prevent further loss
- modification of the patient's environment for safety
- signs and symptoms that require immediate medical attention, such as sudden vision change or eye pain
- the importance of glaucoma screening for early detection and prevention.

Glomerulonephritis

Overview

Description

○ Bilateral inflammation of the glomeruli, typically following a streptococcal infection
○ Also called *acute poststreptococcal glomerulonephritis*

Pathophysiology

○ Epithelial or podocyte layer of the glomerular membrane is disturbed, resulting in a loss of negative charge.
○ Acute post-streptococcal glomerulonephritis results from the entrapment and collection of antigen-antibody complexes in the glomerular capillary membranes, after infection with group A beta-hemolytic streptococcus.
○ Antigens stimulate the formation of antibodies.
○ Circulating antigen-antibody complexes become lodged in the glomerular capillaries.
○ Complexes initiate complement activation and the release of immunologic substances that lyse cells and increase membrane permeability.
○ Antibody damage to basement membranes causes crescent formation.
○ Antibody or antigen-antibody complexes in the glomerular capillary wall activate biochemical mediators of inflammation — complement, leukocytes, and fibrin.
○ Activated complement attracts neutrophils and monocytes, which release lysosomal enzymes that damage the glomerular cell walls and cause a proliferation of the extracellular matrix, affecting glomerular blood flow.
○ Membrane permeability increases and causes a loss of negative charge across the glomerular membrane as well as enhanced protein filtration.
○ Membrane damage leads to platelet aggregation, and platelet degranulation releases substances that increase glomerular permeability.

Causes

○ Streptococcal infection of the respiratory tract
○ Impetigo
○ Immunoglobulin A nephropathy (Berger's disease)
○ Lipoid nephrosis
Chronic glomerulonephritis
○ Membranoproliferative glomerulonephritis
○ Membranous glomerulopathy
○ Focal glomerulosclerosis
○ Rapidly progressive glomerulonephritis (RPGN)
○ Poststreptococcal glomerulonephritis
○ Systemic lupus erythematosus
○ Goodpasture's syndrome
○ Hemolytic uremic syndrome

Incidence

○ Acute glomerulonephritis is most common in boys ages 3 to 7, but it can occur at any age.
○ RPGN most commonly occurs between ages 50 and 60.

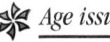 *Age issue*

Goodpasture's syndrome, a type of RPGN, is rare, but occurs most commonly in men ages 20 to 30.

Common characteristics

○ Decreased urination or oliguria
○ Smoky or coffee-colored urine
○ Dyspnea and orthopnea
○ Periorbital edema
○ Mild to severe hypertension

 Alert

The presenting features of glomerulonephritis in children may be encephalopathy with seizures and local neurologic deficits. An elderly patient with glomerulonephritis may report vague, nonspecific symptoms such as nausea, malaise, and arthralgia.

Complications

○ Pulmonary edema
○ Heart failure
○ Sepsis
○ Renal failure
○ Severe hypertension
○ Cardiac hypertrophy

Assessment

History

○ Decreased urination
○ Recent streptococcal infection of the respiratory tract

Physical findings

○ Smoky or coffee-colored urine
○ Dyspnea
○ Periorbital edema
○ Increased blood pressure

Test results

Laboratory
○ Throat culture showing group A beta-hemolytic streptococcus
○ Elevated electrolyte, blood urea nitrogen, and creatinine levels
○ Decreased serum protein level
○ Decreased hemoglobin levels (chronic glomerulonephritis)
○ Elevated antistreptolysin-O titers

- Elevated streptozyme and anti-DNase B
- Low serum complement levels
- Urine showing red blood cells, white blood cells, mixed cell casts, protein, fibrin-degradation products, and C3 protein.

Imaging
- Kidney-ureter-bladder X-ray shows bilateral kidney enlargement (acute glomerulonephritis).
- X-ray reveals symmetric contraction with normal pelves and calyces (chronic glomerulonephritis).

Diagnostic procedures
- Renal biopsy confirms diagnosis.

Treatment

- Treatment of the primary disease
- Bed rest
- Fluid restriction
- Sodium-restricted diet
- Correction of electrolyte imbalance
- Dialysis
- Plasmapheresis

Medication

- Antibiotics
- Anticoagulants
- Diuretics
- Vasodilators
- Corticosteroids

Surgery

- Kidney transplant

Nursing considerations

Key outcomes

The patient will:
- maintain adequate fluid balance
- identify risk factors that exacerbate the condition, and modify lifestyle accordingly
- maintain hemodynamic stability
- have laboratory values return to normal.

Nursing interventions

- Provide appropriate skin care and oral hygiene.
- Encourage the patient to express his feelings about the disorder.
- Give prescribed drugs.

Monitoring

- Vital signs
- Intake and output
- Daily weight
- Laboratory studies
- Signs of renal failure

Patient teaching

Be sure to cover:
- taking prescribed drugs
- how to assess ankle edema
- reporting signs of infection
- recording daily weight.

Goiter

Overview

Description

- Thyroid gland enlargement not caused by inflammation or a neoplasm
- Commonly classified as toxic (associated with hyperthyroidism) or nontoxic (not associated with hyperthyroidism or hypothyroidism)

Pathophysiology

- Thyroid gland can't produce enough thyroid hormone to meet metabolic requirements
- Thyroid gland enlarges to compensate for inadequate hormone synthesis

Causes

- Thyroid growth-stimulating immunoglobulins
- Inherited defects
- Inadequate dietary intake of iodine
- Ingestion of large amounts of goitrogenic foods (such as rutabagas, cabbage, soybeans, peanuts, peaches, peas, strawberries, spinach, and radishes)

Understanding simple goiter

A simple (nontoxic) goiter is any enlargement of the thyroid gland not caused by inflammation or neoplasm. The thyroid mass increases to compensate for inadequate hormone synthesis. It's most common in females, occurring when thyroid hormone secretion fails to meet metabolic needs.

Sporadic goiter follows ingestion of goitrogenic drugs (such as propylthiouracil) and iodides or foods (such as rutabagas and cabbage). Endemic goiter results from geographically related nutritional factors such as iodine-depleted soil. Inherited defects may contribute to either type of goiter.

The patient may report respiratory distress and dysphagia from compression of the trachea and esophagus and dizziness or syncope when raising her arms over her head. A firm, irregular enlargement and stridor caused by tracheal compression may be found.

Diagnostic tests reveal normal serum thyroid hormone levels; abnormalities rule out this diagnosis. Thyroid antibody titers are usually normal. Iodine 131 uptake is usually normal but may increase with iodine deficiency or a biosynthetic defect. Urinalysis may show low urinary excretion of iodine.

Treatment to reduce thyroid hyperplasia involves thyroid hormone replacement. Iodide administration commonly relieves goiters caused by iodine deficiency. Sporadic goiter requires avoidance of goitrogenic drugs and food. Radioiodine ablation therapy aids some patients. Rarely, partial thyroidectomy is needed to relieve pressure on the surrounding structures.

---

or the use of goitrogenic drugs (such as propylthiouracil, methimazole, iodides, and lithium)

Incidence

- Decreases with age
- More common in women than in men

Common characteristics

- Mildly enlarged gland to a massive, multinodular goiter

Complications

- Tracheal compression
- Hyperthyroidism
- Lymphoma
- Abscess

Assessment

History

- Respiratory distress
- Dysphagia

Physical findings

- Swelling and distention of the neck, which may be mildly to massively enlarged (see *Understanding simple goiter*)

Test results

Laboratory
- Thyroid-stimulating hormone — high or normal
- Serum thyroxine concentrations — low normal or normal
- Iodine 131 uptake — normal or increased (50% of the dose at 24 hours)

Other
- Patient history and physical examination

Treatment

General

- Avoidance of known goitrogenic drugs and foods

Medication

- Thyroid hormone replacement
- Small doses of iodine

Surgery

- Subtotal thyroidectomy

Nursing considerations

Key outcomes

The patient will:
- remain hemodynamically stable
- have a reduced goiter
- express feelings of increased comfort

○ not demonstrate respiratory or swallowing difficulty.

Nursing interventions

○ Give prescribed drugs.
○ Encourage the patient to express feelings and concerns.

Monitoring

○ Neck circumference
○ Response to therapy

Patient teaching

Be sure to cover:
○ drug administration and dosage
○ symptoms of thyroid toxicosis
○ use of iodized salt.

Gonadotropin deficiency

Overview

Description
○ Lack of hormones (follicle-stimulating hormone [FSH] and luteinizing hormone [LH]) that stimulate the sex glands, primarily the testes and ovaries
○ If chronic and untreated, can cause infertility and osteopenia

Pathophysiology
○ Gonadotropin-releasing hormone (Gn-RH) is secreted by the hypothalamus and causes the anterior pituitary to secrete the gonadotropins — testosterone, estrogen, FSH, and LH.
○ Estrogen, progesterone, and testosterone, produced by the gonads, function in a negative-feedback loop that regulates Gn-RH secretion.
○ Mechanisms that cause Gn-RH deficiency include:
  – pituitary tumor producing another hormone that impinges on the gonadotropin-producing cells and physically impairs Gn-RH biosynthesis
  – medical treatments such as radiation (impairs Gn-RH–producing cells)
  – oversecretion of estrogen, progesterone, or testosterone by dysfunctional target glands, causing Gn-RH inhibition through the negative-feedback loop
  – prolactin (inhibits pituitary secretion of Gn-RH; prolactin-secreting tumors can cause Gn-RH deficiency)
  – reduced Gn-RH secretion due to response of hypothalamus to physical stress, obesity, or starvation.

Causes
○ Pituitary tumor or hemorrhage
○ Oversecretion of target gland hormone, such as estrogen, progesterone, or testosterone
○ Prolactin-secreting tumor
○ Hypothalamic suppression of Gn-RH during periods of physical or emotional stress, obesity, and starvation
○ Genetics

Incidence
○ Can occur at any age
○ Affects men more commonly than women

Common characteristics
○ Decreased libido, strength, and body hair, and fine wrinkles around the eyes and lips (adults)
○ Amenorrhea; vaginal, uterine, and breast atrophy; clitoral enlargement; voice deepening; and beard growth (women)
○ Testicular atrophy, reduction in beard growth, and erectile dysfunction (men)
○ Mood and behavior changes
○ Anosmia

○ Depending on age of onset: inadequate sexual differentiation, microphallus and partial or complete lack of testicular descent, poor secondary sex characteristics and muscle development

Complications
○ Infertility
○ Sexual dysfunction

Assessment

History
○ Illness that affects testes
○ Underdeveloped secondary sex characteristics
○ Mood and behavior changes
○ Sexual dysfunction
○ Infertility

Physical findings
○ Testicular atrophy
○ Underdeveloped secondary characteristics
○ Decreased body hair
○ Fine wrinkles around eyes and lips

Test results
Laboratory
○ Low testosterone and high Gn-RH levels (primary testicular failure)
○ Low estrogen and high Gn-RH levels (primary ovarian failure)
○ Low Gn-RH and testosterone or estrogen levels (hypothalamic or pituitary dysfunction)
○ Abnormal human chorionic gonadotropin (hCG) stimulation test
○ Gn-RH stimulation test revealing insufficient elevation of LH or FSH levels

Treatment

General
○ Stress reduction
○ Weight gain or loss

Medication
○ Gonadotropin, estrogen, or testosterone replacement

Surgery
○ Removal of tumors

Nursing considerations

Key outcomes
The patient will:
○ relate an understanding of the disorder and its treatment
○ express positive feelings regarding body image
○ seek appropriate support measures.

Nursing interventions

○ Give prescribed drugs.
○ Provide emotional support.

Monitoring

○ Laboratory results

Patient teaching

Be sure to cover:
○ the disorder and treatment
○ taking prescribed drugs.

Discharge planning

○ Stress to the patient the importance of obtaining on-going follow-up care.

Gonorrhea

Overview

Description

- Common venereal disease that usually starts as infection of the genitourinary tract; can also begin in rectum, pharynx, or eyes
- Left untreated, spreads through the blood to the joints, tendons, meninges, and endocardium
- In women, can lead to chronic pelvic inflammatory disease (PID) and sterility

Pathophysiology

- Gonococci infect mucus-secreting epithelial surfaces and penetrate through or between the cells to the connective tissue.
- Inflammation and spread of the infection results.

Causes

- Transmission of *Neisseria gonorrhoea,* the causative organism, through sexual contact with an infected person
- For a child born to an infected mother, acquisition of gonococcal ophthalmia neonatorum during passage through the birth canal
- Acquisition of gonococcal conjunctivitis by touching the eyes with a contaminated hand

Incidence

- Among sexually active individuals, incidence highest in those with multiple partners, teenagers, nonwhites, the poor, the poorly educated, city dwellers, and unmarried people who live alone
- Reinfection common

Common characteristics

- Possible dysuria in males
- Possible absence of symptoms (in both sexes) or symptoms related to the area infected
- Most common infection site in female children older than age 1 is vagina

Complications

- PID
- Acute epididymitis
- Proctitis
- Salpingitis
- Septic arthritis
- Dermatitis
- Perihepatitis
- Corneal ulceration
- Blindness
- Meningitis
- Osteomyelitis
- Pneumonia
- Acute respiratory distress syndrome

Assessment

History

- Unprotected sexual contact (vaginal, oral, or anal) with an infected person, an unknown partner, or multiple sex partners
- History of sexually transmitted disease

Physical findings

- Fever
- Purulent discharge from urethral meatus
- Female urethral meatus possibly red and edematous
- Friable cervix and a greenish yellow discharge
- Engorged, red, swollen vagina with profuse purulent discharge
- Rectal infection
- Ocular infection
- Pharyngeal infection
- Papillary skin lesions on hands and feet
- PID
- Perihepatitis
- Pain and a cracking noise when moving an involved joint

Test results

Laboratory

- Culture from the infection site of the urethra, cervix, rectum, or pharynx, usually establishing the diagnosis
- Culture of conjunctival scrapings confirming gonococcal conjunctivitis
- In males, a Gram stain showing gram-negative diplococci possibly confirming gonorrhea
- Gonococcal arthritis requiring identification of gram-negative diplococci on smear from joint fluid and skin lesions
- Complement fixation and immunofluorescent assays of serum revealing antibody titers four times the normal rate
- Venereal Disease Research Laboratory test possibly reactive in a patient with syphilis
- Rapid plasma reagin test possibly reactive in a patient with syphilis

Treatment

General

- Follow-up cultures 4 to 7 days after treatment and again in 6 months
- For a pregnant patient, final follow-up before delivery
- Effective therapy (ends communicability within hours)
- Abstinence from sexual activity until infection is treated

Medication

- Ceftriaxone plus doxycycline
- Azithromycin

Preventing gonorrhea

Monitoring

○ Response to treatment
○ Adverse drug effects
○ Complications
○ Follow-up culture results

Patient teaching

Be sure to cover:
○ the disorder, diagnosis, and treatment
○ informing all sexual partners of the infection so that they can seek treatment
○ avoiding sexual contact until cultures are negative and infection is eradicated
○ being careful when coming into contact with any bodily discharges to avoid contaminating the eyes
○ safe sex practices
○ taking anti-infective drugs for the time prescribed
○ the importance of returning for follow-up testing. (see *Preventing gonorrhea*).

○ 1% silver nitrate drops or erythromycin ointment in neonates to prevent gonococcal ophthalmia neonatorum

Nursing considerations

Key outcomes

The patient will:
○ express concern about self-concept, esteem, and body image
○ state infection risk factors
○ identify signs and symptoms of infection
○ remain free from all signs and symptoms of infection
○ practice safe sex.

Nursing interventions

○ Practice standard precautions.
○ Isolate the patient if his eyes are infected.
○ With gonococcal arthritis, apply moist heat to ease pain in affected joints.
○ Give prescribed drugs.
○ Report all cases of gonorrhea to the local public health authorities as required.
○ Report all cases of gonorrhea in children to child abuse authorities.
○ Routinely instill prophylactic drugs, according to facility protocol, in the eyes of all neonates on admission to the nursery.
○ Check the neonate of an infected mother for signs of infection, and obtain specimens for culture from the neonate's eyes, pharynx, and rectum.

Goodpasture's syndrome

Overview

Description
○ Pulmonary renal syndrome characterized by hemoptysis and rapidly progressive glomerulonephritis

Pathophysiology
○ Abnormal production and deposition of antibodies against glomerular basement membrane (GBM) and alveolar basement membrane activate the complement and inflammatory responses.
○ This results in glomerular and alveolar tissue damage.

Causes
○ Unknown
○ May be associated with exposure to hydrocarbons or with type II hypersensitivity reaction
○ Possible genetic predisposition

Incidence
○ Occurs at any age; most commonly in men between ages 20 and 30

Common characteristics
○ Hemoptysis
○ Rapidly progressive glomerulonephritis

Complications
○ Renal failure
○ Pulmonary edema and hemorrhage

Assessment

History
○ Possible complaint of malaise, fatigue, and pallor
○ Possible pulmonary bleeding for months or years before developing overt hemorrhage and signs of renal disease

Physical findings
○ Hematuria
○ Decreased urine output
○ Dyspnea, tachypnea, orthopnea
○ Restlessness
○ Hemoptysis, ranging from a cough with blood-tinged sputum to frank pulmonary hemorrhage
○ Pulmonary crackles and rhonchi

Test results
Laboratory
○ Immunofluorescence of alveolar basement membrane showing linear deposition of immunoglobulins as well as C3 and fibrinogen
○ Immunofluorescence of GBM showing linear deposition of immunoglobulins
○ Serum anti-GBM antibody revealing the presence of circulating anti-GBM antibodies that distinguishes Goodpasture's syndrome from other pulmonary-renal syndromes, such as Wegener's granulomatosis, polyarteritis, and systemic lupus erythematosus
○ Serum creatinine and blood urea nitrogen (BUN) levels typically increased to two to three times normal
○ Urinalysis possibly revealing red blood cells and cellular casts, which typify glomerular inflammation; possibly also showing granular casts and proteinuria
Imaging
○ Chest X-rays reveal pulmonary infiltrates in a diffuse, nodular pattern.
Diagnostic procedures
○ Lung biopsy shows interstitial and intra-alveolar hemorrhage with hemosiderin-laden macrophages.
○ Renal biopsy usually shows focal necrotic lesions and cellular crescents.

Treatment

General
○ Plasmapheresis
○ Dialysis
○ Low-protein, low-sodium diet
○ Activity, as tolerated

Medication
○ High-dose I.V. corticosteroids

Surgery
○ Kidney transplantation

Nursing considerations

Key outcomes
The patient will:
○ maintain a patent airway and adequate ventilation
○ maintain adequate fluid balance
○ express feelings of increased energy
○ avoid complications.

Nursing interventions
○ Elevate the head of the bed and administer humidified oxygen, as ordered.
○ Encourage the patient to conserve his energy.
○ Assist with range-of-motion exercises.
○ Assist with activities of daily living, and provide frequent rest periods.
○ Transfuse blood and administer corticosteroids, as ordered. Watch closely for signs of adverse reactions.

Monitoring
○ Respiratory status
○ Vital signs
○ Arterial blood gas levels

○ Intake and output
○ Daily weight
○ Creatinine clearance, BUN, and serum creatinine levels
○ Hematocrit and coagulation studies

Patient teaching

Be sure to cover:
○ the disorder, diagnosis, and treatment
○ the importance of conserving energy
○ an explanation that fluid intake may be restricted
○ the name, dosage, purpose, and adverse effects of all medications
○ how to effectively deep-breathe and cough
○ how to recognize the signs of respiratory or genitourinary bleeding and the need to report such signs to the physician at once.

Discharge planning

○ If dialysis or kidney transplantation is required, refer the patient to a renal support group.
○ Encourage regular follow-up care.

Gout

○ Hypertension
○ Infection when tophi rupture

Overview

Description

○ Inflammatory arthritis caused by uric acid and crystal deposits
○ Red, swollen, and acutely painful joints
○ Mostly affects feet, great toe, ankle, and midfoot
○ Primary gout patient symptom-free for years between attacks
○ First acute attack strikes suddenly and peaks quickly
○ Delayed attacks associated with olecranon bursitis
○ Chronic polyarticular gout — the final, unremitting stage of the disease marked by persistent painful polyarthritis

Pathophysiology

○ Uric acid crystallizes in blood or body fluids, and the precipitate accumulates in connective tissue (tophi).
○ Crystals trigger an immune response.
○ Neutrophils secrete lysosomes for phagocytosis.
○ Lysosomes damage tissue and exacerbate the immune response.

Causes

○ Exact cause unknown
○ Decreased renal excretion of uric acid
○ Genetic defect in purine metabolism (hyperuricemia)
○ Secondary gout that develops with other diseases:
  – Obesity
  – Diabetes mellitus
  – Hypertension
  – Polycythemia
  – Leukemia
  – Myeloma
  – Sickle cell anemia
  – Renal disease
○ Secondary gout that follows treatment with drugs (hydrochlorothiazide or pyrazinamide)

Incidence

○ Primary gout typically in men older than age 30 and postmenopausal women who take diuretics

Common characteristics

○ Extreme pain in affected joints
○ Redness and swelling in joints
○ Tophi in great toe, ankle, or pinna of ear
○ Elevated skin temperature

Complications

○ Renal calculi
○ Atherosclerotic disease
○ Cardiovascular lesions
○ Stroke
○ Coronary thrombosis

Assessment

History

○ Sedentary lifestyle
○ Hypertension
○ Renal calculi
○ Waking during the night with pain in great toe
○ Initial moderate pain that grows intense
○ Chills; mild fever

Physical findings

○ Swollen, dusky red or purple joint
○ Limited movement of joint
○ Tophi, especially in the outer ears, hands, and feet (see *Recognizing gouty tophi*)
○ Skin over tophi that may ulcerate and release chalky white exudate or pus
○ Secondary joint degeneration
○ Erosions, deformity, and disability
○ Warmth over joint
○ Extreme tenderness
○ Fever
○ Hypertension

Test results

Laboratory
○ Elevated serum uric acid levels with a gout attack
○ Elevated white blood cell count in acute attack
○ Elevated urine uric acid level in 20% of patients
Imaging
○ X-ray of the articular cartilage and subchondral bone shows evidence of chronic gout.
Diagnostic procedures
○ Needle aspiration of synovial fluid shows needlelike intracellular crystals.

Treatment

General

○ Termination of acute attack
○ Protection of inflamed, painful joints
○ Treatment for hyperuricemia
○ Local application of cold
○ Prevention of recurrent gout
○ Prevention of renal calculi
○ Weight loss program, if indicated
○ Avoidance of alcohol
○ Sparing use of purine-rich foods (such as anchovies, liver, and sardines)
○ Bed rest (in acute attack)
○ Immobilization of joint

Medication

○ Analgesics
○ Nonsteroidal anti-inflammatory drugs

Recognizing gouty tophi

In advanced gout, urate crystal deposits develop into hard, irregular, yellow-white nodules called tophi. These bumps commonly protrude from the great toe and ear.

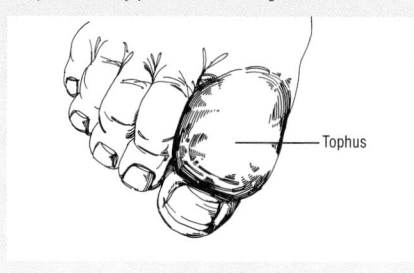

Tophus

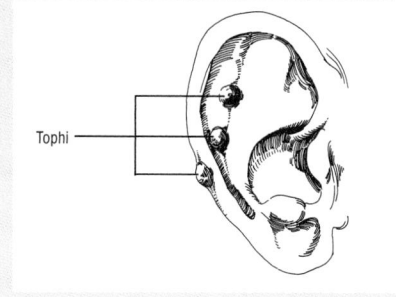

Tophi

○ Colchicine
○ Allopurinol
○ Probenecid or sulfinpyrazone

Nursing considerations

Key outcomes

The patient will:
○ express feelings of increased comfort and decreased pain
○ maintain joint mobility and range of motion
○ perform activities of daily living within confines of the disease
○ demonstrate knowledge of the condition and treatment regimen.

Nursing interventions

○ Allow adequate time for self-care.
○ Institute bed rest.
○ Use a bed cradle, if appropriate.
○ Give pain medication as needed.
○ Apply cold packs to affected areas.
○ Identify techniques and activities that promote rest and relaxation.
○ Administer anti-inflammatory medication.
○ Provide a purine-poor diet.

Monitoring

○ Intake and output
○ Serum uric acid levels
○ Acute gout attacks 24 to 96 hours after surgery

Patient teaching

Be sure to cover:
○ the disorder, diagnosis, and treatment
○ the need to drink plenty of fluids (up to 2 L per day)
○ relaxation techniques
○ compliance with the prescribed drug regimen
○ dietary adjustments
○ the need to control hypertension.

Discharge planning

○ Refer the patient to a weight-reduction program if appropriate.

Graft rejection syndrome

Overview

Description

○ Rejection of a donated organ occurring when the host's immune responses are directed against the graft
○ Three subtypes based on time of onset and mechanisms involved:
  – Hyperacute rejection
  – Acute rejection
  – Chronic rejection

Pathophysiology

○ Hyperacute rejection occurs within minutes to hours after graft transplantation.
○ Circulating host antibodies recognize and bind to graft antigens.
○ Binding of these antibodies leads to initiation of the complement cascade, recruitment of neutrophils, platelet activation, damage to graft endothelial cells, and stimulation of coagulation reactions.
○ Acute rejection may occur several hours to days (even weeks) after transplantation.
○ Alloantigen-reactive T cells from the host infiltrate the graft and are activated by contact with foreign, graft-related proteins that are presented to them by antigen-presenting cells.
○ These T cells may cause graft tissue damage.
○ Chronic rejection is characterized by the development of blood vessel luminal occlusion due to progressive thickening of the intimal layers of medium and large arterial walls.
○ Large amounts of intimal matrix are produced, leading to increasingly occlusive vessel wall thickening.
○ A slowly progressing reduction in blood flow results in regional tissue ischemia, cell death, and tissue fibrosis.

Causes

○ Immune system response to a graft

Incidence

○ Hyperacute rejection rare; affects less than 1% of transplant recipients
○ Acute rejection in 50% of transplant patients (only 10% progress to graft loss)
○ Chronic rejection in 50% of transplant patients within 10 years after transplantation

Common characteristics

○ Rapid or gradual progression of organ dysfunction

Complications

○ Rapid thrombosis
○ Loss of graft function

Assessment

History

○ Signs and symptoms that vary markedly, depending on type of rejection, underlying illnesses, and type of organ transplanted

Physical findings

○ Oliguria and increasing serum creatinine and blood urea nitrogen levels with kidney transplant
○ Elevated transaminase levels, decreased albumin levels, and hypocoagulability with liver transplant
○ Hypotension, heart failure, and edema with heart transplant

Test results

Diagnostic procedures
○ Biopsy of the transplanted tissue confirms rejection.
○ Hyperacute rejection is characterized by large numbers of polymorphonuclear leukocytes in the graft blood vessels, widespread microthrombi, platelet accumulation, and interstitial hemorrhage. There's little or no interstitial inflammation.

Treatment

General

○ Close monitoring of function of grafted organ
○ Surveillance, with prophylactic measures against opportunistic infections
○ Dietary restrictions based on organ system affected
○ Activity, as tolerated

Medication

○ Immunosuppressants
○ Antirejection therapies
○ Antibiotics

Nursing considerations

Key outcomes

The patient will:
○ not experience fever, chills, and other signs and symptoms of illness
○ use support systems to assist with coping
○ express his feelings about the condition
○ comply with the treatment regimen.

Nursing interventions

○ Give prescribed immunosuppressants.
○ Give prescribed antirejection therapies.
○ Give prescribed antibiotics for infection.

Monitoring

○ Vital signs
○ Function of the transplanted organ
○ Signs and symptoms of infection
○ Signs and symptoms of rejection

Patient teaching

Be sure to cover:
○ the disorder, diagnosis, and treatment
○ how to recognize signs and symptoms of organ dysfunction
○ the need to immediately report fever, chills, and other symptoms of infection
○ the need for lifelong medication compliance.

Discharge planning
○ Refer the patient and his family to social support, including psychological support services, as indicated.

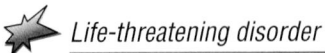 *Life-threatening disorder*

Guillain-Barré syndrome

Overview

Description
- A form of polyneuritis
- Acute, rapidly progressive, and potentially fatal
- Three phases:
  - *Acute:* beginning from first symptom, ending in 1 to 3 weeks
  - *Plateau:* lasting several days to 2 weeks
  - *Recovery:* coincides with remyelination and axonal process regrowth; extends over 4 to 6 months and may take up to 2 to 3 years; recovery possibly not complete

Pathophysiology
- Segmented demyelination of peripheral nerves occurs, preventing normal transmission of electrical impulses.
- Sensorimotor nerve roots are affected; autonomic nerve transmission may also be affected. (See *Understanding sensorimotor nerve degeneration.*)

Causes
- Unknown

Risk factors
- Surgery
- Rabies or swine influenza vaccination
- Viral illness
- Hodgkin's or some other malignant disease
- Lupus erythematosus

Incidence
- Occurs equally in both sexes
- Occurs between ages 30 and 50

Common characteristics
- Symmetrical muscle weakness initially in lower extremities and progressing to upper extremities
- Paresthesia
- Diplegia
- Dysphagia
- Hypotonia
- Areflexia

Complications
- Thrombophlebitis
- Pressure ulcers
- Contractures
- Muscle wasting
- Aspiration
- Respiratory tract infections
- Life-threatening respiratory and cardiac compromise

Assessment

History
- Minor febrile illness 1 to 4 weeks before current symptoms
- Tingling and numbness (paresthesia) in the legs
- Progression of symptoms to arms, trunk and, finally, the face
- Stiffness and pain in the calves

Physical findings
- Muscle weakness (the major neurologic sign)
- Sensory loss, usually in the legs (spreads to arms)
- Difficulty talking, chewing, and swallowing
- Paralysis of the ocular, facial, and oropharyngeal muscles
- Loss of position sense
- Diminished or absent deep tendon reflexes

Test results
Diagnostic procedures
- Cerebrospinal fluid (CSF) analysis may show a normal white blood cell count, an elevated protein count and, in severe disease, increased CSF pressure.

Other
- Electromyography may demonstrate repeated firing of the same motor unit instead of widespread sectional stimulation.
- Nerve conduction studies show marked slowing of nerve conduction velocities.

Treatment

General
- Supportive measures
- Possible endotracheal intubation or tracheotomy
- Fluid volume replacement
- Plasmapheresis
- Possible tube feedings with endotracheal intubation
- Adequate caloric intake
- Exercise program to prevent contractures
- Emotional support
- Maintenance of skin integrity

Medication
- I.V. beta-adrenergic blockers
- Parasympatholytics
- I.V. immune globulin

Surgery
- Possible tracheostomy
- Possible gastrostomy or jejunotomy feeding tube insertion

Understanding sensorimotor nerve degeneration

Guillain-Barré syndrome attacks the peripheral nerves so that they can't transmit messages to the brain correctly. Here's what goes wrong:

The myelin sheath degenerates for unknown reasons. This sheath covers the nerve axons and conducts electrical impulses along the nerve pathways. With degeneration comes inflammation, swelling, and patchy demyelination. As this disorder destroys myelin, the nodes of Ranvier (at the junctures of the myelin sheaths) widen. This delays and impairs impulse transmission along the dorsal and ventral nerve roots.

Because the dorsal nerve roots handle sensory function, the patient may experience sensations, such as tingling and numbness, when the nerve root is impaired. Similarly, because the ventral roots are responsible for motor function, impairment causes varying weakness, immobility, and paralysis.

○ the appropriate home care plan
○ instructions about medications
○ adverse drug reactions.

Discharge planning

○ Refer the patient to physical rehabilitation sources as indicated.
○ Refer the patient to occupational and speech rehabilitation resources as indicated.
○ Refer the patient to the Guillain-Barré Syndrome Foundation.

Nursing considerations

The patient will:
○ maintain a patent airway and adequate ventilation
○ develop alternate means of communication
○ maintain required caloric intake daily
○ maintain joint mobility and range of motion (ROM).

Nursing interventions

○ Establish a means of communication before intubation is required, if possible.
○ Turn and reposition the patient.
○ Encourage coughing and deep breathing.
○ Provide meticulous skin care.
○ Provider passive ROM exercises.
○ In case of facial paralysis, provide eye and mouth care.
○ Provide emotional support.
○ Give prescribed drugs.
○ Provide emotional support.

Monitoring

○ Vital signs
○ Respiratory status
○ Arterial blood gas measurements
○ Level of consciousness
○ Pulse oximetry
○ Signs of thrombophlebitis
○ Signs of urine retention
○ Response to medications
○ Skin integrity

Patient teaching

Be sure to cover:
○ the disorder, diagnosis, and treatment
○ effective means of communication

Gynecomastia

Overview

Description

○ Enlargement of breast tissue in males
○ Usually bilateral, but in men older than age 50, usually unilateral
○ Usually resolves spontaneously in 6 to 12 months

Pathophysiology

○ Disturbance in the normal ratio of active androgen to estrogen results in proliferation of the fibroblastic stroma and the duct system of the breast.

Causes

○ Testicular tumors
○ Obesity
○ Pituitary tumors
○ Some hypogonadism syndromes
○ Liver disease causing inability to break down normal male estrogen secretions
○ Chronic renal failure
○ Chronic obstructive lung disease
○ Other causes (see *Drugs and treatments causing gynecomastia*)

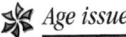 *Age issue*

In neonates, gynecomastia may be associated with galactorrhea ("witch's milk"). This sign usually disappears within a few weeks but may persist until age 2.

Drugs and treatments causing gynecomastia

In addition to the common causes of gynecomastia, various drugs and treatments may also cause this disorder.

Drugs
When gynecomastia is an effect of drugs, it's typically painful and unilateral. Estrogens used to treat prostate cancer, including diethylstilbestrol (DES), estramustine, and chlorotrianisene, directly affect the estrogen-androgen ration. Drugs that have an estrogen-like effect, such as cardiac glycosides and human chorionic gonadotropin, may do the same.

Regular use of alcohol, marijuana, or heroin reduces plasma testosterone levels, causing gynecomastia. Other drugs—such as flutamide, cyproterone, spironolactone, cimetidine, and ketoconazole—produce this sign by interfering with androgen production or action. Some common drugs, including phenothiazines, tricyclic antidepressants, and antihypertensives, produce gynecomastia, but it isn't known how.

Treatments
Gynecomastia may develop within weeks of starting hemodialysis for chronic renal failure. It may also follow major surgery or testicular irradiation.

Incidence

○ Affects 4% to 40% of males based on autopsy studies

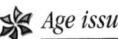 *Age issue*

Most males have physicologic gynecomastia at some time during adolescence, usually around age 14. This gynecomastia is usually asymmetrical and tender; it commonly resolves within 2 years and rarely persists beyond age 20.

Common characteristics

○ Enlarged breast tissue (at least 2 cm in diameter), either unilateral or bilateral, beneath the areola

Complications

○ Malignancy
○ Complications of surgery:
  – Infection
  – Scarring
  – Sensory change
  – Hematoma
  – Breast asymmetry

Assessment

History

○ Causative tumor
○ Change in size of breast tissue
○ History of causative factors
○ Breast pain

Physical findings

○ Enlarged breast tissue beneath the areola
○ Further physical findings depend on cause

Test results

Laboratory
○ Excessively high estrogen levels and normal testosterone levels (in drug- and tumor-induced hyperestrogenism)
○ Very low testosterone levels and normal estrogen levels (hypergonadism)
Diagnostic procedures
○ Biopsy to rule out malignancy
Other
○ Physical examination findings

Treatment

General

○ Treatment of cause

Medication

○ Antiestrogens
○ Testosterone therapy
○ Androgen therapy

Surgery

○ Resection of extra breast tissue for cosmetic reasons
○ Liposuction-assisted mastectomy

Nursing considerations

Key outcomes

The patient will:
○ express understanding of the condition and its cause
○ express positive feelings concerning body image.

Nursing interventions

○ Apply cold compresses.
○ Encourage verbalization of feelings and concerns.
○ Provide emotional support.

Monitoring

○ Breast size
After surgery
○ Pain control
○ Wound site

Patient teaching

Be sure to cover:
○ cause of condition and related treatment
○ drug administration, dosage, and adverse effects
○ preoperative teaching, if appropriate.

Haemophilus influenzae infection

Overview

Description

○ Infection that most commonly attacks respiratory system
○ Common cause of epiglottiditis, laryngotracheobronchitis, pneumonia, bronchiolitis, otitis media, and meningitis
○ Infrequent cause of bacterial endocarditis, conjunctivitis, facial cellulitis, septic arthritis, and osteomyelitis

Pathophysiology

○ Antigenic response occurs with invasion of bacteria.
○ Systemic disease results from invasion and hematogenous spread to distant sites (meninges, bones, and joints).
○ Local invasion occurs on the mucosal surfaces.
○ Otitis media occurs when bacteria reach the middle ear through the eustachian tube.

Causes

○ *H. influenzae,* a gram-negative, pleomorphic aerobic bacillus
○ Transmission by direct contact with secretions or airborne droplets

Incidence

○ *H. influenzae* type B (Hib) infection predominantly affects children at a rate of 3% to 5%; incidence lower when vaccine is administered at ages 2, 4, 6, and 15 months
○ *H. influenza* epiglottiditis most common in children between ages 3 and 7 but can occur at any age
○ Higher incidence of meningitis due to Hib in black children
○ Ten times higher incidence in Native Americans, possibly due to exposure, socioeconomic conditions, and genetic differences in immune response

Common characteristics

○ Generalized malaise
○ High fever

Complications

○ Permanent neurologic sequelae from meningitis
○ Complete upper airway obstruction from epiglottiditis
○ Cellulitis
○ Pericarditis, pleural effusion
○ Respiratory failure from pneumonia

Assessment

History

○ Possible report of recent viral infection
○ Malaise
○ Fatigue
○ Fever

Physical findings

Epiglottiditis
○ Restlessness and irritability
○ Use of accessory muscles, inspiratory retractions, stridor
○ Sitting up, leaning forward with mouth open, tongue protruding, and nostrils flaring
○ Expiratory rhonchi; diminishing breath sounds as the condition worsens
○ Pharyngeal mucosa that may look reddened (rarely, with soft yellow exudate)
○ Epiglottis that appears cherry red with considerable edema
○ Severe pain that makes swallowing difficult or impossible
Pneumonia
○ Shaking chills
○ Tachypnea
○ Productive cough
○ Impaired or asymmetrical chest movement caused by pleuritic pain
○ Dullness over areas of lung consolidation
Meningitis
○ Altered level of consciousness
○ Seizures and coma as disease progresses
○ Positive Brudzinski's and Kernig's signs
○ Exaggerated and symmetrical deep tendon reflexes
○ Nuchal rigidity
○ Opisthotonos

Test results

Laboratory
○ Isolation of the organism in blood culture confirming infection
○ Hib meningitis detected in cerebrospinal fluid cultures

Treatment

General

○ Airway maintenance (critical in epiglottiditis)
○ Diet based on respiratory status (possible need for small frequent meals)
○ Nothing by mouth with inability to swallow adequately
○ Activity, as tolerated

Medication

○ Cephalosporin
○ Chloramphenicol and ampicillin (alternate regimen)
○ Glucocorticoids

Nursing considerations

Key outcomes

The patient will:
- ❍ have no adventitious breath sounds
- ❍ maintain adequate gas exchange
- ❍ have arterial blood gas (ABG) levels that return to normal
- ❍ have no pathogens that appear in cultures
- ❍ remain free from all signs and symptoms of infection.

Nursing interventions

- ❍ Maintain respiratory isolation.
- ❍ Maintain adequate respiratory function through cool humidification, oxygen, as needed, and croup or face tents.
- ❍ Keep emergency resuscitation equipment readily available.
- ❍ Suction, as needed.
- ❍ Give prescribed drugs.
- ❍ Maintain adequate nutrition and elimination.

Monitoring

- ❍ Pulse oximetry
- ❍ ABG results
- ❍ Complete blood count for signs of bone marrow depression when therapy includes ampicillin or chloramphenicol
- ❍ Intake and output
- ❍ Respiratory status
- ❍ Neurologic status
- ❍ Vital signs

Patient teaching

Be sure to cover:
- ❍ the disorder, diagnosis, and treatment
- ❍ the importance of continuing the prescribed antibiotic until the entire prescription is finished
- ❍ using a room humidifier or breathing moist air from a shower or bath, as necessary, for home treatment of a respiratory infection
- ❍ coughing and deep-breathing exercises to clear secretions
- ❍ the disposal of secretions and use of proper hand-washing technique.

Discharge planning

- ❍ Refer the patient to an infectious disease specialist, if necessary.
- ❍ Encourage the patient to receive vaccinations to prevent future infections.

Hantavirus pulmonary syndrome

Overview

Description

○ Viral disease that causes flulike symptoms
○ Rapidly progresses to respiratory failure

Pathophysiology

○ Rodents shed virus in stool, urine, and saliva.
○ Human infection occurs from inhalation, ingestion (of contaminated food or water, for example), contact with rodent excrement, or rodent bites. (See *Sin Nombre virus.*)

Causes

○ Hantaviruses
○ Transmission with exposure to infected rodents (deer mice, pinion mice, brush mice, and western chipmunks)
○ Farming, hiking, or camping in rodent-infested areas and occupying rodent-infested dwellings

Incidence

○ Occurs mainly in southwestern United States
○ More commonly affects whites
○ Affects males more than females

Common characteristics

○ Noncardiogenic pulmonary edema
○ Myalgia

Sin Nombre virus

This illustration shows the Sin Nombre virus, the most common cause of *Hantavirus* pulmonary syndrome in the United States and Canada. It exists primarily in western states and provinces.

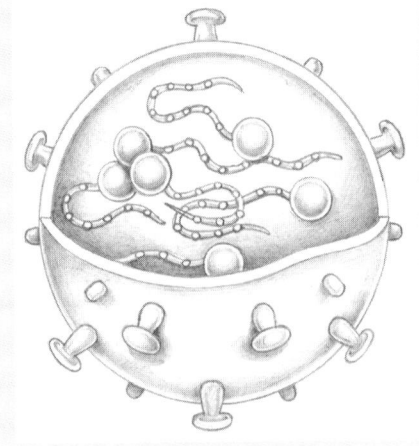

○ Fever
○ Headache
○ Nausea
○ Vomiting
○ Cough

Complications

○ Respiratory failure
○ Death (in 80% of cases)

Assessment

History

○ Rodent exposure (2 weeks before symptoms)
○ Fever
○ Myalgia
○ Abdominal discomfort
○ Dizziness

Physical findings

○ Cough
○ Hypotension
○ Tachycardia
○ Tachypnea
○ Severe hypoxemia and respiratory failure

Test results

○ The Centers for Disease Control and Prevention and state health departments can perform definitive testing for hantavirus exposure and antibody formation.
Laboratory
○ Elevated white blood cell count with a predominance of neutrophils, myeloid precursors, and atypical lymphocytes
○ Elevated hematocrit level
○ Decreased platelet count
○ Elevated partial thromboplastin time
○ Normal fibrinogen level
○ Serum creatinine levels no greater than 2.5 mg/dl
Imaging
○ Chest X-rays eventually show bilateral diffuse infiltrates in almost all patients (findings consistent with acute respiratory distress syndrome).

Treatment

General

○ Intubation and aggressive respiratory management
○ Adequate oxygenation
○ Stabilization of heart rate and blood pressure
○ Cautious fluid volume replacement
○ Nothing by mouth until recovery begins
○ Activity, as tolerated, with frequent rest periods

Medication

○ Vasopressors
○ Ribavirin

Nursing considerations

Key outcomes

The patient will:
- maintain a respiratory rate within 5 breaths/minute of baseline
- maintain adequate gas exchange
- cough effectively
- expectorate mucus.

Nursing interventions

- Maintain a patent airway by suctioning.
- Ensure adequate humidification, and check mechanical ventilator settings frequently.
- Give prescribed drugs.
- Provide I.V. fluid therapy based on results of hemodynamic monitoring.
- Provide emotional support.
- Report cases of *Hantavirus* pulmonary syndrome to your state health department.

Monitoring

- Serum electrolyte levels
- Respiratory status
- Neurologic status

Patient teaching

Be sure to cover:
- the disorder, diagnosis, and treatment
- the need to immediately report signs or symptoms of respiratory distress
- prevention guidelines, with a focus on rodent control.

Discharge planning

- Refer the patient for follow-up with a pulmonologist, if indicated.

Headache

Overview

Description

- Head pain that may be a symptom of an underlying disorder
- Classified as primary (headaches having no organic or structural cause) or secondary (indicative of an underlying structural or organic disease)

Pathophysiology

Headache
- Sustained muscle contractions directly deform pain receptors.
- Inflammation or direct pressure affects the cranial nerves.
- Pain-sensitive structures respond, including the skin, scalp, muscles, arteries, and veins; cranial nerves V, VII, IX, and X; and cervical nerves 1, 2, and 3.

Migraine
- Biochemical abnormalities occur, including local leakage of a vasodilator polypeptide through the dilated arteries and a decreased plasma level of serotonin.

Causes

Headache
- Underlying intracranial disorder
- Systemic disorder
- Psychological disorders
- Allergy
- Tension (muscle contraction)
- Emotional stress
- Fatigue
- Menstruation
- Environmental stimuli
- Glaucoma
- Inflammation of the eyes or mucosa of the nasal or paranasal sinuses
- Disorder of the scalp, teeth, extracranial arteries, or external or middle ear
- Muscle spasms of the face, neck, or shoulders
- Vasodilators
- Hypoxia
- Hypertension
- Head trauma and tumors
- Intracranial bleeding, abscess, or aneurysm
- Caffeine withdrawal
- Overuse of over-the-counter headache medications (rebound headache)

Migraine
- Constriction and dilation of intracranial and extracranial arteries
- Associated with:
  - Epilepsy
  - Hereditary hemorrhagic telangiectasia
  - Tourette syndrome
  - Ischemic stroke
  - Depression

Incidence

Headache
- Affects 60% to 80% of people in the United States at any point in time

Migraine
- Appears in childhood or adolescence
- Recurs throughout adulthood
- Affects 17% of females and 6% of males in the United States
- Strong familial incidence

Common characteristics

- Pain that's aching or tight
- Hatbandlike pattern around head
- Nausea
- Photophobia
- Phonophobia
- Blurred vision

Complications

- Worsening of existing hypertension
- Photophobia
- Emotional lability
- Motor weakness
- Loss of work

Assessment

History

Headache
- Location (frontal, temporal, or cervical), characteristics (frequency and intensity), onset and duration (continuous or intermittent)
- Precipitating factors may include tension, menstruation, loud noises, menopause, alcohol consumption, stress, and food allergies
- Aggravating factors may include coughing, sneezing, and sunlight
- Associated symptoms may include nausea or vomiting, weakness, facial pain, and scotomas
- Use of headache-inducing medications
- Familial history of headaches

Migraine
- Unilateral, pulsating pain that gradually becomes more generalized
- May be preceded by scintillating scotoma, hemianopsia, unilateral paresthesias, or speech disorders
- May be accompanied by irritability, anorexia, nausea or vomiting, and photophobia

Physical findings

Headache
- Findings based on cause
- If no underlying problem, normal physical findings
- Possible crepitus or tender spots of the head and neck

Migraine
- Pallor
- Possible extraocular muscle palsies
- Possible ptosis
- Possible neurologic deficits

Test results
Imaging
- Skull X-rays may show skull fracture (with trauma).
- Computed tomography scan may show tumor or subarachnoid hemorrhage or other intracranial pathology; may show pathology of sinuses.
- Magnetic resonance imaging may also show tumor.
Diagnostic procedures
- Lumbar puncture may show increased intracranial pressure, suggesting tumor, edema, or hemorrhage.
Other
- EEG may show alterations in the brain's electrical activity, suggesting intracranial lesion, head injury, meningitis, or encephalitis.
- Sinus X-rays may show sinusitis.
- Patient questionnaire tool evaluates functional status and quality of life.

Treatment

General
- Yoga, meditation, or other relaxation therapy
- Identification and elimination of causative factors (including environmental)
- Psychotherapy, if emotional stress involved
- For migraine patient, adequate oral fluid intake and avoidance of dietary triggers
- For migraine patient, bed rest in dark, quiet room

Medication
Headache
- Analgesics
- Tranquilizers
- Muscle relaxants
Migraine
- Ergotamine preparations
- Preventive drugs
- Triptan agents
- Serotonin receptor agonists

Nursing considerations

Key outcomes
The patient will:
- express feelings of increased comfort and decreased pain
- demonstrate methods of promoting relaxation and inner well-being
- express an increased sense of well-being
- use support systems to assist with coping
- understand causative factors or triggers.

Nursing interventions
- Encourage the use of relaxation techniques.
- Keep the patient's room dark and quiet.
- Place ice packs on the patient's forehead or a cold cloth over his eyes.
- Give prescribed drugs for pain.

Monitoring
- Pain control
- Response to alternative treatment
- Vital signs, especially blood pressure
- Neurologic status

Patient teaching

Be sure to cover:
- the disorder, diagnosis, and treatment
- migraine prevention
- avoidance of migraine triggers
- lifestyle changes
- nonpharmacologic strategies
- monitoring of headaches with headache diary
- appropriate use of preventive medications
- potential adverse reactions to prescribed drugs.

Discharge planning
- Refer the patient to the National Headache Foundation.

Hearing loss

Overview

Description

- Mechanical or nervous impediment to the transmission of sound waves to the brain
- Classified as sensorineural, conductive, or central
- Presbycusis: most common type of sensorineural hearing loss
- Congenital hearing loss: may be conductive or sensorineural
- Sudden hearing loss: may be conductive, sensorineural, or mixed; usually affects only one ear
- Depending on the cause, with prompt treatment (within 48 hours), hearing possibly restored
- Noise-induced hearing loss possibly transient or permanent

Pathophysiology

- In conductive hearing loss, sound wave transmission is interrupted between the external canal and inner ear (junction of the stapes and oval window).
- In sensorineural hearing loss, sound wave transmission is interrupted between the inner ear and brain, and there's cochlea or acoustic nerve dysfunction.
- In mixed hearing loss, a combination of dysfunction of conduction and sensorineural transmission is involved.

Causes

Conductive hearing loss
- Cerumen impaction
- Blockage of the external ear
- Tympanic membrane thickening, retraction, scarring, or perforation
- Otitis media, otitis externa
- Otosclerosis
- Serous otitis

Sensorineural hearing loss
- Impairment of the cochlea, eighth cranial or acoustic nerve
- Loss of hair cells and nerve fibers in the cochlea
- Drug toxicity
- Vascular occlusion of the anterior cerebellar artery
- Infectious diseases
- Arteriosclerosis
- Otospongiosis
- Head or ear trauma
- Organ of Corti degeneration
- Prolonged exposure to loud noise (85 to 90 dB)
- Perilymphatic fistula
- Brief exposure to extremely loud noise (greater than 90 dB)
- Acoustic neuroma

Congenital hearing loss
- Sensorineural or conductive
- May be transmitted as a dominant, autosomal dominant, autosomal recessive, or sex-linked recessive trait

Hearing loss in neonates
- Trauma during delivery
- Toxicity
- Infection during pregnancy or delivery
- Known hereditary disorders
- Maternal exposure to rubella or syphilis during pregnancy
- Use of ototoxic drugs during pregnancy
- Prolonged fetal anoxia during delivery
- Congenital abnormalities of the ears, nose, or throat

Sudden hearing loss
- Occlusion of internal auditory artery by spasm or thrombosis
- Subclinical mumps
- Bacterial and viral infections
- Acoustic neuroma
- Ménière's disease
- Metabolic, vascular, or neurologic disorders
- Blood dyscrasias
- Ototoxic drugs

Risk factors

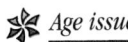 *Age issue*

Premature or low-birth-weight neonates with congenital hearing loss are most likely to have structural or functional hearing impairments.

- Neonates with serum bilirubin levels greater than 20 mg/dl (toxic effects on the brain)
- Erythroblastosis fetalis
- Maternal infection or drug abuse
- Frequent ear infections
- Use of headphones with loud music

Incidence

- Most common disability in the United States
- Third most prevalent disorder in adults older than age 65
- Presbycusis prevalent in adults older than age 50

Common characteristics

- Hearing loss
- Tinnitus

Complications

- Tympanic membrane perforation
- Cholesteatoma
- Permanent hearing loss

Assessment

History

- Deficient response to auditory stimuli within 2 to 3 days after birth

- Older child with hearing loss that impairs speech development
- Recent upper respiratory tract infection
- Use of ototoxic substances

Sudden deafness
- Recent exposure to loud noise
- Brief exposure to extremely loud noise
- Persistent tinnitus
- Transient vertigo

Physical findings
- Obvious hearing difficulty

Test results
Imaging
- Computed tomography scan shows vestibular and auditory pathways.
- Magnetic resonance imaging shows acoustic tumors and brain lesions.

Diagnostic procedures
- Auditory brain response shows activity in auditory nerve and brain stem.
- Pure tone audiometry shows presence and degree of hearing loss.
- Electronystagmography shows vestibular function.
- Otoscopic or microscopic examination shows middle ear disorders; removes debris.
- Rinne and Weber's tests show whether hearing loss is conductive or sensorineural.

Others
- Hearing evaluation

Treatment

General
- Varies with the type and cause of impairment
- Hearing aids or other effective means of aiding communication
- Avoidance of activities that allow water to enter ear, if eardrum perforated

Medication
- Antibiotics
- Agents to dissolve cerumen
- Decongestants
- Analgesics
- Antipyretics
- Sedatives
- Antibiotic steroids

Surgery
- Correction of tympanic membrane perforation

Nursing considerations

Key outcomes
The patient will:
- express understanding of the condition and treatment

- exhibit adequate coping mechanisms
- regain hearing or develop alternate means of communication.

Nursing interventions
- Face the patient when speaking and enunciate words clearly, slowly, and in a normal tone.
- Provide an alternative method of communication.

Monitoring
- Response to medications
- Progression of hearing loss
- Adaptation to hearing aid

Patient teaching

Be sure to cover:
- hearing loss, its causes, and treatments
- tests and procedures
- preoperative and postoperative instructions
- operation and maintenance of a hearing aid
- lip-reading lessons, which may increase the effectiveness
- the danger of excessive noise exposure
- the use of protective devices in a noisy environment
- the danger of exposure to drugs, chemicals, and infection (with pregnancy)
- the proper technique for ear cleaning or irrigation
- how to instill otic medications
- medication use and possible adverse effects.

Discharge planning
- If hearing deteriorates, refer the patient for speech and hearing rehabilitation.
- Refer a child to an audiologist or otolaryngologist for further evaluation, as indicated.
- Refer to community resources, as appropriate.

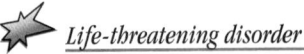

Heart failure

Overview

Description
- Fluid buildup in the heart from myocardium that can't provide sufficient cardiac output
- Usually occurs in a damaged left ventricle, but it may happen in right ventricle primarily, or secondary to left-sided heart failure

Pathophysiology
Left-sided heart failure
- Pumping ability of the left ventricle fails and cardiac output falls.
- Blood backs up into the left atrium and lungs, causing pulmonary congestion.

Right-sided heart failure
- Ineffective contractile function of the right ventricle leads to blood backing up into the right atrium and the peripheral circulation, which results in peripheral edema and engorgement of the kidneys and other organs.

Causes
- Mitral stenosis secondary to rheumatic heart disease, constrictive pericarditis, or atrial fibrillation
- Mitral or aortic insufficiency
- Arrhythmias
- Hypertension
- Atherosclerosis with myocardial infarction
- Myocarditis
- Ventricular and atrial septal defects
- Constrictive pericarditis
- Pregnancy
- Thyrotoxicosis
- Pulmonary embolism
- Infections
- Anemia
- Emotional stress
- Increased salt or water intake

Incidence
- Affects 1% of people older than age 50
- Affects 10% of people older than age 80

Common characteristics
- Reduced cardiac output
- Shortness of breath
- Peripheral edema
- Dyspnea on exertion

Complications
- Pulmonary edema
- Organ failure, especially the brain and kidneys
- Myocardial infarction

Assessment

History
- A disorder or condition that can precipitate heart failure
- Dyspnea or paroxysmal nocturnal dyspnea
- Peripheral edema
- Fatigue
- Weakness
- Insomnia
- Anorexia
- Nausea
- Sense of abdominal fullness (particularly in right-sided heart failure)
- Substance abuse (alcohol, drugs, tobacco)

Physical findings
- Cough that produces pink, frothy sputum
- Cyanosis of the lips and nail beds
- Pale, cool, clammy skin
- Diaphoresis
- Jugular vein distention
- Ascites
- Tachycardia
- Pulsus alternans
- Hepatomegaly and, possibly, splenomegaly
- Decreased pulse pressure
- S_3 and S_4 heart sounds
- Moist, bibasilar crackles, rhonchi, and expiratory wheezing
- Decreased pulse oximetry
- Peripheral edema
- Decreased urinary output

Test results
Laboratory
- B-type natriuretic peptide immunoassay is elevated.

Imaging
- Chest X-rays show increased pulmonary vascular markings, interstitial edema, or pleural effusion and cardiomegaly.

Diagnostic procedures
- Electrocardiography reflects heart strain or enlargement or ischemia. It may also reveal atrial enlargement, tachycardia, extrasystole, or atrial fibrillation.
- Pulmonary artery pressure monitoring typically shows elevated pulmonary artery and pulmonary artery wedge pressures, left ventricular end-diastolic pressure in left-sided heart failure, and elevated right atrial or central venous pressure in right-sided heart failure.

Treatment

General

- Antiembolism stockings
- Elevation of lower extremities
- Sodium-restricted diet
- Fluid restriction
- Calorie restriction, if indicated
- Low-fat diet, if indicated
- Walking program
- Activity, as tolerated

Medication

- Diuretics
- Oxygen
- Inotropic drugs
- Vasodilators
- Angiotensin converting enzyme inhibitors
- Angiotensin receptor blockers
- Cardiac glycosides
- Diuretics
- Potassium supplements
- Beta-adrenergic blockers
- Anticoagulants

Surgery

- For valvular dysfunction with recurrent acute heart failure, surgical replacement
- Heart transplantation
- Ventricular assist device
- Stent placement

Nursing considerations

Key outcomes

The patient will:
- maintain hemodynamic stability
- maintain adequate cardiac output
- carry out activities of daily living without excess fatigue or decreased energy
- maintain adequate ventilation
- maintain adequate fluid balance.

Nursing interventions

- Place the patient in Fowler's position, and give supplemental oxygen.
- Provide continuous cardiac monitoring during acute and advanced stages.
- Assist the patient with range-of-motion exercises.
- Apply antiembolism stockings. Check for calf pain and tenderness.

Monitoring

- Daily weight for peripheral edema and other signs and symptoms of fluid overload
- Cardiac rhythm
- Intake and output

- Response to treatment
- Vital signs
- Mental status
- Peripheral edema

 Alert

Auscultate for abnormal heart and breath sounds, and report changes immediately.

- Blood urea nitrogen and serum creatinine, potassium, sodium, chloride, and magnesium levels

Patient teaching

Be sure to cover:
- the disorder, diagnosis, and treatment
- signs and symptoms of worsening heart failure
- when to notify the physician
- the importance of follow-up care
- the need to avoid high-sodium foods
- the need to avoid fatigue
- instructions about fluid restrictions
- the need to weigh himself every morning, at the same time, before eating, and after urinating; keeping a record of his weight, and reporting a weight gain of 3 to 5 lb (1.5 to 2.5 kg) in 1 week
- the importance of smoking cessation, if appropriate
- weight reduction, as needed
- medication dosage, administration, potential adverse effects, and monitoring needs.

Discharge planning

- Encourage follow-up care.
- Refer the patient to a smoking-cessation program, if appropriate.

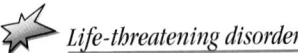 *Life-threatening disorder*

Heat syndrome

Overview

Description

○ Heat exhaustion — acute heat injury with hyperthermia caused by dehydration
○ Heat stroke — extreme hyperthermia with thermoregulatory failure

Pathophysiology

○ Normal regulation of temperature is by evaporation (30% of body's heat loss) or vasodilation. When heat is generated or gained by the body faster than it can dissipate, the thermoregulatory mechanism is stressed and eventually fails.
○ Hyperthermia accelerates.
○ Cerebral edema and cerebrovascular congestion occurs.
○ Cerebral perfusion pressure increases and cerebral perfusion decreases.
○ Tissue damage occurs when temperature exceeds 107.6° F (42° C), resulting in tissue necrosis, organ dysfunction, and failure.

Causes

○ Illness
○ Heart disease
○ Endocrine disorders
○ Neurologic disorder
○ Infection (fever)
○ Dehydration
○ Behavior
○ Excessive physical activity
○ Excessive clothing
○ Lack of acclimatization
○ Hot environment without ventilation
○ Inadequate fluid intake
○ Drugs, such as phenothiazines, anticholinergics, and amphetamines
○ Sudden discontinuation of Parkinson's disease medications

Risk factors

○ Obesity
○ Salt and water depletion
○ Alcohol use
○ Poor physical condition
○ Age
○ Socioeconomic status

Incidence

○ Affects men and women equally
○ Increased incidence among elderly patients and neonates during excessively hot summer days

Common characteristics

○ Temperature in excess of 105.8° F (41° C)
○ Tachycardia greater than 130 beats/minute
○ Widened pulse pressure
○ Changes in level of consciousness
○ Tonic-dystonic contractions of the muscles
○ Coma
○ Tachypnea
○ Hypoxia

Complications

○ Hypovolemic shock
○ Cardiogenic shock
○ Cardiac arrhythmias
○ Renal failure
○ Disseminated intravascular coagulation
○ Hepatic failure

Assessment

History

Heat exhaustion
○ Prolonged activity in a very warm or hot environment
○ Muscle cramps
○ Nausea and vomiting
○ Thirst
○ Weakness
○ Headache
○ Fatigue
Heat stroke
○ Exposure to high temperature and humidity without air circulation
○ Same signs as heat exhaustion
○ Blurred vision
○ Confusion
○ Hallucinations
○ Decreased muscle coordination
○ Syncope

Physical findings

Heat exhaustion
○ Rectal temperature over 100° F (37.8° C)
○ Pale skin
○ Thready, rapid pulse
○ Cool, moist skin
○ Decreased blood pressure
○ Irritability
○ Syncope
○ Impaired judgment
○ Hyperventilation
Heat stroke
○ Rectal temperature of at least 104° F (40° C)
○ Red, diaphoretic, hot skin in early stages
○ Gray, dry, hot skin in later stages
○ Tachycardia
○ Slightly elevated blood pressure in early stages
○ Decreased blood pressure in later stages
○ Signs of central nervous system dysfunction
○ Altered mental status
○ Hyperpnea

○ Cheyne-Stokes respirations
○ Anhydrosis (late sign)

Test results

Laboratory
○ Elevated serum electrolytes possibly showing hyponatremia and hypokalemia
○ Arterial blood gas levels possibly showing respiratory alkalosis
○ Complete blood count possibly showing leukocytosis and thrombocytopenia
○ Coagulation studies possibly showing increased bleeding and clotting times
○ Urinalysis possibly showing concentrated urine and proteinuria with tubular casts and myoglobinuria
○ Possibly elevated blood urea nitrogen
○ Possibly decreased serum calcium
○ Possibly decreased serum phosphorus

Treatment

General

Heat exhaustion
○ Cool environment
○ Oral or I.V. fluid administration

Heat stroke
○ Lowering the body temperature as rapidly as possible
○ Evaporation, hypothermia blankets, and ice packs to the groin, axillae, and neck
○ Supportive respiratory and cardiovascular measures
○ Increased hydration; cool liquids only
○ Avoidance of caffeine and alcohol
○ Rest periods, as needed

Nursing considerations

Key outcomes
The patient will:
○ maintain adequate ventilation
○ maintain a normal body temperature
○ prevent recurrent episodes of hyperthermia
○ express understanding of the need to maintain adequate fluid intake.

Nursing interventions
○ Perform rapid cooling procedures.
○ Provide supportive measures.
○ Provide adequate fluid intake.
○ Give prescribed drugs.

Monitoring
○ Vital signs
○ Pulse oximetry readings
○ Complications
○ Level of consciousness
○ Cardiac rhythm
○ Intake and output
○ Myoglobin test results

Patient teaching

Be sure to cover:
○ the disorder, diagnosis, and treatment
○ how to avoid reexposure to high temperatures
○ the need to maintain adequate fluid intake
○ the need to wear loose clothing
○ limiting activity in hot weather.

Discharge planning
○ Refer the patient to social services, if appropriate.

Hemophilia

Overview

Description
- Hereditary bleeding disorder
- Characterized by greatly prolonged coagulation time
- Results from deficiency of specific clotting factors
- Hemophilia A (classic hemophilia): affects more than 80% of hemophiliacs; results from factor VIII deficiency
- Hemophilia B (Christmas disease): affects 15% of hemophiliacs; results from factor IX deficiency
- Incurable

Pathophysiology
- Low level or absence of the blood protein necessary for clotting causes disruption of normal intrinsic co-agulation cascade.
- Abnormal bleeding, which may be mild, moderate, or severe, depending on the degree of protein factor deficiency, is produced.
- After a platelet plug at a bleeding site, the lack of clotting factors impairs formation of a stable fibrin clot.
- Immediate hemorrhage isn't prevalent; delayed bleeding is common.

Causes
- Hemophilia A and B inherited as X-linked recessive traits
- Spontaneous mutation
- Acquired immunologic process

Incidence
- Most common X-linked genetic disease
- Occurs in about 1.25 of 10,000 live male births

Common characteristics
- Abnormal tendency to bleed
- Painful and swollen joints

Complications
- Pain, swelling, extreme tenderness, and permanent joint and muscle deformity
- Peripheral neuropathies, pain, paresthesia, and muscle atrophy
- Ischemia and gangrene
- Shock and death

Assessment

History
- Familial history of bleeding disorders
- Prolonged bleeding with circumcision
- Concomitant illness
- Pain and swelling in a weight-bearing joint, such as the hip, knee, or ankle
- With mild hemophilia or after minor trauma, lack of spontaneous bleeding, but prolonged bleeding with major trauma or surgery
- Moderate hemophilia producing only occasional spontaneous bleeding episodes
- Severe hemophilia causing spontaneous bleeding
- Prolonged bleeding after surgery or trauma or joint pain in spontaneous bleeding into muscles or joints
- Signs of internal bleeding, such as abdominal, chest, or flank pain; episodes of hematuria or hematemesis; and tarry stools
- Activity or movement limitations and need for assistive devices, such as splints, canes, or crutches

Physical findings
- Hematomas on extremities, torso, or both
- Joint swelling in episodes of bleeding into joints
- Limited and painful joint range of motion in episodes of bleeding into joints

Test results
Laboratory
HEMOPHILIA A
- Factor VIII assay 0% to 25% of normal
- Prolonged partial thromboplastin time (PTT)
- Normal platelet count and function, bleeding time, and prothrombin time

HEMOPHILIA B
- Deficient factor IX assay
- Baseline coagulation results similar to those of hemophilia A, with normal factor VIII

HEMOPHILIA A OR B
- Degree of factor deficiency defines severity:
  - Mild hemophilia—factor levels 5% to 25% of normal
  - Moderate hemophilia—factor levels 1% to 5% of normal
  - Severe hemophilia—factor levels less than 1% of normal

Treatment

General
- Correct treatment to quickly stop bleeding by increasing plasma levels of deficient clotting factors
- Diet consisting of foods high in vitamin K
- Activity guided by degree of factor deficiency

Medication
- Aminocaproic acid
Hemophilia A
- Cryoprecipitated antihemophilic factor (AHF), lyophilized AHF, or both
- Desmopressin
Hemophilia B
- Factor IX concentrate

Nursing considerations

Key outcomes

The patient will:
- maintain hemodynamic stability
- have peripheral pulses that remain palpable and strong
- express feelings of increased comfort and decreased pain
- maintain range of motion and joint mobility
- demonstrate adequate coping skills
- verbalize understanding of disease process and treatment regimen.

Nursing interventions

- Follow standard precautions.
- Provide emotional support, and reassurance when indicated.

During bleeding episodes
- Apply pressure to bleeding sites.
- Give the deficient clotting factor or plasma, as ordered, until bleeding stops.
- Apply cold compresses or ice bags, and elevate the injured part.
- To prevent recurrence of bleeding, restrict activity for 48 hours after bleeding is under control.
- Control pain with prescribed analgesics.
- Avoid I.M. injections.
- Avoid aspirin and aspirin-containing drugs.

During bleeding into a joint
- Immediately elevate the joint.
- To restore joint mobility, begin range-of-motion exercises at least 48 hours after the bleeding is controlled.
- Restrict weight bearing until bleeding stops and swelling subsides.
- Give prescribed analgesics for pain.
- Apply ice packs and elastic bandages to alleviate pain.

Monitoring

- PTT
- Adverse reactions to blood products
- Signs and symptoms of decreased tissue perfusion
- Vital signs
- Bleeding from the skin, mucous membranes, and wounds

Patient teaching

Be sure to cover:
- the benefits of regular isometric exercises
- how parents can protect their child from injury while avoiding unnecessary restrictions that impair normal development
- the need to avoid contact sports
- if an injury occurs, directions for parents to apply cold compresses or ice bags and to elevate the injured part or apply light pressure to bleeding

- the need to notify the physician immediately after even a minor injury
- the need for parents to watch for signs of internal bleeding
- the importance of avoiding aspirin, combination medications that contain aspirin, and over-the-counter anti-inflammatory agents (use acetaminophen instead)
- the importance of good dental care and the need to check with the physician before dental extractions or surgery
- the need to wear medical identification jewelry at all times
- how to administer blood factor components at home, if appropriate
- the need to keep blood factor concentrate and infusion equipment available at all times
- adverse reactions that can result from replacement factor procedures
- signs, symptoms, and treatment of anaphylaxis
- the need for the patient or parents to watch for early signs of hepatitis
- the need to follow standard precautions.

Discharge planning

- Refer new patients to a hemophilia treatment center for evaluation.
- For more information, refer the patient's family to the National Hemophilia Foundation.

Hemorrhoids

Overview

Description

- Varicosities found in the superior or inferior hemorrhoidal venous plexus
- Classified as first, second, third, or fourth degree, depending on their severity
- First-degree hemorrhoids are confined to the anal canal
- Second-degree hemorrhoids prolapse during straining but reduce spontaneously
- Third-degree hemorrhoids are prolapsed hemorrhoids that require manual reduction after each bowel movement
- Fourth-degree hemorrhoids are irreducible

Pathophysiology

- Dilation and enlargement of the superior plexus of the superior hemorrhoidal veins above the dentate line cause internal hemorrhoids.
- Enlargement of the plexus of the inferior hemorrhoidal veins below the dentate line causes external hemorrhoids, which may protrude from the rectum. (See *Comparing types of hemorrhoids.*)

Causes

- Prolonged sitting
- Straining at defecation
- Constipation, low-fiber diet
- Pregnancy
- Obesity

Incidence

- Occur in both sexes
- Most cases occur in people ages 20 and 50

Common characteristics

- Painless, intermittent bleeding during defecation

Complications

- Constipation
- Local infection
- Thrombosis of hemorrhoids
- Secondary anemia from severe or recurrent bleeding

Assessment

History

- Bright red blood on stool or toilet tissue
- Anal itching
- Vague feeling of anal discomfort
- Pain

Physical findings

- Prolapse of rectal mucosa
- Anal tenderness on palpation
- Internal hemorrhoids (with digital examination)

Comparing types of hemorrhoids

Covered by mucosa, internal hemorrhoids bulge into the rectal lumen and may prolapse during defecation. Covered by skin, external hemorrhoids protrude from the rectum and are more likely to thrombose than internal hemorrhoids. The illustrations below show both frontal and cross-sectional views.

INTERNAL HEMORRHOIDS

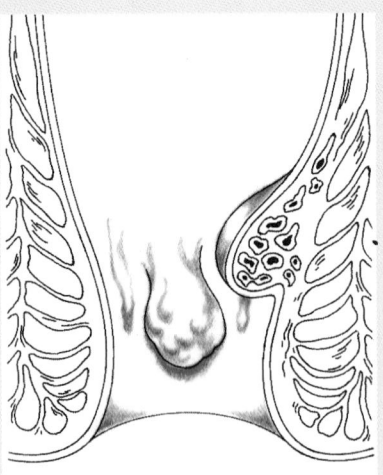

EXTERNAL HEMORRHOIDS

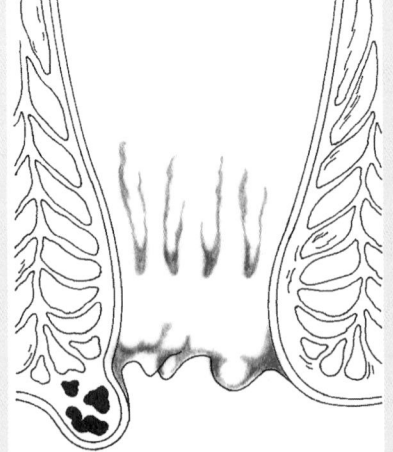

Test results

Diagnostic procedures
- ○ Anoscopy and flexible sigmoidoscopy visualize internal hemorrhoids.

Others
- ○ Physical examination findings

Treatment

General

- ○ High-fiber diet, increased fluid intake
- ○ Avoidance of prolonged sitting
- ○ Warm sitz baths to relieve pain

Medication

- ○ Local anesthetic agents
- ○ Hydrocortisone cream and suppositories

Surgery

- ○ Injection sclerotherapy or rubber band ligation
- ○ Hemorrhoidectomy by cauterization or excision

Nursing considerations

Key outcomes

The patient will:
- ○ express feelings of increased comfort
- ○ have reduced occurrence of hemorrhoids
- ○ express understanding of the disorder and treatment regimen.

Nursing interventions

- ○ Administer enemas preoperatively.
- ○ Give prescribed drugs.
- ○ Keep the wound site clean.
- ○ Provide sitz baths.

Monitoring

- ○ Bleeding
- ○ Pain

Patient teaching

Be sure to cover:
- ○ avoiding stool softeners after surgery
- ○ the importance of regular bowel habits and good anal hygiene
- ○ avoiding too-vigorous wiping with washcloths and use of harsh soaps
- ○ the use of medicated astringent pads and white, unscented toilet paper.

Hemothorax

Overview

Description

- Blood in the pleural cavity
- May result in lung collapse

Pathophysiology

- Damaged intercostal, pleural, mediastinal, and sometimes lung parenchymal vessels cause blood to enter the pleural cavity.
- The amount of bleeding and the cause is associated with varying degrees of lung collapse and mediastinal shift.

Causes

- Damaged intercostal, pleural, or mediastinal vessels
- Damaged parenchymal vessels
- Blunt or penetrating chest trauma
- Pulmonary infarction
- Necrotizing infections
- Pulmonary arteriovenous fistulas
- Hereditary hemorrhagic telangiectasis
- Heart or thorax surgery
- Neoplasm
- Dissecting thoracic aneurysm
- Anticoagulant therapy
- Thoracic endometriosis
- Central venous catheter insertion
- Tuberculosis

Incidence

- Occurs in about 25% of patients with chest trauma

Common characteristics

- Chest pain
- Sudden shortness of breath

Complications

- Mediastinal shift
- Ventilatory compromise
- Lung collapse
- Cardiopulmonary arrest
- Pneumothorax
- Empyema

Assessment

History

- Recent trauma
- Recent thoracic surgery
- Metastatic disease

Physical findings

- Tachypnea
- Dusky skin color
- Diaphoresis
- Hemoptysis
- Restlessness
- Anxiety
- Cyanosis
- Stupor
- Affected side may expand and stiffen
- Unaffected side may rise with gasping respirations
- Dullness over affected side
- Decreased or absent breath sounds over affected side
- Symptoms associated with blunt trauma
- Tachycardia
- Hypotension

Test results

Laboratory
- Pleural fluid analysis showing hematocrit greater than 50% of serum hematocrit
- Arterial blood gas (ABG) analysis possibly showing increased partial pressure of carbon dioxide and decreased partial pressure of oxygen
- Serum hemoglobin level possibly decreased, depending on blood loss

Imaging
- Chest X-rays and computed tomography scan of the thorax show the presence and extent of hemothorax and help to evaluate treatment.

Diagnostic procedures
- Thoracentesis: may yield blood or serosanguineous fluid

Treatment

General

- Stabilization of the patient's clinical condition
- Stoppage of bleeding
- Thoracentesis
- Insertion of chest tube
- Autotransfusion if blood loss approaches or exceeds 1 L (see *Using autotransfusion for chest wounds*)
- Diet, as tolerated
- I.V. therapy
- Activity, as tolerated

Medication

- Oxygen
- Analgesics

Surgery

- Thoracotomy if chest tube doesn't improve condition

Nursing considerations

Key outcomes

The patient will:
- maintain adequate ventilation
- maintain fluid volume balance
- express feelings of increased comfort and decreased pain
- verbalize understanding of the illness.

Autotransfusion is used most often in patients with chest wounds, especially those that involve hemothorax. Through autotransfusion, a patient's own blood is collected, filtered, and reinfused. The procedure may also be used when two or three units of pooled blood can be recovered, such as in cardiac or orthopedic surgery.

Autotransfusion eliminates the patient's risk of transfusion reaction or blood-borne disease, such as cytomegalovirus, hepatitis, and human immunodeficiency virus. It's contraindicated in patients with sepsis or cancer.

How autotransfusion works

A large-bore chest tube connected to a closed drainage system is used to collect the patient's blood from a wound or chest cavity. This blood passes through a filter, which catches most potential thrombi, including clumps of fibrin and damaged red blood cells (RBCs). The filtered blood passes into a collection bag. From the bag, the blood is reinfused immediately, or it may be processed in a commercial cell washer that reduces anticoagulated whole blood to washed RBCs for later infusion.

Assisting with autotransfusion

Set up the blood collection system as you would any closed chest drainage system. Attach the collection bag according to the manufacturer's instructions.

If ordered, inject an anticoagulant, such as heparin or acid-citrate-dextrose solution, into the self-sealing port on the connector of the patient's drainage tubing.

During reinfusion, monitor the patient for complications, such as blood clotting, hemolysis, coagulopathies, thrombocytopenia, particulate and air emboli, sepsis, and citrate toxicity (from the acid-citrate-dextrose solution).

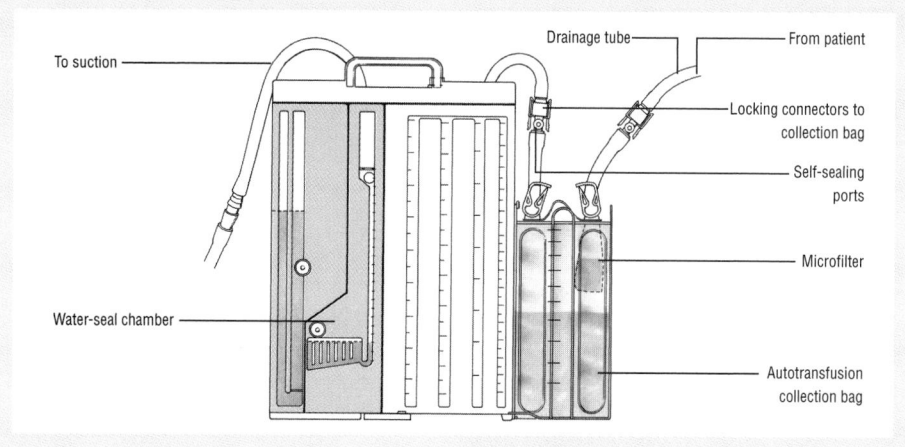

To suction
Water-seal chamber
Drainage tube
From patient
Locking connectors to collection bag
Self-sealing ports
Microfilter
Autotransfusion collection bag

Nursing interventions

- Give prescribed drugs.
- Promote comfort and relaxation.
- Give prescribed oxygen.
- Give prescribed I.V. fluids and blood transfusions.
- Assist with thoracentesis.
- Prepare the patient for surgery, if needed.
- Change the chest tube dressing, and provide chest tube care, as needed.

Monitoring

- Vital signs
- Intake and output
- Chest tube drainage
- Central venous pressure
- ABG results
- Chest X-ray results
- Complete blood count results
- Respiratory status
- Complications
- Signs and symptoms of infection

Patient teaching

Be sure to cover:
- the disorder, diagnosis, and treatment
- prescribed drugs and potential adverse effects
- when to notify the physician
- preoperative and postoperative care, if needed
- mechanical ventilation, if needed
- deep-breathing exercises
- smoking cessation, if appropriate.

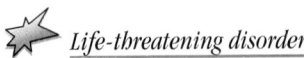 *Life-threatening disorder*

Hepatic encephalopathy

Overview

Description

- A neurologic syndrome that develops as a complication of aggressive fulminant hepatitis or chronic hepatic disease
- Most common in patients with cirrhosis
- In advanced stages, prognosis extremely poor despite vigorous treatment
- Acute form occurs with acute fulminant hepatic failure and may be fatal
- Chronic form occurs with chronic liver disease and is often reversible
- Also called *hepatic coma*

Pathophysiology

- Normally, the ammonia produced by protein breakdown in the bowel is metabolized to urea in the liver. When portal blood shunts past the liver, ammonia directly enters the systemic circulation and is carried to the brain.
- Such shunting may result from the collateral venous circulation that develops in portal hypertension or from surgically created portal-systemic shunts.
- Cirrhosis further compounds this problem because impaired hepatocellular function prevents conversion of ammonia that reaches the liver.

Causes

- Ammonia intoxication of the brain
- Exact cause unknown

Risk factors

- Excessive protein intake
- Sepsis
- Excessive accumulation of nitrogenous body wastes (from constipation or GI hemorrhage)
- Bacterial action on protein and urea to form ammonia
- Hepatitis
- Diuretic therapy
- Alcoholism
- Fluid and electrolyte imbalance (especially metabolic alkalosis)
- Hypoxia
- Azotemia
- Impaired glucose metabolism
- Infection
- Use of sedatives, opioids, and general anesthetics

Incidence

- Occurs in approximately 4 of 100,000 people
- Observed in 70% of patients with cirrhosis

Common characteristics

- Changes in mental status and personality
- Jaundice
- Muscle tremors
- Fruity breath odor

Complications

- Irreversible coma
- Death

Assessment

History

Prodromal stage
- Slight personality changes, such as agitation, belligerence, disorientation, and forgetfulness
- Trouble concentrating or thinking clearly
- Fatigue
- Mental changes, such as confusion and disorientation
- Sleep-wake reversal

Impending stage
- Mental changes, such as confusion and disorientation

Stuporous stage
- Marked mental confusion

Comatose stage
- Unable to arouse

Physical findings

Prodromal stage
- Slurred or slowed speech
- Slight tremor

Impending stage
- Tremors that have progressed to asterixis
- Lethargy
- Aberrant behavior
- Apraxia
- Possible incontinence

Stuporous stage
- Drowsy and stuporous
- Noisy and abusive when aroused
- Hyperventilation
- Muscle twitching
- Asterixis

Comatose stage
- Obtunded
- Seizures
- Hyperactive reflexes
- Positive Babinski's sign
- Fetor hepaticus (musty, sweet breath odor)

Test results

Laboratory
- Serum ammonia levels elevated and, together with characteristic clinical features, strongly suggest hepatic encephalopathy
- Serum bilirubin elevated and prothrombin time prolonged

○ EEG shows slowing waves as the disease progresses

Treatment

General

○ Elimination of underlying cause
○ I.V. fluid administration
○ Control of GI bleeding
○ Life-support measures, if appropriate
○ Bowel cleansing
○ Limited protein intake
○ Nothing by mouth with decreased responsiveness
○ Parenteral or enteric feedings, if appropriate
○ Bed rest until condition improves
○ No alcohol use

Medication

○ Lactulose
○ Neomycin
○ Potassium supplements
○ Salt-poor albumin
○ Sorbitol-induced catharsis

Surgery

○ Possible liver transplant

Nursing considerations

Key outcomes

The patient will:
○ express feelings of increased comfort
○ maintain orientation to environment
○ maintain stable vital signs
○ maintain normal fluid volume
○ maintain skin integrity.

Nursing interventions

○ Promote rest, comfort, and a quiet atmosphere.
○ Give prescribed drugs.
○ Use appropriate safety measures to protect the patient from injury.
○ Maintain skin integrity.
○ Perform passive range-of-motion exercises.
○ Provide emotional support.

Monitoring

○ Level of consciousness
○ Intake and output
○ Fluid and electrolyte balance
○ Weight and abdominal girth
○ Signs of anemia, alkalosis, GI bleeding, and infection
○ Serum ammonia level
○ Changes in handwriting for progression of neurologic involvement

Discharge planning

○ Refer the patient to social services, as indicated.

Patient teaching

Be sure to cover:
○ the disorder, diagnosis, and treatment
○ signs of complications or worsening symptoms
○ dietary modifications
○ drug administration, dosage, and possible adverse effects.

Hepatitis, nonviral

Overview

Description
- Inflammation of the liver
- Classified as toxic or drug-induced (idiosyncratic)

Pathophysiology
- Hepatocellular damage and necrosis usually caused by toxins
- Dose-dependent
- Occurs primarily in connection with acetaminophen overdose

Causes
- Alcohol overuse
- Direct hepatotoxicity
- Lack of bile excretion
- Possibly direct hepatotoxicity from hormonal contraceptives or anabolic steroids
- Hypersensitivity to phenothiazine derivatives such as chlorpromazine
- Antibiotics
- Thyroid medications
- Antidiabetic drugs
- Cytotoxic drugs
- Cholestatic reactions
- Metabolic and autoimmune disorders
- Infectious agents

Incidence
- Can affect males and females (autoimmune affects females more commonly)
- Can occur at any age

Common characteristics
- Clinical features of toxic and drug-induced hepatitis vary with the severity of the liver damage and the causative agent
- Symptoms resemble those of viral hepatitis

 Alert

Carbon tetrachloride poisoning also produces headache, dizziness, drowsiness, and vasomotor collapse; halothane-related hepatitis produces fever, moderate leukocytosis, and eosinophilia; chlorpromazine produces a rash, abrupt fever, arthralgias, lymphadenopathy, and epigastric or right upper quadrant pain.

Complications
- Fulminant hepatic failure
- Renal failure
- Liver fibrosis
- Cirrhosis

Assessment

History
- Causative agent
- Anorexia
- Nausea
- Vomiting
- Possibly abdominal pain
- Pruritus

Physical findings
- Jaundice
- Dark urine
- Hepatomegaly
- Clay-colored stools

Test results
Laboratory
- Elevated serum aspartate aminotransferase and alanine aminotransferase levels
- Elevated total and direct bilirubin (with cholestasis) levels
- Elevated alkaline phosphatase level
- Elevated white blood cell count
- Elevated eosinophil count (possible in the drug-induced type)

Diagnostic procedures
- Liver biopsy may help identify the underlying pathology.

Treatment

General
- Removal of causative agent by lavage, catharsis, or hyperventilation, depending on the route of exposure
- Nutritious diet and adequate fluid intake
- Activity, as tolerated

Medication
- Acetylcysteine (acetaminophen poisoning)
- Corticosteroids (drug-induced hepatitis)

Nursing considerations

Key outcomes
The patient will:
- demonstrate an understanding of the disorder and treatment regimen
- remain free from complications
- express feelings of increased comfort.

Nursing interventions
- Give prescribed drugs.
- Provide emotional support.

Monitoring
○ Response to treatment
○ Laboratory values
○ Vital signs
○ Complications

Patient teaching

Be sure to cover:
○ the disorder, diagnosis, and treatment
○ drug administration, dosage, and possible adverse effects
○ proper handling of cleaning agents and solvents.

Discharge planning
○ Encourage follow-up care.

Hepatitis, viral

Overview

Description

- Infection and inflammation of the liver caused by a virus
- Six types recognized (A, B, C, D, E, and G), and a seventh suspected
- Marked by hepatic cell destruction, necrosis, and autolysis, leading to anorexia, jaundice, and hepatomegaly
- In most patients, hepatic cells eventually regenerate with little or no residual damage, allowing recovery
- Complications more likely with old age and serious underlying disorders
- Prognosis poor if edema and hepatic encephalopathy develop

Pathophysiology

- Hepatic inflammation caused by virus leads to diffuse injury and necrosis of hepatocytes.
- Hypertrophy and hyperplasia of Kupffer cells and sinusoidal lining cells occurs.
- Bile obstruction may occur.

Causes

- Infection with the causative viruses for each of six major forms of viral hepatitis

Type A
- Transmittal by the fecal-oral or parenteral route
- Ingestion of contaminated food, milk, or water

Type B
- Transmittal by contact with contaminated human blood, secretions, and stool

Type C
- Transmittal primarily by sharing of needles by I.V. drug users, through blood transfusions, or tattoo needles

Type D
- Found only in patients with an acute or a chronic episode of hepatitis B

Type E
- Transmittal by parenteral route and commonly waterborne

Type G
- Thought to be blood-borne, with transmission similar to that of hepatitis B and C

Incidence

Hepatitis A
- Occurs in nationwide epidemics

Hepatitis B
- Estimated 1.25 million chronically infected Americans
- Highest rate of disease occurs in people ages 20 to 49

Hepatitis C
- Estimated 3.9 million chronically infected Americans

Common characteristics

- Malaise, fatigue
- Dark-colored urine
- Clay-colored stools
- Abdominal tenderness
- Fever
- Jaundice
- Nausea
- Loss of appetite

Complications

- Life-threatening fulminant hepatitis
- Chronic active hepatitis (in hepatitis B)
- Syndrome resembling serum sickness, characterized by arthralgia or arthritis, rash, and angioedema; can lead to misdiagnosis of hepatitis B as rheumatoid arthritis or lupus erythematosus (in hepatitis B)
- Primary liver cancer (in hepatitis B or C)
- In hepatitis D, mild or asymptomatic form of hepatitis B that flares into severe, progressive chronic active hepatitis and cirrhosis

Assessment

History

- 50% to 60% of people with hepatitis B have no signs or symptoms
- 80% of people with hepatitis C have no signs or symptoms
- Revelation of a source of transmission

Prodromal stage
- Patient easily fatigued, with generalized malaise
- Anorexia, mild weight loss
- Depression
- Headache, photophobia
- Weakness
- Arthralgia, myalgia (hepatitis B)
- Nausea or vomiting
- Changes in the senses of taste and smell

Clinical jaundice stage
- Pruritus
- Abdominal pain or tenderness
- Indigestion
- Anorexia
- Possible jaundice of sclerae, mucous membranes, and skin

Posticteric stage
- Most symptoms decreasing or subsided

Physical findings

Prodromal stage
- Fever (100° to 102° F [37.8° to 38.9° C])
- Dark-colored urine
- Clay-colored stools

Clinical jaundice stage
- Rashes, erythematous patches, or hives
- Abdominal tenderness in the right upper quadrant
- Enlarged and tender liver
- Splenomegaly
- Cervical adenopathy

Posticteric stage
○ Decrease in liver enlargement

Test results
Laboratory
○ In suspected viral hepatitis, hepatitis profile routinely performed; result identifying antibodies specific to the causative virus and establishing the type of hepatitis:
○ Type A — detection of an antibody to hepatitis A confirming the diagnosis
○ Type B — presence of hepatitis B surface antigens and hepatitis B antibodies confirming the diagnosis
○ Type C — diagnosis depending on serologic testing for the specific antibody one or more months after the onset of acute illness; until then, diagnosis principally established by obtaining negative test results for hepatitis A, B, and D
○ Type D — detection of intrahepatic delta antigens or immunoglobulin (Ig) M antidelta antigens in acute disease (or IgM and IgG in chronic disease) establishing the diagnosis
○ Type E — detection of hepatitis E antigens supporting the diagnosis; however, diagnosis possibly also ruling out hepatitis C
○ Type G — detection of hepatitis G ribonucleic acid supporting the diagnosis (serologic assays are being developed)
○ Additional findings from liver function studies supporting the diagnosis:
  – Serum aspartate aminotransferase and serum alanine aminotransferase levels increased in the prodromal stage of acute viral hepatitis
  – Serum alkaline phosphatase levels slightly increased
  – Serum bilirubin levels elevated; levels possibly remaining elevated late in the disease, especially with severe disease
  – Prothrombin time (PT) prolonged (PT more than 3 seconds longer than normal, indicating severe liver damage)
  – White blood cell counts commonly revealing transient neutropenia and lymphopenia followed by lymphocytosis
Diagnostic procedures
○ Liver biopsy shows chronic hepatitis.

Treatment

General
For hepatitis C
○ Aimed at clearing hepatitis C from the body, stopping or slowing of hepatic damage, and symptom relief
○ Symptomatic
○ Small, high-calorie, high-protein meals (reduced protein intake if signs of precoma — lethargy, confusion, mental changes — develop)
○ Parenteral feeding, if appropriate
○ Alcohol cessation

○ Frequent rest periods, as needed
○ Avoidance of contact sports and strenuous activity

Medication
○ Standard immunoglobulin
○ Vaccine
○ Alfa-2b interferon (hepatitis B and C)
○ Antiemetics
○ Cholestyramine
○ Lamivudine (hepatitis B)
○ Ribavirin (hepatitis C)

Surgery
○ Possible liver transplant (hepatitis C)

Nursing considerations

Key outcomes
The patient will:
○ develop no complications
○ maintain stable vital signs
○ perform activities of daily living within the confines of the disease process
○ express understanding of the disorder and treatment regimen.

Nursing interventions
○ Observe standard precautions to prevent transmission of the disease.
○ Provide rest periods throughout the day.
○ Give prescribed drugs.
○ Encourage oral fluid intake.

Monitoring
○ Hydration and nutritional status
○ Daily weight
○ Intake and output
○ Stool for color, consistency, amount, and frequency
○ Signs of complications

Patient teaching

Be sure to cover:
○ the disorder, diagnosis, and treatment
○ measures to prevent the spread of disease
○ the importance of rest and a proper diet
○ the need to abstain from alcohol
○ drug administration, dosage, and possible adverse effects
○ the need to avoid over-the-counter medications unless approved by the physician
○ the need for follow-up care.

Discharge planning
○ Refer the patient to Alcoholics Anonymous, if indicated.

Hereditary hemorrhagic telangiectasia

Overview

Description
- Inherited vascular disorder of the blood vessels that can cause excessive bleeding
- Also called *Osler-Weber-Rendu disease*

Pathophysiology
- Venules and capillaries dilate to form fragile masses of thin convoluted vessels (telangiectases), resulting in an abnormal tendency to hemorrhage.

Causes
- Transmitted by autosomal dominant inheritance

Incidence
- Affects both sexes but may cause less severe bleeding in females
- Occurs in 1 in 50,000 births

Common characteristics
- Recurrent epistaxis
- Telangiectases

Complications
- Secondary iron deficiency anemia
- Vascular malformation causing pulmonary arteriovenous fistulas (rare)
- Recurring cerebral embolism and brain abscess
- Hemorrhagic shock
- Intracranial hemorrhage

Assessment

History
- Established familial pattern of bleeding disorders
- Epistaxis, hemoptysis, or tarry stools
- Appearance of telangiectasia during late childhood or adolescence

Physical findings
- Localized aggregations of dilated capillaries on the skin of the face, ears, tongue, lips, conjunctivae, scalp, hands, arms, and feet and under the nails
- Characteristic telangiectases: violet, bleed spontaneously, flat or raised, blanch on pressure, and nonpulsatile
- Signs of capillary fragility (may exist without overt telangiectasia): Spontaneous bleeding, petechiae, ecchymoses, and spider hemangiomas of varying size (see *Typical lesions of hereditary hemorrhagic telangiectasia*)
- Clubbing of the digits

Test results

Laboratory
- Platelet count possibly abnormal
- Complete blood count and anemia panel possibly showing hypochromic, microcytic anemia

Imaging
- Chest X-rays possibly showing arteriovenous malformation
- Echocardiogram possibly showing "high-output" cardiac failure

---

Typical lesions of hereditary hemorrhagic telangiectasia

The illustrations below show the commonly encountered lesions of hereditary hemorrhagic telangiectasia.

Dilated capillaries, either flat or raised, appear in localized aggregations, as on the fingers.

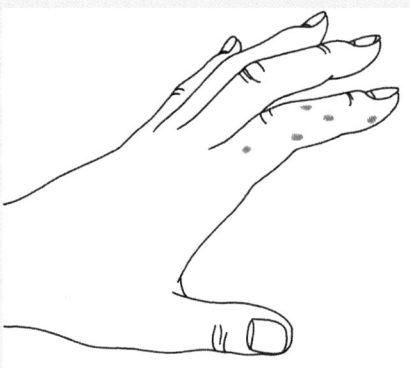

On the face, spider hemangiomas reflect capillary fragility.

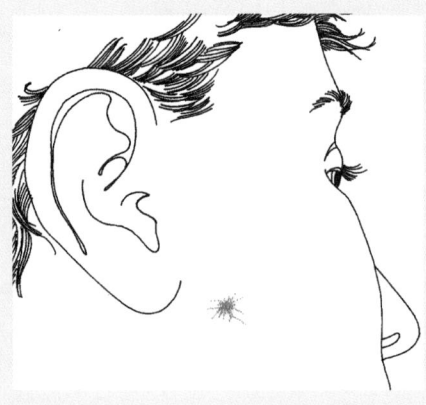

◯ Bone marrow aspiration shows depleted iron stores and confirms secondary iron deficiency anemia.

Treatment

General

◯ Supportive therapy, including blood transfusions and supplemental iron administration
◯ Ancillary treatment consisting of applying pressure and topical hemostatic agents to bleeding sites, cauterizing bleeding sites not readily accessible, and protecting the patient from trauma and unnecessary bleeding
◯ Laser treatment to destroy vessel
◯ Avoidance of activities with the potential for trauma

Medication

◯ Parenteral iron
◯ Antipyretics or antihistamines

Nursing considerations

Key outcomes

The patient will:
◯ maintain hemodynamic stability
◯ have laboratory values that return to normal
◯ demonstrate positive signs of coping
◯ exhibit no signs or symptoms of infection.

Nursing interventions

◯ Provide emotional and psychological support.
◯ Give prescribed blood transfusions.
◯ Encourage fluid intake if the patient is bleeding or hypovolemic.
◯ Provide meticulous skin care and hygiene.
◯ Use aseptic technique when caring for the patient.

Monitoring

◯ Vital signs
◯ Intake and output
◯ Signs of febrile or allergic transfusion reaction
◯ Indications of GI bleeding
◯ Laboratory values to detect possible renal, hepatic, or respiratory failure

Patient teaching

Be sure to cover:
◯ the disorder, signs and symptoms, and treatment
◯ iron supplements, including the importance of following dosage instructions and of taking oral iron with meals to minimize GI irritation
◯ a warning that iron turns stools dark green or black and may cause constipation

◯ the management of minor bleeding episodes, especially recurrent epistaxis
◯ how to recognize major bleeding episodes that require emergency intervention.

Discharge planning

◯ Refer the patient for genetic counseling, as appropriate.

Hernia, hiatal

Overview

Description
- Defect in the diaphragm that permits a portion of the stomach to pass through the diaphragmatic opening into the chest
- Three types: sliding hernia, paraesophageal (rolling) hernia, and mixed hernia (sliding and rolling hernia)

Pathophysiology
Sliding hernia
- The muscular collar around the esophageal and diaphragmatic junction loosens.
- Increased intra-abdominal pressure causes the lower portion of the esophagus and the upper portion of the stomach to rise into the chest.

Paraesophageal hernia
- The stomach isn't properly anchored below the diaphragm.
- Increased intra-abdominal pressure causes the upper portion of the stomach to slide through the esophageal hiatus.

Causes
Sliding hernia
- Normal aging
- Secondary to esophageal carcinoma, kyphoscoliosis, trauma, or surgery
- Diaphragmatic malformations that can cause congenital weakness
- Chronic esophagitis

Paraesophageal hernia
- Not fully understood

Risk factors
- Obesity
- Smoking
- Pregnancy
- Presence of ascites

Incidence
- Sliding hernia 3 to 10 times more common than paraesophageal and mixed hernias combined
- Increases with age
- 60% of people have hiatal hernias by age 60
- Higher prevalence in women than in men

Common characteristics
- May produce no symptoms
- Heartburn

Complications
- Esophageal stricture
- Incarceration (with paraesophageal hernia)
- In association with gastroesophageal reflux disease:
  - Esophagitis
  - Esophageal ulceration and perforation
  - Hemorrhage
  - Peritonitis
  - Mediastinitis
  - Aspiration
  - Strangulation and gangrene of herniated portion of stomach
- Iron deficiency anemia
- Chronic cough
- Dysphagia

Assessment

History
- Heartburn 1 to 4 hours after eating; aggravated by reclining, belching, or conditions that increase intra-abdominal pressure
- Regurgitation or vomiting
- Retrosternal or substernal chest pain (typically after meals or at bedtime)
- Feeling of fullness after eating
- Feeling of breathlessness or suffocation
- Chest pain resembling angina pectoris
- Reflux
- Chronic cough
- Belching

Physical findings
- Possibly none
- Dysphagia

Test results
Laboratory
- Decreased serum hemoglobin level and hematocrit in patients with paraesophageal hernia, if bleeding from esophageal ulceration is present
- Fecal occult blood test possibly positive
- Analysis of gastric contents possibly revealing blood

Imaging
- Chest X-rays reveal an air shadow behind the heart in a large hernia; lower lobe infiltrates with aspiration.
- Barium swallow with fluoroscopy detects a hiatal hernia and diaphragmatic abnormalities.

Diagnostic procedures
- Endoscopy and biopsy results identify the mucosal junction and the edge of the diaphragm indenting the esophagus; differentiate hiatal hernia, varices, erosions, ulcers, Barrett's esophagus, and other small gastroesophageal lesions; and rule out malignant tumors.
- Esophageal motility studies reveal esophageal motor or lower esophageal pressure abnormalities before surgical repair of the hernia.
- pH studies identify reflux of gastric contents.
- Acid perfusion (Bernstein) test identifies esophageal reflux.

Treatment

General

- Smoking cessation (smoking stimulates gastric acid production)
- Six small meals per day
- No fluids or food 1 to 2 hours before bedtime
- Elimination of spicy or irritating foods, alcohol, and coffee
- Weight reduction, as appropriate
- Upright posture for 2 to 3 hours after eating
- Restriction of activities that increase intra-abdominal pressure

Medication

- Antacids
- Histamine-2 receptor antagonists
- Cholinergic agent
- Motility agent
- Antiemetics
- Cough suppressants

Surgery

- Hernia repair (rare)

Nursing considerations

Key outcomes

The patient will:
- avoid or have minimal complications
- show no evidence of aspiration
- maintain a patent airway
- express feelings of increased comfort
- express understanding of the disorder and treatment regimen.

Nursing interventions

- Prepare the patient for diagnostic tests.
- Teach positional therapy.
- If surgery is necessary, provide appropriate preoperative and postoperative care.

Monitoring

 Alert

After endoscopy, watch for signs of perforation, including decreasing blood pressure, rapid pulse, shock, and sudden pain.

- Patient response to prescribed antacids and other drugs

Patient teaching

Be sure to cover:
- the disorder, diagnosis, and treatment
- the development of a dietary plan
- the need to sit upright after meals and snacks

- situations or activities that increase intra-abdominal pressure
- desired drug actions and potential adverse effects
- the need to sleep with the head of the bed elevated about 6″ (15 cm).

Discharge planning

- Refer the patient to a smoking-cessation program, if appropriate.
- Refer the patient to a weight-reduction program, if appropriate.

Herniated intervertebral disk

Overview

Description

○ Rupture of fibrocartilaginous material that surrounds the intervertebral disk, allowing protrusion of the nucleus pulposus
○ Results in pressure on spinal nerve roots or spinal cord that causes back pain and other symptoms of nerve root irritation
○ Most common site for herniation is L4-L5 disk space; other sites include L5-S1, L2-L3, L3-L4, C6-C7, and C5-C6
○ Clinical manifestations determined by:
  – Location and size of the herniation into the spinal canal
  – Amount of space that exists inside the spinal canal
○ Also known as *herniated nucleus pulposus, slipped disk,* or *ruptured disk*

Pathophysiology

○ The ligament and posterior capsule of the disk are usually torn, allowing the nucleus pulposus to extrude, compressing the nerve root.
○ Occasionally, the injury tears the entire disk loose, causing protrusion onto the nerve root or compression of the spinal cord.
○ Large amounts of extruded nucleus pulposus or complete disk herniation of the capsule and nucleus pulposus may compress the spinal cord.

Causes

○ Improper lifting or twisting
○ Direct injury
○ Degenerative disk disease

Risk factors

○ Advanced age
○ Congenitally small lumbar spinal canal
○ Osteophytes along the vertebrae
○ Work environment

Incidence

○ About 90% affect lumbar (L) and lumbosacral spine; 8% in cervical (C) spine; 1% to 2% in thoracic (T) spine
○ Lumbar herniation more common in people ages 20 to 45
○ Cervical herniation more common in people ages 45 and older
○ Herniated disks more common in men than in women

Common characteristics

○ Pain
○ Limited range of motion (ROM)
○ Paresthesias
○ Motor weakness
○ Peripheral neuropathy

Complications

○ Neurologic deficits
○ Bowel and bladder dysfunction
○ Sexual dysfunction

Assessment

History

○ Previous traumatic injury or back strain
○ Unilateral, low back pain
○ Pain that may radiate to the buttocks, legs, and feet
○ Pain that may begin suddenly, subside in a few days, and then recur at shorter intervals with progressive intensity
○ Sciatic pain beginning as a dull ache in the buttocks, worsening with Valsalva's maneuver, coughing, sneezing, or bending
○ Pain that may subside with rest
○ Muscle spasms
○ Chronic repetitive injury

Physical findings

○ Limited ability to bend forward
○ Posture favoring the affected side
○ Muscle atrophy, in later stages
○ Tenderness over the affected region
○ Radicular pain with straight leg raising in lumbar herniation
○ Increased pain with neck movement in cervical herniation
○ Referred upper trunk pain with cervical neck compression

Test results

Imaging
○ X-rays of the spine show degenerative changes.
○ Myelography shows the level of the herniation.
○ Computed tomography scan shows bone and soft-tissue abnormalities; can also show spinal canal compression.
○ Magnetic resonance imaging shows soft-tissue abnormalities.

Other
○ Electromyography measures muscle response to nerve stimulation.
○ Nerve conduction studies show sensory and motor loss.

Treatment

General

○ Initial treatment conservative and symptomatic, unless neurologic impairment progresses rapidly
○ Possible traction
○ Supportive devices such as a brace

- Heat or ice applications
- Transcutaneous electrical nerve stimulation
- Chemonucleolysis
- Avoidance of repetitive activity
- Diet, as tolerated
- Bed rest, initially
- Prescribed exercise program
- Physical therapy

Medication

- Nonsteroidal anti-inflammatory drugs
- Steroids
- Muscle relaxants
- Analgesics

Surgery

- Laminectomy
- Spinal fusion
- Microdiskectomy

Nursing considerations

Key outcomes

The patient will:
- express feelings of increased comfort
- demonstrate adequate joint mobility and ROM
- perform activities of daily living within the confines of the disorder
- achieve the highest level of mobility possible
- demonstrate strategies to prevent self-injury.

Nursing interventions

- Give prescribed drugs.
- Plan a pain-control regimen.
- Offer supportive care.
- Provide encouragement.
- Help the patient cope with chronic pain and impaired mobility.
- Include the patient and his family in all phases of his care.
- Encourage the patient to express his concerns.
- Encourage performance of self-care.
- Help the patient to identify activities that promote rest and relaxation.
- Prepare the patient for myelography, if indicated.
- Periodically remove traction to inspect skin.
- Prevent deep vein thrombosis.
- Prevent footdrop.
- Ensure a consistent regimen of leg- and back-strengthening exercises.
- Encourage adequate oral fluid intake.
- Encourage coughing and deep-breathing exercises.
- Provide meticulous skin care.
- Provide a fracture bedpan for the patient on complete bed rest.

 Alert

During conservative treatment, watch for a deterioration in neurologic status, especially during the first 24 hours after admission, which may indicate an urgent need for surgery.

After surgery
- Enforce bed rest, as ordered.
- Use the logrolling technique to turn the patient.
- Assist the patient during his first attempt to walk.
- Provide a straight-backed chair for the patient to sit in briefly.

Monitoring

- Vital signs
- Intake and output
- Pain control
- Mobility
- Motor strength
- Deep vein thrombosis
- Bowel and bladder function

After surgery
- Blood drainage system
- Drainage
- Incisions
- Dressings
- Neurovascular status
- Bowel sounds and abdominal distention

Patient teaching

Be sure to cover:
- the disorder, diagnosis, and treatment
- prescribed drugs and potential adverse effects
- when to notify the physician
- bed rest
- traction
- heat application
- the exercise program
- myelography, if indicated
- preoperative and postoperative care, if indicated
- relaxation techniques
- proper body mechanics
- skin care.

Discharge planning

- Refer the patient to physical therapy, if indicated.
- Refer the patient to occupational therapy, if indicated.
- Refer the patient to a weight-reduction program, if appropriate.

Herpes simplex

Overview

Description

- Common viral infection that may be latent for years
- After initial herpes simplex virus (HSV) infection, patient becomes carrier susceptible to recurrent attacks
- Recurrent infections may be provoked by fever, menses, stress, heat, cold, lack of sleep, sun exposure, and contact with reactivated disease (kissing, sharing cosmetics, sexual intercourse)

Pathophysiology

- Virus enters mucosal surfaces or abraded skin sites and initiates replication in cells of the epidermis and dermis.
- Replication continues to permit infection of sensory or autonomic nerve endings.
- Virus enters the neuronal cell and is transported intra-axonally to nerve cell bodies in ganglia (where the virus establishes latency) and spreads by the peripheral sensory nerves. (See *Understanding the genital herpes cycle.*)

Causes

- Type 1 (HSV-1) — *Herpesvirus hominis* transmitted primarily by contact with oral secretions; mainly affects oral, labial, ocular, or skin tissues
- Type 2 (HSV-2) — *Herpesvirus hominis* transmitted primarily by contact with genital secretions; mainly affects genital structures

Incidence

- Occurs worldwide and equally in males and females
- Lower socioeconomic groups infected more often, probably because of crowded living conditions
- Infection with HSV-1 more common and occurs earlier in life than infection with HSV-2

Common characteristics

- Fever, malaise, and headache
- Tender inguinal adenopathy
- Typical primary lesions erupt following prodromal tingling and itching
- Ruptured vesicles produce painful ulcers followed by yellow crusting

Complications

- Primary (or initial) HSV infection during pregnancy leading to abortion, premature labor, microcephaly, and uterine growth retardation
- Congenital herpes transmitted during vaginal birth, producing a subclinical neonatal infection or severe infection with seizures, chorioretinitis, skin vesicles, and hepatosplenomegaly
- HSV-1 causing life-threatening nonepidemic encephalitis in infants
- Gingivostomatitis in children ages 1 to 3
- Blindness from ocular infection
- Increased risk for cervical cancer
- Urethral stricture from recurrent genital herpes
- Perianal ulcers
- Colitis
- Esophagitis (more frequent in the impaired host)
- Pneumonitis
- Neurologic disorders
- Uremia with multiple organ involvement

Assessment

History

- Oral, vaginal, or anal sexual contact with an infected person or other direct contact with lesions
- With recurrent infection, various precipitating factors identified

Physical findings

Primary perioral HSV
- Sore throat, fever, anorexia, adenopathy
- Increased salivation
- Severe mouth pain, halitosis
- Small vesicles on an erythematous base possibly present on pharyngeal and oral mucosa

Primary genital HSV
- Malaise, tender inguinal adenopathy
- Dysuria, leukorrhea
- Dyspareunia
- Fluid-filled vesicles on the cervix, labia, perianal skin, vulva, and vagina; glans penis, foreskin, and penile shaft
- Extragenital lesions possibly seen on the mouth or anus

Primary ocular infection
- Photophobia, excessive tearing
- Follicular conjunctivitis, chemosis
- Blepharitis, vesicles on eyelids
- Lethargy and fever
- Regional adenopathy

Test results

Laboratory
- Tissue culture showing isolation of virus (gold standard)
- Staining of scrapings from the base of the lesion demonstrating characteristic giant cells or intranuclear inclusions of herpes virus infection
- Tissue analysis showing HSV antigens or deoxyribonucleic acid in scrapings from lesions

Treatment

General

- Symptomatic and supportive therapy
- Ophthalmologist treatment for eye infections
- Avoidance of acidic foods (with stomatitis)

○ Abstinence from sexual activity during active phase (with genital lesions)

Medication

○ Antipyretics and analgesics
○ Anesthetic mouthwashes
○ Bicarbonate-based mouth rinse
○ Drying agents
○ Ophthalmic drugs
○ Antivirals
○ Docosanol

Nursing considerations

Key outcomes

The patient will:
○ exhibit improved or healed lesions or wounds
○ express feelings of increased comfort and decreased pain
○ exhibit no complications related to trauma to oral mucous membranes
○ voice feelings about potential or actual changes in sexuality.

Nursing interventions

○ Observe standard precautions.
○ Give prescribed drugs.
○ Encourage the patient to express his feelings, and provide support.

Monitoring

○ Response to treatment
○ Adverse reactions to medications
○ Complications
○ Lesions
○ Fluid and electrolyte balance

Patient teaching

Be sure to cover:
○ the disorder, diagnosis, and treatment
○ proper hand-washing technique
○ the recommended use of lip balm with sunscreen (with oral lesions)
○ instructions to keep lesions dry, except for applying prescribed topical drugs
○ information about drugs, administration, dosage, and possible adverse effects
○ the use of sunscreen to prevent skin-induced recurrences
○ the recommendation that sexual partners be screened for sexually transmitted diseases (with genital herpes)
○ for a patient with genital herpes, the recommendation to use warm compresses or take sitz baths several times per day and avoid all sexual contact during outbreaks of active infection.

Understanding the genital herpes cycle

After a patient is infected with genital herpes, a latency period follows. The virus takes up permanent residence in the nerve cells surrounding the lesions, and intermittent viral shedding may take place.

Repeated outbreaks may develop at any time, again followed by a latent stage during which the lesions heal completely. Outbreaks may recur as often as three to eight times yearly.

Although the cycle continues indefinitely, some people remain symptom-free for years.

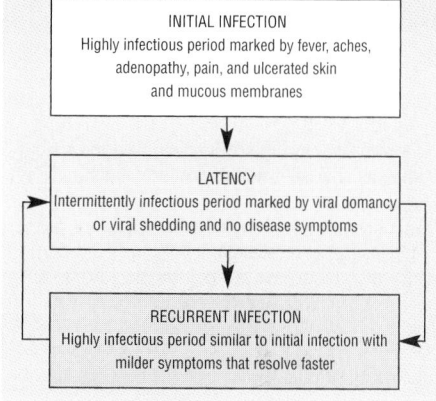

INITIAL INFECTION
Highly infectious period marked by fever, aches, adenopathy, pain, and ulcerated skin and mucous membranes

LATENCY
Intermittently infectious period marked by viral domancy or viral shedding and no disease symptoms

RECURRENT INFECTION
Highly infectious period similar to initial infection with milder symptoms that resolve faster

Discharge planning

○ Refer the patient with an eye infection to an ophthalmologist.
○ Refer the patient to a support group such as the Herpes Resource Center, as appropriate.
○ If child abuse is suspected, make a report to local authorities and social services.

Herpes zoster

Overview

Description

○ Acute unilateral and segmental inflammation of dorsal root ganglia that remains in people who have had chickenpox
○ Also called *shingles*

Pathophysiology

○ Herpes zoster erupts when the virus reactivates after dormancy in the cerebral ganglia (extramedullary ganglia of the cranial nerves) or the ganglia of posterior nerve roots.
○ The virus may multiply as it reactivates, and antibodies remaining from the initial infection may neutralize it.
○ Without opposition from effective antibodies, the virus continues to multiply in the ganglia, destroys neurons, and spreads down the sensory nerves to the skin, causing localized vascular eruptions.

Causes

○ Dormant varicella-zoster virus (herpesvirus that also causes chickenpox) that reactivates

Incidence

○ Most common in adults ages 50 to 70
○ Bone marrow transplant patients especially at risk

A look at herpes zoster

These characteristic herpes zoster lesions are fluid-filled vesicles that dry and form scabs after about 10 days. Unilateral vesicular lesions in a dermatomal pattern should rapidly lead to a diagnosis of herpes zoster.

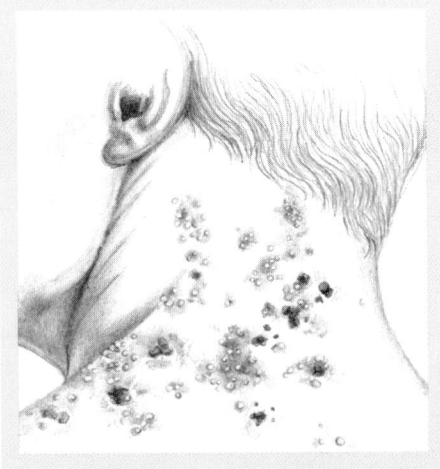

○ Possibly more prevalent in people who had chickenpox at a young age

Common characteristics

○ Localized vesicular skin lesions, confined to a dermatome; thoracic, cervical and ophthalmic dermatomes most commonly involved
○ Severe neuralgic pain in peripheral areas innervated by the nerves arising in the inflamed root ganglia
○ Pain generally precedes rash by 2 to 3 days
○ Lesions pustulate, crust, and heal in 3 to 4 weeks

Complications

○ Deafness
○ Bell's palsy
○ Secondary skin infection
○ Postherpetic neuralgia
○ Meningoencephalitis
○ Cutaneous dissemination
○ Ocular involvement with facial zoster
○ Hepatitis
○ Pneumonitis
○ Peripheral motor weakness
○ Guillain-Barré syndrome
○ Cranial nerve syndrome

Assessment

History

○ Typically no history of exposure to others with the varicella-zoster virus
○ Fever
○ Malaise
○ Pain that mimics appendicitis
○ Pleurisy
○ Musculoskeletal pain
○ Severe, deep pain
○ Pruritus
○ Paresthesia or hyperesthesia (usually affecting the trunk and occasionally the arms and legs)

Physical findings

○ Small, red, vesicular skin lesions spread unilaterally around the thorax or vertically over the arms or legs
○ May see vesicles filled with clear fluid or pus
○ Vesicles dry, forming scabs or even becoming gangrenous (see *A look at herpes zoster*)
○ Enlarged regional lymph nodes
Geniculate involvement
○ Vesicle formation in the external auditory canal and ipsilateral facial palsy
○ Hearing loss, dizziness, and loss of taste
Trigeminal involvement
○ Eye pain
○ Corneal and scleral damage and impaired vision
○ Conjunctivitis, extraocular weakness, ptosis, and paralytic mydriasis
○ Secondary glaucoma

Test results

Laboratory

○ Vesicular fluid and infected tissue analyses showing eosinophilic intranuclear inclusions and varicella virus

○ Staining antibodies from vesicular fluid and identification under fluorescent light aiding differentiation of herpes zoster from herpes simplex virus

○ Specific antibody immune globulin measurement of varicella antibodies elevated

○ Cerebrospinal fluid analysis demonstrating increased protein levels and, possibly, pleocytosis

Diagnostic procedures

○ Lumbar puncture indicating increased pressure

Treatment

General

○ Transcutaneous peripheral nerve stimulation for postherpetic neuralgia

○ Soothing baths

○ Cold compresses

Medication

○ Antivirals
○ Antipruritics
○ Analgesics
○ Tricyclic antidepressants
○ Demulcent and skin protectant
○ Systemic antibiotic
○ Corticosteroids
○ Tranquilizers and sedatives
○ Patient-controlled analgesia

Nursing considerations

Key outcomes

The patient will:

○ exhibit improved or healed lesions or wounds

○ express feelings of increased comfort and decreased pain

○ acknowledge change in body image

○ demonstrate effective social interaction skills in one-on-one and group settings.

Nursing interventions

○ Give prescribed drugs.

○ Maintain meticulous hygiene to prevent spreading the infection to other parts of the patient's body.

○ With open lesions, follow contact isolation precautions to prevent the spread of infection.

Monitoring

○ Response to treatment
○ Adverse reaction to medications
○ Lesions
○ Signs and symptoms of infection

Patient teaching

Be sure to cover:

○ the use of a soft toothbrush, eating soft foods, and using a saline- or bicarbonate-based mouthwash and oral anesthetics to decrease discomfort from oral lesions

○ the need for meticulous hygiene to prevent spreading infection to other body parts

○ the need to avoid scratching lesions

○ advice to apply a cold compress if vesicles rupture

○ local treatment of vesicles.

Discharge planning

○ Refer the patient to an ophthalmologist for ocular involvement.

○ Refer the patient to a pain management specialist for postherpetic neuralgia.

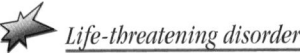 *Life-threatening disorder*

Hip fracture

Overview

Description

- Break in the head or neck of the femur (usually the head)
- Most common fall-related injury resulting in hospitalization
- Leading cause of disability among older adults
- May permanently change level of functioning and independence
- Almost 25% of patients die within 1 year following hip fracture

Pathophysiology

- With bone fracture, the periosteum and blood vessels in the marrow, cortex, and surrounding soft tissues are disrupted.
- This results in bleeding from the damaged ends of the bone and from the neighboring soft tissue.
- Clot formation occurs within the medullary canal, between the fractured bone ends, and beneath the periosteum.
- Bone tissue immediately adjacent to the fracture dies, and the necrotic tissue causes an intense inflammatory response.
- Vascular tissue invades the fracture area from surrounding soft tissue and marrow cavity within 48 hours, increasing blood flow to the entire bone.
- Bone-forming cells in the periosteum, endosteum, and marrow are activated to produce subperiosteal procallus along the outer surface of the shaft and over the broken ends of the bone.
- Collagen and matrix, which become mineralized to form callus, are synthesized by osteoblasts within the procallus.
- During the repair process, remodeling occurs; unnecessary callus is resorbed, and trabeculae are formed along stress lines.
- New bone, not scar tissue, is formed over the healed fracture.

Causes

- Falls
- Trauma
- Cancer metastasis
- Osteoporosis
- Skeletal disease

Incidence

- Affects more than 200,000 people each year
- Occurs in one of five women by age 80
- More common in females than in males
- More common in white females

Common characteristics

- Impaired function
- Deformity
- Edema
- Muscle spasm
- Pain and tenderness
- Impaired sensation

Complications

- Pneumonia
- Venous thrombosis
- Pressure ulcers
- Social isolation
- Depression
- Bladder dysfunction
- Deep vein thrombosis
- Pulmonary embolus
- Hip dislocation
- Death

Assessment

History

- Falls or trauma to the bones
- Pain in the affected hip and leg
- Pain exacerbated by movement

Physical findings

- Outward rotation of affected extremity
- Affected extremity possibly appearing shorter
- Limited or abnormal range of motion (ROM)
- Edema and discoloration of the surrounding tissue
- In an open fracture, bone protruding through the skin

Test results
Imaging
- X-rays showing the location of the fracture
- Computed tomography scan showing abnormalities in complicated fractures

Treatment

General

- Depends on age, comorbidities, cognitive functioning, support systems, and functional ability
- Possible skin traction
- Physical therapy
- Non–weight-bearing transfers
- Well-balanced diet
- Foods rich in vitamin C and A, calcium, and protein
- Adequate vitamin D
- Bed rest, initially
- Ambulation as soon as possible after surgery

Medication

- Analgesics

Surgery

○ Total hip arthroplasty
○ Hemiarthroplasty
○ Percutaneous pinning
○ Internal fixation using a compression screw and plate

Nursing considerations

Key outcomes

The patient will:
○ identify factors that increase the potential for injury
○ maintain muscle strength and tone and joint ROM
○ verbalize feelings of increased comfort
○ attain the highest degree of mobility possible within the confines of the injury
○ maintain skin integrity.

Nursing interventions

○ Give prescribed drugs.
○ Give prescribed prophylactic anticoagulation after surgery.
○ Maintain traction.
○ Maintain proper body alignment.
○ Use logrolling techniques to turn the patient in bed.
○ Maintain non–weight-bearing status.
○ Increase the patient's activity level, as prescribed.
○ Consult physical therapy as early as possible.
○ Assist with active ROM exercises to unaffected limbs.
○ Encourage coughing and deep-breathing exercises.
○ Keep the patient's skin clean and dry.
○ Prevent skin breakdown.
○ Encourage good nutrition; offer high-protein, high-calorie snacks.
○ Perform daily wound care.

 Alert

Don't massage the patient's legs and feet to promote circulation because this could increase the risk of thromboembolism.

Monitoring

○ Vital signs
○ Intake and output
○ Pain
○ Mobility and ROM
○ Incision and dressings
○ Complications
○ Coagulation study results
○ Signs of bleeding
○ Neurovascular status
○ Skin integrity
○ Signs and symptoms of infection

Alert

Following surgery, assess the patient for complications, such as deep vein thrombosis, pulmonary embolus, and hip dislocation.

Patient teaching

Be sure to cover:
○ the disorder, diagnosis, and treatment
○ prescribed drugs and potential adverse effects
○ ROM exercises
○ meticulous skin care
○ proper body alignment
○ wound care
○ signs of infection
○ coughing and deep-breathing exercises and incentive spirometry
○ assistive devices
○ activity restrictions and lifestyle changes
○ safe ambulation practices
○ nutritious diet and adequate fluid intake.

Discharge planning

○ Refer the patient to physical and occupational therapy programs, as indicated.
○ Refer the patient to home health or intermediate care.

Hirschsprung's disease

Overview

Description

- Congenital disorder of the large intestine characterized by the absence or marked reduction of parasympathetic ganglion cells in the colorectal wall
- Usually coexists with other congenital anomalies, particularly trisomy 21 and anomalies of the urinary tract such as megaloureter
- Also called *congenital megacolon* and *congenital aganglionic megacolon*

Pathophysiology

- Parasympathetic ganglion cells in the colorectal wall are absent or markedly reduced in number.
- The aganglionic bowel segment contracts without the reciprocal relaxation needed to propel feces forward.
- Impaired intestinal motility causes severe, intractable constipation.
- Colonic obstruction can ensue, causing bowel dilation and subsequent occlusion of surrounding blood and lymphatics.
- Ensuing mucosal edema, ischemia, and infarction draw large amounts of fluid into the bowel, causing copious amounts of liquid stool.
- Continued infarction and destruction of the mucosa can lead to infection and sepsis.

Causes

- Familial congenital defect

Incidence

- Occurs in 1 in 2,000 to 1 in 5,000 live births
- Up to seven times more common in males than in females (although the aganglionic segment is usually shorter in males)
- Most prevalent in whites
- Both sexes equally affected by total aganglionosis
- Females with Hirschsprung's disease at higher risk for having affected children

Common characteristics

In neonates
- Failure to pass meconium within 24 to 48 hours because of inability to propel intestinal contents forward
- Bile-stained or fecal vomiting as a result of bowel obstruction
- Abdominal distention caused by to retention of intestinal contents and bowel obstruction
- Irritability caused by resultant abdominal distention
- Feeding difficulties and failure to thrive caused by to retention of intestinal contents and abdominal distention
- Dehydration caused by subsequent feeding difficulties and inability to ingest adequate fluids

- Overflow diarrhea caused by increased water secretion into bowel with bowel obstruction

In children
- Intractable constipation caused by decreased GI motility
- Abdominal distention caused by retention of stool
- Easily palpated fecal masses caused by retention of stool
- Wasted extremities (in severe cases) caused by impaired intestinal motility and its effects on nutrition and intake
- Loss of subcutaneous tissue (in severe cases) caused by malnutrition
- Large protuberant abdomen caused by retention of stool and consequent changes in fluid and electrolyte homeostasis

In adults
- Abdominal distention from decreased bowel motility and constipation
- Chronic intermittent constipation caused by impaired intestinal motility

Complications

- Bowel perforation
- Electrolyte imbalances
- Nutritional deficiencies
- Enterocolitis
- Hypovolemic shock
- Sepsis

Assessment

History

- Familial history of difficult stool passage
- Failure to pass meconium within the first 24 to 48 hours after birth
- Vomiting of bile-stained or fecal contents
- Anorexia
- Nausea
- Lethargy
- Constipation

Physical findings

- Distended abdomen
- Tachypnea
- Rectum without stools

Test results

Imaging
- Barium enema reveals a narrowed segment of distal colon with a saw-toothed appearance and a funnel-shaped segment above it.
- Upright plain abdominal X-rays show marked colonic distention.

Diagnostic procedures
- Rectal biopsy confirms diagnosis by showing the absence of ganglion cells.
- Rectal manometry detects failure of the internal anal sphincter to relax and contract.

Treatment

General

○ Daily colonic lavage (to empty the infant's bowel until the time of surgery)
○ Oral feeding with breast milk or predigested formula when bowel sounds return (infants)

 Alert

Without prompt treatment, an infant with colonic obstruction may die within 24 hours from enterocolitis that leads to severe diarrhea and hypovolemic shock.

Surgery

○ Corrective surgery to pull the normal ganglionic segment through to the anus (usually delayed until the infant is at least age 10 months)
○ Temporary colostomy or ileostomy to compress the colon in instances of total bowel obstruction

Nursing considerations

Key outcomes

The patient will:
○ maintain adequate caloric intake
○ avoid complications
○ have bowel function return to normal patterns
○ maintain fluid balance.

Nursing interventions

○ Maintain fluid and electrolyte balance and prevent shock.
○ Provide adequate nutrition and hydrate with I.V. fluids, as needed.
○ Relieve respiratory distress by keeping the patient in an upright position.

After colostomy or ileostomy
○ Place the infant in a heated incubator, with the temperature set at 98° to 99° F (36.7° to 37.2° C), or in a radiant warmer.

Monitoring

○ Vital signs
○ Signs of sepsis and enterocolitis
○ Intake and output
○ Laboratory values

Patient teaching

Be sure to cover:
○ recognizing the signs of fluid loss, dehydration, and enterocolitis
○ withholding foods that have increased the number of stools previously

○ that complete continence may take several years to develop and that constipation may recur at times
○ participating in the child's care as much as possible, if appropriate.

Discharge planning

○ Refer the parents to an enterostomal therapist for information on ostomy care.

Histoplasmosis

Overview

Description
- Fungal infection
- Three forms in the United States
  - Primary acute histoplasmosis
  - Progressive disseminated histoplasmosis (acute disseminated or chronic disseminated disease)
  - Chronic pulmonary (cavitary) histoplasmosis
- Also known as *Ohio Valley disease, Central Mississippi Valley disease, Appalachian Mountain disease,* and *Darling's disease*

Pathophysiology
- Spores reach alveoli and are transformed into budding forms, carried to regional lymphatics, and then disseminated throughout the body.
- Intense granulomatous reaction occurs and caseation necrosis or calcification (resembling tuberculosis) occurs.
- Transient dissemination can leave granulomas in the spleen.

Causes
- Caused by *Histoplasma capsulatum,* which is found in the stool of birds and bats and in soil contaminated by their stool (near roosts, chicken coops, barns, caves, and underneath bridges)
- Transmitted to humans by inhalation of *H. capsulatum* or *H. capsulatum* var. *duboisii* spores or invasion of spores after minor skin trauma

Incidence
- Occurs worldwide, but especially in temperate areas of Asia, Africa, Europe, and North and South America
- In the United States, most prevalent in southeastern, mid-Atlantic, and central states
- Primary acute histoplasmosis most common in infants, young children, and immunocompromised patients

Common characteristics
- Incubation period ranges from 3 to 17 days, although chronic pulmonary histoplasmosis may progress slowly for many years
- Chronic pulmonary infections occur more often in males older than 40, particularly with a history of cigarette smoking or chronic lung disease

Complications
- Vascular or bronchial obstruction
- Acute pericarditis
- Pleural effusion
- Mediastinal fibrosis or granuloma
- Intestinal ulceration
- Addison's disease
- Endocarditis
- Meningitis

Assessment

History
- Possible history of an immunocompromised condition
- Exposure to contaminated soil in an endemic area

Physical findings
- Fever, which may rise as high as 105° F (40.6° C)

Primary acute histoplasmosis
- Usually no characteristic signs
- Mild respiratory illness, cough
- Malaise, headache, myalgia, anorexia
- Chest pain

Progressive disseminated histoplasmosis
- Anorexia and weight loss
- Pain
- Hoarseness, tachypnea in later stages
- Ulceration of the oropharynx, dysphagia
- Pallor from anemia
- Jaundice and ascites
- Hepatosplenomegaly
- Lymphadenopathy

Chronic pulmonary histoplasmosis
- Productive cough, dyspnea, hemoptysis
- Shortness of breath, cyanosis
- Extreme weakness, weight loss
- Upper lobe fibrocavitary pneumonia

Test results

Laboratory
- Blood cultures done by lysis-centrifugation technique revealing organism causing the infection
- In disseminated forms, culture of bone marrow, mucosal lesions, liver, and bronchoalveolar lavage helpful in showing organisms in disseminated histoplasmosis
- Sputum cultures preferred in chronic pulmonary histoplasmosis; may take 2 to 4 weeks to culture, showing growth of the organism
- Radioactive assay for histoplasma antigen in blood or urine showing presence of histoplasma antigen

Imaging
- Chest X-rays show lung damage.

Treatment

General
- Oxygen for respiratory distress
- Parenteral fluids for dysphagia caused by oral or laryngeal ulcerations
- Smoking cessation
- Cool mist humidifier

○ Soft, bland foods (with oropharyngeal ulceration)
○ Small, frequent meals
○ Frequent rest periods

Medication

○ Antifungal therapy
○ Glucocorticoids

Surgery

○ Lung resection to remove pulmonary nodules
○ Shunt for increased intracranial pressure
○ Cardiac repair for constrictive pericarditis

Nursing considerations

Key outcomes

The patient will:
○ be free from pain
○ maintain adequate ventilation
○ express feelings of increased comfort in maintaining air exchange
○ experience no further weight loss
○ maintain hemodynamic stability.

Nursing interventions

○ Give prescribed drugs.
○ Provide oxygen therapy, if needed.
○ Plan rest periods.
○ Consult with the dietitian and patient concerning food preferences.

Monitoring

○ Hypoglycemia and hyperglycemia, which indicate adrenal dysfunction
○ Respiratory status
○ Neurologic status

Patient teaching

Be sure to cover:
○ the disorder, diagnosis, and treatment
○ information about drug administration, dosage, and possible adverse effects
○ cardiac and pulmonary signs that could indicate effusions
○ the need to watch for early signs of this infection and to seek treatment promptly to help prevent histoplasmosis for people in endemic areas
○ the need for people who risk occupational exposure to contaminated soil to wear face masks.

Discharge planning

○ Stress the need for follow-up care on a regular basis for at least 1 year.
○ Refer the patient with chronic pulmonary or disseminated histoplasmosis for psychological support to cope with long-term treatment, if needed.

○ Refer the patient to a social worker or an occupational therapist, as needed.
○ Help the parents of a child with this disease arrange for a visiting teacher.

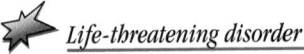
Life-threatening disorder

Hodgkin's disease

Overview

Description
○ Neoplastic disorder characterized by painless, progressive enlargement of lymph nodes, spleen, and other lymphoid tissue
○ With appropriate treatment, 5-year survival rate about 90%

Pathophysiology
○ Enlarged lymphoid tissue results from proliferation of lymphocytes, histiocytes, eosinophils, and Reed-Sternberg cells.
○ Untreated Hodgkin's disease follows a variable but relentlessly progressive and ultimately fatal course.

Causes
○ Exact cause unknown

Risk factors
○ Genetic factors
○ Viral factors
○ Environmental factors

Common characteristics
○ Painless swelling of lymph nodes
○ Fever, night sweats

Incidence
○ Occurs in all races; slightly more common in whites
○ Peaks in two age-groups: ages 15 to 38 and people older than 50
○ Most common in young adults, except in Japan (exclusively in people older than age 50)
○ Greater incidence in men than in women

Complications
○ Multiple organ failure

Assessment

History
○ Painless swelling of one of the cervical, axillary, or inguinal lymph nodes
○ Persistent fever and night sweats
○ Weight loss despite an adequate diet, with resulting fatigue and malaise
○ Increasing susceptibility to infection

Physical findings
○ Edema of the face and neck and jaundice

○ Enlarged, rubbery lymph nodes in the neck (these nodes enlarge during periods of fever and then revert to normal size)

Test results
Laboratory
○ Hematologic tests showing mild to severe normocytic anemia, normochromic anemia in 50% of patients, and elevated, normal, or reduced white blood cell count and differential, showing any combination of neutrophilia, lymphocytopenia, monocytosis, and eosinophilia
○ Serum alkaline phosphatase levels elevated, indicating liver or bone involvement
Diagnostic procedures
○ Tests must first rule out other disorders that enlarge the lymph nodes.
○ Lymph node biopsy confirms the presence of Reed-Sternberg cells, abnormal histiocyte proliferation, and nodular fibrosis and necrosis. Lymph node biopsy is also used to determine lymph node and organ involvement.
○ A staging laparotomy is necessary for patients younger than age 55 and for those without obvious stage III or IV disease, lymphocyte predominance subtype histology, or medical contraindications.

Treatment

General
○ For patient with stage I or II disease, radiation therapy alone
○ For patient with stage III disease, radiation therapy and chemotherapy
○ For patient with stage IV disease, chemotherapy alone (or chemotherapy and radiation therapy to involved sites), sometimes inducing complete remission
○ Autologous bone marrow transplantation or autologous peripheral blood sternal transfusions and immunotherapy
○ Well-balanced diet
○ Frequent rest periods

Medication
○ Chemotherapy
○ Antiemetics
○ Sedatives
○ Antidiarrheals

Nursing considerations

Key outcomes
The patient will:
○ have no further weight loss
○ express feelings of increased energy
○ demonstrate adequate skin integrity

○ demonstrate effective coping mechanisms
○ express feelings of increased comfort and decreased
  pain.

Nursing interventions

○ Provide a well-balanced, high-calorie, high-protein
  diet.
○ Provide for periods of rest.
○ Give prescribed drugs.
○ Provide emotional support.

Monitoring

○ Complications of treatment
○ Pain control
○ Lymph node enlargement
○ Body temperature
○ Fatigue
○ Daily weight
○ Signs and symptoms of infection
○ Response to treatment
○ Signs and symptoms of dehydration

Patient teaching

Be sure to cover:
○ the disorder, diagnosis, and treatment
○ signs and symptoms of infection
○ the importance of maintaining good nutrition
○ the pacing of activities to counteract therapy-induced
  fatigue
○ the importance of good oral hygiene
○ the avoidance of crowds and people with known
  infection
○ the importance of checking the lymph nodes
○ all prescribed drugs, including administration,
  dosage, and possible adverse effects.

Discharge planning

○ Refer the patient to resource and support services.

Hookworm disease

Overview

Description

- Infection of the upper intestine caused by *Ancylostoma duodenale* (found in the Eastern Hemisphere) or *Necator americanus* (in the Western Hemisphere)
- Occurs mostly in tropical and subtropical climates
- Also called *uncinariasis* or *ground itch*

Pathophysiology

- Disease is transmitted to humans through direct skin penetration (usually in the foot) by hookworm larvae in soil contaminated with feces containing hookworm ova.
- These ova develop into infectious larvae in 1 to 3 days
- The larvae travel through the lymphatics to the pulmonary capillaries, where they penetrate alveoli and move up the bronchial tree to the trachea and epiglottis. There they are swallowed and enter the GI tract.
- When they reach the small intestine, they mature, attach to the jejunal mucosa, and suck blood, oxygen, and glucose from the intestinal wall.
- These mature worms then deposit ova, which are excreted in the stool, starting the cycle anew. Hookworm larvae mature in approximately 5 to 6 weeks.

Causes

- Transmission of *Ancylostoma duodenale* (found in the Eastern Hemisphere) or *Necator americanus* (in the Western Hemisphere)

Incidence

- May produce no symptoms
- Affects one billion people worldwide
- More common in whites
- Children more at risk because of playing or walking barefoot in contaminated soil

Common characteristics

- Irritation, pruritus, and edema at the site of entry
- Secondary bacterial infection with pustule formation
- Pneumonitis and hemorrhage with fever, sore throat, crackles, and cough (larvae in lungs)
- Fatigue, nausea, weight loss, dizziness, melena, and uncontrolled diarrhea (larvae in intestines)

Complications

- Anemia
- Cardiomegaly
- Heart failure
- Generalized massive edema

Assessment

History

- Recent walking (barefoot) in an area with contaminated soil
- Irritation and pruritus at entry site
- Fatigue
- Cough, hoarseness
- Abdominal pain
- Fever
- Nausea
- Weight loss
- Dizziness
- Diarrhea

Physical findings

- Papulovasicular rash
- Crackles (with lung involvement)
- Irregular respirations
- Bloody sputum
- Black, tarry stools
- Edema

Test results

Laboratory

- Stool specimen revealing larvae
- Decreased hemoglobin level as low as 5 to 9 g/dl (in severe case)
- Increased leukocyte count as high as 47,000/µl
- Increased eosinophil count as high as 500 to 700/µl

Treatment

General

- Blood transfusions (if anemia is severe)
- Nutritious high-protein, high-iron diet
- Activity, as tolerated, with frequent rest periods

Medication

- Mebendazole
- Pyrantel pamoate
- Albendazole
- Iron supplements
- Topical thiabendazole (cutaneous larva migrans)

Nursing considerations

Key outcomes

The patient will:
- experience no further weight loss
- report having increased energy levels
- have decreased episodes of diarrhea
- maintain a normal respiratory rate.

Nursing interventions

- Follow standard precautions
- Isolate the incontinent patient.

○ Teach proper hand-washing technique.
○ For severe anemia, administer oxygen, if ordered, at low to moderate flow.
○ Encourage coughing and deep breathing.
○ Allow frequent rest periods.
○ Reposition frequently.
○ Assess family members for symptoms.

Monitoring

○ Intake and output
○ Nutritional status
○ Quantity and frequency of stools
○ Daily weight
○ Skin integrity

Patient teaching

Be sure to cover:
○ proper hand-washing technique
○ the need to wear shoes when outdoors
○ nutritious diet
○ proper hygiene after toileting
○ use of prescribed iron supplements and how this treatment affects stools
○ the need to start another course of treatment if stool examination remain positive for lavae.

Huntington's disease

Overview

Description
○ Degenerative disease of the brain that causes dementia
○ Death usually 10 to 15 years after onset
○ Also called *Huntington's chorea, hereditary chorea, chronic progressive chorea,* and *adult chorea*

Pathophysiology
○ Degeneration in the cerebral cortex and basal ganglia leads to chronic progressive chorea (dancelike movements).
○ The final stage is mental deterioration, which ends in dementia.

Causes
○ Genetic link
○ Transmitted as autosomal dominant trait (either sex can transmit and inherit it)

Incidence
○ Most common between ages 35 and 44
○ 2% of cases in children
○ 5% of cases as late as age 60
○ Each child of a parent with this disease has 50% chance of inheritance
○ Child who doesn't inherit it can't pass it on
○ Affects men and women equally

Common characteristics
○ Chorea
○ Emotional changes, irritability
○ Clumsiness, bradykinesia
○ Incontinence
○ Increased appetite
○ Bouts of anger
○ Purposeless movements
○ Grimacing
○ Dysarthria
○ Writhing and twitching
○ Loss of motor control; rigidity
○ Dysphagia
○ Oral apraxia, aprosody

Complications
○ Choking and aspiration
○ Pneumonia
○ Heart failure
○ Infections
○ Suicide

Assessment

History
Findings vary depending on disease progression.
○ Familial history
○ Emotional and mental changes
○ Insidious onset
○ Total dependency through:
  – Intellectual decline
  – Emotional disturbances
  – Loss of musculoskeletal control
○ Described as clumsy, irritable, or impatient
○ Subject to fits of anger
○ Periods of suicidal depression, apathy, or elation
○ Ravenous appetite, especially for sweets
○ Loss of bladder and bowel control in later stages

Physical findings
○ Choreic movements
○ Rapid, often violent, and purposeless movements
○ Cognitive decline
Early stages
○ Mild fidgeting
○ Grimacing, tongue smacking
○ Dysarthria
○ Athetoid movements related to emotional state
○ Torticollis
○ Deficits in short-term memory
Later stages
○ Constant writhing and twitching
○ Unintelligible speech
○ Difficulty chewing and swallowing
○ Ambulation impossible
○ Appears emaciated and exhausted

Test results
Laboratory
○ Deoxyribonucleic acid analysis possibly showing disease
Imaging
○ Positron emission tomography possibly showing disease
○ Magnetic resonance imaging showing characteristic butterfly dilation of the brain's lateral ventricles
○ Computed tomography scan showing brain atrophy

Treatment

General
○ No known cure
○ Supportive and symptomatic treatment
○ Psychotherapy
○ Possibly soft diet
○ Safety measures
○ Electroconvulsive therapy

Medication

○ Tranquilizers
○ Dopamine agonists
○ Neuroleptics
○ Selective serotonin reuptake inhibitors
○ Antidepressants

Nursing considerations

Key outcomes

The patient will:
○ maintain a patent airway without evidence of aspiration
○ maintain joint mobility and range of motion
○ remain free from infection
○ express positive feelings about self
○ perform activities of daily living
○ develop alternative means of communication to express self.

Nursing interventions

○ Provide psychological support.
○ Identify self-care deficits.
○ Encourage the patient to be independent.
○ Provide communication aids.
○ Help the patient with difficulty walking.
○ Maintain a turning schedule.
○ Elevate the head of the bed during eating.
○ Give prescribed drugs.
○ Protect the patient from infections.

Monitoring

○ Response to prescribed drugs
○ Possible suicide ideation
○ Temperature
○ White blood cell count

Patient teaching

Be sure to cover:
○ the disorder, diagnosis, and treatment
○ prescribed drugs and possible adverse effects
○ aspiration precautions
○ signs and symptoms of infection
○ communication strategies.

Discharge planning

○ Refer the patient to the Huntington's Disease Society of America.
○ Refer the patient to appropriate community organizations.
○ Refer the family for genetic counseling.
○ Refer the patient for psychotherapy, as appropriate.

Hydrocele

Overview

Description

○ A collection of fluid between the visceral and parietal layers of the testicle's tunica vaginalis or along the spermatic cord
○ The most common cause of scrotal swelling
○ Described as communicating or noncommunicating

Pathophysiology

Communicating
○ A patency between the scrotal sac and the peritoneal cavity allows peritoneal fluids to collect in the scrotum.
Noncommunicating
○ Fluid accumulation may be caused by infection, trauma, tumor, an imbalance between the secreting and absorptive capacities of scrotal tissue, or an obstruction of lymphatic or venous drainage in the spermatic cord.
○ This leads to a displacement of fluid in the scrotum, outside the testes.
○ Subsequent swelling results, leading to reduced blood flow to the testes.

Causes

○ Congenital malformation (infants)
○ Trauma to the testes or epididymis
○ Infection of the testes or epididymis
○ Testicular tumor

Incidence

○ Apparent in 6% of full-term male neonates
○ Incidence in adult males unknown

Common characteristics

○ Scrotal swelling and feeling of heaviness
○ Inguinal hernia (often present in congenital hydrocele)
○ Size varies from slightly larger than the testes to the size of a grapefruit or larger
○ Fluid collection with either flaccid or tense mass
○ Pain with acute epididymal infection or testicular torsion
○ Scrotal tenderness due to severe swelling

Complications

○ Epididymitis
○ Testicular atrophy

Assessment

History

○ Scrotal tenderness
○ Inguinal hernia

Physical findings

○ Soft, nontender fullness within the hemiscrotum
○ Transillumination of the scrotum revealing a homogenous glow without internal shadows

Test results

Imaging
○ Abdominal X-rays distinguish acute hydrocele from an incarcerated hernia
○ Ultrasound distinguishes spermatoceles from hydroceles and identifies torsion or tumor
Other
○ Transillumination to distinguish fluid-filled from solid mass (a tumor doesn't transilluminate)

Treatment

General

○ Frequently resolves spontaneously
○ Scrotal elevation
○ No dietary restrictions
○ Activity, as tolerated
○ Postoperatively avoidance of vigorous activity for short time.

Medication

○ Nonsteroidal anti-inflammatory drugs
○ Nonopioid analgesics

Surgery

○ Operative exploration if underlying pathology is suspected
○ Surgical repair to avoid strangulation of the bowel (inguinal hernia with bowel present in the sac)
○ Aspiration of fluid and injection of sclerosing drug into the scrotal sac for a tense hydrocele that impedes blood circulation or causes pain
○ Excision of the tunica vaginalis for recurrent hydroceles
○ Suprainguinal excision for testicular tumor detected by ultrasound

Nursing considerations

Key outcomes

The patient (or his parents) will:
○ express feeling of comfort and relief from pain
○ express understanding of disorder, diagnosis, and treatment.

Nursing interventions

○ Place a rolled towel between the patient's legs and elevate the scrotum to help reduce severe swelling.
○ Apply heat or ice packs to the scrotum.
○ Provide preoperative teaching.
○ Provide postoperative wound care, if appropriate.

Monitoring
○ Swelling
○ Worsening of condition

Patient teaching

Be sure to cover:
○ the need to wear a loose-fitting athletic supporter lined with soft cotton dressings
○ how to take a sitz bath
○ the need to avoid tub baths postoperaively for 5 to 7 days
○ the possibility that the hydrocele may reaccumulate for 1 month postoperatively because of edema.

Discharge planning
○ Follow-up visits may be required biweekly, monthly, or every 2 to 3 months, depending on recovery rate.

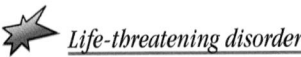

Hydrocephalus

Overview

Description

- A variety of conditions characterized by an excess of fluid within the cranial vault, subarachnoid space, or both
- Occurs because of interference with cerebrospinal fluid (CSF) flow caused by increased fluid production, obstruction within the ventricular system, or defective reabsorption of CSF
- Types include:
  - Noncommunicating hydrocephalus: obstruction within the ventricular system
  - Communicating hydrocephalus: impaired absorption of CSF

Pathophysiology

- The obstruction of CSF flow associated with hydrocephalus produces dilation of the ventricles proximal to the obstruction.
- The obstructed CSF is under pressure, causing atrophy of the cerebral cortex and degeneration of the white matter tracts. There's selective preservation of gray matter.
- When excess CSF fills a defect caused by atrophy, a degenerative disorder, or a surgical excision, the fluid isn't under pressure, and atrophy and degenerative changes aren't induced.

Causes

Noncommunicating hydrocephalus
- Congenital abnormalities in the ventricular system
- Mass lesions such as a tumor that compresses one of the structures of the ventricular system
- Aqueduct stenosis
- Arnold-Chiari malformation

Communicating hydrocephalus
- Adhesions from inflammation, such as with meningitis or subarachnoid hemorrhage
- Compression of the subarachnoid space by a mass such as a tumor
- Congenital abnormalities of the subarachnoid space
- High venous pressure within the sagittal sinus
- Head injury
- Cerebral atrophy

Incidence

- Rare cases of congenital hydrocephalus
- Noncommunicating hydrocephalus more common in children
- Communicating hydrocephalus more common in adults

Common characteristics

- Enlargement of head clearly disproportionate to growth
- Distended scalp veins
- Thin, shiny, fragile-looking scalp skin
- Underdeveloped neck muscles
- Depressed orbital roof
- Downward displacement of eyes
- High-pitched, shrill cry; irritability
- Projectile vomiting
- Skull widening

Complications

- Mental retardation
- Impaired motor function
- Vision loss
- Death (increased intracranial pressure [ICP])
- Infection and malnutrition (more common in infants)

Assessment

History

Infants
- History that may disclose cause
- High-pitched, shrill cry; irritability
- Anorexia
- Episodes of projectile vomiting

Adults and older children
- Frontal headaches
- Nausea and vomiting (may be projectile)
- Symptoms causing wakening or occurring on awakening
- Diplopia
- Restlessness

Physical findings

Infants
- Enlarged head clearly disproportionate to the infant's growth
- Head possibly appearing normal in size with bulging fontanels
- Distended scalp veins
- Thin, fragile, and shiny scalp skin
- Underdeveloped neck muscles
- Depression of the roof of the eye orbit
- Displacement of the eyes downward
- Prominent sclera (sunset sign)
- Abnormal leg muscle tone

Adults and older children
- Decreased level of consciousness
- Ataxia
- Impaired intellect
- Incontinence
- Signs of increased ICP

Test results

Imaging

○ Skull X-rays show thinning of the skull with separation of sutures and widening of the fontanels in infants.
○ Angiography, computed tomography scan, and magnetic resonance imaging show differentiation between hydrocephalus and intracranial lesions and Arnold-Chiari deformity.

Treatment

General

○ Shunting of CSF directly from the ventricular system to some point beyond the obstruction
○ Small, frequent feedings
○ Slow feeding of infant
○ Decreased movement during and immediately after meals

Medication

○ Possible preoperative and postoperative antibiotics

Surgery

○ Surgical correction (the only treatment for hydrocephalus) includes:
  – removal of obstruction to CSF flow
  – implantation of a ventriculoperitoneal shunt to divert CSF flow from the brain's lateral ventricle into the peritoneal cavity
  – with concurrent abdominal problem, ventriculoatrial shunt to divert CSF flow from the brain's lateral ventricle into the right atrium of the heart.

Nursing considerations

Key outcomes

The patient will:
○ maintain adequate ventilation
○ develop no signs and symptoms of infection
○ maintain and improve current level of consciousness
○ develop no signs and symptoms of increased ICP.

Nursing interventions

○ Elevate the head of the bed to 30 degrees or put an infant in an infant seat.
○ Give prescribed oxygen, as needed.
○ Provide small, frequent feedings.
○ Decrease the patient's movement during and immediately after meals.
○ Provide skin care.

After shunt surgery

○ Place the patient on the side opposite the operative site.
○ Give prescribed I.V. fluids.
○ Give prescribed analgesics.

Monitoring

○ Fontanels for tension or fullness
○ Head circumference
○ Signs and symptoms of increased ICP
○ Complications
○ Growth and development
○ Neurologic status
○ Intake and output

After surgery

○ Signs and symptoms of meningitis
○ Redness, swelling, and other signs and symptoms of local infection
○ Dressing for drainage
○ Response to analgesics

 Alert

Monitor the patient for vomiting, which may be an early sign of shunt malfunction.

Patient teaching

Be sure to cover:
○ the disorder, diagnosis, and treatment
○ shunt surgery: hair loss and the visibility of a mechanical device
○ postoperative shunt care
○ signs and symptoms of increased ICP or shunt malfunction
○ signs and symptoms of infection
○ signs and symptoms of paralytic ileus
○ the need for periodic shunt surgery to lengthen the shunt as the child grows older.

Discharge planning

○ Refer the patient to special education programs, as appropriate.

Hydronephrosis

Overview

Description

- Abnormal dilation of the renal pelvis and calyces of one or both kidneys
- Caused by obstruction of urine flow in the genitourinary tract
- May be acute or chronic

Pathophysiology

- With obstruction in the urethra or bladder, hydronephrosis is usually bilateral.
- With obstruction in a ureter, hydronephrosis is usually unilateral.
- Obstructions distal to the bladder cause the bladder to dilate, acting as a buffer zone, delaying hydronephrosis.
- Total obstruction of urine flow with dilation of the collecting system ultimately causes complete cortical atrophy and glomerular filtration ceases.

Causes

- Benign prostatic hyperplasia (BPH)
- Urethral strictures
- Renal calculi
- Strictures or stenosis of the ureter or bladder outlet
- Congenital abnormalities
- Bladder, ureteral, or pelvic tumors
- Blood clots
- Neurogenic bladder
- Ureterocele
- Tuberculosis
- Gram-negative infection
- Neurogenic bladder

Incidence

- About 1 in 100 people affected by unilateral hydronephrosis
- About 1 in 200 people affected by bilateral hydronephrosis

Common characteristics

- Decreased urine output
- Flank pain

Complications

- Renal calculi
- Sepsis
- Renovascular hypertension
- Obstructive nephropathy
- Infection
- Pyelonephritis
- Paralytic ileus
- Renal failure

Assessment

History

- Possibly no initial symptoms, but increasing pressure behind the obstruction eventually results in renal dysfunction
- Varies depending on cause of obstruction
- No symptoms or complaint of only mild pain and slightly decreased urine flow
- Severe, colicky renal pain or dull flank pain that radiates to the groin
- Hematuria
- Pyuria
- Dysuria
- Alternating oliguria and polyuria, anuria
- Nausea
- Vomiting
- Abdominal fullness
- Pain on urination
- Dribbling
- Urinary hesitancy
- Change in voiding pattern

Physical findings

- Hematuria
- Pyuria
- Urinary tract infection
- Palpable kidney
- Lower extremity edema
- Distended bladder
- Costovertebral angle tenderness

Test results

Laboratory
- Abnormal renal function study results
- Urine studies confirming inability to concentrate urine, decreased glomerular filtration rate, and pyuria if infection is present
- Leukocytosis indicating infection

Imaging
- Excretory urography, retrograde pyelography, and renal ultrasonography confirm diagnosis.
- I.V. urogram may show site of obstruction.
- Nephrogram may show delayed appearance time.
- Radionuclide scan may show site of obstruction.
- Computed tomography may indicate cause.

Treatment

General

- For inoperable obstructions, decompression and drainage of the kidney, using a nephrostomy tube placed temporarily or permanently in the renal pelvis
- If renal function affected, low-protein, low-sodium, and low-potassium diet
- Urinary catheterization

Medication
○ Antibiotic therapy
○ Analgesics
○ Oral alkalinization therapy (for uric acid calculi)
○ Steroid therapy (for retroperitoneal fibrosis)

Surgery
○ Dilatation for urethral stricture
○ Prostatectomy for BPH
○ Placement of percutaneous nephrostomy tube

Nursing considerations

Key outcomes
The patient will:
○ avoid or have minimized complications
○ maintain fluid balance
○ report increased comfort
○ maintain hemodynamic stability
○ demonstrate skill in managing urinary elimination.

Nursing interventions
○ Give prescribed drugs.
○ Give prescribed I.V. fluids.
○ Allow the patient to express his fears and anxieties.

Monitoring
○ Renal function studies
○ Intake and output
○ Vital signs
○ Fluid and electrolyte status
○ Nephrostomy tube function and drainage, if appropriate
○ Wound site (postoperatively)

Patient teaching

Be sure to cover:
○ the disorder, diagnosis, and treatment
○ the procedure and postoperative care, if surgery is scheduled
○ nephrostomy tube care, if appropriate
○ medication administration, dosage, and possible adverse effects
○ dietary changes
○ hydronephrosis symptom recognition and reporting.

Discharge planning
○ Follow-up imaging studies may be required to evaluate recovery.
○ Follow-up laboratory studies may be needed to assess renal function.

Hyperaldosteronism

Overview

Description

○ Hypersecretion of the mineralocorticoid aldosterone by the adrenal cortex
○ Causes excessive reabsorption of sodium and water and excessive renal excretion of potassium
○ May be primary (uncommon) or secondary

Pathophysiology

In primary hyperaldosteronism (Conn's syndrome)

○ Chronic excessive secretion of aldosterone is independent of the renin-angiotensin system and suppresses plasma renin activity.
○ This aldosterone excess enhances sodium and water reabsorption and potassium loss by the kidneys, which leads to mild hypernatremia and, simultaneously, hypokalemia and increased extracellular fluid volume.
○ Expansion of intravascular fluid volume also occurs and results in volume dependent hypertension and increased cardiac output.

 Alert

Excessive ingestion of English black licorice or licorice-like substances can produce a syndrome similar to primary hyperaldosteronism because of the mineralocorticoid action of glycyrrhizic acid.

In secondary hyperaldosteronism

○ Results from an extra-adrenal abnormality that stimulates the adrenal gland to increase aldosterone production

Causes

○ Benign aldosterone-producing adrenal adenoma (in 70% of patients)
○ Bilateral adrenocortical hyperplasia (in children) or carcinoma (rarely)
○ Conditions that reduce renal blood flow and extracellular fluid volume (renal artery stenosis)
○ Conditions that produce a sodium deficit (Wilms' tumor)
○ Nephrotic syndrome
○ Bartter's syndrome
○ Hepatic cirrhosis with ascites
○ Heart failure

Incidence

○ Three times more common in women than in men
○ Most common between ages 30 and 50

Common characteristics

○ Muscle weakness
○ Intermittent, flaccid paralysis
○ Fatigue
○ Headaches
○ Paresthesia
○ Possibly tetany (resulting from metabolic alkalosis), which can lead to hypocalcemia

Complications

○ Neuromuscular irritability, tetany, paresthesia
○ Seizures
○ Left ventricular hypertrophy, heart failure, death
○ Metabolic alkalosis, nephropathy, azotemia

Assessment

History

○ Vision disturbances
○ Nocturnal polyuria
○ Polydipsia
○ Fatigue
○ Headaches

Physical findings

○ Muscle weakness
○ Intermittent, flaccid paralysis
○ Paresthesia
○ High blood pressure

Test results

Laboratory

○ Persistently low serum potassium levels
○ Low plasma renin level that fails to increase appropriately during volume depletion (upright posture, sodium depletion) and high plasma aldosterone level during volume expansion by salt loading (confirm primary hyperaldosteronism in a hypertensive patient without edema)
○ Elevated serum bicarbonate level
○ Markedly increased urine aldosterone levels
○ Increased plasma aldosterone levels
○ Increased plasma renin levels (secondary)
○ Suppression test differentiating between primary and secondary hyperaldosteronism

Imaging

○ Chest X-rays show left ventricular hypertrophy from chronic hypertension.
○ Adrenal angiography or computed tomography scan localizes tumor.

Diagnostic procedures

○ Electrocardiogram shows signs of hypokalemia (ST-segment depression and U waves).

Treatment

General

○ Treatment of underlying cause (secondary)
○ Low-sodium, high-potassium diet

Medication

○ Potassium-sparing diuretics (primary)

Surgery
○ Unilateral adrenalectomy (primary)

Nursing considerations

Key outcomes
The patient will:
○ maintain hemodynamic stability
○ express feelings of increased comfort
○ maintain adequate fluid balance
○ express understanding of the condition and treatment modalities.

Nursing interventions
○ Watch for signs of tetany (muscle twitching, Chvostek's sign, Trousseau's sign).
○ Give potassium replacement, and keep I.V. calcium gluconate available.
○ After adrenalectomy, watch for weakness, hyponatremia, rising serum potassium levels, and signs of adrenal hypofunction, especially hypotension.

Monitoring
○ Intake and output
○ Vital signs
○ Weight
○ Serum electrolyte levels
○ Cardiac arrhythmias

Patient teaching

Be sure to cover:
○ adverse effects of spironolactone, including hyperkalemia, impotence, and gynecomastia, if appropriate
○ the importance of wearing medical identification jewelry while taking steroid hormone replacement therapy.

Hyperbilirubinemia, unconjugated

Overview

Description

- Excessive serum bilirubin levels and mild jaundice
- The result of hemolytic processes in the neonate
- Can be physiologic (with jaundice the only symptom) or pathologic (resulting from an underlying disease)
- Also called *neonatal jaundice*

Pathophysiology

- As erythrocytes break down at the end of their neonatal life cycle, hemoglobin separates into globin (protein) and heme (iron) fragments.

Causes of hyperbilirubinemia

The infant's age at onset of hyperbilirubinemia may provide clues as to the sources of this jaundice-causing disorder.
Day 1
- Blood type incompatibility (Rh, ABO, other minor blood groups)
- Intrauterine infection (rubella, cytomegalic inclusion body disease, toxoplasmosis, syphilis and, occasionally, bacteria such as *Escherichia coli, Staphylococcus, Pseudomonas, Klebsiella, Proteus,* and *Streptococcus*)
Day 2 or 3
- Infection (usually from gram-negative bacteria)
- Polycythemia
- Enclosed hemorrhage (skin bruises, subdural hematoma)
- Respiratory distress syndrome (hyaline membrane disease)
- Heinz body anemia from drugs and toxins (vitamin K_3, sodium nitrate)
- Transient neonatal hyperbilirubinemia
- Abnormal red blood cell morphology
- Red cell enzyme deficiencies (glucose-6-phosphate dehydrogenase, hexokinase)
- Physiologic jaundice
- Blood group incompatibilities
Day 4 and 5
- Breast-feeding, respiratory distress syndrome, maternal diabetes
- Crigler-Najjar syndrome (congenital nonhemolytic icterus)
- Gilbert syndrome
Day 7 and later
- Herpes simplex
- Pyloric stenosis
- Hypothyroidism
- Neonatal giant cell hepatitis
- Infection (usually acquired in neonatal period)
- Bile duct atresia
- Galactosemia
- Choledochal cysts.

- Heme fragments form unconjugated (indirect) bilirubin, which binds with albumin for transport to liver cells to conjugate with glucuronide, forming direct bilirubin.
- Because unconjugated bilirubin is fat-soluble and can't be excreted in the urine or bile, it may escape to extravascular tissue, especially fatty tissue and the brain, resulting in hyperbilirubinemia.
- Hyperbilirubinemia may develop when:
  - certain factors disrupt conjugation and usurp albumin-binding sites, including drugs (such as aspirin, tranquilizers, and sulfonamides) and conditions (such as hypothermia, anoxia, hypoglycemia, and hypoalbuminemia)
  - decreased hepatic function results in reduced bilirubin conjugation
  - increased erythrocyte production or breakdown results from hemolytic disorders or Rh or ABO incompatibility
  - biliary obstruction or hepatitis results in blockage of normal bile flow
  - maternal enzymes present in breast milk inhibit the infant's glucuronyl-transferase conjugating activity.

Causes

See *Causes of hyperbilirubinemia.*

Incidence

- Common in neonates
- More common in males than females
- Less common in Black infants than in White infants

Common characteristics

- Jaundice

Complications

- Kernicterus
- Cerebral palsy
- Epilepsy
- Mental retardation

Assessment

History

- Previous sibling with neonatal jaundice
- Familial history of anemia, bile stones, splenectomy, liver disease
- Maternal illness suggestive of viral or other infection
- Maternal drug intake
- Delayed cord clamping
- Birth trauma with bruising

Physical findings

- Yellowish skin, particularly in the sclerae

Test results

Laboratory
- Elevated serum bilirubin levels

Treatment

General

○ Phototherapy
○ Exchange transfusions

Medication

○ Albumin
○ Phenobarbital (rarely used)
○ $Rh_0(D)$ immune globulin (human) (to Rh-negative mother)

Nursing considerations

Key outcomes

The patient will:
○ exhibit normal body temperature
○ maintain normal fluid balance
○ maintain skin integrity
○ have a reduced bilirubin level.

Nursing interventions

○ Reassure parents that most infants experience some degree of jaundice.
○ Keep emergency equipment available when transfusing blood.
○ Administer $Rh_0(D)$ immune globulin (human), to an Rh-negative mother after amniocentesis, or — to prevent hemolytic disease in subsequent infants — to an Rh-negative mother during the third trimester, after the birth of an Rh-positive infant, or after spontaneous or elective abortion.

Monitoring

○ Jaundice
○ Bilirubin levels
○ Body temperature
○ Intake and output
○ Bleeding and complications

Patient teaching

Be sure to cover:
○ the disorder, diagnosis, and treatment
○ that the infant's stool contains some bile and may be greenish.

Hypercalcemia

Overview

Description

○ Excessive levels of serum calcium

Pathophysiology

○ Together with phosphorus, calcium is responsible for the formation and structure of bones and teeth.
○ Calcium helps to maintain cell structure and function.
○ It plays a role in cell membrane permeability and impulse transmission.
○ It affects the contraction of cardiac muscle, smooth muscle, and skeletal muscle.
○ It participates in the blood-clotting process.

Causes

○ Hyperparathyroidism
○ Hypervitaminosis D
○ Certain cancers
○ Multiple fractures and prolonged immobilization
○ Certain drugs (see *Drugs causing hypercalcemia*)

Incidence

○ Considerably higher in women than in men
○ No gender predominance in elevated calcium levels related to cancer
○ Increases with age

Common characteristics

See *Clinical effects of hypercalcemia.*

Complications

○ Renal calculi
○ Coma
○ Cardiac arrest

Assessment

History

○ Underlying cause
○ Lethargy
○ Weakness
○ Anorexia
○ Constipation

Drugs causing hypercalcemia

These drugs can cause or contribute to hypercalcemia:
○ antacids that contain calcium
○ calcium preparations (oral or I.V.)
○ lithium
○ thiazide diuretics
○ vitamin A
○ vitamin D.

○ Nausea, vomiting
○ Polyuria

Physical findings

○ Confusion
○ Muscle weakness
○ Hyporeflexia
○ Decreased muscle tone

Test results

Laboratory
○ Serum calcium levels greater than 10.5 mg/dl
○ Ionized calcium levels less than 5.3 mg/dl
Diagnostic procedures
○ Electrocardiogram shows shortened QT interval and ventricular arrhythmias

Treatment

General

○ Treatment of the underlying cause
○ Activity, as tolerated

Medication

○ Normal saline solution
○ Loop diuretics

Nursing considerations

Key outcomes

The patient will:
○ maintain stable vital signs
○ maintain adequate cardiac output
○ express an understanding of the disorder and treatment regimen.

Nursing interventions

○ Provide safety measures and institute seizure precautions, if appropriate.
○ Give prescribed I.V. solutions.
○ Watch for signs of heart failure.

Clinical effects of hypercalcemia

Dysfunction	*Effects*
Cardiovascular	● Signs of heart block, cardiac arrest, hypertension
Gastrointestinal	● Anorexia, nausea, vomiting, constipation, dehydration, polydipsia
Musculoskeletal	● Weakness, muscle flaccidity, bone pain, pathologic fractures
Neurologic	● Drowsiness, lethargy, headaches, depression or apathy, irritability, confusion
Other	● Renal polyuria, flank pain and, eventually, azotemia

Monitoring

○ Cardiac rhythm
○ Seizures
○ Calcium levels

Patient teaching

Be sure to cover:
○ avoiding nonprescription drugs that are high in calcium
○ increasing fluid intake
○ following a low-calcium diet.

Discharge planning

○ Refer the patient to a dietitian and social services, if indicated.

Hyperchloremia

Overview

Description

- Excessive serum levels of the chloride anion
- Usually accompanied by sodium and water retention

Pathophysiology

- Chloride accounts for two-thirds of all serum anions.
- Chloride is secreted by stomach mucosa as hydro-chloric acid; it provides an acid medium that aids digestion and activation of enzymes.
- Chloride helps to maintain acid-base and body water balances, influences the osmolality or tonicity of extracellular fluid, plays a role in the exchange of oxygen and carbon dioxide in red blood cells, and helps activate salivary amylase (which, in turn, activates the digestive process).
- An inverse relationship exists between chloride and bicarbonate. When the level of one goes up the level of the other goes down. (See *Anion gap and metabolic acidosis.*)

Causes

- Hyperparathyroidism
- Renal tubular acidosis
- Metabolic acidosis
- Hypernatremia
- Prolonged diarrhea
- Loss of pancreatic secretion
- Certain drugs (see *Drugs causing hyperchloremia*)

Common characteristics

- Agitation, tachycardia, hypertension, pitting edema, dyspnea
- Deep, rapid breathing; weakness; diminished cognitive ability; and, ultimately, coma (if in metabolic acidosis)

Complications

- Coma

Assessment

History

- Risk factors for high chloride level
- Altered level of consciousness

Physical findings

- Agitation
- Pitting edema
- Dyspnea
- Rapid deep breathng (Kussmaul's respirations)
- Weakness
- Tachypnea
- Hypertension

Test results

- Serum chloride level above 108 mEq/L
- With metabolic acidosis, serum pH below 7.35 and serum carbon dioxide level below 22 mEq/L and a normal anion gap
- Serum sodium level above 145 mEq/L

Treatment

General

- Treatment of underlying cause
- Activity, as tolerated
- Restoring fluid, electrolyte, and acid base balance
- Restricted sodium and chloride intake

Medication

- Sodium bicarbonate I.V.
- Lactated Ringer's solution
- Diuretics

Nursing considerations

Key outcomes

The patient will:
- maintain adequate cardiac output
- maintain stable vital signs
- maintain adequate fluid volume
- avoid complications.

Nursing interventions

- Provide a safe environment.
- Give prescribed I.V. fluids.

Drugs causing hyperchloremia

These drugs can cause or contribute to hyperchloremia:
- acetazolamide
- ammonium chloride
- phenylbutazone
- sodium polystyrene sulfonate (Kayexalate)
- salicylates (overdose)
- triamterene.

○ Evaluate muscle strength and adjust activity level.
○ Reorient the confused patient when necessary.

Monitoring

○ Serum electrolyte levels
○ Respiratory status
○ Signs of metabolic alkalosis
○ Intake and output
○ Neurologic status
○ Cardiac rhythm
○ Arterial blood gas levels

Patient teaching

Be sure to cover:
○ the disorder, diagnosis, and treatment
○ dietary or fluid restrictions, as indicated
○ drug administration, dosage, and possible adverse effects.

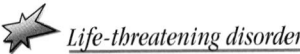
Life-threatening disorder

Hyperkalemia

Overview

Description

- Excessive serum levels of the potassium anion
- Commonly induced by other treatments

Pathophysiology

- Potassium facilitates contraction of both skeletal and smooth muscles, including myocardial contraction.
- Potassium figures prominently in nerve impulse conduction, acid-base balance, enzyme action, and cell membrane function.
- Often induced by other treatments
- Slight deviation in serum levels can produce profound clinical consequences.
- Potassium imbalance can lead to muscle weakness and flaccid paralysis because of an ionic imbalance in neuromuscular tissue excitability.

Causes

- Renal dysfunction or failure
- Use of potassium-sparing diuretics such as triamterene by patients with renal disease
- Burns
- Crushing injuries
- Adrenal gland insufficiency
- Dehydration
- Diabetic acidosis
- Increased intake of potassium
- Decreased urinary excretion of potassium
- Severe infection
- Large quantities of blood transfusions
- Certain drugs (see *Drugs causing hyperkalemia*)

Incidence

- Affects males and females equally
- Diagnosed in up to 8% of hospitalized patients in the United States

Common characteristics

See *Clinical effects of hyperkalemia.*

Drugs causing hyperkalemia

These drugs may increase potassium levels:
- angiotensin-converting enzyme inhibitors
- antibiotics
- beta-adrenergic blockers
- chemotherapeutic drugs
- nonsteroidal anti-inflammatory drugs
- potassium (in excessive amounts)
- spironolactone.

Complications

- Cardiac arrhythmia
- Metabolic acidosis
- Cardiac arrest

Assessment

History

- Irritability
- Paresthesia
- Muscle weakness
- Nausea
- Abdominal cramps
- Diarrhea

Physical findings

- Hypotension
- Irregular heart rate
- Cardiac arrhythmia (possible)

Test results

Laboratory
- Serum potassium levels greater than 5 mEq/L
- Decreased arterial pH

Diagnostic procedures
- Electrocardiogram shows a tall, tented T wave.

Treatment

General

- Treatment of the underlying cause
- Hemodialysis or peritoneal dialysis
- Activity, as tolerated

Clinical effects of hyperkalemia

Dysfunction	Effects
Acid-base balance	• Metabolic acidosis
Cardiovascular	• Tachycardia and later bradycardia, ECG changes (tented and elevated T waves, widened QRS complex, prolonged PR interval, flattened or absent P waves, depressed ST segment), cardiac arrest (with levels > 7.0 mEq/L)
Gastrointestinal	• Nausea, diarrhea, abdominal cramps
Genitourinary	• Oliguria, anuria
Musculoskeletal	• Muscle weakness, flaccid paralysis
Neurologic	• Hyperreflexia progressing to weakness, numbness, tingling, flaccid paralysis

Medication

○ Rapid infusion of 10% calcium gluconate (decreases myocardial irritability)
○ Insulin and 10% to 50% glucose I.V.
○ Sodium polystyrene sulfonate with 70% sorbitol

Nursing considerations

Key outcomes

The patient will:
○ maintain hemodynamic stability
○ maintain a normal potassium level
○ understand potential adverse effects of prescribed drugs.

Nursing interventions

○ Check the serum sample. (See *Avoiding false results.*)
○ Give prescribed drugs.
○ Insert an indwelling urinary catheter.
○ Implement safety measures.
○ Be alert for signs of hypokalemia after treatment.

Monitoring

○ Serum potassium levels
○ Cardiac rhythm
○ Intake and output

Patient teaching

Be sure to cover:
○ prescribed drugs and potential adverse effects
○ monitoring intake and output
○ preventing future episodes of hyperkalemia
○ need for potassium-restricted diet.

Hyperlipoproteinemia

Overview

Description

- ○ Increased plasma concentrations of one or more lipoproteins
- ○ Primary form includes at least five distinct and inherited metabolic disorders
- ○ May occur secondary to other conditions such as diabetes mellitus
- ○ Clinical changes range from relatively mild symptoms, managed by diet, to potentially fatal pancreatitis

Pathophysiology

- ○ Increased low-density lipoprotein (LDL) and decreased high-density lipoprotein (HDL) levels
- ○ Accelerated development of atherosclerosis

Causes

- ○ Primary hyperlipoproteinemia
  - Types I and III transmitted as autosomal recessive traits
  - Types II, IV, and V transmitted as autosomal dominant traits
- ○ Secondary hyperlipoproteinemia
  - Diabetes mellitus
  - Pancreatitis
  - Hypothyroidism
  - Renal disease

Incidence

Type I
- ○ Relatively rare and present at birth

Type II
- ○ Onset between ages 10 and 30

Type III
- ○ Uncommon and usually occurring after age 20

Type IV
- ○ Relatively common, especially in middle-aged men

Type V
- ○ Uncommon and usually occurring in late adolescence or early adulthood

Common characteristics

- ○ Increased plasma concentrations of one or more lipoproteins

Complications

- ○ Coronary artery disease (CAD)
- ○ Pancreatitis

Assessment

History

Type I
- ○ Recurrent attacks of severe abdominal pain
- ○ Abdominal pain usually preceded by fat intake
- ○ Malaise and anorexia

Type II
- ○ History of premature and accelerated coronary atherosclerosis
- ○ Symptoms typically develop in 20s or 30s

Type III
- ○ No clinical symptoms until after age 20
- ○ Aggravating factors, such as obesity, hypothyroidism, and diabetes mellitus

Type IV
- ○ Atherosclerosis
- ○ Early CAD
- ○ Excessive alcohol consumption
- ○ Poorly controlled diabetes mellitus
- ○ Birth control pills containing estrogen (can precipitate severe hypertriglyceridemia)
- ○ Hypertension
- ○ Hyperuricemia

Type V
- ○ Abdominal pain associated with pancreatitis
- ○ Complaints related to peripheral neuropathy

Physical findings

Type I
- ○ Papular or eruptive xanthomas over pressure points and extensor surfaces
- ○ Ophthalmoscopic examination: lipemia retinalis (reddish white retinal vessels)
- ○ Abdominal spasm, rigidity, or rebound tenderness
- ○ Hepatosplenomegaly, with liver or spleen tenderness
- ○ Fever possibly present

Type II
- ○ Tendinous xanthomas on the Achilles tendons and tendons of the hands and feet
- ○ Tuberous xanthomas, xanthelasma
- ○ Juvenile corneal arcus

Type III
- ○ Tuberoeruptive xanthomas over elbows and knees
- ○ Palmar xanthomas on the hands, particularly the fingertips

Type IV
- ○ Obesity
- ○ Xanthomas possibly noted during exacerbations

Type V
- ○ Eruptive xanthomas on extensor surface of arms and legs
- ○ Ophthalmoscopic examination: lipemia retinalis
- ○ Hepatosplenomegaly

Test results

Laboratory
- ○ Serum lipid profiles showing elevated levels of total cholesterol, triglycerides, very low-density lipoproteins, LDLs, or HDLs

Treatment

General

- Weight reduction
- Elimination or treatment of aggravating factors, such as diabetes mellitus, alcoholism, and hypothyroidism
- Reduction of risk factors for atherosclerosis
- Smoking cessation
- Treatment of hypertension
- Avoidance of hormonal and estrogen-containing contraceptive drugs
- Restriction of cholesterol and saturated animal fat intake
- Avoidance of alcoholic beverages to decrease plasma triglyceride levels
- Inclusion of polyunsaturated vegetable oils (reduces plasma LDLs)
- Maintenance of exercise and physical fitness program

Type I
- Restricted fat intake (less than 20 g/day); 20- to 40-g/day, medium-chain triglyceride diet to supplement calorie intake

Type II
- Restriction of cholesterol intake to less than 300 mg/day for adults and less than 150 mg/day for children; restricted triglyceride intake (to less than 100 mg/day for children and adults); and diet high in polyunsaturated fats

Type III
- Restricted cholesterol intake (to less than 300 mg/day) and carbohydrates; increased polyunsaturated fats

Type IV
- Restricted cholesterol intake; increased polyunsaturated fats

Type V
- Long-term maintenance of a low-fat diet; 20- to 40-g/day medium-chain triglyceride diet

Medication

- Nicotinic acid
- Clofibrate and niacin
- Niacin, clofibrate, gemfibrozil

Surgery

- If unable to tolerate drug therapy, surgical creation of an ileal bypass
- For severely affected homozygote children, portacaval shunt as a last resort to reduce plasma cholesterol levels

Nursing considerations

Key outcomes

The patient will:
- develop no complications
- maintain stable vital signs
- verbalize understanding of the disorder and treatment regimen.

Nursing interventions

- Give prescribed antilipemics.
- Prevent or minimize adverse reactions.
- Urge the patient to adhere to the prescribed diet.
- Assist the patient with additional lifestyle changes.
- Encourage verbalization of fears related to premature CAD.

Monitoring

- Vital signs
- Adverse reactions
- Serum lipoproteins
- Response to treatment
- Signs and symptoms related to CAD or its sequelae

Patient teaching

Be sure to cover:
- the disorder, diagnosis, and treatment
- the need to maintain a steady weight and strictly adhere to the prescribed diet (for the 2 weeks preceding serum cholesterol and serum triglyceride tests), and to fast for 12 hours before the test
- the need to avoid excessive sugar intake and alcoholic beverages
- minimized intake of saturated fats (higher in meats and coconut oil)
- increased intake of polyunsaturated fats (vegetable oils)
- avoiding hormonal contraceptives or drugs that contain estrogen
- foods high in cholesterol and saturated fats
- the prescribed drug regimen and potential adverse effects
- signs and symptoms requiring medical evaluation.

Discharge planning

- Refer the patient for a medically supervised exercise program.
- Refer the patient to a smoking-cessation program, if indicated.
- Refer the patient to a dietitian, if necessary.

Hypermagnesemia

Overview

Description
○ Excessive serum levels of the magnesium cation

Pathophysiology
○ Magnesium enhances neuromuscular integration and stimulates parathyroid hormone secretion, thus regulating intracellular fluid calcium levels.
○ Magnesium may also regulate skeletal muscles through its influence on calcium utilization by depressing acetylcholine release at synaptic junctions.
○ Magnesium activates many enzymes for proper carbohydrate and protein metabolism, aids in cell metabolism and the transport of sodium and potassium across cell membranes, and influences sodium, potassium, calcium, and protein levels.
○ About one-third of magnesium taken into the body is absorbed through the small intestine and is eventually excreted in the urine; remaining unabsorbed magnesium is excreted in the stool.

Causes
○ Chronic renal insufficiency
○ Use of laxatives (magnesium sulfate, milk of magnesia, and magnesium citrate solutions), especially with renal insufficiency (see *Drugs and supplements causing hypermagnesemia*)
○ Overuse of magnesium-containing antacids
○ Severe dehydration (resulting oliguria can cause magnesium retention)
○ Overcorrection of hypomagnesemia
○ Addison's disease
○ Adrenocortical insufficiency
○ Untreated diabetic ketoacidosis

Risk factors
○ Advanced age
○ Pregnancy
○ Neonates whose mothers received magnesium sulfate during labor
○ Patients receiving magnesium sulfate to control seizures

Incidence
○ Rarely occurs in the United States

Common characteristics
See *Clinical effects of hypermagnesemia*.

Complications
○ Respiratory depression
○ Cardiac arrhythmia
○ Cardiac arrest

Assessment

History
○ Nausea
○ Vomiting
○ Drowsiness
○ Confusion

Physical findings
○ Flushed appearance
○ Hypotension
○ Weak pulse
○ Muscle weakness
○ Hyporeflexia (see *Testing the patellar reflex*)

Test results
Laboratory
○ Serum magnesium levels greater than 2.5 mEq/L
Diagnostic procedures
○ Electrocardiogram showing prolonged PR interval, widened QRS complex, and tall T waves

Treatment

General
○ Identification and correction of the underlying cause
○ Increased fluid intake
○ Peritoneal dialysis or hemodialysis

Medication
○ Loop diuretics, such as furosemide, with impaired renal function
○ Calcium gluconate (10%)

Drugs and supplements causing hypermagnesemia

Monitor your patient's magnesium level closely if he's receiving:
○ an antacid (Di-Gel, Gaviscon, Maalox)
○ a laxative (Milk of Magnesia, Haley's M-O, magnesium citrate)
○ a magnesium supplement (magnesium oxide, magnesium sulfate).

Clinical effects of hypermagnesemia

Dysfunction	Effects
Cardiovascular	● Bradycardia, weak pulse, hypotension, heart block, cardiac arrest
Neurologic	● Drowsiness, flushing, lethargy, confusion, diminished sensorium
Neuromuscular	● Diminished reflexes, muscle weakness, flaccid paralysis, respiratory muscle paralysis that may cause respiratory embarrassment

Testing the patellar reflex

One way to gauge your patient's magnesium status is to test his patellar reflex, one of the deep tendon reflexes that the magnesium level affects. To test the reflex, strike the patellar tendon just below the patella with the patient sitting or lying in a supine position, as shown. Look for leg extension or contraction of the quadriceps muscle in the front of the thigh.

If the patellar reflex is absent, notify the physician immediately. This finding may mean your patient's magnesium level is 7 mEq/L or higher.

Sitting
Have the patient sit on the side of the bed with his legs dangling freely, as shown here. Then test the reflex.

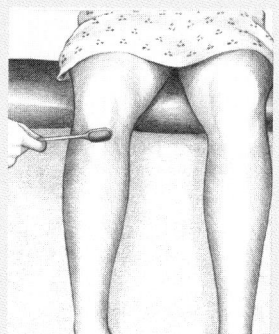

Supine position
Flex the patient's knee at a 45-degree angle, and place your nondominant hand behind it for support. Then test the reflex

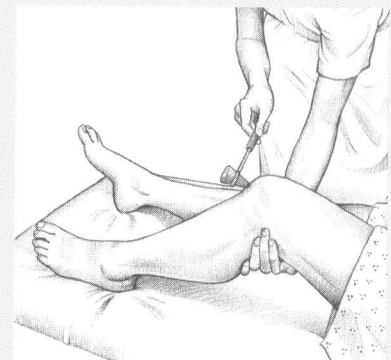

Nursing considerations

Key outcomes
The patient will:
○ maintain hemodynamic stability
○ attain and maintain a normal magnesium level
○ understand the causes of high magnesium levels
○ have a normal ECG.

Nursing interventions
○ Provide sufficient fluids for adequate hydration and maintenance of renal function.
○ Give prescribed drugs.
○ Report abnormal serum electrolyte levels immediately.
○ Watch patients receiving a cardiac glycoside and calcium gluconate simultaneously because calcium excess enhances the cardiac glycoside.

Monitoring
○ Vital signs
○ Magnesium levels
○ Electrolyte levels
○ Intake and output
○ Cardiac rhythm
○ Neuromuscular system
○ Level of consciousness
○ Respiratory status

Patient teaching

Be sure to cover:
○ avoidance of abusing laxatives and antacids containing magnesium, particularly in the elderly or those patients with compromised renal function
○ hydration requirements
○ prescribed drugs.

Hypernatremia

Overview

Description

○ Excessive serum levels of the sodium cation relative to body water

Pathophysiology

○ Sodium is the major cation (90%) in extracellular fluid; potassium, the major cation in intracellular fluid.
○ During repolarization, the sodium-potassium pump continually shifts sodium into the cells and potassium out of the cells; during depolarization, it does the reverse.
○ Sodium cation functions include maintaining tonicity and concentration of extracellular fluid, acid-base balance (reabsorption of sodium ion and excretion of hydrogen ion), nerve conduction and neuromuscular function, glandular secretion, and water balance.
○ Increased sodium causes high serum osmolality (increased solute concentrations in the body), which stimulates the hypothalmus and intiates the sensation of thirst.

Causes

○ Decreased water intake
○ Excess adrenocortical hormones, as in Cushing's syndrome
○ Antidiuretic hormone deficiency (diabetes insipidus)
○ Salt intoxication (less common), which may be produced by excessive table salt ingestion
○ Excessive I.V. administration of sodium solutions
○ Certain drugs (see *Drugs causing hypernatremia*)

Risk factors

○ People who can't drink voluntarily

Drugs causing hypernatremia

Ask your patient if he's taking any of these drugs that can elevate his sodium level:
○ antacids with sodium bicarbonate
○ antibiotics such as ticarcillin disodium-clavulanate potassium (Timentin)
○ salt tablets
○ sodium bicarbonate injections (such as those given during cardiac arrest)
○ I.V. sodium chloride preparations
○ sodium polystyrene sulfonate (Kayexalate).

Incidence

○ Occurs in approximately 1% of hospitalized patients (usually elderly patients)
○ Affects males and females equally

Common characteristics

○ Pulmonary edema
○ Circulatory disorders
○ Decreased level of consciousness (see *Clinical effects of hypernatremia*)

Complications

○ Seizures
○ Coma
○ Permanent neurologic damage

Assessment

History

○ Fatigue
○ Restlessness, agitation
○ Weakness
○ Disorientation
○ Lethargy

Physical findings

○ Flushed skin
○ Dry, swollen tongue
○ Sticky mucous membranes
○ Low-grade fever
○ Twitching
○ Hypertension, dyspnea (with hypervolemia)
○ Orthostatic hypotension and oliguria (with hypovolemia)

Test results

Laboratory
○ Serum sodium level greater than 145 mEq/L
○ Urine sodium level less than 40 mEq/24 hours, with high serum osmolality

Clinical effects of hypernatremia

Dysfunction	Effects
Cardiovascular	● Hypertension, tachycardia, pitting edema, excessive weight gain
Cutaneous	● Flushed skin; dry, sticky membranes
Gastrointestinal	● Rough, dry tongue; intense thirst
Genitourinary	● Oliguria
Neurologic	● Fever, agitation, restlessness, seizures
Respiratory	● Dyspnea, respiratory arrest, death (from dramatic rise in osmotic pressure)

Treatment

General

○ Treatment of underlying cause
○ Administration of salt-free solutions (such as dextrose in water) followed by infusion of half-normal saline solution to prevent hyponatremia
○ Discontinuation of drugs that promote sodium retention
○ Sodium-restricted diet
○ Activity, as tolerated

Nursing considerations

Key outcomes

The patient will:
○ maintain adequate fluid volume
○ maintain a normal sodium level
○ maintain stable vital signs
○ remain alert and oriented to his environment.

Nursing interventions

○ Obtain a drug history to check for drugs that promote sodium retention.
○ Assist with oral hygiene.
○ Observe for signs of cerebral edema during fluid replacement therapy.

Monitoring

○ Serum sodium levels
○ Intake and output
○ Neurologic status

Patient teaching

Be sure to cover:
○ the disorder and treatment
○ the importance of sodium restriction
○ low-sodium diet
○ prescribed drugs
○ signs and symptoms of hypernatremia
○ avoiding over-the-counter medications that contain sodium.

Hyperparathyroidism

Overview

Description

- Characterized by a greater than normal secretion of parathyroid hormone (PTH)
- Classified as either primary or secondary

Pathophysiology

- In primary hyperparathyroidism, one or more of the parathyroid glands enlarges, increasing PTH secretion and elevating serum calcium levels or an adenoma secretes PTH, unresponsive to negative feedback of serum calcium.
- In secondary hyperparathyroidism, excessive compensatory production of PTH stems from a hypocalcemia-producing abnormality outside the parathyroid gland, which isn't responsive to PTH such as decreased intestinal absorption of calcium or vitamin D.
- Increased PTH levels act directly on the bone and the kidney tubules, resulting in an increase in extracellular calcium.
- Renal excretion and uptake into the soft tissues or skeleton can't compensate for increased calcium.

Causes

- Adenoma
- Genetic disorders
- Multiple endocrine neoplasia
- Dietary vitamin D or calcium deficiency
- Decreased intestinal absorption of vitamin D or calcium
- Chronic renal failure
- Osteomalacia
- Ingestion of drugs such as phenytoin
- Laxative ingestion
- Idiopathic

Incidence

- More common in women than in men
- Increased incidence in postmenopausal women
- Onset usually between ages 35 and 65

Common characteristics

- Bone pain and tenderness
- Renal calculi
- Abdominal distress
- Anxiety and depression

Complications

- Osteoporosis
- Subchondral fractures
- Traumatic synovitis
- Renal calculi and colic
- Renal insufficiency and failure
- Peptic ulcers
- Cholelithiasis
- Cardiac arrhythmias
- Vascular damage
- Heart failure
- Muscle atrophy
- Depression

Assessment

History

- Recurring nephrolithiasis
- Polyuria
- Hematuria
- Chronic lower back pain
- Easy fracturing
- Osteoporosis
- Constant, severe epigastric pain that radiates to the back
- Abdominal pain
- Anorexia, nausea, and vomiting
- Constipation
- Polydipsia
- Muscle weakness, particularly in the legs
- Lethargy
- Personality disturbances
- Depression
- Overt psychosis
- Cataracts
- Anemia

Physical findings

- Muscle weakness and atrophy
- Psychomotor disturbances
- Stupor and, possibly, coma
- Skin necrosis
- Subcutaneous calcification

Test results

Laboratory

IN PRIMARY DISEASE

- Alkaline phosphatase increased
- Osteocalcin increased
- Tartrate-resistant acid phosphatase increased
- Serum PTH increased
- Serum calcium increased
- Serum phosphorus levels decreased
- Urine and serum calcium and serum chloride increased
- Creatinine levels possibly increased
- Basal acid secretion possibly increased
- Serum amylase possibly increased

IN SECONDARY DISEASE

- Serum calcium normal or slightly decreased
- Serum phosphorus level variable
- Serum PTH increased

Imaging

- X-rays show diffuse bone demineralization, bone cysts, outer cortical bone absorption, and subperiosteal erosion of the phalanges and distal clavicles in primary disease.
- X-ray spectrophotometry shows increased bone turnover in primary disease.

❍ Esophagography, thyroid scan, parathyroid thermography, ultrasonography, thyroid angiography, computed tomography scan, and magnetic resonance imaging may show location of parathyroid lesions.

Treatment

General

❍ In primary disease, treatment to decrease calcium levels
❍ In renal failure, dialysis
❍ In secondary disease, treatment to correct underlying cause of parathyroid hypertrophy
❍ Increased oral fluid intake
❍ Activity, as tolerated

Medication

Primary disease
❍ Bisphosphonates
❍ Oral sodium or potassium phosphate
❍ Calcitonin
❍ Plicamycin, if primary disease is metastatic
Secondary disease
❍ Vitamin D therapy
❍ Aluminum hydroxide
❍ Glucocorticoids
Postoperatively
❍ I.V. magnesium and phosphate
❍ Sodium phosphate
❍ Supplemental calcium
❍ Vitamin D or calcitriol

Surgery

❍ With primary hyperparathyroidism, removal of adenoma or all but one-half of one gland

Nursing considerations

Key outcomes

The patient will:
❍ maintain current weight
❍ express feelings of increased comfort
❍ maintain adequate cardiac output
❍ maintain balanced fluid volume status
❍ perform activities of daily living without excessive fatigue
❍ express positive feelings about self.

Nursing interventions

❍ Obtain baseline serum potassium, calcium, phosphate, and magnesium levels before treatment.
❍ Provide at least 3 L of fluid per day.
❍ Institute safety precautions.
❍ Schedule frequent rest periods.
❍ Provide comfort measures.
❍ Give prescribed drugs.
❍ Help the patient turn and reposition every 2 hours.
❍ Support affected extremities with pillows.
❍ Offer emotional support.

❍ Help the patient develop effective coping strategies.
After parathyroidectomy
❍ Keep a tracheotomy tray and endotracheal tube setup at the bedside.
❍ Maintain seizure precautions.
❍ Place the patient in semi-Fowler's position.
❍ Support the patient's head and neck with sandbags.
❍ Have the patient ambulate as soon as possible.

 Alert

Watch for complaints of tingling in the hands and around the mouth. If these symptoms don't subside quickly, they may be prodromal signs of tetany, so keep I.V. calcium gluconate or calcium chloride available for emergency administration.

Monitoring

❍ Vital signs
❍ Intake and output
❍ Serum calcium levels
❍ Respiratory status
❍ Cardiovascular status
After parathyroidectomy
❍ Increased neuromuscular irritability
❍ Complications
❍ Neck edema
❍ Chvostek's sign
❍ Trousseau's sign

Patient teaching

Be sure to cover:
❍ the disorder, diagnosis, and treatment
❍ prescribed drugs and possible adverse effects
❍ when to notify the physician
❍ the signs and symptoms of tetany, respiratory distress, and renal dysfunction
❍ the need for periodic blood tests
❍ avoidance of calcium-containing antacids and thiazide diuretics
❍ the need to wear medical identification jewelry.

Hyperphosphatemia

Overview

Description
- Excessive serum levels of phosphate
- Reflects the kidney's inability to excrete excess phosphorus

Pathophysiology
- Phosphorus exists primarily in inorganic combination with calcium in teeth and bones.
- In extracellular fluid, the phosphate ion supports several metabolic functions: utilization of B vitamins, acid-base homeostasis, bone formation, nerve and muscle activity, cell division, transmission of hereditary traits, and metabolism of carbohydrates, proteins, and fats.
- Renal tubular reabsorption of phosphate is inversely regulated by calcium levels—an increase in phosphorus causes a decrease in calcium. An imbalance causes hypophosphatemia or hyperphosphatemia.

Causes
- Hypocalcemia
- Hypervitaminosis D
- Hypoparathyroidism
- Renal failure
- Overuse of laxatives with phosphates or phosphate enemas
- Certain drugs (see *Drugs and supplements causing hyperphosphatemia*)
- Acid-base imbalance

Risk factors
- Muscle necrosis
- Infection
- Heat stroke
- Trauma
- Chemotherapy

Incidence
- Occurs most commonly in children, who tend to consume more phosphorus-rich foods and beverages than adults
- Greater incidence in children and adults with renal insufficiency

---

Drugs and supplements causing hyperphosphatemia

These drugs may cause hyperphosphatemia:
- enemas such as Fleet enemas
- laxatives containing phosphorus or phosphate
- oral phosphorus supplements
- parenteral phosphorus supplements (sodium phosphate, potassium phosphate)
- vitamin D supplements.

Common characteristics
- Usually remains asymptomatic
- May result in hypocalcemia with tetany and seizures

Complications
- Soft tissue calcifications
- Hypocalcemia
- Bone fractures

Assessment

History
- Anorexia
- Decreased mental status
- Nausea and vomiting

Physical findings
- Hyperreflexia
- Hypocalcemic electrocardiogram changes
- Muscle weakness and cramps
- Papular eruptions
- Paresthesia
- Presence of Chvostek's or Trousseau's sign
- Abdominal spasm
- Tetany
- Visual impairment
- Conjunctivitis

Test results
Laboratory
- Serum phosphorus level over 4.5 mg/dl
- Serum calcium level below 8.9 mg/dl
- Increased blood urea nitrogen and creatinine levels

Imaging
- X-ray studies may reveal skeletal changes caused by osteodystrophy in chronic hyperphosphatemia

Diagnostic procedures
- Electrocardiogram may show changes characteristic of hypercalcemia

Treatment

General
- Treatment of the underlying cause
- Peritoneal dialysis or hemodialysis (if severe)
- Discontinuation of drugs associated with hyperphosphatemia
- Low-phosphorus diet
- Activity, as tolerated
- I.V. saline solution

Medication
- Aluminum
- Magnesium
- Calcium gel
- Phosphate-bindng antacids

Foods high in phosphorus

These foods have a high phosphorus content:
- beans
- bran
- cheese
- chocolate
- dark-colored sodas
- ice cream
- lentils
- milk
- nuts
- peanut butter
- seeds
- yogurt.

Nursing considerations

Key outcomes

The patient will:
- maintain a patent airway
- maintain adequate vital signs
- have a normal phosphorus level
- express understanding of condition and treatment
- maintain a low phosphorus diet.

Nursing interventions

- Provide safety measures.
- Be alert for signs of hypocalcemia.
- Give prescribed drugs.
- Give antacids with meals to increase their effectiveness.
- Prepare the patient for dialysis, if appropriate.
- Assist with selecting a low-phosphorus diet.

Monitoring

- Vital signs
- Phosphorus and calcium levels
- Intake and output
- Renal studies

Patient teaching

Be sure to cover:
- the disorder and treatment
- prescribed drugs
- avoidance of preparations that contain phosphorus
- avoidance of high-phosphorus foods. (See *Foods high in phosphorus.*)

Discharge planning

- Refer the patient to a dietitian and social services, if indicated.

Hyperpituitarism

Overview

Description

○ Chronic, progressive disease marked by hormonal dysfunction and startling skeletal overgrowth
○ Prognosis dependent on cause
○ Life expectancy usually reduced
○ Appears in two forms: acromegaly and gigantism
○ Also referred to as *growth hormone (GH) excess*

Pathophysiology

○ Progressive excessive secretion of pituitary GH occurs.
○ Acromegaly occurs after epiphyseal closure, causing bone thickening and transverse growth and visceromegaly.
○ Gigantism occurs before epiphyseal closure with excess GH, causing proportional overgrowth of all body tissues.
○ A large tumor may cause loss of other trophic hormones, such as thyroid-stimulating hormone, luteinizing hormone, follicle-stimulating hormone, and corticotropin, which may cause dysfunction of target organs.

Causes

○ GH-producing adenoma of the anterior pituitary gland
○ Excessive GH secretion
○ Excessive GH-releasing hormone
○ Possible genetic cause

Incidence

Acromegaly
○ Occurs equally in men and women
○ Usually occurs between ages 30 and 50
Gigantism
○ Affects infants and children

Common characteristics

○ Progressive enlargement of the face, hands and feet, thorax, and soft tissue
○ Coarsening of features
○ Headache
○ Menstrual disturbances

Complications

○ Arthritis
○ Carpal tunnel syndrome
○ Osteoporosis
○ Kyphosis
○ Hypertension
○ Arteriosclerosis
○ Cardiomegaly and heart failure
○ Blindness
○ Severe neurologic disturbances
○ Glucose intolerance
○ Diabetes mellitus
○ Severe psychological stress

Assessment

History

○ Gradual onset of acromegaly
○ Relatively abrupt onset of gigantism
○ Soft-tissue swelling
○ Hypertrophy of the face and extremities
○ Diaphoresis, oily skin
○ Fatigue, sleep disturbances
○ Weight gain
○ Headaches, decreased vision
○ Decreased libido, impotence
○ Oligomenorrhea, infertility
○ Joint pain
○ Hypertrichosis
○ Irritability, hostility, and other psychological disturbances

Physical findings

○ Enlarged jaw, thickened tongue
○ Enlarged and weakened hands
○ Coarsened facial features
○ Oily or leathery skin
○ Prominent supraorbital ridge
○ Deep, hollow-sounding voice
○ Cartilaginous and connective tissue overgrowth
○ Skeletal abnormalities

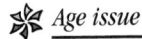 *Age issue*

In infants, inspection reveals a highly arched palate, muscular hypotonia, slanting eyes, and exophthalmos.

Test results

Laboratory
○ GH radioimmunoassay showing increased plasma GH levels and levels of insulin-like growth factor I
○ Glucose suppression test failing to suppress the hormone level to below the accepted norm of 2 ng/ml
Imaging
○ Skull X-rays, computed tomography scan, or magnetic resonance imaging showing location of pituitary tumor
○ Bone X-rays showing a thickening of the cranium and long bones and osteoarthritis in the spine

Treatment

General

○ Treatment to curb overproduction of GH
○ Pituitary radiation therapy

Medication

○ Replacement of thyroid, cortisone, and gonadal hormones postoperatively if entire pituitary removed
○ GH synthesis inhibitor
○ Long-acting analogue of somatostatin

Surgery

○ Transsphenoidal hypophysectomy

Nursing considerations

Key outcomes

The patient will:
○ demonstrate age-appropriate skills and behaviors to the extent possible
○ express feelings of increased comfort
○ express positive feelings about self
○ maintain joint mobility and range of motion (ROM).

Nursing interventions

○ Provide emotional support.
○ Provide reassurance that mood changes result from hormonal imbalances and can be reduced with treatment.
○ Give prescribed drugs.
○ Provide comfort measures.
○ Perform or assist with ROM exercises.
○ Evaluate muscle weakness.
○ Institute safety precautions.
○ Provide meticulous skin care.
○ Assist with early postoperative ambulation.

 Alert

Report large increases in urine output after surgery, which may indicate diabetes insipidus.

Monitoring

○ Vital signs
○ Intake and output
○ Serum glucose levels
○ Signs and symptoms of hyperglycemia
After surgery
○ Signs and symptoms of increased intracranial pressure (ICP) and intracranial bleeding
○ Respiratory status
○ Surgical incisions and dressings
○ Complications
○ Signs and symptoms of infection
○ Signs and symptoms of hormonal deficiency

Patient teaching

Be sure to cover:
○ the disorder, diagnosis, and treatment
○ prescribed drugs and potential adverse effects
○ when to notify the physician
○ avoidance of activities that increase ICP

○ deep breathing through the mouth if nasal packing is in place postoperatively
○ hormone replacement therapy, if ordered
○ the need to wear a medical identification bracelet
○ follow-up examinations
○ possible tumor recurrence.

Discharge planning

○ Refer the patient for psychological counseling to help deal with body image changes and sexual dysfunction, as needed.

Hypersplenism

Overview

Description

○ Exaggerated splenic activity and, possibly, splenomegaly
○ Results in peripheral blood cell deficiency as the
spleen traps and destroys peripheral blood cells
○ May be primary or secondary

Pathophysiology

○ The spleen's normal filtering and phagocytic functions accelerate indiscriminately, automatically removing antibody-coated, aging, and abnormal cells,
even though some cells may be functionally normal.
○ The spleen may also temporarily sequester normal
platelets and red blood cells (RBCs), withholding
them from circulation. In this manner, the enlarged
spleen may trap as many as 90% of the body's
platelets and up to 45% of its RBC mass.

Causes

○ Idiopathic (see *Causes of splenomegaly*)
○ An extrasplenic disorder, such as chronic malaria,
polycythemia vera, or rheumatoid arthritis

Incidence

○ Affects all ages
○ Affects males and females equally

Common characteristics

○ Anemia
○ Leukopenia
○ Thrombocytopenia
○ Splenomegaly
○ Easy bruising

Complications

○ Bleeding
○ Postsplenectomy infection and thromboembolic
disease

Causes of splenomegaly

Congestive
○ Cirrhosis, thrombosis
Cystic or neoplastic
○ Cysts, leukemia, lymphoma, myelofibrosis
Hyperplastic
○ Hemolytic anemia, polycythemia
Infectious
○ Acute (abscesses, subacute infective endocarditis),
chronic (tuberculosis, malaria, Felty's syndrome)
Infiltrative
○ Gaucher's disease, Niemann-Pick disease

Assessment

History

○ Frequent bacterial infection
○ Frequent bruising
○ Spontaneous hemorrhaging from the mucous mem-
branes and GI or genitourinary tract
○ Fever
○ Weakness
○ Palpitations
○ Weight loss

Physical findings

○ Ulcerations of the mouth, legs, and feet
○ Bruising
○ Splenomegaly
○ Jaundice
○ Pallor

Test results

Laboratory
○ A high spleen-liver ratio of radioactivity indicates
splenic destruction or sequestration
○ Decreased hemoglobin level (as low as 4 g/dl)
○ Decreased white blood cell count (less than
4,000/µl)
○ Decreased platelet count (less than 125,000/µl)
○ Elevated reticulocyte count (more than 75,000/µl)
Imaging
○ Ultrasound or splenic scan shows enlarged spleen or
possible underlying cause such as a tumor.

Treatment

General

○ Treatment of underlying disease (secondary)
○ Limited activity—noncontact
○ Nothing by mouth if surgery is indicated

Medication

○ Antibiotics if infection present
○ Pneumococcal vaccine (after splenectomy)

Surgery

○ Splenectomy indicated only in transfusion-dependent
patients who are refractory to medical therapy

Nursing considerations

Key outcomes

The patient will:
○ express understanding of the disorder and treatment
○ maintain stable vital signs
○ understand restrictions imposed by illness
○ not show signs of bleeding.

Nursing interventions
- If splenectomy is scheduled, administer preoperative transfusions of blood or blood products (fresh frozen plasma and platelets) to replace deficient blood elements.
- Treat symptoms or complications of any underlying disorder.
- Provide emotional support.

Monitoring
- Vital signs
- Signs of bleeding
- Complete blood cell count
- Signs of infection

After surgery
- Pain conrol
- Wound site

Patient teaching

Be sure to cover:
- the disorder, diagnosis and treatment
- signs and symptoms of infection
- activity restrictions.

Hypertension

Overview

Description

○ Intermittent or sustained elevation of diastolic or systolic blood pressure
○ Usually begins as benign disease, slowly progressing to accelerated or malignant state
○ Two major types: essential (also called primary or idiopathic) hypertension and secondary hypertension, which results from renal disease or another identifiable cause
○ Malignant hypertension, a medical emergency, is a severe, fulminant form commonly arising from both types

Pathophysiology

Several theories
○ Changes in arteriolar bed, causing increased peripheral vascular resistance
○ Abnormally increased tone in the sympathetic nervous system originating in the vasomotor system centers, causing increased peripheral vascular resistance
○ Increased blood volume resulting from renal or hormonal dysfunction
○ Increase in arteriolar thickening caused by genetic factors, leading to increased peripheral vascular resistance
○ Abnormal renin release, resulting in the formation of angiotensin II, which constricts the arterioles and increases blood volume

Causes

○ Unknown

Risk factors

○ Family history
○ Blacks in the United States
○ Stress
○ Obesity
○ High-sodium, high-saturated fat diet
○ Use of tobacco
○ Use of hormonal contraceptives
○ Excess alcohol intake
○ Sedentary lifestyle
○ Aging

Incidence

○ Affects 15% to 20% of adults in the United States
○ Essential hypertension accounts for 90% to 95% of cases

Common characteristics

○ Serial blood pressure measurements:

– prehypertension: systolic blood pressure (SBP) 120 to 139 mm Hg or diastolic blood pressure (DBP) 80 to 89 mm Hg
– stage 1: SBP 140 to 159 mm Hg or DBP 90 to 99 mm Hg
– stage 2: SBP ≥ 160 mm Hg or DBP ≥ 100 mm Hg

Complications

○ Cardiac disease
○ Renal failure
○ Blindness
○ Stroke

Assessment

History

○ In many cases, no symptoms, and disorder revealed incidentally during evaluation for another disorder or during a routine blood pressure screening program
○ Symptoms that reflect the effect of hypertension on the organ systems
○ Awakening with a headache in the occipital region, which subsides spontaneously after a few hours
○ Dizziness, fatigue, and confusion
○ Palpitations, chest pain, dyspnea
○ Epistaxis
○ Hematuria
○ Blurred vision

Physical findings

○ Bounding pulse
○ S_4
○ Peripheral edema in late stages
○ Hemorrhages, exudates, and papilledema of the eye in late stages if hypertensive retinopathy present
○ Pulsating abdominal mass, suggesting an abdominal aneurysm
○ Elevated blood pressure on at least two consecutive occasions after initial screenings
○ Bruits over the abdominal aorta and femoral arteries or the carotids

Test results

Laboratory
○ Urinalysis possibly showing protein, red blood cells, or white blood cells, suggesting renal disease, or glucose, suggesting diabetes mellitus
○ Serum potassium levels less than 3.5 mEq/L, possibly indicating adrenal dysfunction (primary hyperaldosteronism)
○ Blood urea nitrogen levels normal or elevated to more than 20 mg/dl and serum creatinine levels normal or elevated to more than 1.5 mg/dl, suggesting renal disease

Imaging
○ Excretory urography may reveal renal atrophy, indicating chronic renal disease; one kidney more than

⅝″ (1.6 cm) shorter than the other suggests unilateral renal disease.
○ Chest X-rays may demonstrate cardiomegaly.
○ Renal arteriography may show renal artery stenosis.

Diagnostic procedures
○ Electrocardiography may show left ventricular hypertrophy or ischemia.
○ An oral captopril challenge may be done to test for renovascular hypertension.
○ Ophthalmoscopy reveals arteriovenous nicking and, in hypertensive encephalopathy, edema.

Treatment

General

○ Lifestyle modification, such as weight control, limiting alcohol, regular exercise, and smoking cessation
○ For a patient with secondary hypertension, correction of the underlying cause and control of hypertensive effects
○ Low-saturated fat and low-sodium diet
○ Adequate calcium, magnesium, and potassium in diet
○ Regular exercise program

Medication

○ Diuretics
○ Beta-adrenergic blockers
○ Calcium channel blockers
○ Angiotensin-converting enzyme inhibitors
○ Alpha-receptor antagonists
○ Vasodilators
○ Angiotensin-receptor blockers
○ Aldosterone antagonist

Nursing considerations

Key outcomes

The patient will:
○ maintain adequate cardiac output
○ maintain hemodynamic stability
○ develop no arrhythmias
○ express feelings of increased energy
○ comply with the therapy regimen.

Nursing interventions

○ Give prescribed drugs.
○ Encourage dietary changes, as appropriate.
○ Help the patient identify risk factors and modify his lifestyle, as appropriate.

Monitoring

○ Vital signs, especially blood pressure
○ Signs and symptoms of target end-organ damage
○ Complications
○ Response to treatment
○ Risk factor modification
○ Adverse effects of antihypertensive agents

Patient teaching

Be sure to cover:
○ the disorder, diagnosis, and treatment
○ how to use a self-monitoring blood pressure cuff and to record the reading in a journal for review by the physician
○ the importance of compliance with antihypertensive therapy and establishing a daily routine for taking prescribed drugs
○ the need to report adverse effects of drugs
○ the need to avoid high-sodium antacids and over-the-counter cold and sinus medications containing harmful vasoconstrictors
○ examining and modifying lifestyle, including diet
○ the need for a routine exercise program, particularly aerobic walking
○ dietary restrictions
○ the importance of follow-up care.

Discharge planning

○ Refer the patient to stress-reduction therapies or support groups, as needed.

Hyperthyroidism

Overview

Description

- An alteration in thyroid function in which thyroid hormones (TH) exert greater than normal responses
- Management determined by cause
- Hyperthyroidism: a form of thyrotoxicosis in which excess thyroid hormones are secreted by the thyroid gland
- Thyrotoxicoses not associated with hyperthyroidism: subacute thyroiditis, ectopic thyroid tissue, and ingestion of excessive TH
- Graves' disease: (also known as *toxic diffuse goiter*) an autoimmune disease, the most common form of hyperthyroidism
- Also known as *thyrotoxicosis*

Pathophysiology

- In Graves' disease, thyroid-stimulating antibodies bind to and stimulate the thyroid-stimulating hormone (TSH) receptors of the thyroid gland.
- The trigger for this autoimmune disease is unclear.
- It's associated with the production of autoantibodies possibly caused by a defect in suppressor-T-lymphocyte function that allows the formation of these autoantibodies.

Causes

- Diseases that can cause hyperthyroidism:
  - Graves' disease
  - Toxic multinodular goiter
  - Thyroid cancer
  - Increased TSH secretion
  - Genetic and immunologic factors
- Precipitating factors:
  - Excessive iodine intake
  - Stress
  - Surgery
  - Infection
  - Toxemia of pregnancy
  - Diabetic ketoacidosis

Incidence

- Graves' disease: most common between ages 30 and 60; more common in women than in men
- Increased among monozygotic twins
- More common with family history of thyroid abnormalities
- Only 5% of hyperthyroid patients younger than age 15

Common characteristics

- Increased metabolic rate
- Heat intolerance
- Increased tissue sensitivity to sympathetic nervous system stimulation
- Goiter (almost always present)
- Exophthalmos

Complications

- Arrhythmias
- Left ventricular hypertrophy
- Heart failure
- Muscle weakness and atrophy
- Paralysis
- Osteoporosis
- Vitiligo
- Skin hyperpigmentation
- Corneal ulcers
- Myasthenia gravis
- Impaired fertility
- Decreased libido
- Gynecomastia
- Thyrotoxic crisis or thyroid storm
- Hepatic or renal failure

Assessment

History

Graves' disease

- Nervousness, tremor
- Heat intolerance
- Weight loss despite increased appetite
- Sweating
- Frequent bowel movements
- Palpitations
- Poor concentration
- Shaky handwriting
- Clumsiness
- Emotional instability and mood swings
- Thin, brittle nails
- Hair loss
- Nausea and vomiting
- Weakness and fatigue
- Oligomenorrhea or amenorrhea
- Fertility problems
- Diminished libido
- Diplopia

Physical findings

Graves' disease

- Enlarged thyroid (goiter)
- Exophthalmos
- Tremor
- Smooth, warm, flushed skin
- Fine, soft hair
- Premature graying and increased hair loss
- Friable nails and onycholysis
- Pretibial myxedema
- Thickened skin
- Accentuated hair follicles
- Tachycardia at rest
- Full, bounding pulses
- Arrhythmias, especially atrial fibrillation
- Wide pulse pressure
- Possible systolic murmur
- Dyspnea
- Hepatomegaly
- Hyperactive bowel sounds

- Weakness, especially in proximal muscles, and atrophy
- Possible generalized or localized paralysis
- Gynecomastia in males
- Increased tearing

Test results

Laboratory
- Radioimmunoassay showing increased serum triiodothyronine and thyroxine concentrations
- Increased serum protein-bound iodine
- Decreased serum cholesterol and total lipid levels
- Decreased TSH

Imaging
- Thyroid scan showing increased uptake of radioactive iodine (^{131}I)
- Ultrasonography showing subclinical ophthalmopathy

Treatment

General
- Adequate caloric intake
- Activity, as tolerated

Medication
- Treatment with ^{131}I: a single oral dose; treatment of choice for women past reproductive age or men and women not planning to have children
- Thyroid hormone antagonists
- Beta-adrenergic antagonists
- Corticosteroids
- Sedatives

Surgery
- Subtotal (partial) thyroidectomy
- Surgical decompression

Nursing considerations

Key outcomes
The patient will:
- maintain stable vital signs
- maintain normal cardiac output
- maintain balanced fluid status
- have normal bowel movements
- remain normothermic.

Nursing interventions
- Minimize physical and emotional stress.
- Balance rest and activity periods.
- Keep the patient's room cool and quiet and the lights dim.
- Encourage the patient to dress in loose-fitting, cotton clothing.
- Consult a dietitian to ensure a nutritious diet with adequate calories and fluids.
- Offer small, frequent meals.
- Provide meticulous skin care.

- Reassure the patient and his family that mood swings and nervousness usually subside with treatment.
- Encourage verbalization of feelings.
- Help the patient identify and develop coping strategies.
- Offer emotional support.
- Give prescribed drugs.
- Avoid excessive palpation of the thyroid.

After thyroidectomy
- Change dressings and perform wound care, as ordered.
- Keep the patient in semi-Fowler's position.
- Support the patient's head and neck with sandbags.

Monitoring
- Vital signs
- Daily weight
- Intake and output
- Daily neck circumference
- Serum electrolyte results
- Hyperglycemia and glycosuria
- Electrocardiogram for arrhythmias and ST-segment changes
- Complete blood count results
- Signs and symptoms of heart failure
- Frequency and characteristics of stools

After thyroidectomy
- Dressings
- Signs and symptoms of hemorrhage into the neck
- Surgical incision
- Dysphagia or hoarseness
- Signs and symptoms of hypocalcemia

Patient teaching

Be sure to cover:
- the disorder, diagnosis, and treatment
- prescribed drugs and potential adverse effects
- when to notify the physician
- the need for regular medical follow-up visits
- the need for lifelong thyroid hormone replacement
- the importance of wearing medical identification jewelry
- precautions with ^{131}I therapy
- signs and symptoms of hypothyroidism and hyperthyroidism
- eye care for ophthalmopathy.

Hypocalcemia

Overview

Description
○ Deficient serum levels of calcium

Pathophysiology
○ Together with phosphorous, calcium is responsible for the formation and structure of bones and teeth.
○ Calcium helps maintain cell structure and function.
○ It plays a role in cell membrane permeability and impulse transmission.
○ It affects the contraction of cardiac muscle, smooth muscle, and skeletal muscle.
○ It also participates in the blood-clotting process.

Causes
○ Inadequate dietary intake of calcium and vitamin D
○ Hypoparathyroidism
○ Malabsorption or loss of calcium from the GI tract
○ Severe infections or burns
○ Overcorrection of acidosis
○ Pancreatic insufficiency
○ Renal failure
○ Hypomagnesemia

Incidence
○ Occurs equally in males and females
○ Affects persons of all ages

Common characteristics
See *Clinical effects of hypocalcemia.*

Complications
○ Laryngeal spasm
○ Seizures
○ Cardiac arrhythmia
○ Respiratory arrest

Clinical effects of hypocalcemia

Dysfunction	Effects
Cardiovascular	● Arrhythmias, hypotension
Gastrointestinal	● Increased GI motility, diarrhea
Musculoskeletal	● Paresthesia, tetany or painful tonic muscle spasms, facial spasms, abdominal cramps, muscle cramps, spasmodic contractions
Neurologic	● Anxiety, irritability, twitching around mouth, laryngospasm, seizures, Chvostek's sign, Trousseau's sign
Other	● Blood-clotting abnormalities

Assessment

History
○ Underlying cause
○ Anxiety
○ Irritability
○ Seizures
○ Muscle cramps
○ Diarrhea

Physical findings
○ Twitching
○ Carpopedal spasm
○ Tetany
○ Hypotension
○ Confusion
○ Positive Chvostek's and Trousseau's sign (see *Eliciting signs of hypocalcemia*)

Test results
Laboratory
○ Serum calcium levels less than 8.5 mg/dl
○ Ionized calcium levels less than 4.5 mg/dl
Diagnostic procedures
○ Electrocardiogram shows lengthened QT interval, prolonged ST segment, and arrhythmias.

Treatment

General
○ Treatment of the underlying cause
○ Diet high in calcium and vitamin D
○ Activity, as tolerated

Medication
○ Oral calcium and vitamin D supplements
○ Calcium gluconate I.V.

Nursing considerations

Key outcomes
The patient will:
○ maintain stable vital signs
○ maintain adequate cardiac output
○ express an understanding of the disorder and treatment.

Nursing interventions
○ Provide safety measures; institute seizure precautions, if appropriate.
○ Give prescribed calcium replacement.
○ Assess I.V. sites if administering calcium I.V. (infiltration causes sloughing).

Eliciting signs of hypocalcemia

When the patient complains of muscle spasms and paresthesia in his limbs, try eliciting Chvostek's and Trousseau's signs—indications of tetany associated with calcium deficiency.

Follow the procedures described here, keeping in mind the discomfort they typically cause. If you detect these signs, notify the physician immediately. During these tests, watch the patient for laryngospasm, monitor his cardiac status, and have resuscitation equipment nearby.

Chvostek's sign

To elicit this sign, tap the patient's facial nerve just in front of the earlobe and below the zygomatic arch or between the zygomatic arch and the corner of the mouth, as shown below.

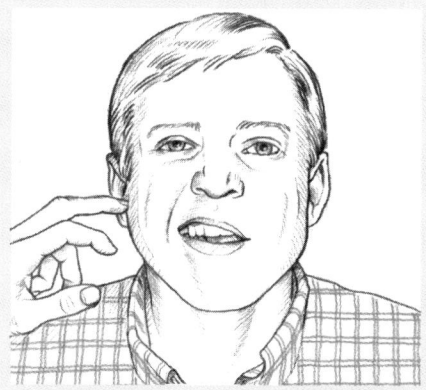

A positive response (indicating latent tetany) ranges from simple mouth-corner twitching to twitching of all facial muscles on the side tested. Simple twitching may be normal in some patients. However, a more pronounced response usually confirms Chvostek's sign.

Trousseau's sign

In this test, occlude the brachial artery by inflating a blood pressure cuff on the patient's upper arm to a level between diastolic and systolic blood pressure. Maintain this inflation for 3 minutes while observing the patient for carpal spasm (shown above), which is Trousseau's sign.

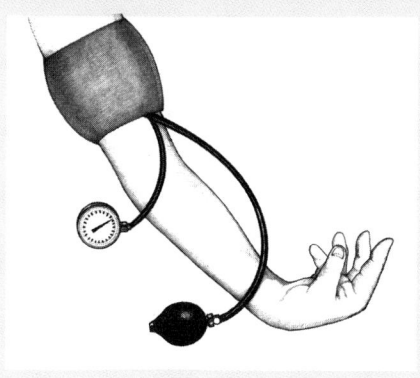

Monitoring
○ Cardiac rhythm
○ Seizures
○ Calcium levels

Patient teaching

Be sure to cover:
○ proper administration of calcium supplements
○ the need to follow a high-calcium diet.

Discharge planning
○ Refer the patient to a dietitian and social services, if indicated.

Hypochloremia

Overview

Description

- Deficient serum levels of the chloride anion
- When serum chloride levels drop, levels of sodium, potassium, calcium, and other electrolytes may be affected
- When chloride levels decrease, bicarbonate levels rise to compensate

Pathophysiology

- Chloride accounts for two-thirds of all serum anions.
- Chloride is secreted by the stomach's mucosa as hydrochloric acid; it provides an acid medium that aids digestion and activation of enzymes.
- It participates in maintaining acid-base and body water balances, influences the osmolality or tonicity of extracellular fluid, plays a role in the exchange of oxygen and carbon dioxide in red blood cells, and helps activate salivary amylase (which, in turn, activates the digestive process).

Causes

- Untreated diabetic ketoacidosis
- Addison's disease
- Chloride-deficient formula (for infants)
- Salt-restricted diets
- Prolonged use of mercurial diuretics
- Administration of dextrose I.V. without electrolytes
- Prolonged diarrhea or diaphoresis
- Loss of hydrochloric acid in gastric secretions due to vomiting, gastric suctioning, or gastric surgery
- Certain drugs (see *Drugs causing hypochloremia*)

Risk factors

- Cystic fibrosis
- Pyloric obstruction
- Draining fistula
- Ileostomy
- Heart failure

Common characteristics

- Muscle weakness and twitching
- Muscle hypertonicity
- Tetany
- Shallow, depressed breathing (if metabolic alkalosis occurs)

Complications

- Respiratory arrest
- Seizures
- Coma

Assessment

History

- Risk factors for low chloride levels
- Agitation
- Irritability

Physical findings

- Muscle weakness
- Twitching
- Tetany
- Shallow, depressed breathing
- Hyperactive deep tendon reflexes
- Muscle cramps
- Cardiac arrhythmias

Test results

Laboratory
- Serum chloride level less than 98 mEq/L
- Serum sodium level below 135 mEq/L
- Supportive values in metabolic alkalosis:
  - Serum pH above 7.45
  - Serum carbon dioxide level above 32 mEq/L

Treatment

General

- Treatment of underlying condition
- High-sodium diet
- Activity, as tolerated
- Treatment of associated metabolic acidosis or electrolyte imbalances

Medication

- Normal saline I.V. solution
- Ammonium chloride
- Potassium chloride (for metabolic acidosis)

Drugs causing hypochloremia

These kinds of diuretics may cause hypochloremia:
- loop (such as furosemide)
- osmotic (such as mannitol)
- thiazide (such as hydrochlorothiazide).

Dietary sources of chloride

These foods provide chloride:
- fruits
- vegetables
- table salt
- salty foods
- processed meats
- canned vegetables.

Nursing considerations

Key outcomes

The patient will:
○ maintain adequate cardiac output
○ maintain stable vital signs
○ maintain adequate fluid volume
○ avoid complications.

Nursing interventions

○ Offer foods high in chloride. (See *Dietary sources of chloride.*)
○ Provide environmental safety.
○ Give prescribed I.V. fluids and drugs.

Monitoring

○ Level of consciousness
○ Muscle strength and movement
○ Cardiac rhythm
○ Arterial blood gas levels
○ Serum electrolyte levels
○ Respiratory status
○ Signs of metabolic alkalosis

Patient teaching

Be sure to cover:
○ the disorder, diagnosis, and treatment
○ signs and symptoms of electrolyte imbalance
○ dietary supplements
○ prescribed drugs.

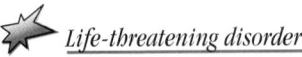 *Life-threatening disorder*

Hypokalemia

Overview

Description

○ Deficient serum levels of the potassium anion
○ Normal range for a serum potassium level narrow (3.5 to 5 mEq/L); a slight decrease can have a profound consequence

Pathophysiology

○ Potassium facilitates contraction of both skeletal and smooth muscles, including myocardial contraction.
○ Potassium figures prominently in nerve impulse conduction, acid-base balance, enzyme action, and cell membrane function.
○ A slight deviation in serum levels can produce profound clinical consequences.
○ Potassium imbalance can lead to muscle weakness and flaccid paralysis because of an ionic imbalance in neuromuscular tissue excitability.

Causes

○ Excessive GI or urinary losses, such as vomiting, gastric suction, diarrhea, dehydration, anorexia, or chronic laxative abuse
○ Trauma (injury, burns, or surgery)
○ Chronic renal disease, with tubular potassium wasting
○ Certain drugs, especially potassium-wasting diuretics, steroids, and certain sodium-containing antibiotics (carbenicillin) (see *Drugs causing hypokalemia*)
○ Acid-base imbalances
○ Prolonged potassium-free I.V. therapy
○ Hyperglycemia
○ Cushing's syndrome
○ Primary hyperaldosteronism
○ Excessive ingestion of licorice
○ Severe serum magnesium deficiency
○ Low-potassium diet

Drugs causing hypokalemia

These drugs can deplete potassium and cause hypokalemia:
○ adrenergics, such as albuterol and epinephrine
○ antibiotics, such as amphotericin B, carbenicillin, and gentamicin
○ cisplatin
○ corticosteroids
○ diuretics, such as furosemide and thiazide
○ insulin
○ laxatives (when used excessively).

Incidence

○ Affects up to 20% of hospitalized patients (significant in only about 4% to 5% of these patients)
○ Affects up to 14% of outpatients mildly
○ Approximately 80% of patients who receive diuretics become hypokalemic
○ Males and females affected equally

Common characteristics

See *Clinical effects of hypokalemia.*

Complications

○ Cardiac arrhythmia
○ Cardiac arrest
○ Rhabdomyolysis

Assessment

History

○ Muscle weakness
○ Paresthesia
○ Abdominal cramps
○ Anorexia
○ Nausea, vomiting
○ Constipation
○ Polyuria

Physical findings

○ Hyporeflexia
○ Weak, irregular pulse
○ Orthostatic hypotension
○ Decreased bowel sounds

Clinical effects of hypokalemia

Dysfunction	Effects
Acid-base balance	● Metabolic alkalosis
Cardiovascular	● Dizziness, hypotension, arrhythmias, electrocardiogram changes (flattened T waves, elevated U waves, decreased ST segments), cardiac arrest (with levels < 2.5 mEq/L)
Gastrointestinal	● Nausea, vomiting, anorexia, diarrhea, abdominal distention, paralytic ileus or decreased peristalsis
Genitourinary	● Polyuria
Musculoskeletal	● Muscle weakness and fatigue, leg cramps
Neurologic	● Malaise, irritability, confusion, mental depression, speech changes, decreased reflexes, respiratory paralysis

Test results

Laboratory
- Serum potassium levels less than 3.5 mEq/L
- Elevated pH and bicarbonate levels
- Slightly elevated serum glucose level

Diagnostic procedures
- Characteristic ECG changes — flattened T wave, depressed ST segment and U wave

Treatment

General

- Treatment of the underlying cause
- High-potassium diet
- Activity, as tolerated

Medication

- Potassium chloride (I.V. or orally)

 Alert

A patient taking a diuretic may be switched to a potassium-sparing diuretic to prevent excessive urinary loss of potassium.

Nursing considerations

Key outcomes

The patient will:
- maintain hemodynamic stability
- maintain a normal potassium level
- understand potential adverse effects of medications
- express understanding of high-potassium foods.

Nursing interventions

- Give prescribed drugs.
- Insert an indwelling urinary catheter.
- Implement safety measures.
- Be alert for signs of hyperkalemia after treatment.
- Administer I.V. fluids.

Monitoring

- Serum potassium levels
- Cardiac rhythm
- Intake and output
- Vital signs
- Respiratory status

 Alert

A patient taking a cardiac glycoside, especially if he's also taking a diuretic, should be monitored closely for hypokalemia, which can potentiate the action of the cardiac glycoside and cause toxicity.

Patient teaching

Be sure to cover:
- the disorder and treatment
- prescribed drugs and potential adverse effects
- monitoring intake and output
- preventing future episodes of hypokalemia
- need for a high-potassium diet
- warning signs and symptoms to report to the physician.

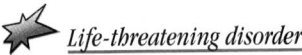 *Life-threatening disorder*

Hypomagnesemia

Overview

Description

○ Deficient serum levels of the magnesium cation
○ Relatively common imbalance

Pathophysiology

○ Magnesium enhances neuromuscular integration and stimulates parathyroid hormone secretion, thus regulating intracellular fluid calcium levels.
○ Magnesium may also regulate skeletal muscles through its influence on calcium utilization by depressing acetylcholine release at synaptic junctions.
○ It activates many enzymes for proper carbohydrate and protein metabolism, aids in cell metabolism and the transport of sodium and potassium across cell membranes, and influences sodium, potassium, calcium, and protein levels.
○ Approximately one-third of magnesium taken into the body is absorbed through the small intestine and is eventually excreted in the urine; the remaining unabsorbed magnesium is excreted in the stool.

Causes

○ Malabsorption syndrome
○ Chronic diarrhea
○ Postoperative complications after bowel resection
○ Chronic alcoholism
○ Prolonged diuretic therapy
○ Nasogastric suctioning
○ Administration of parenteral fluids without magnesium salts
○ Starvation or malnutrition
○ Severe dehydration
○ Diabetic acidosis
○ Hyperaldosteronism
○ Hypoparathyroidism

○ Hyperparathyroidism
○ Hypercalcemia
○ Excessive release of adrenocortical hormones
○ Certain drugs (see *Drugs causing hypomagnesemia*)

Risk factors

○ Sepsis
○ Serious burns
○ Wounds requiring debridement

Incidence

○ Occurs in 10% to 20% of hospitalized patients (50 to 60% of patients in the intensive care unit)
○ Occurs in 25% of outpatients with diabetes
○ Occurs in 30% to 80% of alcoholics
○ Affects males and females equally

Common characteristics

See *Clinical effects of hypomagnesemia.*

Complications

○ Laryngeal stridor
○ Seizures
○ Respiratory depression
○ Cardiac arrhythmia
○ Cardiac arrest

Assessment

History

○ Dysphagia
○ Nausea
○ Vomiting
○ Drowsiness
○ Confusion
○ Leg and foot cramps

Physical findings

○ Tachycardia
○ Hypertension
○ Muscle weakness, tremors, twitching
○ Hyperactive deep tendon reflexes
○ Chvostek's and Trousseau's signs
○ Cardiac arrhythmia

Drugs causing hypomagnesemia

Monitor your patient's magnesium level if he's taking any of these drugs that can cause or contribute to hypomagnesemia:

○ aminoglycoside antibiotic, such as amikacin, gentamicin, streptomycin, or tobramycin
○ amphotericin B
○ cisplatin
○ cyclosporine
○ insulin
○ laxative
○ loop or thiazide diuretic, such as bumetanide, furosemide, or torsemide
○ pentamidine isethionate.

Clinical effects of hypomagnesemia

Dysfunction	Effects
Cardiovascular	● Arrhythmias, vasomotor changes (vasodilation and hypotension) and, occasionally, hypertension
Neurologic	● Confusion, delusions, hallucinations, seizures
Neuromuscular	● Hyperirritability, tetany, leg and foot cramps, Chvostek's sign (facial muscle spasms induced by tapping the branches of the facial nerve)

Test results

Laboratory
- Serum magnesium levels less than 1.5 mEq/L
- Other electrolyte abnormalities, such as below normal serum potassium or calcium level

Diagnostic procedures
- Electrocardiogram shows abnormalities, such as prolonged QT interval and atrioventricular block.

Treatment

General
- Treatment of the underlying cause
- Dietary replacement of magnesium
- Activity, as tolerated

Medication
- Magnesium oxide
- Magnesium sulfate (I.M. or I.V.)

Nursing considerations

Key outcomes
The patient will:
- maintain hemodynamic stability
- maintain a normal magnesium level
- understand the causes of high magnesium levels.

Nursing interventions
- Institute seizure precautions.
- Give prescribed drugs.
- Report abnormal serum electrolyte levels immediately.

 Alert

A low magnesium level may increase the body's retention of a cardiac glycoside. Be alert for signs of digoxin toxicity if your patient is taking digoxin.

- Ensure patient safety.
- Reorient the patient as needed.

Monitoring
- Vital signs
- Magnesium levels
- Electrolyte levels
- Intake and output
- Cardiac rhythm
- Level of consciousness
- Respiratory status

Patient teaching

Be sure to cover:
- the disorder and treatment
- prescribed drugs

- avoidance of drugs that deplete magnesium, such as diuretics and laxatives
- the need to adhere to a high-magnesium diet
- danger signs and when to report them.

Discharge planning
- Refer the patient to Alcoholics Anonymous if appropriate.

Hyponatremia

Overview

Description

○ Deficient serum levels of the sodium cation in relation to body water

Pathophysiology

○ Sodium is the major cation (90%) in extracellular fluid; potassium, the major cation in intracellular fluid.
○ During repolarization, the sodium-potassium pump continually shifts sodium into the cells and potassium out of the cells; during depolarization, it does the reverse.
○ Sodium cation functions include maintaining tonicity and concentration of extracellular fluid, acid-base balance (reabsorption of sodium ion and excretion of hydrogen ion), nerve conduction and neuromuscular function, glandular secretion, and water balance.

Causes

○ Vomiting
○ Suctioning
○ Diarrhea
○ Excessive perspiration or fever
○ Use of potent diuretics
○ Tap water enemas
○ Excessive water intake
○ Infusion of I.V. dextrose in water without other solutes
○ Malnutrition or starvation
○ Low-sodium diet, usually in combination with one of the other causes
○ Trauma, surgery (wound drainage), or burns
○ Adrenal gland insufficiency (Addison's disease) or hypoaldosteronism
○ Cirrhosis of the liver with ascites
○ Syndrome of inappropriate antidiuretic hormone (SIADH), resulting from brain tumor, stroke, pulmonary disease, or neoplasm with ectopic ADH production
○ Certain drugs, such as chlorpropamide and clofibrate (see *Drugs causing hyponatremia*)

Incidence

○ Occurs in about 1% of hospitalized patients
○ More common in the very young and very old
○ Affects males and females equally

Common characteristics

○ Pulmonary edema
○ Circulatory disorders
○ Decreased level of consciousness (see *Clinical effects of hyponatremia*)

Complications

○ Seizures
○ Coma
○ Permanent neurologic damage

Assessment

History

○ Altered level of consciousness
○ Nausea
○ Headache
○ Muscle weakness
○ Abdominal cramps

Physical findings

○ Orthostatic hypotension
○ Dry mucous membranes
○ Poor skin turgor
○ Rapid, bounding pulse
○ Muscle twitching

Drugs causing hyponatremia

Drugs can contribute to the development of hyponatremia by potentiating the action of antidiuretic hormone, by causing syndrome of inappropriate antidiuretic hormone secretion, or by inhibiting sodium reabsorption in the kidney (diuretics).

Anticonvulsants
○ carbamazepine
Antidiabetics
○ chlorpropamide
○ tolbutamide (rarely)
Antineoplastics
○ cyclophosphamide
○ vincristine
Antipsychotics
○ fluphenazine
○ thioridazine
○ thiothixene

Diuretics
○ bumetanide
○ ethacrynic acid
○ furosemide
○ thiazides
Sedatives
○ barbiturates
○ morphine

Clinical effects of hyponatremia

Dysfunction	Effects
Cardiovascular	● Hypotension; tachycardia; with severe deficit, vasomotor collapse, thready pulse
Cutaneous	● Cold, clammy skin; decreasing skin turgor
Gastrointestinal	● Nausea, vomiting, abdominal cramps
Genitourinary	● Oliguria or anuria
Neurologic	● Anxiety, headaches, muscle twitching and weakness, seizures
Respiratory	● Cyanosis with severe deficiency

Test results

Laboratory

- Serum sodium level lower than 135 mEq/L
- Urine specific gravity less than 1.010
- Serum osmolality less than 280 mOsm/kg (dilute blood)
- Increased urine specific gravity and elevated urine sodium (0.20 mEq/L) in patients with SIADH

Treatment

General

- Treatment of the underlying cause
- Restricted fluid intake
- High-sodium diet
- Activity, as tolerated

Medication

- Oral sodium supplements
- Demeclocycline or lithium
- Administration of normal saline solution
- Hypertonic (3% or 5%) saline solutions (with serum sodium levels below 110 mEq/L)

Nursing considerations

Key outcomes

The patient will:
- maintain adequate fluid volume
- maintain a normal sodium level
- maintain stable vital signs
- remain alert and oriented to his environment.

Nursing interventions

- Restrict fluid intake.
- Give prescribed I.V. fluids.
- Provide a safe environment.

Monitoring

- Vital signs
- Serum sodium levels
- Urine specific gravity
- Intake and output
- Neurologic status

Patient teaching

Be sure to cover:
- the disorder and treatment
- drug therapy and possible adverse effects
- dietary changes and fluid restrictions
- monitoring daily weight
- signs and symptoms to report to the physician.

Hypoparathyroidism

Overview

Description

- Deficiency in parathyroid hormone (PTH) secretion by the parathyroid glands or the decreased action of PTH in the periphery
- Because parathyroid glands primarily regulate calcium balance, neuromuscular symptoms range from paresthesia to tetany
- May be acute or chronic
- Classified as idiopathic, acquired, or reversible

Pathophysiology

- PTH normally maintains serum calcium levels by increasing bone resorption and by stimulating renal conversion of vitamin D to its active form, which enhances GI absorption of calcium and bone resorption.
- PTH also maintains the inverse relationship between serum calcium and phosphate levels by inhibiting phosphate reabsorption in the renal tubules and enhancing calcium reabsorption.
- Abnormal PTH production in hypoparathyroidism disrupts this delicate balance.

Causes

- Autoimmune genetic disorder
- Congenital absence or malformation of the parathyroid glands
- Accidental removal of or injury to one or more parathyroid glands during surgery
- Ischemia or infarction of the parathyroid glands during surgery
- Hemochromatosis
- Sarcoidosis
- Amyloidosis
- Tuberculosis
- Neoplasms
- Trauma
- Massive thyroid irradiation
- Hypomagnesemia-induced impairment of hormone secretion
- Suppression of normal gland function due to hypercalcemia
- Delayed maturation of parathyroid function
- Abnormalities of the calcium-sensor receptor

Incidence

- Idiopathic and reversible forms most common in children
- Acquired form most common in older patients who have undergone thyroid gland surgery

Common characteristics

- Muscle spasms
- Hyperreflexia
- Neuromuscular excitability

Complications

- Heart failure
- Cataracts
- Tetany
- Increased intracranial pressure
- Irreversible calcification of basal ganglia
- Bone deformities
- Laryngospasm, respiratory stridor, anoxia
- Vocal cord paralysis
- Seizures
- Death

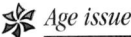 *Age issue*

Hypoparathyroidism that develops during childhood results in malformed teeth.

Assessment

History

- Neck surgery or irradiation
- Malabsorption disorders
- Alcoholism
- Tingling in the fingertips, around the mouth and, occasionally, in the feet
- Muscle tension and spasms
- Feeling like throat is constricted
- Dysphagia
- Difficulty walking and a tendency to fall
- Nausea, vomiting, abdominal pain
- Constipation or diarrhea
- Personality changes
- Fatigue

Physical findings

- Brittle nails
- Dry skin
- Coarse hair, alopecia
- Transverse and longitudinal ridges in the fingernails
- Loss of eyelashes and fingernails
- Stained, cracked, and decayed teeth
- Tetany
- Positive Chvostek's and Trousseau's signs
- Increased deep tendon reflexes
- Irregular, slow or rapid pulse

Test results

Laboratory
- Radioimmunoassay for PTH decreased
- Serum and urine calcium levels decreased
- Serum phosphate levels increased
- Urine creatinine levels decreased

Imaging
○ Computed tomography scan may show frontal lobe and basal ganglia calcifications.
○ X-rays may show increased bone density and bone malformation.
Diagnostic procedures
○ Electrocardiogram shows a prolonged QT interval.

Treatment

General
○ To restore the calcium and associated mineral balance within the body
○ Supportive care necessary for an acute, life-threatening attack or hypoparathyroid tetany
○ High-calcium, low-phosphorus diet
○ Activity, as tolerated

Medication
○ Vitamin D
○ Supplemental calcium
○ Calcitriol
Acute, life-threatening tetany
○ I.V. administration of 10% calcium gluconate, 10% calcium glucepate, or 10% calcium chloride
○ Sedatives
○ Anticonvulsants

Surgery
○ To treat underlying cause such as tumor

Nursing considerations

Key outcomes
The patient will:
○ maintain normal cardiac output
○ maintain stable vital signs
○ maintain adequate ventilation
○ maintain intact skin integrity
○ verbalize an understanding of the disorder and treatment regimen.

Nursing interventions
○ Give prescribed drugs.
○ Maintain a patent I.V. line.
○ Keep emergency equipment readily available.
○ Maintain seizure precautions.
○ Provide meticulous skin care.
○ Institute safety precautions.
○ Encourage the patient to express his feelings.
○ Offer emotional support.
○ Help the patient develop effective coping strategies.

Monitoring
○ Vital signs
○ Intake and output
○ Serum calcium and phosphorus levels

○ Electrocardiogram for QT interval changes and arrhythmias
○ Signs and symptoms of decreased cardiac output
○ Chvostek's sign
○ Trousseau's sign

 Alert

Closely monitor the patient receiving digoxin and calcium because calcium potentiates the effect of digoxin. Stay alert for signs of digoxin toxicity.

Patient teaching

Be sure to cover:
○ the disorder, diagnosis, and treatment
○ prescribed drugs and potential adverse effects
○ when to notify the physician
○ follow-up care
○ complications
○ periodic checks of serum calcium levels.

Discharge planning
○ Refer the patient to a mental health professional for additional counseling, if necessary.

Hypophosphatemia

Overview

Description

○ Deficient serum phosphate levels

Pathophysiology

○ Phosphorus exists primarily in inorganic combination with calcium in teeth and bones.
○ In extracellular fluid, the phosphate ion supports several metabolic functions: utilization of B vitamins, acid-base homeostasis, bone formation, nerve and muscle activity, cell division, transmission of hereditary traits, and metabolism of carbohydrates, proteins, and fats.
○ Renal tubular reabsorption of phosphate is inversely regulated by calcium levels — an increase in phosphorus causes a decrease in calcium. An imbalance causes hypophosphatemia or hyperphosphatemia.

Causes

○ Inadequate dietary intake
○ Often related to malnutrition resulting from a prolonged catabolic state or chronic alcoholism
○ Intestinal malabsorption
○ Chronic diarrhea
○ Hyperparathyroidism with resultant hypercalcemia
○ Hypomagnesemia
○ Vitamin D deficiency
○ Chronic use of antacids containing aluminum hydroxide
○ Use of parenteral nutrition solution with inadequate phosphate content
○ Renal tubular defects
○ Tissue damage in which phosphorus is released by injured cells
○ Diabetic acidosis

Incidence

○ Varies according to the underlying cause

Common characteristics

○ Anorexia
○ Muscle weakness
○ Tremor
○ Paresthesia
○ Osteomalacia (when persistent)
○ Peripheral hypoxia

Complications

○ Heart failure
○ Shock
○ Arrhythmias
○ Rhabdomyolysis
○ Seizures
○ Coma

Assessment

History

○ Anorexia
○ Memory loss
○ Muscle and bone pain
○ Fractures
○ Chest pain

Physical findings

○ Tremor and weakness in speaking voice
○ Confusion
○ Bruising and bleeding

Test results

○ Serum phosphorus levels less than 2.5 mg/dl

Treatment

General

○ Treatment of the underlying cause
○ Discontinuation of drugs that may cause hypophosphatemia (see *Drugs that may cause hypophosphatemia*)
○ High-phosphorus diet
○ Activity, as tolerated

Medication

○ Phosphate salt tablets or capsules
○ Potassium phosphate I.V.

Nursing considerations

Key outcomes

The patient will:
○ maintain a patent airway
○ maintain adequate vital signs
○ maintain a normal phosphorus level.

Nursing interventions

○ Provide safety measures.
○ Give prescribed phosphorus replacement.
○ Assist with ambulation and activities of daily living.

Drugs that may cause hypophosphatemia

The following drugs may cause hypophosphatemia:
○ acetazolamide, thiazide diuretics (chlorothiazide and hydrochlorothiazide), loop diuretics (bumetanide and furosemide), and other diuretics
○ antacids, such as aluminum carbonate, aluminum hydroxide, calcium carbonate, and magnesium oxide
○ insulin
○ laxatives.

Monitoring
○ Respiratory status
○ Neurologic status
○ Phosphorus and calcium levels
○ Intake and output

Patient teaching

Be sure to cover:
○ proper administration of phosphorus supplements
○ the need to adhere to a high-phosphorus diet. (See *Foods high in phosphorus,* page 395.)

Discharge planning
○ Refer the patient to a dietitian and social services, if indicated.

Hypopituitarism

Overview

Description

- Partial or complete failure of the anterior pituitary gland to produce its vital hormones: corticotropin, thyroid-stimulating hormone (TSH), luteinizing hormone (LH), follicle-stimulating hormone (FSH), growth hormone (GH), and prolactin
- May be primary or secondary, resulting from dysfunction of the hypothalamus
- Development of clinical features typically slow and not apparent until 75% of the pituitary gland is destroyed
- Total loss of all hormones fatal without treatment
- Prognosis good with adequate replacement therapy and correction of the underlying causes
- Panhypopituitarism: absence of all hormones

Pathophysiology

- The pituitary gland is extremely vulnerable to ischemia and infarction because it's highly vascular.
- Any event that leads to circulatory collapse and compensatory vasospasm may result in gland ischemia, tissue necrosis, or edema.
- Expansion of the pituitary within the fixed compartment of the sella turcica further impedes blood supply to the pituitary.

Causes

- Tumor
- Congenital defects
- Pituitary gland hypoplasia or aplasia
- Pituitary infarction
- Partial or total hypophysectomy by surgery, irradiation, or chemical agents
- Granulomatous disease
- Deficiency of hypothalamus releasing hormones
- Idiopathic
- Infection
- Trauma

Incidence

- Relatively rare
- Occurs in adults and children
- Affects males and females equally

Common characteristics

- Metabolic dysfunction
- Sexual immaturity
- Growth retardation
- Fatigue

Complications

- Any combination of deficits in the production of the six major hormones
- GH deficiency
- TSH deficiency
- Corticotropin deficiency
- Gonadotropin and prolactin deficiency
- Pituitary apoplexy (a medical emergency)
- High fever, shock, coma, and death
- Diabetes insipidus

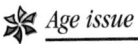 Age issue

In children, hypopituitarism can cause dwarfism and pubertal delay.

Assessment

History

- Signs and symptoms depend on which pituitary hormones are deficient, patient's age, and severity of disorder.

Gonadotropin (FSH and LH) deficiency in women
- Amenorrhea
- Dyspareunia
- Infertility
- Reduced libido

Gonadotropin (FSH and LH) deficiency in men
- Impotence
- Reduced libido

TSH deficiency
- Cold intolerance
- Constipation
- Menstrual irregularity
- Lethargy
- Severe growth retardation in children despite treatment

Corticotropin deficiency
- Fatigue
- Nausea, vomiting, anorexia
- Weight loss

Prolactin deficiency
- Absent postpartum lactation
- Amenorrhea

Physical findings

GH deficiency
- Physical signs possibly not apparent in neonate
- Growth retardation usually apparent at age 6 months
  In children:
- Chubbiness from fat deposits in the lower trunk
- Short stature
- Delayed secondary tooth eruption
- Delayed puberty
- Average height of 4′ (1.2 m), with normal proportions
- More subtle signs in adults (fine wrinkles near the mouth and eyes)

Gonadotropin (FSH and LH) deficiency in women
- Breast atrophy
- Sparse or absent axillary and pubic hair
- Dry skin

Gonadotropin (FSH and LH) deficiency in men
○ Decreased muscle strength
○ Testicular softening and shrinkage
○ Retarded secondary sexual hair growth

TSH deficiency
○ Dry, pale, puffy skin
○ Slow thought processes
○ Bradycardia

Corticotropin deficiency
○ Depigmentation of skin and nipples
○ Hypothermia and hypotension during periods of stress

Prolactin deficiency
○ Sparse or absent growth of pubic and axillary hair

Panhypopituitarism
○ Mental abnormalities, including lethargy and psychosis
○ Physical abnormalities, including orthostatic hypotension and bradycardia

Test results

Laboratory
○ Serum thyroxin levels decreased in diminished thyroid gland function due to lack of TSH
○ Radioimmunoassay showing decreased plasma levels of some or all of the pituitary hormones
○ Increased prolactin levels possibly indicating a lesion in the hypothalamus or pituitary stalk

Imaging
○ CT scans, magnetic resonance imaging, or cerebral angiography may show the presence of intrasellar or extrasellar tumors.

Other
○ Oral administration of metyrapone may show the source of low hydroxycorticosteroid levels.
○ Insulin administration shows low levels of corticotropin, indicating pituitary or hypothalamic failure.
○ Dopamine antagonist administration evaluates prolactin secretory reserve.
○ I.V. administration of gonadotropin-releasing hormone may distinguish pituitary and hypothalamic causes of gonadotropin deficiency.
○ Provocative testing shows persistently low GH and insulin-like growth factor-1 levels, confirming GH deficiency.

Treatment

General
○ If caused by a lesion or tumor, removal, radiation, or both, followed by possible lifelong hormone replacement therapy
○ Endocrine substitution therapy for affected organs
○ High-calorie, high-protein diet
○ Regular exercise program
○ Rest periods for fatigue

Medication
○ Hormone replacement

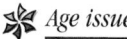 *Age issue*

Children with hypopituitarism may also need adrenal and thyroid hormone replacement and, as they approach puberty, sex hormones.

Surgery
○ For pituitary tumor

Nursing considerations

Key outcomes
The patient will:
○ maintain body weight
○ maintain normal body temperature
○ demonstrate age-appropriate skills and behavior to the extent possible
○ verbalize feelings of positive self-esteem.

Nursing interventions
○ Give prescribed drugs.
○ Encourage maintenance of adequate calorie intake.
○ Offer small, frequent meals.
○ Keep the patient warm.
○ Institute safety precautions.
○ Provide emotional support.
○ Encourage the patient to express his feelings.

Monitoring
○ Laboratory tests for hormonal deficiencies
○ Calorie intake
○ Daily weight
○ Vital signs
○ Neurologic status
○ Signs and symptoms of pituitary apoplexy, a medical emergency
○ Signs and symptoms of hypoglycemia

Patient teaching

Be sure to cover:
○ the disorder, diagnosis, and treatment
○ long-term hormonal replacement therapy and adverse reactions
○ when to notify the physician
○ regular follow-up appointments
○ energy-conservation techniques
○ the need for adequate rest
○ the need for a balanced diet.

Discharge planning
○ Refer the parents for psychological counseling or to community resources.

Hypothyroidism

Overview

Description

- Clinical condition characterized by either decreased circulating levels of or resistance to free thyroid hormone (TH)
- Classified as primary or secondary
- Severe hypothyroidism known as myxedema

Pathophysiology

- In primary hypothyroidism, a decrease in TH production is a result of the loss of thyroid tissue.
- This results in an increased secretion of thyroid-stimulating hormone (TSH) that leads to a goiter.
- In secondary hypothyroidism, the pituitary typically fails to synthesize or secrete adequate amounts of TSH, or target tissues fail to respond to normal blood levels of TH.
- Either type may progress to myxedema, which is clinically more severe and considered a medical emergency.

Causes

- Autoimmune thyroiditis (Hashimoto's) (most common cause)
- Thyroid gland surgery
- Radioactive iodine therapy
- Inflammatory conditions
- Endemic iodine deficiency
- Antithyroid drugs
- Congenital defects
- Amyloidosis
- Sarcoidosis
- External radiation to the neck
- Drugs, such as iodides and lithium
- Pituitary failure to produce TSH
- Hypothalamic failure to produce thyrotropin-releasing hormone
- Postpartum pituitary necrosis
- Pituitary tumor
- Idiopathic

Incidence

- Most prevalent in women
- In the United States, increased incidence in people older than age 40

Common characteristics

- Decreased energy metabolism
- Decreased heat production

Complications

Cardiovascular complications
- Hypercholesterolemia
- Arteriosclerosis
- Ischemic heart disease
- Peripheral vascular disease
- Cardiomegaly
- Heart failure
- Pleural and pericardial effusion

GI complications
- Achlorhydria
- Anemia
- Dynamic colon
- Megacolon
- Intestinal obstruction
- Bleeding tendencies

Other complications
- Conductive or sensorineural deafness
- Psychiatric disturbances
- Carpal tunnel syndrome
- Benign intracranial hypertension
- Impaired fertility
- Myxedema coma

Assessment

History

- Vague and varied symptoms that developed slowly over time
- Energy loss, fatigue
- Forgetfulness
- Sensitivity to cold
- Unexplained weight gain
- Constipation
- Anorexia
- Decreased libido
- Menorrhagia
- Paresthesia
- Joint stiffness
- Muscle cramping

Physical findings

- Slight mental slowing to severe obtundation
- Thick, dry tongue
- Hoarseness; slow, slurred speech
- Dry, flaky, inelastic skin
- Puffy face, hands, and feet
- Periorbital edema; drooping upper eyelids
- Dry, sparse hair with patchy hair loss
- Loss of outer third of eyebrow
- Thick, brittle nails with transverse and longitudinal grooves
- Ataxia, intention tremor; nystagmus
- Doughy skin that feels cool
- Weak pulse and bradycardia
- Muscle weakness
- Sacral or peripheral edema
- Delayed reflex relaxation time
- Possible goiter
- Absent or decreased bowel sounds
- Hypotension
- A gallop or distant heart sounds
- Adventitious breath sounds
- Abdominal distention or ascites

Test results

Laboratory

○ Radioimmunoassay showing decreased serum levels of T_3 and T_4
○ Serum TSH level increased with thyroid insufficiency; decreased with hypothalamic or pituitary insufficiency
○ Serum cholesterol, alkaline phosphatase, and triglycerides levels elevated
○ Serum electrolytes showing low serum sodium levels in myxedema coma
○ Arterial blood gases showing decreased pH and increased partial pressure of carbon dioxide in myxedema coma

Imaging

○ Skull X-rays, computed tomography scan, and magnetic resonance imaging may show pituitary or hypothalamic lesions.

Treatment

General

○ To restore and maintain a normal thyroid state
○ Need for long-term thyroid replacement
○ Low-fat, low-cholesterol, high-fiber, low-sodium diet
○ Possibly fluid restriction
○ Activity, as tolerated

Medication

○ Synthetic hormone levothyroxine
○ Synthetic liothyronine

Surgery

○ For underlying cause such as pituitary tumor

Nursing considerations

Key outcomes

The patient will:
○ maintain adequate cardiac output
○ maintain stable vital signs
○ demonstrate normal laboratory values
○ maintain balanced fluid volume status
○ consume adequate daily calorie requirements
○ express positive feelings about self.

Nursing interventions

○ Give prescribed drugs.
○ Provide adequate rest periods.
○ Apply antiembolism stockings.
○ Encourage coughing and deep-breathing exercises.
○ Maintain fluid restrictions and a low-salt diet.
○ Provide a high-bulk, low-calorie diet.
○ Reorient the patient, as needed.
○ Offer support and encouragement.
○ Provide meticulous skin care.
○ Keep the patient warm, as needed.
○ Encourage the patient to express his feelings.
○ Help the patient develop effective coping strategies.

Monitoring

○ Vital signs
○ Intake and output
○ Daily weight
○ Cardiovascular status
○ Pulmonary status
○ Edema
○ Bowel sounds, abdominal distention, frequency of bowel movements
○ Mental and neurologic status
○ Signs and symptoms of hyperthyroidism

Patient teaching

Be sure to cover:
○ the disorder, diagnosis, and treatment
○ prescribed drugs and possible adverse effects
○ when to notify the physician
○ physical and mental changes
○ signs and symptoms of myxedema
○ the need for lifelong hormone replacement therapy
○ the need to wear a medical identification bracelet
○ the importance of keeping accurate records of daily weight
○ the need to adhere to a well-balanced, high-fiber, low-sodium diet
○ energy-conservation techniques.

Discharge planning

○ Refer the patient and family members to a mental health professional for additional counseling, if needed.

Idiopathic thrombocytopenic purpura

Overview

Description

- A deficiency of platelets that occurs when the immune system destroys the body's own platelets
- May be acute, as in postviral thrombocytopenia, or chronic, as in essential thrombocytopenia or autoimmune thrombocytopenia
- Excellent prognosis for acute form; nearly four of five patients recover without treatment
- Good prognosis for chronic form; remissions commonly lasting weeks or years, especially among women

Pathophysiology

- Circulating immunoglobulin (Ig) G molecules react with host platelets, which are then destroyed in the spleen and, to a lesser degree, in the liver.
- Normally, the life span of platelets in circulation is 7 to 10 days. In idiopathic thrombocytopenic purpura (ITP), platelets survive 1 to 3 days or less.

Causes

- Viral infection
- Immunization with a live virus vaccine
- Immunologic disorders
- Drug reactions

Incidence

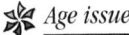 *Age issue*

Acute ITP usually affects children between ages 2 and 6; chronic ITP mainly affects adults younger than age 50, especially women between ages 20 and 40.

Common characteristics

- Epistaxis
- Bleeding gums
- Hemorrhages into the skin, mucous membranes, and other tissues causing red discoloration of skin (purpura)
- Small, purplish hemorrhagic spots on skin (petechiae)
- Excessive menstrual bleeding

Complications

- Hemorrhage
- Cerebral hemorrhage
- Purpuric lesions of vital organs (such as the brain and kidney)

Assessment

History

- Epistaxis
- Bleeding gums
- Menorrhagia
- Recent viral illness

Physical findings

- Petechiae or ecchymosis
- Bleeding into mucous membranes
- Splenomegaly

Test results

Laboratory
- Platelet count less than 20,000/µl
- Prolonged bleeding time
- Abnormal size and appearance of platelets
- Decreased hemoglobin level (if bleeding occurred)
- Bone marrow studies showing abundant megakaryocytes (platelet precursor cells) and a circulating platelet survival time of only several hours to a few days
- Humoral tests that measure platelet-associated IgG (half of all patients with ITP display elevated IgG levels)

Treatment

General

- Platelet replacement
- Rest periods between activities
- Complete bed rest during active bleeding
- Well-balanced diet

Medication

Acute
- Glucocorticoids to prevent further platelet destruction
- Ig to prevent platelet destruction
- Plasmapheresis
- Platelet pheresis

Chronic
- Vitamin K
- Corticosteroids

Surgery

- Splenectomy (when splenomegaly accompanies the initial thrombocytopenia)

Other

- Immunosuppressants to help stop platelet destruction
- High-dose I.V. immunoglobulin
- Immunoabsorption apheresis using staphylococcal protein A columns

Nursing considerations

Key outcomes

The patient will:
- demonstrate the use of protective measures, including conserving energy, maintaining a balanced diet, and getting plenty of rest
- demonstrate effective coping mechanisms
- express positive feelings about self.

Nursing interventions

- Give prescribed platelets.
- Provide emotional support.
- Protect all areas of petechia and ecchymoses from further injury.

Monitoring

- Signs of bleeding
- Platelet count
- Intake and output
- Vital signs

When receiving immunosuppressants
- Bone marrow depression
- Infection
- Mucositis
- GI ulcers
- Severe diarrhea or vomiting

Patient teaching

Be sure to cover:
- how to observe for petechiae, ecchymoses, and other signs of recurrence
- avoiding aspirin and ibuprofen
- avoiding straining during defecation and coughing.

Discharge planning

- Advise the patient to carry medical identification to alert others about the condition.

Impetigo

Overview

Description

- Contagious, superficial bacterial skin infection
- Nonbullous and bullous forms
- May complicate chickenpox, eczema, and other skin disorders marked by open lesions
- Most commonly appears on face, arms, and legs

Pathophysiology

Nonbullous impetigo
- Eruption occurs when bacteria inoculate traumatized skin cells.
- Lesions begin as small vesicles, which rapidly erode.
- Honey-colored crusts surrounded by erythema are formed.

Bullous impetigo
- Eruption occurs in nontraumatized skin via bacterial toxin or exotoxin.
- Lesions begin as thin-walled bullae and vesicles.
- Lesions contain clear to turbid yellow fluid; some crusting exists. (See *Recognizing impetigo.*)

Causes

- Bacterial infection
- Spread by autoinoculation through scratching

Recognizing impetigo

In impetigo, when the vesicles break, crust forms from the exudate. This infection is especially contagious among young children.

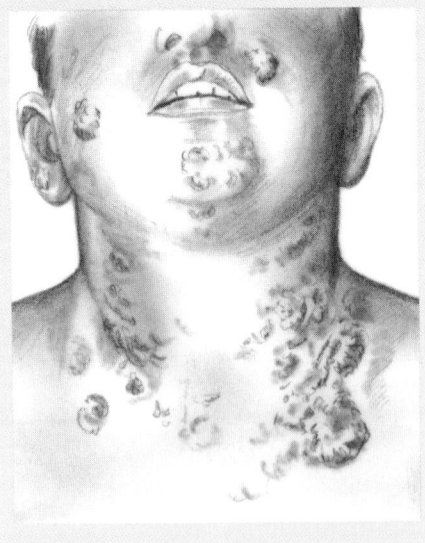

Risk factors

- Poor hygiene
- Untreated minor trauma
- Overcrowded living conditions
- Lesions of preexisting eczema, chickenpox, scabies
- Other skin rashes
- Anemia
- Malnutrition

Incidence

- Most common among infants, children, and young adults
- More common in warm ambient temperatures
- Predominant during late summer and early fall

Common characteristics

- Painlessness
- Tender red macule or papule
- Pustules

Complications

- Acute glomerulonephritis
- Ecthyma (see *Comparing ecthyma and impetigo*)
- Exfoliative eruption (staphylococcal scalded-skin syndrome)

Assessment

History

- Presence of risk factors
- Absence of pain
- Possible pruritus

Physical findings

Nonbullous impetigo
- Small, red macule or vesicle that becomes pustular within a few hours
- Characteristic thick, honey-colored crust formed from the exudate
- Satellite lesions caused by autoinoculation

Bullous impetigo
- Thin-walled vesicle
- Thin, clear crust formed from exudate
- Lesion that appears as a central clearing circumscribed by an outer rim

Test results

Laboratory
- Gram stain of vesicular fluid showing infecting organism
- Culture and sensitivity testing of exudate or denuded crust showing infecting organism
- Elevated white blood cell count

Treatment

General

○ Removal of exudate by washing lesions two to three times per day with soap and water
○ Warm soaks or compresses of normal saline solution or a diluted soap solution for stubborn crusts
○ Prevention by benzoyl peroxide soap

Medication

○ Antibiotics
○ Antihistamines

Nursing considerations

Key outcomes

The patient will:
○ exhibit improved or healed wounds or lesions
○ report feelings of increased comfort
○ demonstrate proper skin care regimen
○ verbalize feelings about changed body image.

Nursing interventions

○ Use meticulous hand-washing technique.
○ Follow standard precautions.
○ Remove crusts by gently washing with bactericidal soap and water.
○ Soften stubborn crusts with cool compresses.
○ Give prescribed drugs.
○ Encourage verbalization of feelings about body image.
○ Comply with local public health standards and guidelines.

Monitoring

○ Response to treatment
○ Adverse drug reactions
○ Complications

Patient teaching

Be sure to cover:
○ the disorder, diagnosis, and treatment
○ meticulous hand-washing technique
○ trimming fingernails short
○ regular bathing with bactericidal soap
○ avoiding sharing clothes and linens
○ identification of characteristic lesions
○ completion of prescribed medications
○ potential adverse reactions
○ lesion care.

Comparing ecthyma and impetigo

Ecthyma is a superficial skin infection that usually causes scarring. It generally results from infection by group A beta-hemolytic streptococci.

Ecthyma differs from impetigo in that its characteristic ulcer results from deeper penetration of the skin by the infecting organism (involving the lower epidermis and dermis), and the overlying crust tends to be raised (⅜″ to 1¼″) [1 to 3 cm]).

These lesions are usually found on the legs after a scratch or an insect bite. Autoinoculation can transmit ecthyma to other parts of the body, especially to sites that have been scratched open.

Therapy for ecthyma is basically the same as for impetigo, beginning with removal of the crust, but the patient's response may be slower. Parenteral antibiotics are also used.

Discharge planning

○ Encourage the patient to schedule follow-up appointments as recommended by his physician.

Infectious mononucleosis

Overview

Description

○ An acute infectious disease that causes fever, sore throat, and cervical lymphadenopathy

Pathophysiology

○ Virus enters and replicates in epithelial cells of the oropharynx and B cells of tonsillar tissue, causing alteration of shape and function of the infected cells.
○ Infected B cells activate cell-mediated immunity with proliferation of abnormal cytotoxic T cells in lymphoid tissues.
○ Lymphoproliferation stops when cytotoxic T cells are able to destroy infected B cells.

Causes

○ Epstein-Barr virus (EBV), a member of the herpes group
○ Spread by contact with oral secretions (kissing)
○ Also transmitted during bone marrow transplantation and blood transfusion

Incidence

○ Primarily affects young adults and children
○ Common and widespread in early childhood in developing countries and socioeconomically depressed populations

Common characteristics

○ Incubation period of about 4 to 6 weeks in young adults
○ Prodromal symptoms include headache, malaise, and profound fatigue
○ After 3 to 5 days, triad of symptoms including sore throat, cervical lymphadenopathy, and temperature fluctuations, with an evening peak of 101° to 102° F (38.3° to 38.9° C)

Complications

○ Splenic rupture
○ Aseptic meningitis
○ Encephalitis
○ Hemolytic anemia
○ Pericarditis
○ Guillain-Barré syndrome

Assessment

History

○ Contact with a person who has infectious mononucleosis
○ Headache
○ Malaise
○ Fatigue
○ Sore throat
○ Fever

Physical findings

○ Exudative tonsillitis, pharyngitis
○ Palatal petechiae
○ Periorbital edema
○ Maculopapular rash that resembles rubella
○ Cervical adenopathy; possible inguinal and axillary adenopathy
○ Splenomegaly, hepatomegaly, jaundice

Test results

Laboratory

○ Increased white blood cell (WBC) count 10,000 to 20,000/µl during the 2nd and 3rd weeks of illness; lymphocytes and monocytes account for 50% to 70% of the total WBC count; 10% of the lymphocytes are atypical
○ Fourfold increase in heterophil antibodies (agglutinins for sheep red blood cells) during the acute phase and at 3- to 4-week intervals
○ Antibodies to EBV and cellular antigens shown by indirect immunofluorescence
○ Abnormal liver function studies

Treatment

General

○ Essentially supportive
○ Nutritious diet
○ Soft food (with throat soreness)
○ Frequent rest periods
○ Avoidance of strenuous activity or contact sports until fully recovered

Medication

○ Aspirin or another salicylate
○ Steroids
○ Antibiotics

Surgery

○ Splenectomy for splenic rupture

Nursing considerations

Key outcomes

The patient will:
○ maintain temperature within normal limits
○ conserve energy while performing daily activities to tolerance level
○ identify factors that intensify pain and change behavior accordingly
○ express needs and communicate whether needs are met.

Nursing interventions

○ Give prescribed drugs.
○ Provide warm saline gargles for symptomatic relief of sore throat.
○ Provide adequate fluids and nutrition.
○ Plan care to provide frequent rest periods.

Monitoring

○ Response to treatment
○ Fatigue
○ Nutritional status
○ Liver function tests
○ Complications

Patient teaching

Be sure to cover:
○ the disorder, diagnosis, and treatment
○ expectation that convalescence may take several weeks
○ need for bed rest during the acute illness
○ explanation that there's a period of prolonged communicability (stress good hand washing and avoidance of salivary contamination)
○ benefits of bland foods, milk shakes, fruit juices, and broths to minimize throat discomfort.

Discharge planning

○ Refer the patient to an otolaryngologist for marked tonsillar swelling or a neurologist for a central nervous system complication.

Influenza

Overview

Description

○ An acute, highly contagious infection of the respiratory tract
○ Has capacity for antigenic variation (ability to mutate into different strains so that no immunologic resistance is present in those at risk)
○ Antigenic variation characterized as antigenic drift (minor changes that occur yearly or every few years) and antigenic shift (major changes that lead to pandemics)
○ Also called the *grippe* or the *flu*

Pathophysiology

○ The virus invades the epithelium of the respiratory tract, causing inflammation and desquamation.
○ After attaching to the host cell, viral ribonucleic acid enters the cell and uses host components to replicate its genetic material and protein, which are then assembled into new virus particles.
○ Newly produced viruses burst forth to invade other healthy cells.
○ Viral invasion destroys host cells, impairing respiratory defenses (especially mucociliary transport system) and predisposing the patient to secondary bacterial infection.

Causes

○ Type A, most prevalent and strikes annually with new serotypes causing epidemics every 3 years
○ Type B also annual but causes epidemics only every 4 to 6 years
○ Type C endemic and causes only sporadic cases
○ Infection transmitted by inhaling a respiratory droplet from an infected person or by indirect contact (drinking from a contaminated glass)

Incidence

○ Affects all age groups; highest incidence among school-age children
○ Greatest severity (may lead to death) in young children, elderly people, and those with chronic diseases
○ Occurs sporadically or in epidemics (usually during colder months) with peak within 2 to 3 weeks after initial cases and lasting 2 to 3 months

Common characteristics

○ After incubation period of 24 to 48 hours, flu symptoms appear
○ Sudden onset of chills, fever (101° to 104° F [38.3° to 40° C]), headache, malaise, myalgia (particularly in the back and limbs), photophobia, a nonproductive cough and, occasionally, laryngitis, hoarseness, rhinitis, and rhinorrhea

Complications

○ Pneumonia
○ Myositis
○ Exacerbation of chronic obstructive pulmonary disease
○ Reye's syndrome
○ Myocarditis
○ Pericarditis
○ Transverse myelitis
○ Encephalitis

Assessment

History

○ Usually, recent exposure (typically within 48 hours) to a person with influenza
○ Patient didn't receive influenza vaccine during the past season
○ Headache
○ Malaise
○ Myalgia
○ Fatigue, listlessness, weakness

Physical findings

○ Fever (usually higher in children)
○ Signs of croup, dry cough
○ Red, watery eyes; clear nasal discharge
○ Erythema of the nose and throat without exudate
○ Tachypnea, shortness of breath, cyanosis
○ With bacterial pneumonia, purulent or bloody sputum
○ Cervical adenopathy and tenderness
○ Breath sounds may be diminished in areas of consolidation

Test results

○ After an epidemic is confirmed, diagnosis requires only observation of clinical signs and symptoms.

Laboratory

○ Inoculation of chicken embryos with nasal secretions from infected patients showing influenza virus
○ Throat swabs, nasopharyngeal washes, or sputum culture showing isolation of the influenza virus
○ Immunodiagnostic techniques showing viral antigens in tissue culture or in exfoliated nasopharyngeal cells obtained by washings
○ Elevated leukocyte counts in secondary bacterial infection
○ Decreased leukocyte counts in overwhelming viral or bacterial infection

Treatment

General

○ Fluid and electrolyte replacements
○ Oxygen and assisted ventilation, if indicated
○ Increased fluid intake
○ Rest periods, as needed

Medication

○ Acetaminophen or aspirin
○ Guaifenesin or expectorant
○ Amantadine
○ Antibiotics

Nursing considerations

Key outcomes

The patient will:
○ report increased energy level
○ maintain a normal temperature
○ express feelings of increased comfort and relief from pain
○ maintain adequate fluid volume
○ maintain respiratory rate within 5 breaths/minute of baseline.

Nursing interventions

○ Give prescribed drugs.
○ Follow standard precautions.
○ Administer oxygen therapy, if warranted.

Monitoring

○ Temperature
○ Signs and symptoms of dehydration
○ Respiratory status
○ Response to treatment
○ Complications

Patient teaching

Be sure to cover:
○ the disorder, diagnosis, and treatment
○ mouthwash or warm saline gargles to ease sore throat
○ importance of increased fluids to prevent dehydration
○ warm bath or a heating pad to relieve myalgia
○ proper hand-washing technique and tissue disposal to prevent the virus from spreading
○ influenza immunization.

Inguinal hernia

Overview

Description

- Part of an internal organ that protrudes through an abnormal opening in the wall of the cavity that surrounds it
- The most common type of hernia (see *Common sites of hernia*)
- May be direct or indirect
- Also called ruptures

Pathophysiology

- In an inguinal hernia, the large or small intestine, omentum, or bladder protrudes into the inguinal canal.
- In an indirect hernia, abdominal viscera leave the abdomen through the inguinal ring and follow the spermatic cord (in males) or round ligament (in females); they emerge at the external ring and extend down into the inguinal canal, often into the scrotum or labia.
- In a direct inguinal hernia, instead of entering the canal through the internal ring, the hernia passes through the posterior inguinal wall, protrudes directly through the transverse fascia of the canal (in an area known as Hesselbach's triangle), and comes out at the external ring.

Causes

- Indirect — weakness in fascial margin of internal inguinal ring
- Direct — weakness in fascial floor of inguinal canal
- Either — weak abdominal muscles (caused by congenital malformation, trauma, or aging) or increased intra-abdominal pressure (caused by heavy lifting, pregnancy, obesity, or straining)

Incidence

- Indirect hernias are more common; they may develop at any age, are three times more common in males, and are especially prevalent in infants.

Identifying a hernia

Palpation of the inguinal area while the patient is performing Valsalva's maneuver confirms the diagnosis of inguinal hernia. To detect a hernia in a male patient, ask the patient to stand with his ipsilateral leg slightly flexed and his weight resting on the other leg. Insert an index finger into the lower part of the scrotum and invaginate the scrotal skin so the finger advances through the external inguinal ring to the internal ring (about ½" to 2" [1 to 5 cm] through the inguinal canal). Tell the patient to cough. If pressure is felt against the fingertip, an indirect hernia exists; if pressure is felt against the side of the finger, a direct hernia exists.

- Direct hernias occur more often in middle-aged and elderly people.

Common characteristics

- A lump appears over the herniated area when the patient stands or strains and disappears when the patient is supine.
- Tension on the herniated contents may cause a sharp, steady pain in the groin, which fades when the hernia is reduced.
- Strangulation produces severe pain and may lead to partial or complete bowel obstruction and intestinal necrosis.

Complications

- Strangulation
- Intestinal obstruction
- Infection (after surgery)

Assessment

History

- Sharp or "catching" pain when lifting or straining

Physical findings

- Obvious swelling or lump in the inguinal area (large hernia) (see *Identifying a hernia*)

Test results

Laboratory
- Elevated white blood cell count (with intestinal obstruction)

Other
- Physical examination

Treatment

General

- Manual reduction
- Truss
- Activity, as tolerated
- Nothing by mouth if surgery is necessary

Medication

- Analgesics
- Antibiotics
- Electrolyte replacement

Surgery

- Herniorrhaphy
- Hernioplasty
- Bowel resection (with strangulation or necrosis)

Nursing considerations

Key outcomes

The patient will:
- express feelings of increased comfort

There are four common sites of hernia: umbilical, incisional, inguinal, and femoral. Here are descriptions of each type with an illustration demonstrating where each type is located.

Umbilical

Umbilical hernia results from abnormal muscular structures around the umbilical cord. This hernia is quite common in neonates but also occurs in women who are obese or who have had several pregnancies. Because most umbilical hernias in infants close spontaneously, surgery is warranted only if the hernia persists for more than 4 or 5 years. Taping or binding the affected area or supporting it with a truss may relieve symptoms until the hernia closes. A severe congenital umbilical hernia, which allows the abdominal viscera to protrude outside the body, must be repaired immediately.

Incisional

Incisional (ventral) hernia develops at the site of previous surgery, usually along vertical incisions. This hernia may result from a weakness in the abdominal wall, caused by an infection, impaired wound healing, inadequate nutrition, extreme abdominal distention, or obesity. Palpation of an inci-

sional hernia may reveal several defects in the surgical scar. Effective repair requires pulling the layers of the abdominal wall together without creating tension or, if this isn't possible, the use of Teflon, Marlex mesh, or tantalum mesh to close the opening.

Inguinal

Inguinal hernia can be direct or indirect. An indirect inguinal hernia causes the abdominal viscera to protrude through the inguinal ring and follow the spermatic cord (in males) or round ligament (in females). A direct inguinal hernia results from a weakness in the fascial floor of the inguinal canal.

Femoral

Femoral hernia occurs where the femoral artery passes into the femoral canal. Typically, a fatty deposit within the femoral canal enlarges and eventually creates a hole big enough to accommodate part of the peritoneum and bladder. A femoral hernia appears as a swelling or bulge at the pulse point of the large femoral artery. It's usually a soft, pliable, reducible, nontender mass but commonly becomes incarcerated or strangulated.

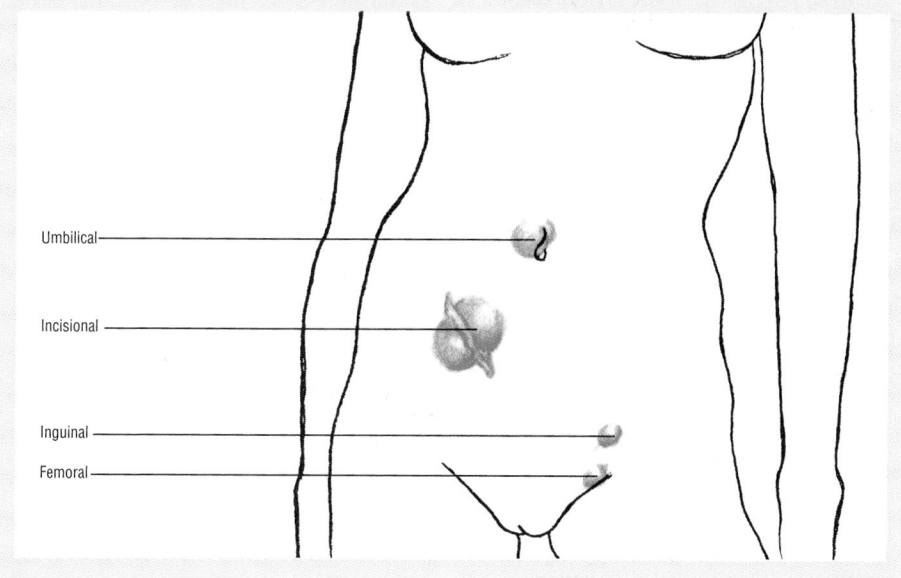

Umbilical

Incisional

Inguinal

Femoral

○ have normal bowel function
○ avoid complications.

Nursing interventions

○ Apply a truss after a hernia has been reduced.
○ Give prescribed drugs for pain.
○ Encourage coughing and deep breathing.

Monitoring

○ Vital signs
○ Pain control
○ Signs of strangulation or incarceration

Patient teaching

Be sure to cover:
○ avoiding lifting heavy objects or straining during bowel movements
○ signs and symptoms of infection (oozing, tenderness, warmth, and redness) at the incision site
○ wound care
○ after surgery, not resuming normal activity or returning to work without the surgeon's permission.

Discharge planning

○ Encourage the patient to schedule follow-up appointments as recommended by the surgeon.

Insect bites and stings

Overview

Description

○ Bite or sting from an insect or other arthropod, such as a tick, brown recluse spider, black widow spider, scorpion, bee, wasp, yellow jacket, or fire ant, that causes pain or a local systemic reaction

Pathophysiology

○ A bite or sting can injure the skin, and secretions released from a bite or sting can cause a physiologic response specific to the insect or arthropod.
○ Reactions to secretion exposure range from barely noticeable to life-threatening.
○ Transmission of disease may result from a bite or sting.
○ Mouth parts of an insect or arthropod are classified as piercing-sucking, sponging, or biting-chewing.

Causes

○ Toxic effects of venom
○ Hypersensitivity response

Incidence

○ Not known

Common characteristics

Local reaction
○ Mild discomfort to moderate or severe pain
○ Erythema and warmth
○ Tenderness
○ Edema of surrounding tissues
○ Severe local reaction
○ Generalized erythema
○ Urticaria
○ Pruritic edema
Systemic response
○ All of the above symptoms
○ Anxiety, disorientation
○ Weakness
○ GI disturbances
○ Dizziness
○ Hypotension
○ Stridor
○ Dyspnea and cough
○ Cardiovascular collapse

Complications

○ Anaphylaxis
○ Hemolytic anemia
○ Rarely, thrombocytopenia (brown recluse spider only)

Assessment

History

Tick bite
○ Itching at the affected site
○ Tick exposure lesion
Brown recluse spider bite
○ Minimal initial pain that increases over time
○ Fever, chills, malaise, weakness
○ Nausea, vomiting
○ Joint pain
Black widow spider bite
○ Pinprick sensation, followed by dull, numbing pain
○ Leg bite: severe pain and large-muscle cramping
○ Vertigo
○ Chills and sweats
Bee, wasp, or yellow jacket sting
○ Pain and pruritus
○ Generalized weakness
○ Chest tightness
○ Dizziness
○ Nausea and vomiting
○ Abdominal cramps
○ Throat constriction
Fire ant sting
○ Immediate pain, itching, and burning

Physical findings

Tick bite
○ Tick paralysis
○ Expanding skin lesion, erythema migrans
Brown recluse spider bite
○ Bleb (blister)
○ Bluish ring around bite
○ Joint pain
○ Seizures
○ Petechiae
Black widow spider bite
○ Rigid, painful abdomen
○ Rigidity and pain in the chest, shoulders, and back (if arm bite)
○ Extreme restlessness (systemic)
○ Pallor
○ Seizures, especially in children
○ Hyperactive reflexes
○ Hypertension
○ Tachycardia with thready pulse
○ Circulatory collapse
Bee, wasp, or yellow jacket sting
○ Raised, reddened wheal, possibly with a protruding stinger from the bee, wasp, or yellow jacket
○ Wheezing
○ Hypotension
Fire ant sting
○ Clear vesicles with surrounding erythema
○ Pustule

Test results

Laboratory
○ Urinalysis showing hematuria (black widow spider bite)
○ Increased white blood cell count (black widow spider bite)
○ Anemia panel showing hemolytic anemia (brown recluse spider bite)
○ Platelet count showing thrombocytopenia (brown recluse spider bite)

Other
○ Identification of the insect is difficult unless stung by a honeybee or bumblebee, which commonly leave a stinger with a venom sac in the lesion.

Treatment

General

Tick bite
○ Tick removal
○ Symptomatic therapy for severe symptoms
Brown recluse spider bite
○ Cool compresses and elevation of extremity
○ I.V. fluids
Black widow spider bite
○ Ice packs
Bee, wasp, yellow jacket, or fire ant sting
○ Ice application
○ Elevation of affected extremity
○ Supportive treatment
○ No dietary restrictions
○ Nothing by mouth if severe, systemic reaction
○ Rest to limit toxic effects of venom

Medication

Tick bite
○ Antipruritics
○ Antibiotics (Lyme disease treatment or Rocky Mountain spotted fever treatment)
Brown recluse spider bite
○ Corticosteroids
○ Antibiotics
○ Antihistamines
○ Tranquilizers
○ Tetanus prophylaxis
Black widow spider bite
○ Antivenin I.V.
○ Calcium gluconate I.V.
○ Muscle relaxants
○ Adrenaline or antihistamines
○ Tetanus immunization
○ Antibiotics
○ Oxygen for respiratory difficulty
Bee, wasp, yellow jacket, or fire ant sting
○ Antihistamines
○ Steroids for severe reactions

Surgery
○ Lesion excision for brown recluse spider bite

Nursing considerations

Key outcomes
The patient will:
○ maintain adequate ventilation and a patent airway
○ express feelings of increased comfort
○ regain skin integrity
○ maintain normal fluid volume.

Nursing interventions
○ Keep the affected part immobile.
○ Clean the bite or sting site with antiseptic.
○ Apply ice.
○ Give prescribed drugs.
○ Provide emergency resuscitation.
Tick bite
○ Remove the tick promptly and carefully.
○ Use tweezers to grasp the tick near its head or mouth, and gently pull to remove the whole tick without crushing it.
○ If possible, seal the tick in a plastic bag and keep it in case the patient needs to see a physician. Otherwise, flush the tick down the toilet or burn it.
Brown recluse spider bite
○ Clean the lesion with a 1:20 Burow's aluminum acetate solution.
○ Apply antibiotic ointment, as ordered.
Black widow spider bite
○ Remove all jewelry.
○ Apply cool compresses.
○ Avoid cutting into the wound or applying suction.
Scorpion sting
○ Wash the bite area thoroughly.
○ Remove all jewelry.
○ Apply cool compresses.
○ Avoid cutting into the wound or applying suction.
Bee, wasp, or yellow jacket sting
○ Scrape stinger off; don't pull or squeeze it, which releases more toxin.
Fire ant sting
○ Apply cool compresses.
○ Gently wash the bite area, leaving the blister intact.
○ Be prepared to intervene for an acute severe allergic reaction (rare).

Monitoring
○ Vital signs
○ Respiratory status
○ General appearance
○ Changes at the bite or sting site

Patient teaching

Be sure to cover:
○ avoidance of insect bites and stings
○ examination of the body for ticks after being outdoors
○ removal of ticks
○ medical identification jewelry or card
○ anaphylaxis kit use
○ insect repellent use.

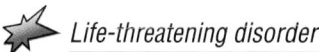 *Life-threatening disorder*

Intestinal obstruction

Overview

Description

- Partial or complete blockage of the lumen of the small or large bowel
- Commonly a medical emergency
- Most likely after abdominal surgery or with congenital bowel deformities
- Without treatment, complete obstruction in any part of bowel can cause death within hours from shock and vascular collapse

Pathophysiology

- Mechanical or nonmechanical (neurogenic) blockage of the lumen occurs.
- Fluid, air, or gas collects near the site.
- Peristalsis increases temporarily in an attempt to break through the blockage.
- Intestinal mucosa is injured, and distention at and above the site of obstruction occurs.
- Venous blood flow is impaired, and normal absorptive processes cease.
- Water, sodium, and potassium are secreted by the bowel into the fluid pooled in the lumen.

Causes

Mechanical obstruction
- Adhesions
- Strangulated hernias
- Carcinomas
- Foreign bodies
- Compression of the bowel wall from stenosis, intussusception, volvulus of the sigmoid or cecum, tumors, and atresia

Nonmechanical obstruction
- Paralytic ileus
- Electrolyte imbalances
- Toxicity, such as that associated with uremia or generalized infection
- Neurogenic abnormalities
- Thrombosis or embolism of mesenteric vessels

Risk factors

- Abdominal surgery
- Radiation therapy
- Gallstones
- Inflammatory bowel disease

Incidence

- Diagnosed in approximately 20% of hospital admissions for abdominal illness
- Occurs equally in men and women

Common characteristics

- Abdominal pain
- Change in bowel habits

Complications

- Perforation
- Peritonitis
- Septicemia
- Secondary infection
- Metabolic alkalosis or acidosis
- Death

Assessment

History

- Recent change in bowel habits
- Hiccups

Mechanical obstruction
- Colicky pain
- Nausea, vomiting
- Constipation

Nonmechanical obstruction
- Diffuse abdominal discomfort
- Frequent vomiting
- Severe abdominal pain (if obstruction results from vascular insufficiency or infarction)

Physical findings

Mechanical obstruction
- Distended abdomen
- Borborygmi and rushes (occasionally loud enough to be heard without a stethoscope)
- Abdominal tenderness
- Rebound tenderness

Nonmechanical obstruction
- Abdominal distention
- Decreased bowel sounds (early), then absent bowel sounds

Test results

Laboratory
- Decreased serum sodium, chloride, and potassium levels
- Elevated white blood cell counts
- Increased serum amylase level if pancreas is irritated by a bowel loop
- Increased blood urea nitrogen (with dehydration)

Imaging
- Abdominal X-rays reveal the presence and location of intestinal gas or fluid. In small-bowel obstruction, a typical "stepladder" pattern emerges, with alternating fluid and gas levels apparent in 3 to 4 hours.
- Barium enema reveals a distended, air-filled colon or a closed loop of sigmoid with extreme distention (in sigmoid volvulus).

Treatment

General

○ Correction of fluid and electrolyte imbalances
○ Decompression of the bowel to relieve vomiting and distention
○ Treatment of shock and peritonitis
○ Nothing by mouth if surgery is planned
○ Parenteral nutrition until bowel is functioning
○ High-fiber diet when obstruction is relieved
○ Bed rest during acute phase
○ Postoperatively, avoidance of lifting and contact sports

Medication

○ Broad-spectrum antibiotics
○ Analgesics
○ Blood replacement

Surgery

○ Usually the treatment of choice (exception is paralytic ileus in which nonoperative therapy is usually attempted first)
○ Type of surgery depends on cause of blockage

Nursing considerations

Key outcomes

The patient will:
○ express feelings of increased comfort
○ maintain normal fluid volume
○ return to normal bowel function
○ maintain caloric requirement
○ maintain stable vital signs.

Nursing interventions

○ Insert a nasogastric (NG) tube and attach to low-pressure, intermittent suction.
○ Maintain the patient in semi-Fowler's position.
○ Provide mouth and nose care.
○ Begin and maintain I.V. therapy, as ordered.
○ Give prescribed drugs.

Monitoring

○ Vital signs
○ Signs and symptoms of shock
○ Bowel sounds and signs of returning peristalsis
○ NG tube function and drainage
○ Pain control
○ Abdominal girth measurement to detect progressive distention
○ Hydration and nutritional status
○ Electrolytes and signs and symptoms of metabolic derangements
○ Wound site (postoperatively)

Patient teaching

Be sure to cover:
○ the disorder (focusing on the patient's type of intestinal obstruction), diagnosis, and treatment
○ techniques for coughing and deep breathing, and use of incentive spirometry
○ colostomy or ileostomy care, if appropriate
○ incision care
○ postoperative activity limitations and why these restrictions are necessary
○ proper use of prescribed medications, focusing on their correct administration, desired effects, and possible adverse reactions
○ importance of following a structured bowel regimen, particularly if the patient had a mechanical obstruction from fecal impaction.

Discharge planning

○ Refer the patient to an enterostomal therapist, if indicated.

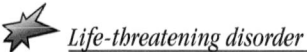
Intussusception

Overview

Description

- Condition in which a portion of the bowel telescopes or invaginates into an adjacent bowel portion (see *Understanding intussusception*)
- Can be fatal if treatment delayed more than 24 hours
- Pediatric emergency

Pathophysiology

- A bowel section invaginates and is propelled by peristalsis.
- More bowel is pulled in, causing edema, obstruction, and pain.

Causes

- Intussusception may be linked to viral infections because of seasonal peaks.

In infants
- Unknown

In older children
- Polyps
- Hemangioma
- Lymphosarcoma

- Lymphoid hyperplasia
- Meckel's diverticulum
- Alterations in intestinal motility

In adults
- Benign or malignant tumors (65% of patients)
- Polyps
- Meckel's diverticulum
- Gastroenterostomy with herniation
- Appendiceal stump

Incidence

- Most common in infants
- Three times more common in males than in females
- About 87% of children with intussusception younger than age 2; about 70% of these children between 4 and 11 months old
- Seasonal peaks in late spring and early summer

Common characteristics

- Intermittent attacks of colicky pain
- Vomiting
- Abdominal guarding

Complications

- Strangulation of the intestine
- Gangrene of the bowel
- Shock
- Bowel perforation
- Peritonitis
- Death

Assessment

History

- Intermittent attacks of colicky pain
- Pain that causes the child to scream, draw his legs up to his abdomen, turn pale and diaphoretic and, possibly, grunt
- Vomiting, initially stomach contents; later, bile-stained or fecal material
- "Currant jelly" stools, which contain mixture of blood and mucus

Physical findings

- Distended, tender abdomen
- Guarding over the intussusception site
- Palpable sausage-shaped abdominal mass in the right upper quadrant or in the midepigastric area if transverse colon is involved
- Bloody mucus found on rectal examination
- In adults, abdominal pain localized in right lower quadrant, radiating to the back, and increasing with eating

Test results

Laboratory
- White blood cell count up to 15,000/μl indicating obstruction; more than 15,000/μl, strangulation; and more than 20,000/μl, bowel infarction

---

Understanding intussusception

In intussusception, a bowel section invaginates and is propelled along by peristalsis, pulling in more bowel. This illustration shows intussusception of a portion of the transverse colon. Intussusception typically produces edema, hemorrhage from venous engorgement, incarceration, and obstruction.

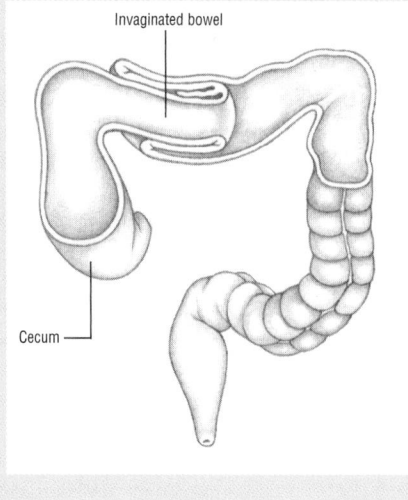

Invaginated bowel

Cecum

○ Barium enema confirms colonic intussusception when it shows the characteristic coiled-spring sign; it also delineates the extent of intussusception.
○ Upright abdominal X-rays may show a soft-tissue mass and signs of complete or partial obstruction, with dilated loops of bowel.

Treatment

General

○ Hydrostatic reduction
○ Bowel decompression
○ Nothing by mouth until bowel functions properly
○ Bed rest until condition is resolved

Medication

○ Analgesics
○ Antibiotics

Surgery

○ Indicated for children with recurrent intussusception, those who show signs of shock or peritonitis, and those in whom symptoms present longer than 24 hours
○ In adults, always the treatment of choice

Nursing considerations

Key outcomes

The patient will:
○ express feelings of increased comfort
○ avoid complications
○ maintain normal fluid volume
○ have family members who understand the disorder and treatment regimen.

Nursing interventions

○ Offer reassurance and emotional support to the patient and, if the patient is a child, to his parents.
○ Give prescribed I.V. fluids.
○ Encourage coughing and deep breathing.
○ Give prescribed antibiotics.

Monitoring

○ Vital signs
○ Intake and output
○ Hydration status
○ Nasogastric tube function and drainage
○ Bowel sounds, stools, abdominal distention
○ Wound site (after surgery)
○ For recurrence in the first 36 to 48 hours after reduction

Patient teaching

Be sure to cover:
○ the disorder, diagnosis, and treatment
○ medication administration, dosage, and possible adverse effects
○ wound care
○ signs and symptoms of infection
○ parental participation in their child's care to minimize the stress of hospitalization (visiting hours should be flexible).

Discharge planning

○ Encourage the patient's family to make follow-up appointments as recommended by his physician.

Irritable bowel syndrome

Overview

Description

- Common condition marked by chronic or periodic diarrhea alternating with constipation
- Accompanied by straining and abdominal cramps
- Initial episodes early in life and late teens to twenties
- Prognosis good
- Also known as *spastic colon, spastic colitis, mucous colitis*

Pathophysiology

- Precise etiology unclear
- Involves a change in bowel motility, reflecting an abnormality in the neuromuscular control of intestinal smooth muscle

Causes

- Anxiety and stress
- Dietary factors, such as fiber, raw fruits, coffee, alcohol, and foods that are cold, highly seasoned, or laxative in nature

Other possible triggers

- Hormones
- Laxative abuse
- Allergy to certain foods or drugs
- Lactose intolerance

Incidence

- Occurs mostly in women, with symptoms first emerging before age 40

Common characteristics

- Chronic constipation or diarrhea
- Lower abdominal pain

Complications

- Diverticulitis and colon cancer
- Chronic inflammatory bowel disease

Assessment

History

- Chronic constipation, diarrhea, or both
- Lower abdominal pain (typically in the left lower quadrant) usually relieved by defecation or passage of gas
- Small stools with visible mucus or pasty, pencil-like stools instead of diarrhea
- Dyspepsia
- Abdominal bloating
- Heartburn
- Faintness and weakness

- Contributing psychological factors, such as a recent stressful life change, that may have triggered or aggravated symptoms
- Anxiety and fatigue

Physical findings

- Normal bowel sounds
- Tympany over a gas-filled bowel

Test results

- Assessment involves studies to rule out other, more serious disorders.

Laboratory

- Negative stool examination for occult blood, parasites, and pathogenic bacteria
- Normal complete blood count, serologic tests, serum albumin, and erythrocyte sedimentation rate

Imaging

- Barium enema may reveal colonic spasm and a tubular appearance of the descending colon. It's also used to rule out certain other disorders, such as diverticula, tumors, and polyps.

Diagnostic procedures

- Sigmoidoscopy may disclose spastic contractions.

Treatment

General

- Stress management
- Lifestyle modifications
- Diet based on the patient's symptoms
- Initially, an elimination diet
- Avoidance of sorbitol, nonabsorbable carbohydrates, and lactose-containing foods
- Increased dietary bulk
- Increased fluid intake
- Regular exercise

Medication

- Anticholinergic, antispasmodic drugs
- Antidiarrheals
- Laxatives
- Antiemetics
- Simethicone
- Mild tranquilizers
- Tricyclic antidepressants

Nursing considerations

Key outcomes

The patient will:
- express feelings of increased comfort
- maintain adequate caloric intake
- have normal bowel function
- express positive feelings about self
- maintain normal laboratory values
- understand the disease process and treatment regimen.

Nursing interventions

○ Because the patient with irritable bowel syndrome isn't hospitalized, nursing interventions almost always focus on patient teaching.

Monitoring

○ Weight
○ Diet
○ Bowel movements

Patient teaching

Be sure to cover:
○ the disorder, diagnosis, and treatment
○ dietary plans and implementation
○ need to drink 8 to 10 glasses of water or other compatible fluids daily
○ proper use of prescribed medication, reviewing desired effects and possible adverse reactions
○ need to implement lifestyle changes that reduce stress
○ smoking cessation
○ need for regular physical examinations. (For patients older than age 40, emphasize the need for colorectal cancer screening, including annual proctosigmoidoscopy and rectal examinations.)

Juvenile rheumatoid arthritis

Overview

Description

○ Several inflammatory conditions characterized by chronic synovitis and joint swelling, pain, and tenderness
○ Major types — systemic (Still's disease or acute febrile type), polyarticular, and pauciarticular

Pathophysiology

○ If juvenile rheumatoid arthritis (JRA) isn't arrested, the inflammatory process in the joints occurs in four stages:
  – Synovitis develops from congestion and edema of the synovial membrane and joint capsule.
  – Pannus covers and invades cartilage and eventually destroys the joint capsule and bone.
  – Fibrous tissue and ankylosis occludes the joint space.
  – Fibrous tissue calcifies, resulting in bony ankylosis and total immobility.

Causes

○ Unknown
○ Suggested link to genetic factors or an abnormal immune response
○ Viral or bacterial (streptococcal) infection, trauma, and emotional stress

Incidence

○ May occur as early as age 6 weeks but seldom before age 6 months; peak onset between ages 1 and 3 and 8 and 12
○ Occurs in an estimated 150,000 to 250,000 children in United States; affects twice as many girls as boys

Common characteristics

○ Joint stiffness in the morning

Complications

○ Flexion contractures
○ Ocular damage and loss of vision
○ Retarded growth and development

Assessment

History

○ Common complaint of joint stiffness in morning or after periods of inactivity
○ In young children, typically irritability and listlessness

Physical findings

Systemic JRA

○ Mild, transient arthritis or frank polyarthritis with fever and rash
○ Behavior may clearly suggest joint pain and fatigue
○ Painful breathing and nonspecific abdominal pain
○ Fatigue, shortness of breath, palpitations, and fever
○ Resting or exertional tachycardia; arrhythmias; jugular vein distention; heart murmurs
○ Hepatic, splenic, and lymph node enlargement
○ Friction rub associated with pericarditis

Polyarticular JRA

○ Pain in the wrists, elbows, knees, ankles, and small joints of the hands and feet
○ Pain in larger joints, including the temporomandibular, cervical spine, hips, and shoulders
○ Tenderness, stiffness, and swelling of joints
○ Possible low-grade fever with daily peaks
○ Weight loss
○ Noticeable developmental retardation
○ Hepatic, splenic, and lymph node enlargement
○ Subcutaneous nodules on the elbows or heels

Pauciarticular JRA

○ Pain in the hips, knees, heels, feet, ankles, and elbows
○ Eye redness, blurred vision, and photophobia
○ Lower back pain

Test results

Laboratory

○ Decreased serum hemoglobin levels and increased neutrophil (neutrophilia) and platelet (thrombocytosis) levels; others include elevated erythrocyte sedimentation rate and elevated C-reactive protein, serum haptoglobin, immunoglobulin, and C3 complement levels
○ Positive antinuclear antibody test in patients with polyarticular JRA and in those with pauciarticular JRA with chronic iridocyclitis
○ Rheumatoid factor (RF) appearing in about 15% of patients with JRA (In contrast, about 85% of patients with RA test positive for RF; patients with polyarticular JRA may test positive for RF.)
○ Human leukocyte antigen-B27 forecasting later development of ankylosing spondylitis

Imaging

○ X-ray studies demonstrate early structural changes associated with JRA. These include soft-tissue swelling, effusion, and periostitis in affected joints. Later evidence includes osteoporosis and accelerated bone growth followed by subchondral erosions, joint-space narrowing, bone destruction, and fusion.

Treatment

General

○ Physical therapy
○ Splints
○ Heat application during passive exercises

- Adequate iron, protein, calcium, and caloric intake
- Activity, as tolerated

Medication

- Aspirin
- Nonsteroidal anti-inflammatory drugs (NSAIDs)
- Gold salts
- Hydroxychloroquine
- Penicillamine
- Low-dose cytotoxic agents

Surgery

- Soft-tissue releases to improve mobility
- Joint replacement (delayed until child matures physically and can tolerate vigorous rehabilitation)

Nursing considerations

Key outcomes

The patient will:
- express feelings of increased comfort and decreased pain
- recognize and express feelings about limitations due to illness
- identify factors that increase risk for injury
- maintain optimum mobility.

Nursing interventions

- Focus nursing care on reducing pain and promoting mobility.
- During inflammatory exacerbations, administer NSAIDs or prescribed medication on a regular schedule.
- Allow the patient to rest frequently throughout the day to conserve energy for times when she must be mobile.
- Arrange the patient's environment for participation in activities of daily living so that she feels capable of accomplishing tasks.

Monitoring

- Pain level
- Response to treatment
- Signs and symptoms of bleeding
- Nutritional status
- Joint mobility
- Adverse drug reactions

Patient teaching

Be sure to cover:
- the disorder, diagnosis, and treatment
- need to encourage the child to be as independent as possible
- need for regular slit-lamp examinations to enable early diagnosis and treatment of iridocyclitis
- signs and symptoms of bleeding caused by aspirin or NSAID therapy (instructing the patient to take these medications with meals or milk to reduce adverse GI reactions)
- signs and symptoms of exacerbation, and the need to notify the pediatrician about these symptoms
- need for proper nutrition and caloric consumption
- child's special needs (tell teachers and the school principal).

Discharge planning

- Consult an occupational therapist to assess the patient's home care needs.

Kaposi's sarcoma

Overview

Description
- Most common acquired immunodeficiency syndrome (AIDS)–related cancer
- Characterized by obvious, colorful lesions
- Most common internal sites are lungs and GI tract (esophagus, oropharynx, and epiglottis)

Pathophysiology
- Kaposi's sarcoma causes structural and functional damage.
- When associated with AIDS, it progresses aggressively, involving the lymph nodes, the viscera and, possibly, GI structures.

Causes
- Exact cause unknown
- May be related to immunosuppression
- Genetic or hereditary predisposition suspected

Risk factors
- Immunosuppression
- Genetic or hereditary predisposition

Incidence
- Originally affected 35% of AIDS patients; now declining with earlier detection of AIDS
- Possibly more common in middle-aged and older Mediterranean, Eastern European, and Jewish men

Common characteristics
- History of AIDS
- Lesions of various shapes, sizes, and colors

Complications
- Severe pulmonary involvement, resulting in respiratory distress
- GI involvement, leading to digestive problems

Assessment

History
- Possible history of AIDS
- Pain (in advanced cases)

Physical findings
- Several lesions of various shapes, sizes, and colors (ranging from red-brown to dark purple) on the skin, buccal mucosa, hard and soft palates, lips, gums, tongue, tonsils, conjunctiva, and sclera (the most common sites)
- In advanced disease, lesions that may merge, becoming one large plaque
- Untreated lesions that may appear as large, ulcerative masses
- Dyspnea
- Edema from lymphatic obstruction
- Wheezing and hypoventilation

Test results
Diagnostic procedures
- Tissue biopsy shows the type and stage of the lesion. (See *Laubenstein's stages in Kaposi's sarcoma.*)

Treatment

General
- Radiation therapy for palliation of symptoms (pain from obstructing lesions in the oral cavity or extremities and edema caused by lymphatic blockage); also for cosmetic improvement
- High-calorie, high-protein diet
- Small meals
- Limited activity
- Frequent rest periods

Medication
- Chemotherapy
- Biological response modifier

Surgery
- Removal of lesion from skin (especially if lesion is small), using local excision, electrodesiccation and curettage, or cryotherapy

---

Laubenstein's stages in Kaposi's sarcoma

L.J. Laubenstein proposed this staging system to evaluate and treat patients with acquired immunodeficiency syndrome and Kaposi's sarcoma:
- Stage I — locally indolent cutaneous lesions
- Stage II — locally aggressive cutaneous lesions
- Stage III — mucocutaneous and lymph node involvement
- Stage IV — visceral involvement.

Within each stage, a patient may have different symptoms further classified as stage subtype A or B, which are:
- Subtype A — no systemic signs or symptoms
- Subtype B — one or more systemic signs and symptoms, including 10% weight loss, fever of unknown origin that exceeds 100° F (37.8° C) for longer than 2 weeks, chills, lethargy, night sweats, anorexia, and diarrhea.

Nursing considerations

Key outcomes

The patient will:
- have no further weight loss
- express positive feelings about self
- maintain adequate ventilation
- maintain a patent airway
- exhibit no signs and symptoms of infection.

Nursing interventions

- Encourage verbalization and offer support.
- Inspect the skin for new lesions and skin breakdown.
- Give prescribed drugs.
- Provide rest periods.

Monitoring

- Adverse effects of treatment
- Vital signs
- Pain control
- Nutritional status
- Respiratory status

Patient teaching

Be sure to cover:
- the disorder, diagnosis, and treatment
- medication administration, dosage, and possible adverse effects
- infection prevention techniques and, if necessary, basic hygiene measures to prevent infection (especially if the patient also has AIDS)
- the need for ongoing treatment and care.

Discharge planning

- Refer the patient to available resources and support services.

Kawasaki syndrome

Overview

Description

- A noncontagious, febrile, self-limited disorder of unknown origin
- Affects the mucus membranes, lymph nodes, blood vessels, and heart
- Occurs in stages: acute, subacute, and convalescent
- Cardiac complications most serious sequelae
- Full recovery expected
- Also known as *mucocutaneous lymph node syndrome* and *infantile polyarteritis*

Pathophysiology

- An infection results in altered immune function.
- Antibodies increase as a result of the infection and cause inflammation of blood vessels.
- Blood vessel inflammation increases platelet accumulation and results in thrombi.
- Thrombi result in obstruction of the heart and blood vessels.

Causes

- Possible genetic role after exposure to an unknown virus, bacteria, or other pathogen

Risk factors

- None known
- No known preventive measures

Incidence

- Peak incidence in boys younger than age 4, but can occur up to puberty
- Affects boys 1½ times more commonly than girls
- Occurs more commonly in late winter and spring
- Most common in Japan or in Japanese or Korean children living elsewhere
- Commonly occurs in clusters within a geographic location
- Rarely occurs twice in the same household

Common characteristics

Acute phase
- High fever for 5 days or more (up to 106.5° F [41.4° C]) that doesn't respond to antipyretics
- Lethargy and irritability
- Reddened, swollen hands and feet
- Inflamed mucous membrane of eyes
- "Strawberry" tongue with red, cracked lips
- Rash in trunk area
- Enlarged cervical lymph nodes
- Abdominal pain, anorexia, and diarrhea resulting from internal lymph node swelling
- Reddened, swollen joints

Subacute phase
- Begins about 10 days after the onset of symptoms
- Skin desquamation, especially in the groin, on the palms of the hands, and soles of the feet
- Possible aneurysms leading to sudden death

Convalescent phase
- Occurs between the 25th and 40th days
- May continue beyond 40 days without distinguishing features

Complications

- Vasculitis leading to aneurysm and myocardial infarction
- Death (2% of patients with Kawasaki syndrome die from coronary vasculitis)
- Future coronary bypass surgery if coronary artery disease develops
- Myocarditis
- Pericarditis
- Cardiac arrhythmias
- Abnormal valve functioning

Assessment

History

- Fever of 5 days or more, unresponsive to antipyretics
- Occurrence of characteristic symptoms

Physical findings

- Reddened, swollen hands and feet
- Inflamed mucous membrane of eyes
- "Strawberry" tongue with red, cracked lips
- Rash in trunk area
- Enlarged cervical lymph nodes
- Reddened, swollen joints
- Possible enlarged gallbladder

Test results

Laboratory
- Elevated white blood cell count and erythrocyte sedimentation rate in acute phase
- Platelet count elevated in the subacute phase
- Aseptic meningitis
- Urethritis
- Elevated liver function tests
- Anemia
- Urinalysis possibly showing pyuria or proteinuria

Imaging
- Sequential echocardiograms detect artery disease.
- Chest X-ray rules out cardiomegaly or subclinical pneumonitis

Treatment

General

- Hospitalization
- Symptomatic
- Prevention of complications
- Soft, nonirritating foods
- Avoidance of citrus (mouth sores)
- Activity, as tolerated

Medication

○ I.V. gamma globulin
○ Aspirin
○ Dipyridamole/Persantine

Nursing considerations

Key outcomes

The patient will:
○ maintain adequate tissue perfusion
○ have normal vital signs
○ have a capillary refill time of less than 5 seconds
○ experience a tolerable pain level
○ experience increased comfort
○ maintain adequate nutrition.

Nursing interventions

○ Observe for signs of heart failure: tachycardia, dyspnea, crackles, edema.
○ Inspect the extremities for color, temperature, and capillary refill.
○ Observe and report joint swelling and redness.
○ Observe and report nature of rash.
○ Keep clothing from constricting or irritating rash.
○ Moisten lips with lip balm to prevent cracking.
○ Offer frequent fluids.
○ Observe for signs of GI upset, such as nausea and vomiting.
○ Avoid pressure on the extremities with edema.
○ Give prescribed drugs.

Monitoring

○ Complications such as chest pain, arrhythmias, and ECG changes
○ Edema changes
○ Intake and output
○ Nutritional status
○ Response to treatment
○ Adverse effects of I.V. immunoglobulin: allergic reactions, fever, chills, headache, transfusion reactions, and pulmonary edema

Patient teaching

Be sure to cover:
○ aspirin therapy during and after hospitalization
○ reporting exposure to viral illnesses, such as influenza or chickenpox, while taking aspirin, in order to prevent Reyes syndrome
○ possibility of long-term management if cardiac complications exist
○ need to delay immunizations (especially the measles-mumps-rubella and chickenpox vaccines) when immunoglobulin is given.

Discharge planning

○ Encourage the patient to schedule a follow-up examination in 2 to 3 weeks.

Keratitis

Overview

Description
○ Infection of the cornea
○ Usually affects only one eye
○ May be acute or chronic

Pathophysiology
○ Inflammation of the cornea results from corneal infection.
○ Inflammation may be deep or superficial.

Causes
○ Viral, bacterial, or fungal infection
○ Tear deficiency
○ Denervation
○ Immune reactions
○ Ischemia
○ Trauma
○ Congenital syphilis

Incidence
○ Fairly common
○ May develop at any age

Common characteristics
○ Photophobia
○ Pain
○ Lacrimation

Examining the eye with a slit lamp

An ophthalmologist uses the slit lamp, an instrument equipped with a special lighting system and a binocular microscope, to view the eyelids, eyelashes, conjunctiva, sclera, cornea, tear film, anterior chamber, iris, crystalline lens, and vitreous face. The examiner may adjust the size, shape, intensity, and depth of the light source as well as the magnification of the microscope, to evaluate normally transparent or near-transparent ocular fluids and tissues. If he notes abnormalities, he can attach special devices to the slit lamp to allow more detailed investigation.

Preparing the patient
○ Tell the patient that the slit-lamp examination evaluates the front portion of the eyes and that it requires that he remain still. Reassure him that the examination is painless.
○ If the patient wears contact lenses, tell him to remove them for the test, unless the test is being performed to evaluate the fit of the lens.
○ If the test calls for dilating eyedrops, check the patient's history for adverse reactions to mydriatics and for the presence of angle-closure glaucoma before giving the drops. Dilating eyedrops aren't used in routine eye examinations, but some diseases require pupillary dilation before slit-lamp examination.

Complications
○ Blindness
○ Corneal scarring or perforation

Assessment

History
○ Recent upper respiratory tract infection, accompanied by cold sores
○ Eye pain
○ Central vision loss
○ Sensitivity to light
○ Sensation of a foreign body in eye
○ Blurred vision

Physical findings
○ Cornea lacks normal luster
○ Characteristic branched lesion of the cornea with herpes simplex virus type 1

Test results
Diagnostic procedures
○ Slit-lamp examination with sodium fluorescein staining may show corneal inflammation or abrasion; small branchlike (dendritic) lesions indicate possible herpes simplex virus infection. (See *Examining the eye with a slit lamp*.)

Treatment

General
○ Eye shield or patch

Medication
Acute dendritic keratitis
○ Trifluridine eyedrops
○ Vidarabine ophthalmic ointment
○ Broad-spectrum antibiotic
Chronic dendritic keratitis
○ Vidarabine therapy
○ Long-term topical therapy may be necessary
Fungal keratitis
○ Natamycin

Surgery
○ Corneal transplantation for severe ulcerations with residual scarring

Nursing considerations

Key outcomes
The patient will:
○ maintain current health status
○ sustain no harm or injury
○ express increased feelings of comfort
○ regain visual function.

Nursing interventions

 Alert

Watch for keratitis in patients predisposed to cold sores. Corneal infection is commonly caused by a virus, such as adenovirus or herpes simplex, the same viruses that cause cold sores. Be sure to tell patients never to touch their eyes after touching their mouths.

○ Wear gloves when in contact with eyes or ocular drainage with herpes simplex virus.
○ Apply warm compresses.
○ Dim the lights in case of photophobia.
○ Give prescribed drugs.

Monitoring
○ Response to treatment
○ Visual acuity

Patient teaching

Be sure to cover:
○ the disorder, diagnosis, and treatment
○ medication and possible adverse effects
○ how stress, traumatic injury, fever, colds, and sun overexposure can trigger flare-up
○ wearing sunglasses for photophobia
○ meticulous hand washing
○ preventing spread of infection.

Kidney cancer

Overview

Description

- Proliferation of cancer cells in the kidney
- 85% originate in kidneys; 15% metastasize from various primary-site carcinomas
- Also called *nephrocarcinoma, renal carcinoma, hypernephroma,* and *Grawitz's tumor*

Pathophysiology

- Most kidney tumors are large, firm, nodular, encapsulated, unilateral, and solitary.
- Kidney cancer may affect either kidney; occasionally tumors are bilateral or multifocal. (See *Unilateral kidney tumor.*)
- Renal cancers arise from the tubular epithelium.
- Tumor margins are usually clearly defined.
- Tumors can include areas of ischemia, necrosis, and focal hemorrhage.
- Tumor cells may be well differentiated to anaplastic.
- Kidney cancer can be separated histologically into clear cell, granular cell, and spindle cell types.
- The prognosis is better for patients with the clear cell type than for the other types; in general, however, the prognosis depends more on the cancer's stage than on its type. The overall prognosis has improved considerably, with a 5-year survival rate of about 50%.

Unilateral kidney tumor

In kidney cancer, tumors such as this one in the upper kidney pole usually occur unilaterally.

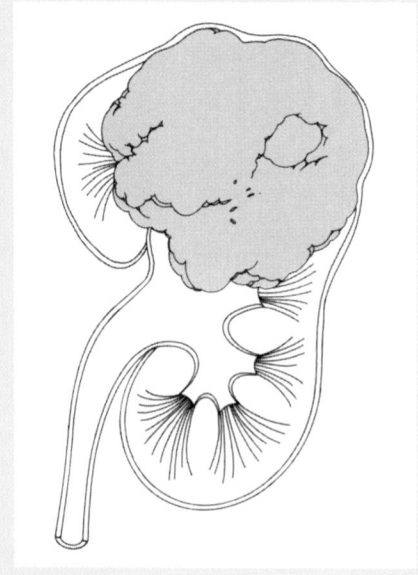

Causes

- Unknown

Risk factors

- Heavy cigarette smoking
- Regular hemodialysis treatments

Incidence

- Twice as common in men as in women
- More common after age 40
- Renal pelvic tumors and Wilms' tumor most common in children

Common characteristics

- Hematuria
- Flank pain

Complications

- Hemorrhage
- Metastasis

Assessment

History

- Hematuria
- Dull, aching flank pain
- Weight loss (rare)

Physical findings

- Palpable smooth, firm, nontender abdominal mass

Test results

Laboratory
- Increased alkaline phosphatase, bilirubin, and transaminase levels
- Prolonged prothrombin time

Imaging
- Renal ultrasonography and computed tomography scan can be used to verify renal cancer.
- Excretory urography, nephrotomography, and kidney-ureter-bladder radiography are used to aid diagnosis and help in staging.

Treatment

General

- Because of radiation resistance, radiation used only when cancer has spread into perinephric region or lymph nodes or when primary tumor or metastatic sites can't be completely excised
- Low-protein diet
- Postoperatively, no heavy lifting or contact sports for 6 to 8 weeks

Medication

- Chemotherapy
- Biotherapy with lymphokine-activated killer cells plus recombinant interleukin-2
- Interferon

Surgery
○ Radical nephrectomy, with or without regional lymph node dissection

Nursing considerations

Key outcomes
The patient will:
○ maintain fluid balance
○ report increased comfort
○ communicate understanding of medical regimen, medications, diet, and activity restrictions
○ maintain ventilation
○ utilize support services.

Nursing interventions
○ Give prescribed drugs.
○ Encourage verbalization and provide support.

Monitoring
○ Wound site
○ Intake and output
○ Complete blood count; serum chemistry results
○ Pain control

Patient teaching

Be sure to cover:
○ the disorder, diagnosis, and treatment
○ medication administration, dosage, and possible adverse effects
○ need for a healthy, well-balanced diet and regular exercise
○ importance of checking with the physician before taking vitamins or other dietary supplements
○ importance of follow-up care.

Discharge planning
○ Refer the patient to support services
○ Refer the patient to a weight-reduction program, if indicated
○ Refer the patient to a smoking-cessation program, if indicated.

Klinefelter syndrome

Overview

Description

○ Relatively common genetic abnormality that results from an extra X chromosome, creating an XXY sex chromosome constitution
○ Affects only males and usually becomes apparent at puberty, when secondary sex characteristics develop
○ Failure of the testicles to mature and degenerative testicular changes that eventually result in irreversible infertility

Pathophysiology

○ The extra chromosome responsible for Klinefelter syndrome probably results from either meiotic nondisjunction during parental gametogenesis or from mitotic nondisjunction in the zygote.

Turner's syndrome

In Turner's syndrome, one of the X chromosomes (or part of the second X chromosome) may be lost from either the ovum or sperm through nondisjunction or chromosome lag. Mixed aneuploidy may result from mitotic nondisjunction.

This disorder occurs in 1 in 2,500 to 7,000 births; up to 95% of affected fetuses are spontaneously aborted.

Signs and symptoms

In utero, the fetus may have a cystic hygroma, seen on ultrasound; however, these may also be seen in fetuses that don't have Turner's syndrome. The mother may have elevated or low levels of serum alpha-fetoprotein.

At birth, 50% of infants with this syndrome measure below the third percentile in length. Many have swollen hands and feet, a wide chest with laterally displaced nipples, and a low hairline that becomes more obvious as they grow. They may have webbing of the neck and coarse, enlarged, prominent ears. Gonadal dysgenesis is seen at birth and typically causes sterility in adult females (unless they have the mosaic form).

Cardiovascular defects, such as a bicuspid aortic valve and coarctation of the aorta, occur in 10% to 40% of patients. Short stature (usually under 59″ [150 cm]) is the most common adult sign.

Most patients have average or slightly below-average intelligence; they commonly exhibit spatial defects, right–left disorientation for extrapersonal space, and defective figure drawing.

Diagnosis and treatment

Turner's syndrome can be diagnosed by chromosome analysis. Differential diagnosis should rule out mixed gonadal dysgenesis, Noonan's syndrome, and other similar disorders.

Treatment should begin in early childhood and may include hormonal therapy (androgens, human growth hormone and, possibly, small doses of estrogen). Later, progesterone and estrogen can induce sexual maturation, but most patients remain sterile.

○ The incidence of meiotic nondisjunction increases with maternal age.

Causes

○ One extra X chromosome creates 47,XXY complement instead of the normal 46,XY.
○ In the rare mosaic form, some cells contain extra X chromosomes; others contain normal XY complement.
○ Turner's syndrome, the lack of one X chromosome (45,X), may also be a cause. (See *Turner's syndrome.*)

Incidence

○ In the United States, approximately 1 in 500 to 1,000 males is born with an extra sex chromosome; over 3,000 affected males are born yearly.
○ The prevalence is 5 to 20 times higher in neonates with mental retardation.

Common characteristics

○ May not be apparent until puberty (or later in mild cases)
○ Behavioral problems in adolescence
○ Infertility

Complications

○ Aspermatogenesis and infertility
○ Learning disabilities and behavioral problems
○ Osteoporosis
○ Breast cancer because of the extra X chromosome

Assessment

History

○ Sexual dysfunction (impotence, lack of libido)
○ In some individuals, behavioral problems beginning in adolescence
○ Increased incidence of pulmonary disease and varicose veins

Physical findings

○ Small penis and prostate gland
○ Small testicles
○ Sparse facial and abdominal hair
○ Feminine distribution of pubic hair (triangular shape)
○ In fewer than 50% of patients, gynecomastia
○ In the mosaic form, delay of pathologic changes and resulting infertility
○ Abnormal body build (long legs with short, obese trunk)
○ Tall stature

Test results

Laboratory

○ A karyotype (chromosome analysis) determined by culturing lymphocytes from the patient's peripheral blood
○ Decreased urinary 17-ketosteroid levels

- ○ Increased excretion of follicle-stimulating hormone
- ○ Decreased levels of plasma testosterone after puberty

Treatment

General

- ○ Activity, as tolerated
- ○ Diet, as tolerated
- ○ Psychological counseling

Medication
- ○ Supplemental testosterone

Surgery
- ○ Mastectomy in patients with persistent gynecomastia to induce secondary sexual characteristics of puberty for body image problems or emotional maladjustment due to sexual dysfunction

Nursing considerations

Key outcomes

The patient will:
- ○ express feelings about disorder
- ○ demonstrate effective coping mechanisms
- ○ comply with prescribed treatment.

Nursing interventions

- ○ Encourage the patient to discuss his feelings of confusion and rejection that may arise, and try to reinforce his male identity.
- ○ Give prescribed drugs.

Monitoring

- ○ Response to treatment

Patient teaching

Be sure to cover:
- ○ the potential benefits and adverse effects of testosterone administration.

Discharge planning

- ○ Send the fertile patient with the mosaic form of the syndrome for genetic counseling.

Labyrinthitis

Overview

Description

○ Inflammation of the labyrinth of the inner ear
○ Typically produces severe vertigo with head movement and sensorineural hearing loss
○ Viral labyrinthitis most prevalent form

Pathophysiology

○ Lesion within vestibular pathways (inner ear to cerebral cortex) results in an imbalance in the vestibular system.

Causes

○ Viral or bacterial infections
○ Cholesteatoma
○ Drug toxicity
○ Head injury
○ Tumor
○ Vasculitis

Incidence

○ Affects all ages beyond infancy
○ Affects males and females equally

Common characteristics

○ Severe vertigo with head movement
○ Nausea and vomiting
○ Sensorineural hearing loss

Complications

○ Meningitis
○ Permanent balance disability
○ Permanent hearing loss

Assessment

History

○ Severe vertigo from any movement of the head
○ Nausea and vomiting
○ Unilateral or bilateral hearing loss
○ Recent upper respiratory tract infection

Managing labyrinthitis

○ Tell the patient to avoid sudden position changes.
○ Help the patient assess how much this disability will affect his daily life.
○ Work with the patient to identify hazards in the home, such as throw rugs and dark stairways.
○ Discuss the patient's anxieties and concerns about vertigo attacks and decreased hearing.
○ Stress the importance of maintaining and resuming normal diversions or social activities when balance disturbance is absent.

○ Loss of balance and falling in the direction of the affected ear

Physical findings

○ Spontaneous nystagmus
○ Jerking movements of eyes toward unaffected ear
○ Purulent drainage

Test results

Laboratory
○ Culture and sensitivity tests showing the infecting organism
Imaging
○ Computed tomography scanning results rule out brain lesion.
Diagnostic procedures
○ Audiometric testing reveals sensorineural hearing loss.
○ A flat tympanogram may suggest fluid in the middle ear, a perforated tympanic membrane, or impacted cerumen. Fluctuations on the tympanogram, synchronous with the patient's pulse, suggest a glomangioma in the middle ear.
○ Electronystagmography may show decreased velocity from one side that indicates hypofunction or canal paresis. An inability to induce nystagmus with ice water denotes a dead labyrinth.

Treatment

General

○ Based on relieving symptoms
○ Increased oral fluids
○ During acute attacks, bed rest in darkened room with head immobilized between pillows

Medication

○ Meclizine to relieve vertigo
○ Antiemetics
○ Antibiotics
○ I.V. fluids for severe dehydration

Surgery

○ Surgical excision of cholesteatoma
○ Drainage of middle and inner ear infected areas
○ Labyrinthectomy

Nursing considerations

Key outcomes

The patient will:
○ express feelings of increased comfort
○ maintain normal fluid volumes
○ incur no injury or harm
○ verbalize understanding of the condition and treatment.

Nursing interventions

○ Offer the patient reassurance when appropriate.

- Maintain bed rest in a darkened room with his head immobilized during acute attacks.
- Give prescribed drugs.
- Encourage oral fluid intake.

For patient with hearing loss
- Encourage expression of concerns about hearing loss.
- Give clear, concise explanations.
- Face him when speaking.
- Enunciate words clearly, slowly, and in a normal tone.
- Provide a pencil and paper to aid communication.
- Alert staff to communication needs.

Monitoring

- Response to medication
- Vital signs
- Signs of dehydration
- Intake and output
- Auditory acuity
- Complications

Patient teaching

Be sure to cover:
- the disorder, diagnosis, and treatment
- limitation of activities to avoid danger from vertigo
- recovery time (up to 6 weeks)
- prompt treatment of upper respiratory tract and systemic infections
- controlling use of salicylates and other potentially toxic substances
- completion of the prescribed medication regimen
- adverse drug reactions
- preoperative and postoperative instructions, as indicated
- management of labyrinthitis (see *Managing labyrinthitis*).

Lactose intolerance

Overview

Description

- Inability to digest and absorb lactose, the main carbohydrate in milk
- Stems from an insufficiency of the enzyme lactase
- May be congenital (rare) or acquired
- Deficiency continues for life

Pathophysiology

See *Understanding lactase insufficiency.*

Causes

- Genetic basis
- Medical conditions that disrupt the intestinal mucosa (secondary)
- Medications that cause GI disturbances
- Ionizing radiation to the abdomen and abdominal surgery

Incidence

- High incidence among certain ethnic groups, including Blacks, Asians, Native Americans, Greek Cypriots, and some Ashkenazic Jews

Common characteristics

- Abdominal pain and distention after ingesting dairy products

Complications

- Dehydration

Assessment

History

- GI signs and symptoms, such as diarrhea, abdominal cramping, discomfort, distention, flatulence, and borborygmus (intestinal rumbling), following ingestion of milk products
- History of a medical disorder or treatment that disrupts the GI mucosa

Physical findings

- Abdominal distention
- Nonverbal signs of patient distress, such as doubling over or holding the abdomen
- Rectal tissue irritation and excoriation related to diarrhea
- Hyperactive bowel sounds

Test results

Laboratory

- Lactose tolerance testing: A blood sample is taken after the patient has fasted overnight. Then the patient ingests a specified oral lactose load. Serum glucose levels are taken on blood samples drawn at specified intervals following lactose ingestion and on the fasting blood sample. A minimal increase (less than 20 mg/dl) in the serum glucose level and GI symptoms (cramping, flatulence and, perhaps, diarrhea) confirm lactase deficiency.
- Breath hydrogen analysis measures excess hydrogen exhalation resulting from bacterial fermentation of lactose in the colon. (Hydrogen from the colon passes to the blood and then to the lungs.) Increased hydrogen content of expired air confirms lactose intolerance.

Other

- Lactose challenge test produces diarrhea and bloating within minutes to hours.
- Lactose-free diet testing eliminates lactose from the patient's diet for a period of time such as 5 days. If he becomes asymptomatic, the diagnosis is upheld.
- Small-bowel biopsy (rarely used) determines whether lactose intolerance is primary or secondary. Only the secondary form shows abnormal epithelium.

Understanding lactase insufficiency

Normally, the enzyme lactase hydrolyzes dietary lactose in the jejunum and proximal ileus. The hydrolysis splits lactose into glucose and galactose, which bind to glucose carriers and eventually pass into the portal vein. If lactase levels are insufficient to split the lactose, a chain of effects is triggered.

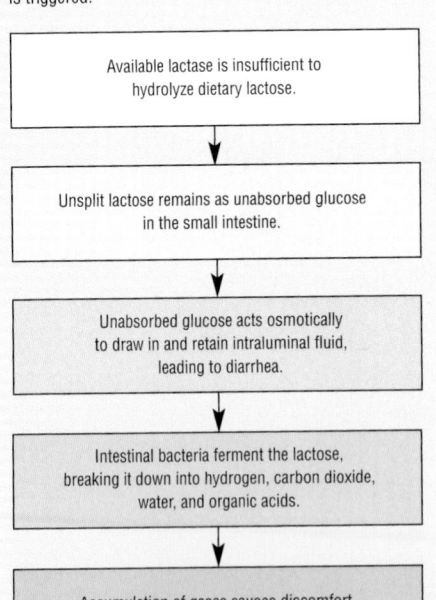

Available lactase is insufficient to hydrolyze dietary lactose.

↓

Unsplit lactose remains as unabsorbed glucose in the small intestine.

↓

Unabsorbed glucose acts osmotically to draw in and retain intraluminal fluid, leading to diarrhea.

↓

Intestinal bacteria ferment the lactose, breaking it down into hydrogen, carbon dioxide, water, and organic acids.

↓

Accumulation of gases causes discomfort, flatulence, and distention.

Treatment

General
○ Lactose-free diet

Medication
○ Lactase enzyme products (LactAid, Lactrase)
○ Antidiarrheal agents

Nursing considerations

Key outcomes
The patient will:
○ express feelings of increased comfort
○ have normal bowel function
○ have fluid volume within normal parameters
○ maintain adequate caloric intake.

Nursing interventions
○ Give prescribed antidiarrheal agents.
○ Give prescribed lactase enzyme products.
○ Assess the patient for abdominal discomfort.
○ Encourage relaxation and diversion techniques to relieve discomfort.
○ Initiate patient care measures to protect the rectal skin and mucous membranes.
○ Assess the patient for signs of dehydration.
○ Offer emotional support.
○ Provide patient privacy.

Monitoring
○ Elimination pattern
○ Diet
○ Skin integrity

Patient teaching

Be sure to cover:
○ lactose intolerance and its associated signs and symptoms, risks, and treatment, especially dietary management
○ avoiding foods that contain lactose, such as milk (whole, low-fat, skim, evaporated, condensed, buttermilk, cream), ice cream, cheese, sour cream, custards, milk-based puddings, butter, drinks prepared with chocolate or malted milk powder, cream sauces and gravies, cream-based soups, chocolate candy, instant potatoes, baked products made with milk, and frozen or canned fruits and vegetables containing lactose
○ checking product labels carefully for lactose content and avoiding products that list milk solids, milk sugars, whey, or casein
○ the need to eliminate all sources of lactose from his diet until he is symptom free
○ how to use lactase enzyme products
○ avoiding vitamin D and calcium deficiencies.

Laryngeal cancer

Overview

Description
○ Malignant cells in the tissues of the larynx or voice box
○ Squamous cell carcinoma: most common form (95% of cases)
○ Adenocarcinoma and sarcoma: rare (5% of cases)
○ Tumor intrinsic (located on the true vocal cords; tends not to spread because underlying connective tissues lack lymph nodes) or extrinsic (located on another part of the larynx; tends to spread easily)

Pathophysiology
○ Laryngeal cancer is classified by its location:
  – supraglottic (on the false vocal cords)
  – glottic (on the true vocal cords)
  – subglottic (rare downward extension from the vocal cords).
○ Malignant cells that proliferate can cause swallowing and breathing impairment.
○ A tumor can decrease mobility of the vocal cords.

Causes
○ Unknown

Risk factors
○ Smoking
○ Alcoholism
○ Chronic inhalation of noxious fumes
○ Familial disposition
○ History of gastroesophageal reflux disease

Incidence
○ About nine times more common in men than women
○ Most victims between ages 50 and 65

Common characteristics
Intrinsic laryngeal cancer
○ Hoarseness lasting longer than 3 weeks
Extrinsic laryngeal cancer
○ Lump in the throat
○ Pain or burning of the throat when drinking hot liquid or citrus drinks
With metastasis
○ Dysphagia
○ Dyspnea
○ Cough
○ Pain, most often radiating to the ear
○ Enlarged cervical lymph nodes

Complications
○ Increased swallowing difficulty and pain
○ Metastasis

Assessment

History
Stage I
○ Complaints of local throat irritation
○ 2-week history of hoarseness
Stages II and III
○ Hoarseness
○ Sore throat
○ Voice volume reduced to whisper
Stage IV
○ Pain radiating to ears
○ Dysphagia
○ Dyspnea

Physical findings
Stage I
○ None
Stage II
○ Possible abnormal movement of vocal cords
Stage III
○ Abnormal movement of vocal cords; possible lymphadenopathy
Stage IV
○ Neck mass or enlarged cervical nodes

Test results
Imaging
○ Xeroradiography, laryngeal tomography, computed tomography scan, and laryngography to confirm the presence of a mass
○ Chest X-ray to rule out metastasis
Diagnostic procedures
○ Laryngoscopy allows definitive staging by obtaining multiple biopsy specimens to establish a primary diagnosis, to determine the extent of the disease, and to identify additional premalignant lesions or second primaries.
Other
○ Biopsy identifies cancer cells.

Treatment

General
○ Precancerous lesions — laser surgery
○ Early lesions — laser surgery or radiation therapy
○ Advanced lesions — radiation therapy and chemotherapy
○ Speech preservation
○ Speech rehabilitation (when speech preservation impossible) — esophageal speech, prosthetic devices, or experimental surgical reconstruction of the voice box
○ Diet based on treatment options
○ May require enteral feeding
○ Frequent rest periods

Medication
○ Chemotherapeutic agents
○ Analgesics

Surgery
○ Cordectomy
○ Partial or total laryngectomy
○ Supraglottic laryngectomy or total laryngectomy with laryngoplasty

Nursing considerations

Key outcomes
The patient will:
○ express feelings regarding illness
○ express feelings of increased comfort
○ maintain a patent airway
○ utilize available support systems.

Nursing interventions
○ Provide supportive psychological, preoperative, and postoperative care.
○ Encourage verbalization and provide support.
○ Assist with establishing a method of communication.
○ Prepare the patient for functional losses (inability to smell, blow his nose, whistle, gargle, sip, or suck on a straw).
○ Provide frequent mouth care.
○ Suction when needed.
○ After total laryngectomy, elevate the head of the bed 30 to 45 degrees and support the back of the neck to prevent tension on sutures and, possibly, wound dehiscence.

Monitoring
After partial laryngectomy
○ Hydration and nutritional status
○ Tracheostomy tube care
○ Use of voice
After total laryngectomy
○ Laryngectomy tube care
○ Vital signs
○ Postoperative complications
○ Pain control
○ Nasogastric (NG) tube placement and function

Patient teaching

Be sure to cover:
○ the disorder, diagnosis, and treatment
○ appropriate oral hygiene practices (before partial or total laryngectomy)
○ postoperative procedures, such as suctioning, NG tube feeding, and laryngectomy tube care
○ preparation for any functional losses.

Discharge planning
○ Arrange for rehabilitation measures (including laryngeal speech, esophageal speech, an artificial larynx, and various mechanical devices).
○ Refer the patient to local resources and support services.

Laryngitis

Overview

Description
- Acute or chronic inflammation of vocal cords
- Isolated infection or part of a generalized bacterial or viral upper respiratory tract infection
- Typical viral infection mild, with limited duration
- Inflammatory changes caused by repeated attacks (associated with chronic laryngitis)

Pathophysiology
- Inflammatory response to cell damage by viruses results in hyperemia and fluid exudation.
- Irritant receptors are triggered.
- Kinins and other inflammatory mediators may induce spasm of upper airway smooth muscle.

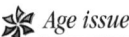 *Age issue*

Developmental differences in the upper airway structures of young children may result in severe narrowing of the upper airways with inflammation, to the degree that respiratory failure may result from hypoventilation.

Causes
- Infection
- Overuse of the voice
- Inhalation of smoke or fumes
- Aspiration of caustic chemicals
- Chronic laryngitis
- Chronic upper respiratory tract disorders
- Mouth breathing
- Smoking
- Constant exposure to dust or other irritants
- Alcohol abuse
- Gastroesophageal reflux
- Reflux esophagitis

Incidence
- Common disorder
- Affects all ages
- Affects males and females equally

Common characteristics
- Hoarseness
- Dry cough

Complications
- Chronic hoarseness
- Permanent laryngeal tissue changes
- Airway obstruction

Assessment

History
- Hoarseness ranging from mild to complete loss of voice
- Feeling of throat rawness
- Throat pain
- Dry cough
- Malaise
- Difficulty swallowing

Physical findings
- Cough
- Fever
- Regional lymphadenopathy
- Stridor (in children)

Test results
Laboratory
- Elevated white blood cell count in bacterial infection
Diagnostic procedures
- Indirect laryngoscopy reveals red, inflamed and, occasionally, hemorrhagic vocal cords exudate.

Treatment

General
- Symptom-based
- Elimination of underlying cause
- Resting the voice (primary treatment)
- Humidification
- Avoidance of smoking
- Avoidance of whispering
- Cold fluids
- Rest during febrile period, with head of bed elevated

Medication
- Analgesics
- Throat lozenges
- Antibiotics (bacterial infection)

Surgery
- Tracheotomy in chronic laryngitis

Nursing considerations

Key outcomes
The patient will:
- express feelings of increased comfort
- exhibit an adequate breathing pattern
- show no signs of infection
- express understanding of the condition and treatment.

Nursing interventions
- Encourage discussion of concerns.
- Keep tracheotomy tray at bedside.
- Encourage modification of predisposing factors.

- Restrict verbal communication.
- Provide alternative communication means.
- Anticipate needs.
- Give prescribed drugs.

Monitoring

- Response to treatment
- Respiratory status

 Alert

In severe, acute laryngitis, monitor the patient for signs and symptoms of airway obstruction.

Patient teaching

Be sure to cover:
- the disorder, diagnosis, and treatment
- why the patient shouldn't talk
- alternate methods of communication
- speaking softly rather than whispering
- maintenance of adequate humidification
- smoking cessation
- medication and potential adverse reactions
- importance of completing prescribed antibiotics
- avoidance of occupational hazards.

Discharge planning

- Refer the patient to a smoking-cessation program, if indicated.

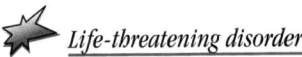

Latex allergy

Overview

Description

- An immunoglobulin (Ig) E–mediated immediate hypersensitivity reaction to products that contain natural latex
- Can range from local dermatitis to life-threatening anaphylactic reaction

Pathophysiology

- Mast cells release histamine and other secretory products.
- Vascular permeability increases and vasodilation and bronchoconstriction occur.
- Chemical sensitivity dermatitis is a type IV delayed hypersensitivity reaction to the chemicals used in processing rather than the latex itself.
- In a cell-mediated allergic reaction, sensitized T lymphocytes are triggered, stimulating the proliferation of other lymphocytes and mononuclear cells, resulting in tissue inflammation and contact dermatitis.

Causes

- Frequent contact with latex-containing products (see *Products that contain latex*)

Risk factors

- Medical and dental professionals
- Workers in latex companies
- Patients with spina bifida or other conditions that require multiple surgeries involving latex material
- History of:
  - asthma or other allergies, especially to bananas, avocados, tropical fruits, or chestnuts
  - multiple intra-abdominal or genitourinary surgeries
  - frequent intermittent urinary catheterization

Incidence

- Present in 1% to 5% of population of the United States
- Affects 10% to 30% of health care workers
- Most prevalent (20% to 68%) in patients with spina bifida and urogenital abnormalities
- Affects males and females equally

Common characteristics

- Hypotension
- Tachycardia
- Urticaria and pruritus
- Difficulty breathing, bronchospasm, wheezing, and stridor
- Angioedema

Complications

- Respiratory obstruction
- Systemic vascular collapse
- Death

Assessment

History

- Exposure to latex

Physical findings

- Signs of anaphylaxis
- Rash
- Angioedema
- Conjunctivitis
- Wheezing, stridor

Test results

Diagnosis of latex allergy is based mainly on history and physical assessment.

Laboratory

- Radioallergosorbent test showing specific IgE antibodies to latex (safest for use in patients with history of type I hypersensitivity)

Products that contain latex

Medical products
- Adhesive bandages
- Airways, Levin tube
- Handheld resuscitation bags
- Blood pressure cuff, tubing, and bladder
- Catheters
- Catheter leg straps
- Dental dams
- Elastic bandages
- Electrode pads
- Fluid-circulating hypothermia blankets
- Hemodialysis equipment
- I.V. catheters
- Latex or rubber gloves
- Medication vials
- Pads for crutches
- Protective sheets
- Reservoir breathing bags
- Rubber airways and endotracheal tubes
- Tape
- Tourniquets

Nonmedical products
- Adhesive tape
- Balloons (excluding Mylar)
- Cervical diaphragms
- Condoms
- Disposable diapers
- Elastic stockings
- Glue
- Latex paint
- Nipples and pacifiers
- Rubber bands
- Tires

Other
- ○ Patch test resulting in hives with itching or redness as a positive response

Treatment

General
- ○ Prevention of exposure, including use of latex-free products to decrease possible exacerbation of hyper-sensitivity
- ○ Maintenance of patent airway

Medication
- ○ Before and after possible exposure to latex
- ○ Corticosteroids
- ○ Antihistamines
- ○ Histamine-2-receptor blockers

Acute treatment
- ○ Epinephrine 1:1,000
- ○ Oxygen therapy
- ○ Volume expanders
- ○ I.V. vasopressors
- ○ Aminophylline and albuterol

Nursing considerations

Key outcomes
The patient will:
- ○ maintain a patent airway
- ○ remain hemodynamically stable
- ○ identify latex products in order to avoid exposure.

Nursing interventions
- ○ Maintain airway, breathing, and circulation.
- ○ Give prescribed drugs.

 Alert

When adding medication to an I.V. bag, inject the drug through the spike port, not the rubber latex port.

- ○ Keep the patient's environment latex free.

Monitoring
- ○ Vital signs
- ○ Respiratory status

Patient teaching

Be sure to cover:
- ○ the disorder, diagnosis, and treatment
- ○ potential for life-threatening reaction
- ○ wearing medical identification jewelry that identifies allergy
- ○ how to use an epinephrine autoinjector.

Legg-Calvé-Perthes disease

Overview

Description

○ Ischemic necrosis leading to eventual flattening of the head of the femur due to vascular interruption
○ Typically unilateral, occurs bilaterally in 20% of patients
○ Also called *coxa plana*
○ Usually runs its course in 3 to 4 years
○ May lead to premature osteoarthritis later in life from misalignment of the acetabulum and flattening of the femoral head

Pathophysiology

Occurs in four stages
○ The first stage, synovitis, is characterized by synovial inflammation and increased joint fluid, and typically lasts 1 to 3 weeks.
○ In the second (avascular) stage, vascular interruption causes necrosis of the ossification center of the femoral head (usually in several months to 1 year).
○ In the third stage, revascularization, a new blood supply causes bone resorption and deposition of immature bone cells. New bone replaces necrotic bone and the femoral head gradually reforms.
○ The final, or residual stage, involves healing and regeneration. Immature bone cells are replaced by normal bone cells, thereby fixing the joint's shape. There may or may not be residual deformity, based on the degree of necrosis that occurred in stage two.

Causes

○ Exact vascular obstructive changes that initiate disease unknown
○ Current etiologic theories include:
  – venous obstruction with secondary intraepiphyseal thrombosis
  – trauma to retinacular vessels
  – vascular irregularities (congenital or developmental)
  – vascular occlusion secondary to increased intracapsular pressure from acute transient synovitis
  – increased blood viscosity resulting in stasis and decreased blood flow.

Incidence

○ Occurs most frequently in boys ages 4 to 10
○ Tends to occur in families

Common characteristics

○ Persistent thigh pain or limp that becomes progressively more severe

○ Mild pain in the hip, thigh, or knee that's aggravated by activity and relieved by rest
○ Muscle spasm
○ Atrophy of muscles in the upper thigh
○ Slight shortening of the leg
○ Severely restricted abduction and internal rotation of the hip

Complications

○ Permanent disability
○ Premature osteoarthritis

Assessment

History

○ Family history
○ Limp that becomes progressively worse
○ Persistent pain in the groin, anterior thigh, or knee that's aggravated by activity and relieved by rest

Physical findings

○ Muscle atrophy
○ Slight shortening of the affected leg
○ Restricted hip abduction and internal rotation
○ Adductor muscle spasm in the affected hip

Test results

Imaging
○ Hip X-rays taken every 3 to 4 months confirm the diagnosis, with findings that vary according to the stage of the disease.
○ Anterior-posterior X-rays and magnetic resonance imaging enhance early diagnosis of necrosis and visualization of articular surface.

Other

○ Physical examination and clinical history

Treatment

○ Protection of the femoral head from further stress and damage by containing it within the acetabulum
○ Reduced weight bearing by means of bed rest in bilateral split counterpoised traction, then application of hip abduction splint or cast, or weight bearing while a splint, cast, or brace holds the leg in abduction (braces may remain in place for 6 to 18 months)
○ Physical therapy with passive and active range-of-motion exercises after cast removal
○ Well-balanced diet

Medication

○ Analgesics

Surgery

○ For a young child in the early stages of the disease, osteotomy and subtrochanteric derotation provide maximum confinement of the epiphysis within the acetabulum to allow return of the femoral head to normal shape and full range of motion. Proper placement of the epiphysis thus allows remolding with ambulation. Postoperatively, the patient requires a spica cast for about 2 months.

Nursing considerations

Key outcomes

The patient will:
○ express feelings of increased comfort and decreased pain
○ perform activities of daily living within the confines of the disease
○ express understanding of the disorder and treatment regimen.

Nursing interventions

○ Provide cast care.
○ Give prescribed analgesics.
○ Provide emotional support.

Monitoring

○ Intake and output
○ Neurovascular status of affected extremity
○ Skin integrity

Patient teaching

Be sure to cover:
○ the disorder, diagnosis, and treatment
○ proper cast care and monitoring of skin integrity.

Legionnaires' disease

Overview

Description

- An acute bronchopneumonia produced by a gram-negative bacillus
- Illness ranging from mild (with or without pneumonitis) to serious multilobed pneumonia with mortality as high as 15%
- Outbreaks (usually in late summer and early fall) epidemic or confined to a few cases

Pathophysiology

- The legionella enter the lungs after aspiration or inhalation.
- Although alveolar macrophages phagocytize the legionella, the organisms aren't killed and proliferate intracellularly.
- The cells rupture, releasing the legionella, and the cycle starts again.
- Lesions develop a nodular appearance and alveoli become filled with fibrin, neutrophils, and alveolar macrophages.

Causes

- *Legionella pneumophila*, an aerobic, gram-negative bacillus that's most likely transmitted by air
- Water distribution systems (such as whirlpool spas and decorative fountains) are a primary reservoir for the organism

Incidence

- Most likely to affect men more than women
- Others at increased risk include:
  - elderly patients
  - immunocompromised patients
  - patients with chronic underlying disease such as diabetes
  - alcoholics
  - cigarette smokers

Common characteristics

- Nonspecific prodromal symptoms
- Initial nonproductive cough that becomes productive

Complications

- Hypoxia and acute respiratory failure
- Hypotension
- Delirium
- Seizures
- Heart failure
- Arrhythmias
- Renal failure
- Shock

Assessment

History

- Presence at a suspected source of infection
- Prodromal symptoms including anorexia, malaise, myalgia, and headache

Physical findings

- Rapidly rising fever with chills
- Grayish or rust-colored, nonpurulent, occasionally blood-streaked sputum
- Tachypnea
- Bradycardia (in about 50% of patients)
- Neurologic signs (altered level of consciousness [LOC])
- Dullness over areas of secretions and consolidation or pleural effusions
- Fine crackles that develop into coarse crackles as the disease progresses

Test results

Laboratory

- Gram staining revealing numerous neutrophils but no organism
- Definitive method of diagnosis involving isolation of the organisms from respiratory secretions or bronchial washings or through thoracentesis
- Definitive tests including direct immunofluorescence of *L. pneumophila* and indirect fluorescent serum antibody testing
- Leukocytosis and increased erythrocyte sedimentation rate
- Decreased partial pressure of arterial oxygen; initially decreased partial pressure of arterial carbon dioxide
- Hyponatremia (serum sodium level less than 131 mg/L)

Imaging

- Chest X-ray typically shows patchy, localized infiltration, which progresses to multilobed consolidation (usually involving the lower lobes) and pleural effusion.
- In fulminant disease, chest X-ray reveals opacification of the entire lung.

Treatment

General

- Fluid replacement
- Oxygen administration

Medication

- Antibiotics
- Antipyretics
- Pressor drugs

Nursing considerations

Key outcomes

The patient will:
○ cough effectively
○ expectorate sputum effectively
○ express feelings of increased comfort in maintaining air exchange
○ regain and maintain normal fluid and electrolyte balance
○ have normal breath sounds.

Nursing interventions

○ Give tepid sponge baths or use hypothermia blankets to lower fever.
○ Provide frequent mouth care. If necessary, apply soothing cream to irritated nostrils.
○ Replace fluids and electrolytes, as needed.
○ Institute seizure precautions.
○ Give prescribed drugs.

Monitoring

○ Vital signs
○ Respiratory status and arterial blood gases
○ LOC

Patient teaching

Be sure to cover:
○ the disorder, diagnosis, and treatment
○ prevention of infection
○ importance of disinfection of water supply
○ purpose of postural drainage, and how to perform coughing and deep-breathing exercises
○ proper hand washing and disposal of soiled tissues to prevent disease transmission.

Discharge planning

○ Refer the patient to a pulmonologist, if necessary.

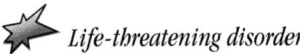 *Life-threatening disorder*

Leukemia, acute

Overview

Description

○ Malignant proliferation of white blood cell (WBC) precursors, or blasts, in bone marrow or lymph tissue; blasts accumulate in peripheral blood, bone marrow, and body tissues
○ Most common form of cancer among children
○ Common forms:
  – Acute lymphoblastic (lymphocytic) leukemia (ALL), characterized by abnormal growth of lymphocyte precursors (lymphoblasts)
  – Acute myeloblastic (myelogenous) leukemia (AML); causes rapid accumulation of myeloid precursors (myeloblasts)
  – Acute monoblastic (monocytic) leukemia, or Schilling's type; results in marked increase in monocyte precursors (monoblasts)
○ ALL: treatment induces remissions in 90% of children (average survival time: 5 years) and 65% of adults (average survival time: 1 to 2 years); children ages 2 to 8 have best survival rate—about 50%—with intensive therapy
○ AML: average survival time is only 1 year after diagnosis, even with aggressive treatment (remissions lasting 2 to 10 months in 50% of children; adult survival, only about 1 year after diagnosis, even with treatment)
○ Without treatment, invariably fatal

Pathophysiology

○ Immature, nonfunctioning WBCs appear to accumulate first in the tissue where they originate, such as lymphocytes in lymph tissue and granulocytes in bone marrow.
○ The immature, nonfunctioning WBCs spill into the bloodstream and overwhelm red blood cells (RBCs) and platelets; from there, they infiltrate other tissues.

Causes

○ Unknown

Risk factors

○ Radiation (especially prolonged exposure)
○ Certain chemicals and drugs
○ Viruses
○ Genetic abnormalities
○ Chronic exposure to benzene
In children
○ Down syndrome
○ Ataxia
○ Telangiectasia
○ Congenital disorders, such as albinism and congenital immunodeficiency syndrome

Incidence

○ More common in males than females
○ More common in whites (especially of Jewish ancestry)
○ More common in children between ages 2 and 5 (80% of leukemias in this age group are ALL), and those who live in urban and industrialized areas

Common characteristics

○ Sudden onset of high fevers
○ Bleeding
○ Night sweats
○ Malaise

Complications

○ Infection
○ Organ malfunction through encroachment or hemorrhage

Assessment

History

○ Sudden onset of high fever
○ Abnormal bleeding
○ Fatigue and night sweats
○ Weakness, lassitude, recurrent infections, and chills
○ Abdominal or bone pain in patients with ALL, AML, or acute monoblastic leukemia

Physical findings

○ Tachycardia, palpitations, and a systolic ejection murmur
○ Decreased ventilation
○ Pallor
○ Lymph node enlargement
○ Liver or spleen enlargement

Test results

Laboratory
○ Blood counts showing thrombocytopenia and neutropenia and a WBC differential showing the cell type
Imaging
○ Computed tomography scan shows the affected organs, and cerebrospinal fluid analysis shows abnormal WBC invasion of the central nervous system.
Diagnostic procedures
○ Bone marrow aspiration that shows a proliferation of immature WBCs confirms acute leukemia; if the aspirate is dry or free from leukemic cells but the patient has other typical signs of leukemia, a bone marrow biopsy, usually of the posterior superior iliac spine, must be performed.
○ Lumbar puncture is used to detect meningeal involvement.

Treatment

General

○ Transfusions of platelets to prevent bleeding
○ Transfusions of RBCs to prevent anemia
○ Bone marrow transplantation in some patients
○ Radiation therapy in case of brain or testicular infiltration
○ Chemotherapeutic and radiation treatment, depending on diagnosis
○ Well-balanced diet
○ Frequent rest periods

Medication

For meningeal infiltration

○ Intrathecal instillation of methotrexate or cytarabine with cranial radiation

For ALL

○ Vincristine, prednisone, high-dose cytarabine, and daunorubicin
○ Intrathecal methotrexate or cytarabine because ALL carries 40% risk of meningeal infiltration

For AML

○ Combination of I.V. daunorubicin and cytarabine (If these fail to induce remission, treatment involves some or all of the following drugs: a combination of cyclophosphamide, vincristine, prednisone, or methotrexate; high-dose cytarabine alone or with other drugs; amsacrine; etoposide; and 5-azacytidine and mitoxantrone.)

For acute monoblastic leukemia

○ Cytarabine and thioguanine with daunorubicin or doxorubicin
○ Anti-infective agents, such as antibiotics, antifungals, and antiviral drugs and granulocyte injections

Nursing considerations

Key outcomes

The patient will:
○ have no further weight loss
○ exhibit intact mucous membranes
○ experience no chills, fever, or other signs and symptoms of illness
○ express feelings of increased comfort
○ utilize available support systems.

Nursing interventions

○ Encourage verbalization and provide comfort.
○ Provide adequate hydration.
○ After bone marrow transplantation, keep the patient in a sterile room, administer antibiotics, and transfuse packed RBCs as necessary.
○ Give prescribed drugs.
○ Control mouth ulceration by checking often for obvious ulcers and gum swelling and by providing frequent mouth care and saline rinses.

Monitoring

○ Complications from treatment
○ Hydration and nutritional status
○ Urine pH (should be above 7.5)
○ Vital signs
○ Signs and symptoms of bleeding

Patient teaching

Be sure to cover:
○ the disorder, diagnosis, and treatment
○ medication, including administration, dosage, and possible adverse effects
○ use of a soft toothbrush and avoidance of hot, spicy foods and commercial mouthwashes
○ signs and symptoms of infection
○ signs and symptoms of abnormal bleeding
○ planned rest periods during the day.

Discharge planning

○ Refer the patient to available resources and support services.

Leukemia, chronic granulocytic

Overview

Description

○ Type of leukemia characterized by abnormal over-growth of granulocytic precursors (myeloblasts, promyelocytes, metamyelocytes, and myelocytes) in bone marrow, peripheral blood, and body tissues
○ Always fatal (average survival time 3 to 4 years after onset of chronic phase and 3 to 6 months after onset of acute phase)
○ Clinical course proceeds in two distinct phases:
  – insidious chronic phase (characterized by anemia and bleeding abnormalities)
  – acute phase (blast crisis, or myeloblasts, the most primitive granulocytic precursors, proliferate rapidly)
○ During acute phase, either lymphoblastic or myeloblastic disease may develop (Despite vigorous treatment, chronic granulocytic leukemia rapidly advances after onset of acute phase.)
○ Also called chronic myelogenous (or myelocytic) leukemia (CML)

Pathophysiology

○ CML is a myeloproliferative disorder, originating in a progenitor stem cell.
○ Malignant transformation is identified in erythroid, megakaryocytic, and macrophage cell lines.
○ Malignant transformation arises from pluripotential stem cells or lymphoid stem cells.

Causes

○ Exact cause unknown

Risk factors

○ Presence of the Philadelphia chromosome (found in almost 90% of patients)
○ Myeloproliferative diseases

Incidence

○ Most common in young and middle-aged adults
○ Slightly more common in men than in women, and rare in children
○ In United States, 3,000 to 4,000 cases annually (about 20% of all leukemias)

Common characteristics

○ Fatigue
○ Weakness
○ Weight loss
○ History of gouty arthritis or renal calculi

Complications

○ Infection
○ Hemorrhage
○ Pain

Assessment

History

○ Renal calculi or gouty arthritis
○ Fatigue, weakness, dyspnea, decreased exercise tolerance, and headache
○ Recent weight loss and anorexia

Physical findings

○ Evidence of bleeding and clotting disorders
○ Low-grade fever and tachycardia
○ Pallor
○ Difficulty breathing
○ Retinal hemorrhage
○ Hepatosplenomegaly with abdominal discomfort and pain
○ Sternal and rib tenderness

Test results

Laboratory
○ Chromosomal studies of peripheral blood or bone marrow showing the Philadelphia chromosome
○ Low leukocyte alkaline phosphatase levels confirming chronic granulocytic leukemia
○ White blood cell (WBC) abnormalities, including:
  – Leukocytosis (WBC count over 50,000/µl, rising as high as 250,000/µl)
  – Occasionally leukopenia (WBC count under 5,000/µl)
  – Neutropenia (neutrophil count under 1,500/µl) despite high WBC count
○ Increased circulating myeloblasts
○ Decreased hemoglobin level (below 10 g/dl) and low hematocrit level (less than 30%)
○ Thrombocytosis (more than 1 million thrombocytes/µl)
○ Serum uric acid level that may exceed 8 mg/dl
Imaging
○ Computed tomography scan may show the affected organs.
Diagnostic procedures
○ Bone marrow aspirate or biopsy (performed only if the aspirate is dry) may be hypercellular, characteristically showing bone marrow infiltration by a significantly increased number of myeloid elements; in the acute phase, myeloblasts predominate.

Treatment

General

○ Bone marrow transplantation (chronic phase, more than 60% of patients who receive transplant achieve remission)
○ Local splenic radiation

- Leukapheresis (selective leukocyte removal) to reduce WBC count
- Well-balanced diet
- Frequent rest periods

Medication

- Busulfan and hydroxyurea
- Aspirin
- Allopurinol
- Antibiotic treatment

Surgery

- Splenectomy

Nursing considerations

Key outcomes

The patient will:
- have no further weight loss
- have intact mucous membranes
- experience no chills, fever, or other signs and symptoms of illness
- express feelings of increased comfort and energy
- utilize available support systems.

Nursing interventions

- Plan care to minimize fatigue.
- Regularly check skin and mucous membranes for pallor, petechiae, and bruising.
- Encourage deep-breathing and coughing exercises.
- Encourage verbalization and provide comfort.
- Give prescribed drugs.
- After bone marrow transplantation, keep the patient in a sterile room and give prescribed antibiotics and packed red blood cells.

Monitoring

- Adverse effects of treatment
- Signs and symptoms of bleeding
- Signs and symptoms of infection
- Complete blood count
- Vital signs
- Hydration and nutritional status

Patient teaching

Be sure to cover:
- the disorder, diagnosis, and treatment
- how to minimize bleeding and infection risks (such as by using a soft-bristled toothbrush, an electric razor, and other safety devices)
- high-calorie, high-protein diet
- if the patient is to undergo bone marrow transplantation, reinforcement of the physician's explanation of the procedure, possible outcome, and potential adverse effects
- medication, including administration, dosage, and possible adverse effects

- signs and symptoms of infection and thrombocytopenia.

Discharge planning

- Refer the patient to available resources and support services.

Leukemia, chronic lymphocytic

Overview

Description

○ The most benign and the most slowly progressive form of leukemia
○ Prognosis poor if anemia, thrombocytopenia, neutropenia, bulky lymphadenopathy, and severe lymphocytosis develop

Pathophysiology

○ Chronic lymphocytic leukemia is a generalized, progressive disease marked by an uncontrollable spread of abnormal, small lymphocytes in lymphoid tissue, blood, and bone marrow.
○ Once these cells infiltrate bone marrow, lymphoid tissue, and organ systems, clinical signs begin to appear.
○ Gross bone marrow replacement by abnormal lymphocytes is the most common cause of death, usually within 4 to 5 years of diagnosis.

Causes

○ Exact cause unknown

Risk factors

○ Hereditary factors
○ Undefined chromosomal abnormalities
○ Certain immunologic defects, such as acquired agammaglobulinemia or ataxia-telangiectasia

Common characteristics

○ Fever, malaise, weakness
○ Enlarged lymph nodes

Incidence

○ Most common in elderly people; nearly all afflicted are men older than age 50
○ Chronic lymphocytic leukemia almost one-third of new leukemia cases annually
○ Higher incidence recorded within families

Complications

○ Infection
○ In end-stage disease: anemia, progressive splenomegaly, leukemic cell replacement of the bone marrow, and profound hypogammaglobulinemia, which usually terminates with fatal septicemia

Assessment

History

○ Fatigue, malaise, fever, weight loss, and frequent infections
○ Weakness, palpitations

Physical findings

○ Macular or nodular eruptions and evidence of skin infiltration
○ Enlarged lymph nodes, liver, and spleen
○ Bone tenderness and edema from lymph node obstruction
○ Pallor, dyspnea, tachycardia, bleeding, and infection from bone marrow involvement
○ Signs of opportunistic fungal, viral, or bacterial infections

Test results

Laboratory
○ Miscellaneous blood tests revealing the disease (Typically, chronic lymphocytic leukemia is an incidental finding during a routine complete blood count that reveals numerous abnormal lymphocytes.)
   – In the early stages, mildly but persistently elevated white blood cell (WBC) count; granulocytopenia the rule, although WBC count climbs as disease progresses
   – Hemoglobin level under 11g/dl
   – WBC differential showing neutropenia (less than 1,500/µl), lymphocytosis (more than 10,000/µl)
   – Platelet count showing thrombocytopenia (less than 150,000/µl)
   – Serum protein electrophoresis showing hypogammaglobulinemia
Imaging
○ Computed tomography scan shows affected organs.
Diagnostic procedures
○ Bone marrow aspiration and biopsy show lymphocytic invasion.

Treatment

General

○ Radiation therapy to relieve symptoms (generally for patient with enlarged lymph nodes, painful bony lesions, or massive splenomegaly)
○ High-calorie, high-protein diet
○ Avoidance of hot and spicy foods for patient with impaired oral membranes
○ Frequent rest periods

Medication

○ Systemic chemotherapy

Nursing considerations

Key outcomes

The patient will:
○ have no further weight loss
○ have intact mucous membranes
○ experience no chills, fever, or other signs and symptoms of illness
○ express feelings of increased comfort and energy
○ utilize available support systems.

Nursing interventions

○ Help establish an appropriate rehabilitation program during remission.
○ Place in reverse isolation, if necessary.
○ Give prescribed drugs.
○ Encourage verbalization and provide support.
○ Administer blood component therapy, as necessary.

Monitoring

○ Signs and symptoms of bleeding and thrombocytopenia
○ Adverse effects of treatment
○ In rectal area, induration, swelling, erythema, skin discoloration, and drainage
○ Pain control
○ Vital signs

Patient teaching

Be sure to cover:
○ the disorder, diagnosis, and treatment
○ use of a soft toothbrush and avoidance of commercial mouthwashes to prevent irritating the mouth ulcers that result from chemotherapy
○ medication, including administration, dosage, and possible adverse effects
○ signs and symptoms of infection, bleeding, and recurrence
○ staying away from anyone with an infection
○ importance of follow-up care
○ signs and symptoms of recurrence.

Discharge planning

○ Refer the patient to available resources and support services.

Listeriosis

Overview

Description

○ An infection caused by the weakly hemolytic, gram-positive bacillus *Listeria monocytogenes* (a non–spore producing, motile gram-positive bacillus with aerobic and anaerobic characteristics)
○ Occurs most commonly in fetuses, in neonates (during the first 3 weeks of life), and in older or immunosuppressed adults; infected fetus usually stillborn or born prematurely, almost always with lethal listeriosis
○ Infection produces milder illness in pregnant women and varying degrees of illness in older and immunosuppressed patients; prognoses depend on the severity of underlying illness.

Pathophysiology

○ *L. Monocytogenes* is a non–spore producing, motile gram-positive bacillus with aerobic and anaerobic characteristics.
○ It grows best at neutral to slightly alkaline pH.
○ Transmission occurs:
  – in utero (through the placenta) or during passage through an infected birth canal
  – by inhaling contaminated dust
  – by drinking contaminated, unpasteurized milk
  – by coming in contact with infected animals, contaminated sewage or mud, or soil contaminated with feces organism.(See *Avoiding listeriosis.*)

Causes

○ Contamination with *L. monocytogenes*

Incidence

○ 7.4 cases per million population
○ Affects women of childbearing age

Common characteristics

○ Transient asymptomatic carrier state
○ Bacteremia and a febrile, generalized illness
○ In a pregnant woman, especially during the third trimester: a mild illness with malaise, chills, fever, and back pain (possibly also severe uterine infection, abortion, premature delivery, or stillbirth)
○ Transplacental infection possibly causing early neonatal death or granulomatosis infantiseptica, which produces organ abscesses in infants

Complications

○ Stillbirth
○ Meningitis
○ Septic arthritis
○ Endocarditis

Assessment

History

○ Ingestion of infected food
○ Eye or skin exposure to laboratory animals or animals seen in veterinary practice
○ Back pain and malaise
○ Fever

Physical findings

○ Skin lesions on trunk and extremities
○ Signs of sepsis

Test results

○ *L. monocytogenes* identified by its diagnostic tumbling motility on a wet mount of the culture
○ Positive culture of blood, spinal fluid, drainage from cervical or vaginal lesions, or lochia from a mother with an infected infant; isolation of the organism from these specimens generally difficult

Treatment

General

○ Symptomatic
○ Activity, as tolerated
○ Diet, as tolerated

Medication

○ Antibiotics

Avoiding listeriosis

Follow these general guidelines to avoid listeriosis:
○ Thoroughly cook raw food from animal sources, such as beef, pork, or poultry.
○ Wash raw vegetables thoroughly before eating.
○ Keep uncooked meats separate from vegetables and from cooked foods and ready-to-eat foods.
○ Avoid unpasteurized (raw) milk or foods made from unpasteurized milk.
○ Wash hands, knives, and cutting boards after handling uncooked foods.

Patients at high risk, such as those with weakened immune systems and pregnant women, should follow the general guidelines, plus:
○ Avoid hot dogs, luncheon meats, and deli meats, unless they are reheated until steaming hot.
○ Avoid cross-contaminating other foods, utensils, and food preparation surfaces with fluid from hot dog packages, and wash hands after handling hot dogs, luncheon meats, and deli meats.
○ Don't eat soft cheeses such as feta, Brie, Camembert, blue-veined cheeses, and Mexican-style cheeses such as "queso blanco fresco."
○ Don't eat refrigerated patés or meat spreads. Canned or shelf-stable pâtés and meat spreads may be eaten.
○ Don't eat refrigerated smoked seafood, such as salmon, trout, whitefish, cod, tuna, or mackerel, unless it's in a cooked dish, such as a casserole.

Nursing considerations

Key outcomes

The patient will:
○ maintain fluid balance
○ maintain stable vital signs
○ show improvement in signs and symptoms.

Nursing interventions

○ Follow standard precautions.
○ Provide adequate nutrition by total parenteral nutrition, nasogastric tube feedings, or a soft diet, as ordered.

Monitoring

○ Neurologic status
○ Fontanels (in neonates)
○ Vital signs
○ Intake and output

Patient teaching

Be sure to cover:
○ the disorder, diagnosis, and treatment
○ how to avoid infective materials on farms where listeriosis is endemic among livestock.

Liver cancer

Overview

Description

- Malignant cells growing in the tissues of the liver
- Rapidly fatal, usually within 6 months
- After cirrhosis, the leading cause of fatal hepatic disease
- Liver metastasis occurring as solitary lesion (the first sign of recurrence after a remission)

Pathophysiology

- Most (90%) primary liver tumors originate in the parenchymal cells and are hepatomas. Others originate in the intrahepatic bile ducts (cholangiomas).
- Approximately 30% to 70% of patients with hepatomas also have cirrhosis.
- Rare tumors include a mixed-cell type, Kupffer cell sarcoma, and hepatoblastoma.
- The liver is one of the most common sites of metastasis from other primary cancers. Cells metastasize to gallbladder, mesentery, peritoneum, and diaphragm by direct extension.

Causes

- Immediate cause unknown
- Environmental exposure to carcinogens
- Possibly androgens and oral estrogens
- Hepatitis B virus
- Hepatitis C virus
- Hepatitis D virus

Risk factors

- Cirrhosis
- Excessive alcohol intake
- Malnutrition

Incidence

- Most prevalent in men older than age 60
- Primary liver cancer roughly 2% of all cancers in North America and 10% to 50% of cancers in Africa and parts of Asia

Common characteristics

- Right upper quadrant pain
- Fatigue

Complications

- GI hemorrhage
- Progressive cachexia
- Liver failure

Assessment

History

- Weight loss
- Weakness, fatigue, and fever
- Initially, dull aching abdominal pain
- Severe pain in the epigastrium or right upper quadrant

Physical findings

- Jaundice
- Dependent edema
- Abdominal bruit, hum, or rubbing sound
- Tender, nodular, enlarged liver
- Ascites
- Palpable mass in the right upper quadrant

Test results

Laboratory
- Abnormal liver function studies
- Alpha-fetoprotein levels greater than 500 mcg/ml
- Abnormal electrolyte study results

Imaging
- Liver scan may show filling defects and lesions in the liver.
- Arteriography may define large tumors.
- Ultrasound and computed tomography scans may reveal lesions in the liver.

Diagnostic procedures
- Liver biopsy by needle or open biopsy reveals cancerous cells.

Treatment

General

- Radiation therapy (alone or with chemotherapy)
- High-calorie, low-protein diet
- Frequent rest periods
- Postoperative avoidance of heavy lifting and contact sports

Medication

- Chemotherapeutic drugs

Surgery

- Resection (lobectomy or partial hepatectomy)
- Liver transplantation

Nursing considerations

Key outcomes

The patient will:
- maintain stable hemodynamic status
- maintain adequate cardiac output
- exhibit adequate coping behaviors
- maintain normal fluid volume
- express feelings of increased comfort.

Nursing interventions

- Give prescribed drugs.
- Provide meticulous skin care.
- Encourage verbalization and provide support.

Monitoring

○ Vital signs
○ Hydration and nutritional status
○ Weight
○ Pain control
○ Neurologic status
○ Complete blood count; liver function tests
○ Postoperative complications
○ Wound site

Patient teaching

Be sure to cover:
○ the disorder, diagnosis, and treatment
○ dietary restrictions
○ relaxation techniques
○ medication, including administration, dosage, and possible adverse effects.

Discharge planning

○ Refer the patient and family members to support services.

Liver failure

Overview

Description

- Inability of the liver to function properly, usually as the end result of any liver disease
- Causes a complex syndrome involving the impairment of many different organs and body functions (see *Understanding liver functions*)
- Two conditions occurring in liver failure — hepatic encephalopathy and hepatorenal syndrome
- Liver transplantation only cure

Pathophysiology

- Manifestations of liver failure include hepatic encephalopathy and hepatorenal syndrome.

Hepatic encephalopathy
- The liver can no longer detoxify the blood.
- Liver dysfunction and collateral vessels that shunt blood around the liver to the systemic circulation permit toxins absorbed from the GI tract to circulate freely to the brain.
- The normal liver transforms ammonia (a by-product of protein metabolism) to urea, which the kidneys excrete.
- When the liver is no longer able to transform ammonia to urea, ammonia blood levels rise and the ammonia is delivered to the brain.
- Short-chain fatty acids, serotonin, tryptophan, and false neurotransmitters may also accumulate in the blood.

Hepatorenal syndrome
- Renal failure is concurrent with liver disease; the kidneys appear to be normal but abruptly cease functioning.
- Blood volume expands, hydrogen ions accumulate, and electrolyte disturbances occur.
- The cause may be the accumulation of vasoactive substances that cause inappropriate constriction of renal arterioles, leading to decreased glomerular filtration and oliguria.
- The vasoconstriction may also be a compensatory response to portal hypertension and the pooling of blood in the splenic circulation.

Causes

- Viral hepatitis
- Nonviral hepatitis
- Cirrhosis
- Liver cancer
- Acetaminophen toxicity

Incidence

- Patients younger than age 10 and older than age 40 fare poorly.

Common characteristics

- Jaundice
- Abdominal pain or tenderness
- Nausea and anorexia
- Fatigue
- Weight loss
- Pruritus
- Oliguria
- Splenomegaly
- Ascites
- Peripheral edema
- Varices of the esophagus, rectum, and abdominal wall
- Bleeding tendencies
- Petechia
- Amenorrhea
- Gynecomastia (in males)

Complications

- Variceal bleeding
- GI hemorrhage
- Coma
- Death

Assessment

History

- Liver disorder
- Fatigue
- Weight loss
- Nausea
- Anorexia
- Pruritus

Physical findings

- Jaundice
- Abdominal tenderness
- Splenomegaly
- Ascites
- Peripheral edema

Understanding liver functions

To understand how liver disease affects the body, you need to understand its main functions. The liver:
- detoxifies poisonous chemicals, including alcohol, and drugs (prescribed and over-the-counter as well as illegal substances)
- makes bile to help digest food
- stores energy by stockpiling sugar (carbohydrates, glucose, and fat) until needed
- stores iron reserves as well as vitamins and minerals
- manufactures new proteins
- produces important plasma proteins necessary for blood coagulation, including prothrombin and fibrinogen
- serves as a site for hematopoiesis during fetal development.

Test results

Laboratory
○ Liver function tests reveal elevated levels of aspartate aminotransferase, alanine aminotransferase, alkaline phosphatase, and bilirubin.
○ Blood studies reveal anemia, impaired red blood cell production, elevated bleeding and clotting times, low blood glucose levels, and increased serum ammonia levels.
○ Urine osmolarity is increased.

Treatment

General
○ Paracentesis to remove ascitic fluid
○ Balloon tamponade to control bleeding varices
○ Low-protein, high-carbohydrate diet
○ Activity, as tolerated

Medication
○ Lactulose
○ Potassium-sparing diuretics (for ascites)
○ Potassium supplements
○ Vasoconstrictor drugs (for variceal bleeding)
○ Vitamin K

Surgery
○ Sclerosis to stop bleeding varices
○ Shunt placement
○ Liver transplantation

Nursing considerations

Key outcomes
The patient will:
○ express feelings of increased comfort
○ maintain stable vital signs
○ stabilize fluid status
○ remain oriented to his surroundings.

Nursing interventions
○ Reorient patient, as needed.
○ Provide a safe environment.
○ Provide emotional support.

Monitoring
○ Level of consciousness
○ Vital signs
○ Laboratory values
○ Intake and output
○ Weight and abdominal girth

Patient teaching

Be sure to cover:
○ the disorder, diagnosis, and treatment
○ signs of complications and when to notify the physician

○ importance of following a low-protein diet
○ importance of avoiding alcohol.

Discharge planning
○ Refer the patient to available support services, as appropriate.

Lung cancer

Overview

Description

- Malignant tumors arising from the respiratory epithelium
- Most common types are epidermoid (squamous cell), adenocarcinoma, small-cell (oat cell), and large-cell (anaplastic)
- Most common site is wall or epithelium of bronchial tree
- For most patients, poor prognosis, depending on extent of cancer when diagnosed and cells' growth rate (Only about 13% of patients with lung cancer survive 5 years after being diagnosed.)

Pathophysiology

- Individuals with lung cancer demonstrate bronchial epithelial changes progressing from squamous cell alteration or metaplasia to carcinoma in situ.
- Tumors originating in the bronchi are thought to be more mucus producing.
- Partial or complete obstruction of the airway occurs with tumor growth, resulting in lobar collapse distal to the tumor.
- Early metastasis occurs to other thoracic structures, such as hilar lymph nodes or the mediastinum.
- Distant metastasis occurs to the brain, liver, bone, and adrenal glands.

Causes

- Exact cause unknown

Risk factors

- Smoking
- Exposure to carcinogenic and industrial air pollutants (asbestos, arsenic, chromium, coal dust, iron oxides, nickel, radioactive dust, and uranium)
- Genetic predisposition

Incidence

- Family susceptibility

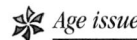 *Age issue*

Lung cancer is the most common cause of death from cancer for men and women ages 50 to 75.

Common characteristics

Epidermoid and small-cell
- Smoker's cough
- Hoarseness
- Wheezing
- Dyspnea
- Hemoptysis
- Chest pain

- Cushing's and carcinoid syndromes
- Hypercalcemia

Adenocarcinoma and large-cell
- Fever
- Weakness
- Weight loss
- Anorexia
- Shoulder pain
- Gynecomastia
- Hypertrophic pulmonary osteoarthropathy

Complications

- Spread of primary tumor to intrathoracic structures
- Tracheal obstruction
- Esophageal compression with dysphagia
- Phrenic nerve paralysis with hemidiaphragm elevation and dyspnea
- Sympathetic nerve paralysis with Horner's syndrome
- Spinal cord compression
- Lymphatic obstruction with pleural effusion
- Hypoxemia
- Anorexia and weight loss, sometimes leading to cachexia, digital clubbing, and hypertrophic osteoarthropathy
- Neoplastic and paraneoplastic syndromes, including Pancoast's syndrome and syndrome of inappropriate secretion of antidiuretic hormone

Assessment

History

- Possibly no symptoms
- Exposure to carcinogens
- Coughing
- Hemoptysis
- Shortness of breath
- Hoarseness
- Fatigue

Physical findings

- Dyspnea on exertion
- Finger clubbing
- Edema of the face, neck, and upper torso
- Dilated chest and abdominal veins (superior vena cava syndrome)
- Weight loss
- Enlarged lymph nodes
- Enlarged liver
- Decreased breath sounds
- Wheezing
- Pleural friction rub

Test results

Laboratory
- Cytologic sputum analysis showing diagnostic evidence of pulmonary malignancy
- Abnormal liver function tests, especially with metastasis

Imaging
- Chest X-rays show advanced lesions and can show a lesion up to 2 years before signs and symptoms appear; findings may indicate tumor size and location.
- Contrast studies of the bronchial tree (chest tomography, bronchography) demonstrate size and location as well as spread of lesion.
- Bone scan is used to detect metastasis.
- Computed tomography (CT) of the chest is used to detect malignant pleural effusion.
- CT of the brain is used to detect metastasis.
- Positron emission tomography aids in the diagnosis of primary and metastatic sites.

Diagnostic procedures
- Bronchoscopy can be used to identify the tumor site. Bronchoscopic washings provide material for cytologic and histologic study.
- Needle biopsy of the lungs (relies on biplanar fluoroscopic visual control to locate peripheral tumors before withdrawing a tissue specimen for analysis) allows firm diagnosis in 80% of patients.
- Tissue biopsy of metastatic sites (including supraclavicular and mediastinal nodes and pleura) is used to assess disease extent. Based on histologic findings, staging describes the disease's extent and prognosis and is used to direct treatment.
- Thoracentesis allows chemical and cytologic examination of pleural fluid.
- Gallium scans of the liver and spleen help to detect metastasis.
- Exploratory thoracotomy is performed to obtain biopsy.

Treatment

General
- Various combinations of surgery, radiation therapy, and chemotherapy to improve prognosis
- Palliative (most treatments)
- Preoperative and postoperative radiation therapy
- Laser therapy (experimental)
- Well-balanced diet
- Activity, as tolerated per breathing capacity

Medication
- Chemotherapy drug combinations
- Immunotherapy (investigational)

Surgery
- Partial removal of lung (wedge resection, segmental resection, lobectomy, radical lobectomy)
- Total removal of lung (pneumonectomy, radical pneumonectomy)

Nursing considerations

Key outcomes
The patient will:
- maintain normal fluid volume
- maintain adequate ventilation
- maintain a patent airway
- express feelings of increased comfort and decreased pain.

Nursing interventions
- Provide supportive care.
- Encourage verbalization.
- Give prescribed drugs.

Monitoring
- Chest tube function and drainage
- Postoperative complications
- Wound site
- Vital signs
- Sputum production
- Hydration and nutrition
- Oxygenation
- Pain control

Patient teaching

Be sure to cover:
- the disorder, diagnosis, and treatment
- postoperative procedures and equipment
- chest physiotherapy
- exercises to prevent shoulder stiffness
- medications, including dosage, administration, and possible adverse effects
- risk factors for recurrent cancer.

Discharge planning
- Refer smokers to local branches of the American Cancer Society or Smokenders.
- Provide information about group therapy, individual counseling, and hypnosis.
- Refer the patient to available resources and support services.

Lupus erythematosus

Overview

Description

○ This chronic inflammatory disorder of the connective tissues appears in two forms: discoid lupus erythematosus, which affects only the skin, and systemic lupus erythematosus (SLE), which affects multiple organ systems as well as the skin and can be fatal.
○ SLE is characterized by recurring remissions and exacerbations, which are especially common during the spring and summer.
○ The prognosis improves with early detection and treatment but remains poor for patients who develop cardiovascular, renal, or neurologic complications, or severe bacterial infections.

Pathophysiology

○ Autoimmunity is believed to be the prime mechanism involved with SLE.
○ The body produces antibodies against components of its own cells such as the antinuclear antibody (ANA), and immune complex disease follows.
○ Patients with SLE may produce antibodies against many different tissue components, such as red blood cells (RBCs), neutrophils, platelets, lymphocytes, or almost any organ or tissue in the body.

Causes

○ Exact cause unknown, but contributing factors include:
  – physical or mental stress
  – streptococcal or viral infections
  – exposure to sunlight or ultraviolet light
  – immunization
  – pregnancy
  – abnormal estrogen metabolism
  – treatment with certain drugs, such as procainamide (Pronestyl), hydralazine (Apresoline), and anticonvulsants

Incidence

○ Affects 14 to 50 people per 100,000 in the United States
○ Affects females more than males
○ Affects all ages, but peak incidence is young adulthood

Common characteristics

See *Signs of systemic lupus erythematosus*.

Complications

○ Concomitant infections
○ Urinary tract infections
○ Renal failure
○ Osteonecrosis of hip from long-term steroid use

Assessment

History

○ History of contributing factor
○ Fever
○ Weight loss
○ Malaise
○ Fatigue
○ Polyarthralgia
○ Abdominal pain
○ Headaches, irritability, and depression (common)
○ Nausea, vomiting, diarrhea, constipation
○ Irregular menstrual periods or amenorrhea during the active phase of SLE

Physical findings

○ Rashes
○ Joint involvement, similar to rheumatoid arthritis (although the arthritis of lupus is usually nonerosive)
○ Skin lesions, most commonly an erythematous rash in areas exposed to light (classic butterfly rash over the nose and cheeks in less than 50% of patients) or a scaly, papular rash (mimics psoriasis), especially in sun-exposed areas
○ Vasculitis (especially in the digits), possibly leading to infarctive lesions, necrotic leg ulcers, or digital gangrene
○ Patchy alopecia and painless ulcers of the mucous membranes
○ Lymph node enlargement (diffuse or local, and nontender)

Test results

Laboratory

○ Anti–double-stranded deoxyribonucleic acid antibody (anti-dsDNA); most specific test for SLE, correlates with disease activity, especially renal involvement, and helps monitor response to therapy; may be low or absent in remission
○ Complete blood count with differential possibly showing anemia and a decreased white blood cell (WBC) count
○ Decreased platelet count
○ Elevated erythrocyte sedimentation rate
○ Hypergammaglobulinemia
○ ANA and lupus erythematosus cell tests showing positive results in active SLE
○ Urine studies possibly showing RBCs and WBCs, urine casts and sediment, and significant protein loss (more than 0.5 g/24 hours)
○ Serum complement blood studies showing decreased serum complement (C3 and C4) levels indicating active disease
○ Lupus anticoagulant and anticardiolipin tests possibly positive in some patients (usually in patients prone to antiphospholipid syndrome of thrombosis, abortion, and thrombocytopenia)

Imaging
○ Chest X-ray possibly showing pleurisy or lupus pneumonitis

Diagnostic procedures
○ Electrocardiography possibly showing a conduction defect with cardiac involvement or pericarditis
○ Kidney biopsy to determine disease stage and extent of renal involvement

Treatment

General
○ Symptomatic
○ Dialysis or kidney transplant for renal failure
○ Diet restrictions based on extent of disorder
○ Activity, as tolerated
○ Frequent rest periods

Medication
○ Nonsteroidal anti-inflammatory compounds, including aspirin
○ Topical corticosteroid creams, such as hydrocortisone buteprate or triamcinolone (Aristocort)
○ Intralesional corticosteroids or antimalarials such as hydroxychloroquine sulfate (Plaquenil)
○ Systemic corticosteroids

Nursing considerations

Key outcomes
The patient will:
○ remain free from infection
○ remain hemodynamically stable
○ express understanding of disease and treatment.

Nursing interventions
○ Provide a balanced diet. Renal involvement may mandate a low-sodium, low-protein diet.
○ Urge the patient to get plenty of rest. Schedule diagnostic tests and procedures to allow adequate rest.
○ Explain all tests and procedures.
○ Apply heat packs to relieve joint pain and stiffness.
○ Encourage regular exercise to maintain full range of motion (ROM) and prevent contractures.

Monitoring
○ Signs and symptoms
○ Vital signs
○ Intake and output
○ Laboratory reports

Patient teaching

Be sure to cover:
○ ROM exercises as well as body alignment and postural techniques
○ expected benefit of prescribed medications, as well as adverse effects

○ cosmetic tips, such as suggesting the use of hypoallergenic makeup and referral to a hairdresser who specializes in scalp disorders.

Discharge planning
○ Arrange for physical therapy and occupational counseling, as appropriate.
○ Refer the patient to the Lupus Foundation of America and the Arthritis Foundation, as necessary.

Lyme disease

Overview

Description
○ A multisystem disorder caused by a spirochete

Pathophysiology
○ A tick injects spirochete-laden saliva into the bloodstream or deposits fecal matter on the skin.
○ After incubating for 3 to 32 days, the spirochetes migrate outward on the skin, causing a rash, and disseminate to other skin sites or organs through the bloodstream or lymph system.
○ Spirochetes may survive for years in the joints or die after triggering an inflammatory response in the host.

Causes
○ The spirochete *Borrelia burgdorferi*, carried by the minute tick *Ixodes dammini* (also called *I. scapularis*) or another tick in the Ixodidae family

Incidence
○ Affects all ages and both sexes
○ Onset during the summer months
○ Occurs in geographic ranges of ixodid ticks

Common characteristics
○ Typically begins with classic skin lesion, erythema migrans (EM)
○ Skin lesions with bright red outer rims and white centers appearing on axilla, thigh, and groin
○ Initial reported symptoms such as fatigue, malaise, migratory myalgia, and arthralgia
○ Cardiac, neurologic, or joint abnormalities that may develop weeks or months later

Complications
○ Myocarditis
○ Pericarditis
○ Arrhythmias
○ Meningitis
If untreated in acute phase
○ Encephalitis
○ Cranial or peripheral neuropathies
○ Arthritis

Differentiating Lyme disease

Lyme disease, or chronic neuroborreliosis, needs to be differentiated from chronic fatigue syndrome or fibromyalgia, which is difficult late in the disease because of chronic pain and fatigue. The other diseases produce more generalized and disabling symptoms; also, patients lack evidence of joint inflammation, have normal neurologic tests, and have a greater degree of anxiety and depression than patients with Lyme disease.

Assessment

History
○ Recent exposure to ticks
○ Onset of symptoms in warmer months
○ Severe headache and stiff neck with rash eruption
○ Fever (up to 104° F [40° C]) and chills

Physical findings
○ Regional lymphadenopathy
○ Tenderness in the skin lesion site or the posterior cervical area
Early stage
○ Tachycardia or irregular heartbeat
○ Mild dyspnea
○ EM
○ Headache
○ Myalgia
○ Arthralgia
Later stage
○ Neurologic signs such as memory impairment
○ Bell's palsy
○ Intermittent arthritis (see *Differentiating Lyme disease*)
○ Cardiac symptoms, such as heart failure, pericarditis, and dyspnea
○ Neurologic symptoms, such as memory impairment and myelitis
○ Fibromyalgia
○ Ocular signs such as conjunctivitis

Test results
Laboratory
○ Assays for anti-*B. burgdorferi* (Anti-B) showing evidence of previous or current infection
○ Enzyme-linked immunosorbent technology (ELISA or EIA) or indirect immunofluorescence microscopy (IFA) showing immunoglobulin (Ig) M levels that peak 3 to 6 weeks after infection; IgG antibodies detected several weeks after infection that may continue to develop for several months and generally persist for years
○ Positive Western blot assay showing serologic evidence of past or current infection with *B. burgdorferi*
○ Polymerase chain reaction (PCR) used when joint and cerebrospinal fluid involvement is present

 Alert

Serologic testing isn't useful early in the course of Lyme disease because of its low sensitivity. However, it may be more useful in later disease stages, when sensitivity and specificity of the test are improved.

Diagnostic procedures
○ Lumbar puncture with analysis of cerebrospinal fluid may show antibodies to *B. burgdorferi*.
○ Skin biopsy may be used to detect *B. burgdorferi*.

Treatment

General

○ Prompt tick removal using proper technique
○ Rest periods when needed

Medication

○ I.V. or oral antibiotics (initiated as soon as possible after infection)

Nursing considerations

Key outcomes

The patient will:
○ maintain hemodynamic stability
○ maintain adequate cardiac output
○ express relief from pain
○ attain the highest degree of mobility possible.

Nursing interventions

○ Plan care to provide adequate rest.
○ Give prescribed drugs.
○ Assist with range-of-motion and strengthening exercises (with arthritis).
○ Encourage verbalization and provide support.

Monitoring

○ Skin lesions
○ Response to treatment
○ Adverse drug reactions
○ Complications

Patient teaching

Be sure to cover:
○ the disorder, diagnosis, and treatment
○ medication administration, dosage, and possible adverse effects
○ importance of follow-up care and reporting recurrent or new symptoms to the physician
○ prevention of Lyme disease, such as avoiding tick-infested areas, covering the skin with clothing, using insect repellants, inspecting exposed skin for attached ticks at least every 4 hours, and removing ticks
○ information about the vaccine for persons at risk for contracting Lyme disease.

Discharge planning

○ If the patient is in the late stages of the disease, refer him to a dermatologist, neurologist, cardiologist, or infectious disease specialist, as indicated.

Lymphocytic choriomeningitis

Overview

Description

○ A mild, biphasic, febrile illness lasting about 2 weeks
○ Asymptomatic in one-third of individuals and re-solves without serious sequelae in most cases
○ Rarely fatal (less than 1% mortality rate)
○ Also known as *LCM* or *lymphocytic meningitis*

Pathophysiology

○ Infected mice or other hosts excrete lymphocytic choriomeningitis virus (LCMV) in saliva, urine, and feces.
○ Human infection is through inhalation of infectious aerosolized particles of host urine, feces, or saliva; food contaminated with virus; or contamination of mucous membranes, skin lesions, or cuts with infect-ed body fluids.
○ The incubation period is 8 to 13 days and is followed by a biphasic, febrile illness.
○ The initial viremia extensively seeds extra-central nervous system tissue and sometimes cortical tissue.
○ The leptomeninges are infiltrated mainly by lympho-cytes and histiocytes, with few neutrophils.
○ The host's immune response to the infected cells produces various symptoms.
○ Natural killer cells are first to respond, then cytotox-ic T cells respond with interferon.
○ Meningeal symptoms appear in 15 to 21 days.

Causes

○ LCMV
○ Arenavirus

Risk factors

○ Handling infected animals or their excreta

Incidence

○ Prevalence of LCM in humans is 2% to 10%, but it's important to note that LCM has historically been un-derreported.
○ Individuals of all ages are susceptible, but young adults are infected more commonly.
○ Cases have been reported in Europe, North America, South America, Australia, and Japan, but most cases occur in the northeast and eastern seaboard areas of the United States.
○ LCM is more common during fall and winter.
○ Infection occurs equally in men and women.

Common characteristics

○ Early characteristics include fever, malaise, anorexia, weakness, muscle aches, retro-orbital headache, nausea, and vomiting. Other symptoms that appear less commonly include sore throat, nonproductive cough, joint pain, chest pain, testicular pain, and parotid (salivary gland) pain.
○ Later characteristics include alopecia and signs and symptoms of meningitis (fever, increased headache, and stiff neck) or encephalitis (drowsiness, confu-sion, sensory disturbances, and motor abnormalities such as paralysis).

Complications

○ Temporary or permanent neurological damage possi-ble (meningitis, paralysis, coma)
○ Possible maternal transmission (Pregnancy-related infection is associated with abortion, congenital hy-drocephalus, chorioretinitis, and mental retarda-tion.)
○ Myelitis presenting with muscle weakness, paralysis, or changes in body sensation
○ Guillain-Barré-type syndrome
○ Orchitis (usually unilateral) or parotitis
○ Cardiac involvement such as myocarditis
○ Psychosis
○ Joint pain and arthritis during convalescence, espe-cially in the metacarpophalangeal and proximal in-terphalangeal joints
○ Prolonged convalescence, with continuing dizziness, somnolence, and fatigue

Assessment

History

○ Exposure to rodents, hamsters, or their excreta 1 to 3 weeks before symptom onset

Physical findings

○ Lymphadenopathy
○ Maculopapular rash
○ Fever
○ Cough
○ Possible bradycardia

Test results

Laboratory
PHASE I
○ Decreased white blood cell (WBC) count (leukope-nia)
○ Decreased platelet count (thrombocytopenia)
○ Mild elevation of liver enzymes
PHASE II
○ Increased protein levels
○ Increased WBC count
○ Decreased glucose levels in cerebrospinal fluid (CSF)

Diagnostic procedures
○ Detection of immunoglobulin M antibodies by en-zyme-linked immunosorbent assay from serum or CSF (the preferred diagnostic test)
○ Lumbar puncture: patients with meningeal signs, CSF typically abnormal, consisting of an increased open-

ing pressure, increased protein levels, and a lymphocytic pleocytosis, usually in the range of several hundred WBCs

Treatment

General

○ Hospitalization and supportive treatment based on severity
○ Activity, as tolerated

Medication

○ No specific treatment
○ Anti-inflammatory drugs possibly useful
○ Ribavirin (effective against LCMV in vitro)
○ Analgesics (for symptom relief)

Surgery

○ Acute hydrocephalus may require surgical shunting to relieve increased intracranial pressure.

Nursing considerations

Key outcomes

The patient will:
○ report acute symptom relief
○ use precautions in handling rodents in the future
○ have a plan to manage potential complications during convalescence
○ understand the importance of follow-up appointments.

Nursing interventions

○ Encourage rest and fluids postlumbar puncture.
○ Give prescribed drugs.
○ Administer total parental care if the patient is paralyzed or in a coma.
○ Encourage diet and activity, as tolerated.

Monitoring

○ Vital signs
○ Acute hydrocephalus
○ Cardiac signs and symptoms
○ Skin integrity
○ If lumbar puncture, complications

Patient teaching

Be sure to cover:
○ rodent control measures
○ basic hygiene practices
○ use of a personal respirator
○ importance of adequate ventilation
○ use of a liquid disinfectant such as a diluted household bleach solution to clean up rodent droppings.

Discharge planning

○ Refer pregnant patients to an obstetrician for monitoring.
○ Refer paralyzed or comatose patients to physical therapy or occupational therapy, as needed.
○ Refer psychotic patients for follow-up with a psychiatrist.

Lymphoma, non-Hodgkin's

Overview

Description

- Heterogeneous group of malignant diseases that originate in lymph glands and other lymphoid tissue
- Usually classified according to histologic, anatomic, and immunomorphic characteristics developed by the National Cancer Institute (Rappaport histologic and Lukes and Collins classifications also used in some facilities)
- New categories of non-Hodgkin's lymphoma, called *mantle zone lymphoma* and *marginal zone lymphoma*, identified recently
- Also called *malignant lymphoma* and *lymphosarcoma*

Pathophysiology

- Non-Hodgkin's lymphoma seems to be similar to Hodgkin's disease, but Reed-Sternberg cells aren't present, and the lymph node destruction is different.
- Lymphoid tissue is defined by the pattern of infiltration as diffuse or nodular. Nodular lymphomas yield a better prognosis than the diffuse form, but in both the prognosis is less hopeful than in Hodgkin's disease.

Causes

- Exact cause unknown

Risk factors

- History of autoimmune disease

Incidence

- Three times more common than Hodgkin's disease
- Incidence increasing, especially in patients with autoimmune disorders and those receiving immunosuppressant treatment or those with acquired immunodeficiency syndrome

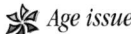 *Age issue*

Men older than age 60 have the highest incidence of non-Hodgkin's lymphoma.

Common characteristics

- Enlarged, painless lymph nodes
- Fever, malaise
- Weight loss

Complications

- Hypercalcemia
- Hyperuricemia
- Lymphomatosis
- Meningitis
- Anemia
- Liver, kidney, and lung problems (with tumor growth)
- Central nervous system involvement can lead to increased intracranial pressure

Assessment

History

- Symptoms mimic those of Hodgkin's disease
- Painless, swollen lymph glands (swelling may have appeared and disappeared over several months)
- Complaints of fatigue, malaise, weight loss, fever, and night sweats
- Trouble breathing, cough (usually children)

Physical findings

- Enlarged tonsils and adenoids
- Rubbery nodes in the cervical and supraclavicular areas

Test results

Laboratory
- Complete blood count showing anemia
- Normal or elevated uric acid levels
- Elevated calcium level resulting from bone lesions

Imaging
- Miscellaneous scans (chest X-rays; lymphangiography; liver, bone, and spleen scans; a computed tomography scan of the abdomen; and excretory urography) show disease progression.

Diagnostic procedures
- Biopsies of lymph nodes; of tonsils, bone marrow, liver, bowel, or skin; or, as needed, of tissue removed during exploratory laparotomy help to differentiate non-Hodgkin's lymphoma from Hodgkin's disease.
- The same staging system used for Hodgkin's disease is used for non-Hodgkin's lymphomas.

Treatment

General

- Radiation therapy mainly during the localized stage of the disease
- Total nodal irradiation usually effective in nodular and diffuse lymphomas
- Well-balanced, high-calorie, high-protein diet
- Increased fluid intake
- Small, frequent meals
- Limited activity
- Frequent rest periods

Medication

- Chemotherapy in combinations

Surgery

○ Perforation (common in patients with gastric lymphomas) usually necessitates debulking procedure (such as subtotal or, in some cases, total gastrectomy) before chemotherapy.

Nursing considerations

Key outcomes

The patient will:
○ have no further weight loss
○ demonstrate effective coping mechanisms
○ express feelings of increased comfort and decreased pain.

Nursing interventions

○ Give prescribed drugs.
○ Provide time for rest periods.
○ Encourage verbalization and provide support.

Monitoring

○ Adverse effects of treatment
○ Vital signs
○ Pain control
○ Hydration and nutritional status

Patient teaching

Be sure to cover:
○ the disorder, diagnosis, and treatment
○ preoperative and postoperative procedures
○ dietary plan
○ mouth care using a soft-bristled toothbrush and avoidance of commercial mouthwashes
○ relaxation and comfort measures
○ medication, including administration, dosage, and possible adverse effects
○ symptoms that require immediate attention.

Discharge planning

○ Refer the patient to available resources and support services.

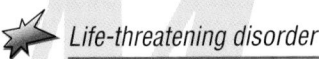

Major depression

Overview

Description

- Persistent sad, dysphoric mood; may be life-threatening
- Unipolar depressive disorder with onset in early adulthood and recurrences throughout life (at least two more episodes in 50% to 60% of patients)
- Recurrences possible after protracted symptom-free period or occurring sporadically, increasing in frequency, or occurring in clusters

Pathophysiology

- Changes occur in the receptor-neurotransmitter relationships in the limbic system.
- Changes in the hypothalamic-pituitary-adrenal regulation system may be an adaptive deregulation of the stress response.
- There's a possible defect on chromosome II or X.

Causes

- Psychological stress
- Genetic, familial, biochemical, physical, psychological, and social causes
- Many physical causes result in secondary depression
- Seasonal depression

Risk factors

- Female sex
- Family history of major depression or bipolar disorder
- Chronic illness
- Chronic pain
- Substance abuse
- Adverse reaction to medication such as beta-adrenergic blockers

Incidence

- Affects approximately 17.6 million Americans each year
- Affects 5% to 20% of general population at some time in their lives
- 6% to 8% of patients in care settings meet diagnostic criteria
- Incidence increases with age
- Twice as common in women as in men, regardless of age

Common characteristics

- Depressed mood daily for 2 weeks or longer
- History of personal loss or severe stress
- Patient expresses doubts about self-worth or ability to cope
- Patient appears unhappy and apathetic

Complications

- Profound alteration of social, family, and occupational functioning
- Suicide

Assessment

History

- Profound loss of pleasure in all enjoyable activities for a full month to 1 or more years
- Life problems or losses
- Physical disorder
- Use of prescription, nonprescription, or illegal drugs
- Change in eating and sleeping patterns
- Lack of interest in sex
- Constipation or diarrhea

Physical findings

- Difficulty concentrating or thinking clearly
- Easily distracted
- Indecisiveness
- Delusions of persecution or guilt
- Agitation
- Psychomotor retardation

DSM-IV-TR criteria

A diagnosis is confirmed when five or more of the following symptoms present during the same 2-week period and represent a change from previous functioning:

- Depressed mood (irritable mood in children and adolescents) most of the day, nearly every day, as indicated by either subjective account or observation by others
- Markedly diminished interest or pleasure in all, or almost all, activities most of the day, nearly every day
- Significant weight loss or weight gain (greater than 5% of the patient's body weight in a month) when not dieting, or a change in appetite nearly every day
- Insomnia or hypersomnia nearly every day
- Psychomotor agitation or retardation nearly every day
- Fatigue or loss of energy nearly every day
- Feelings of worthlessness and excessive or inappropriate guilt nearly every day
- Diminished ability to think or concentrate, or indecisiveness, nearly every day
- Recurrent thoughts of death, recurrent suicidal ideation without a specific plan, or suicide attempt or a specific plan for committing suicide (see *Suicide prevention guidelines*)
- Symptoms not due to a mixed episode, a medical condition, the effects of a medication or other substance, or bereavement

Test results

Laboratory
○ Toxicology screening suggesting a drug-induced depression

Diagnostic procedures
○ Dexamethasone suppression test may show a failure to suppress cortisol secretion.

Other
○ Beck Depression Inventory shows the onset, severity, duration, and progression of depressive symptoms.

Treatment

General

○ Electroconvulsive therapy
○ Short-term psychotherapy (a combination of individual, family, or group psychotherapy)
○ Well-balanced diet
○ Scheduled activities of daily living

Medication

○ Selective serotonin-reuptake inhibitors
○ Maprotiline
○ Tricyclic antidepressants
○ Monoamine oxidase inhibitors

Nursing considerations

Key outcomes

The patient will:
○ voice feelings related to self-esteem
○ make a verbal contract not to harm self
○ engage in social interactions with others
○ verbally and behaviorally demonstrate a positive self-evaluation.

Nursing interventions

○ Encourage participation in individual and group therapy.
○ Encourage verbalization and expression of feelings.
○ Listen attentively and respectfully.
○ Provide a structured routine.
○ Encourage interaction with others.
○ Document observations and significant conversations.
○ Assume an active role in initiating communication.
○ Plan activities for when the patient's energy levels are highest.
○ Provide distraction from self-absorption.

Monitoring

○ Adverse effects of medication
○ Suicidal ideations
○ Self-care
○ Social interaction
○ Functioning level
○ Response to treatment

Suicide prevention guidelines

To help deter potential suicide in the patient with major depression, keep in mind these guidelines.

Assess for clues to suicide
Watch for such clues as communicating suicidal thoughts, threats, and messages; hoarding medication; talking about death and feelings of futility; giving away prized possessions; describing a suicide plan; and changing behavior, especially as depression begins to lift.

Provide a safe environment
Check patient areas and correct dangerous conditions, such as exposed pipes, windows without safety glass, and access to the roof or open balconies.

Remove dangerous objects
Remove such objects as belts, razors, suspenders, light cords, glass, knives, nail files, and clippers from the patient's environment.

Consult with staff
Recognize and document verbal and nonverbal suicidal behaviors, keep the physician informed, share data with all staff, clarify the patient's specific restrictions, assess risk and plan for observation, and clarify day and night staff responsibilities and frequency of consultation.

Observe the suicidal patient
Be alert when the patient is using a sharp object (shaving), taking medication, or using the bathroom (to prevent hanging or other injury). Assign the patient to a room near the nurses' station and with another patient. Continuously observe the acutely suicidal patient.

Maintain personal contact
Help the suicidal patient feel that he isn't alone or without resources or hope. Encourage continuity of care and consistency of primary nurses. Building emotional ties to others is the ultimate technique for preventing suicide.

Patient teaching

Be sure to cover:
○ the disorder, diagnosis, and treatment
○ depression and its effects on daily living
○ prescribed medications
○ need for adherence to medication regimen
○ medication administration, dosage, and possible adverse reactions and interactions with other substances.

Discharge planning

○ Refer the patient to available support services and community assistance.

Malabsorption

Overview

Description

○ Malabsorption is a defect in the gastrointestinal tract in which the intestinal mucosa fails to absorb single or multiple nutrients efficiently.
○ Absorption of amino acids, fat, sugar, or vitamins may be impaired.
○ The result is inadequate movement of nutrients from the small intestine to the bloodstream or lymphatic system.
○ Manifestations depend primarily on what isn't being absorbed.

Pathophysiology

○ The mechanism of malabsorption depends on the cause.
○ In celiac sprue, dietary gluten — a product of wheat, barley, rye, and oats — is toxic to the patient, caus-ing injury to the mucosal villi. The mucosa appears flat and has lost absorptive surface. Symptoms generally disappear when gluten is removed from the diet.
○ Lactase deficiency is a disaccharide deficiency syndrome. Lactase is an intestinal enzyme that splits nonabsorbable lactose (a disaccharide) into the absorbable monosaccharides glucose and galactose. Production may be deficient, or another intestinal disease may inhibit the enzyme.
○ After gastrectomy, poor mixing of chyme with gastric secretions is the cause of postsurgical malabsorption.
○ In Zollinger-Ellison syndrome, increased acidity in the duodenum inhibits release of cholecystokinin, which stimulates pancreatic enzyme secretion. Pancreatic enzyme deficiency leads to decreased breakdown of nutrients and malabsorption.
○ Bacterial overgrowth in the duodenal stump (loop created in the Billroth II procedure) causes malabsorption of vitamin B_{12}.

Causes

○ Prior gastric surgery
○ Pancreatic disorders
○ Hepatobiliary disease
○ Disease of the small intestine such as celiac disease
○ Hereditary disorders
○ Drug toxicity (see *Causes of malabsorption*)

Incidence

○ Depends on cause of malabsorption

Common characteristics

○ Weight loss and generalized malnutrition
○ Diarrhea
○ Steatorrhea
○ Flatulence and abdominal distention
○ Nocturia
○ Weakness and fatigue
○ Edema
○ Amenorrhea
○ Anemia
○ Glossitis, cheilosis
○ Peripheral neuropathy
○ Bruising, bleeding tendency
○ Bone pain, skeletal deformities, fractures
○ Tetany, paresthesias

Complications

○ Fractures
○ Anemias
○ Bleeding disorders
○ Tetany
○ Malnutrition

Assessment

History

○ Fatigue
○ Diarrhea

Causes of malabsorption

Many disorders — from systemic to organ-specific diseases — may lead to malabsorption.

Diseases of the small intestine
Primary small bowel disease
○ Bacterial overgrowth from stasis in afferent loop after Billroth II gastrectomy
○ Massive bowel resection
○ Nontropical sprue (celiac disease)
○ Regional enteritis
○ Tropical sprue
Ischemic small bowel disease
○ Chronic heart failure
○ Mesenteric atherosclerosis
Systemic disease involving small bowel
○ Acute enteritis
○ Giardiasis
Drug-induced malabsorption
○ Calcium carbonate
○ Neomycin
Hepatobiliary disease
○ Biliary fistula
○ Biliary tract obstruction
○ Cirrhosis and hepatitis
Hereditary disorder
○ Primary lactase deficiency
Pancreatic disorders
○ Chronic pancreatitis
○ Cystic fibrosis
○ Pancreatic cancer
○ Pancreatic resection
○ Zollinger-Ellison syndrome
Previous gastric surgery
○ Billroth II gastrectomy
○ Pyloroplasty
○ Total gastrectomy
○ Vagotomy

○ Steatorrhea

Physical findings

○ Orthostatic hypotension
○ Signs of weight loss or muscle wasting
○ Abdominal distention
○ Hyperactive bowel sounds
○ Pallor
○ Ecchymosis
○ Peripheral edema

Test results

Laboratory
○ Stool specimen for fat reveals excretion of greater than 6 g of fat per day.
○ D-xylose absorption test shows less than 20% of 25 g of D-xylose in the urine after 5 hours (reflects disorders of proximal bowel).
○ Schilling test reveals deficiency of vitamin B_{12} absorption.
○ Culture of duodenal and jejunal contents confirms bacterial overgrowth in the proximal bowel.
Imaging
○ GI barium studies show characteristic features of the small intestine.
Diagnostic procedures
○ Small intestine biopsy reveals the atrophy of mucosal villi.

Treatment

General

○ Identification of cause and appropriate correction
○ Gluten-free diet to stop progression of celiac disease and malabsorption
○ Lactose-free diet to treat lactase deficiency

Medication

○ Dietary supplementation
○ Vitamin B_{12} injections

Nursing considerations

Key outcomes

The patient will:
○ have improved absorption of nutrients
○ maintain or improve weight
○ express understanding of cause of disorder.

Nursing interventions

○ Watch for signs of dehydration, such as dry skin and mucous membranes and poor skin turgor.
○ Protect patients with osteomalacia from injury by keeping the side rails up and assisting with ambulation, as necessary.

Monitoring

○ Nutritional status
○ Calorie intake

○ Weight
○ Intake and output
○ Laboratory values

Patient teaching

Be sure to cover:
○ the disorder, diagnosis, and treatment
○ following a gluten-free diet.

Discharge planning

○ Encourage follow-up visits, as ordered.

Malaria

Overview

Description

○ Malaria is an acute infectious disease caused by protozoa of the genus *Plasmodium: P. falciparum, P. vivax, P. malariae, and P. ovale.*
○ Mosquito vectors transmit the disease to humans.
○ Falciparum malaria is the most severe form of the disease.
○ Untreated primary attacks last from a week to a month or longer.
○ Relapses are common and can recur sporadically for several years.
○ Hepatic parasites (*P. vivax, P. ovale, and P. malariae*) may persist for years in the liver and are responsible for the chronic carrier state.

Pathophysiology

○ *Plasmodium* sporozoites are injected by the bite of a mosquito vector.
○ The infective sporozoites migrate by blood circulation to parenchymal cells of the liver; there they form cystlike structures containing thousands of merozoites.
○ Upon release, each merozoite invades an erythrocyte and feeds on hemoglobin.
○ Eventually, the erythrocyte ruptures, releasing heme (malaria pigment), cell debris, and more merozoites, which, unless destroyed by phagocytes, enter other erythrocytes.

Causes

○ Bite of female *Anopheles* mosquitoes

Incidence

○ 300 to 500 million cases annually (internationally)
○ Since 1940, few cases of malaria contracted in the United States; most of these transmitted by blood transfusions or the use of contaminated needles by drug addicts

Common characteristics

○ Chills
○ Fever
○ Headache
○ Myalgia
○ Interspersed periods of well-being (the hallmark of the benign form of malaria)

Acute attack
○ Occurs when erythrocytes rupture
○ Three stages:
– cold stage, lasting 1 to 2 hours, ranging from chills to extreme shaking
– hot stage, lasting 3 to 4 hours, characterized by high fever up to 107° F (41.7° C)
– wet stage, lasting 2 to 4 hours, characterized by profuse sweating

Falciparum malaria
○ Persistent high fever
○ Orthostatic hypotension
○ Red blood cell (RBC) sludging that leads to capillary obstruction at various sites

Complications

○ Renal failure
○ Liver failure
○ Heart failure
○ Pulmonary edema
○ Disseminated intravascular coagulation
○ Circulatory collapse
○ Severe normocytic anemia
○ Seizures
○ Hypoglycemia
○ Splenic rupture
○ Cerebral dysfunction
○ Death

Assessment

History

○ Travel to endemic area
○ Recent blood transfusion

Special considerations for antimalarial drugs

Chloroquine
○ Perform baseline and periodic ophthalmologic examinations, and report blurred vision, increased sensitivity to light, and muscle weakness to the physician.
○ Consult with the physician about altering therapy if muscle weakness appears in a patient on long-term therapy.
○ Monitor the patient for tinnitus and other signs of ototoxicity, such as nerve deafness and vertigo.
○ Caution the patient to avoid excessive exposure to the sun to prevent exacerbating drug-induced dermatoses.

Primaquine
○ Give with meals or antacids.
○ Discontinue administration if you observe a sudden fall in hemoglobin concentration or in erythrocyte or leukocyte count or marked darkening of the urine, suggesting impending hemolytic reaction.

Pyrimethamine
○ Give with meals to minimize GI distress.
○ Check blood counts (including platelets) twice a week. If signs of folic or folinic acid deficiency develop, reduce or discontinue dosage while patient receives parenteral folinic acid until blood counts become normal.

Quinine
○ Use with caution in patients with cardiovascular conditions, asthma, hemolytic anemia, and granulocytosis, in a severe reaction.
○ Monitor blood pressure frequently while administering quinine I.V. infusion. Rapid administration causes marked hypotension.

- I.V. drug abuse
- Chills, fever
- Headache, backache

Physical findings

- Pale skin
- Urticaria
- Jaundice
- Petechial rash
- Hepatosplenomegaly (*P. vivax* and *P. ovale)*

Test results

Laboratory
- Identification of the parasites in RBCs of peripheral blood smears
- Decreased hemoglobin levels
- Possibly decreased leukocyte count (as low as 3,000/µl)
- Protein and leukocytes in urine sediment

FALCIPARUM MALARIA
- Reduced number of platelets (20,000 to 50,000/µl)
- Prolonged prothrombin time (18 to 20 seconds)
- Prolonged partial thromboplastin time (60 to 100 seconds)
- Decreased plasma fibrinogen

Treatment

General

- Symptomatic
- Activity, as tolerated (bed rest during acute phase)
- Increased fluid intake

Medication

- Oral chloroquine (for all forms except chloroquine-resistant *P. falciparum)*
- Oral quinine (for malaria caused by *P. falciparum*) given concurrently with pyrimethamine and a sulfonamide, such as sulfadiazine
- Primaquine phosphate (for hepatic phase) (see *Special considerations for antimalarial drugs*)
- Antipyretics

Nursing considerations

Key outcomes

The patient will:
- have stable vital signs
- have adequate fluid volume
- express feelings and fears about current situation.

Nursing interventions

- Obtain a detailed patient history.
- Follow proper hand-washing and aseptic techniques.
- Follow standard precautions.
- Record symptom pattern, fever, type of malaria, and systemic signs.
- Report all cases of malaria to local public health authorities.

Monitoring

- Vital signs
- Response to treatment
- Intake and output

Patient teaching

Be sure to cover:
- the disorder, diagnosis, and potential for relapse
- proper administration of medication and possible adverse effects.

Mastitis

Overview

Description
- Inflammation of the breast tissue
- Lactating breast infection
- Good prognosis

Pathophysiology
- A pathogen (typically originating in nursing infant's nose or pharynx) invades the breast tissue, entering through a fissured or abraded nipple.
- The result is parenchymatous inflammation of the mammary glands, which disrupts normal lactation.
- Systemic manifestations of inflammation may result.

Causes
- Most common pathogen *Staphylococcus aureus;* less frequently, *S. epidermidis* or beta-hemolytic streptococci
- Disseminated tuberculosis (rare)
- Mumps virus (rare)

Risk factors
- Fissure or abrasion of the nipple
- Blocked milk ducts
- Incomplete letdown reflex
- Tight bra
- Prolonged intervals between breast-feedings

Incidence
- Occurs in about 1% of lactating women
- More common in breast-feeding primiparas
- Occurs occasionally in nonlactating women
- Rare in men

Preventing mastitis

To help your patient prevent mastitis from recurring, follow these guidelines:
- Stress to the patient the importance of emptying the breasts completely because milk stasis can cause infection and mastitis.
- Teach the patient to alternate feeding positions and to rotate pressure areas on the nipples.
- Remind the patient to position the infant properly on the breast with the entire areola in his mouth.
- Advise the patient to expose sore nipples to the air as often as possible.
- Teach the patient proper hand-washing technique and personal hygiene.
- Instruct the patient to get plenty of rest and consume sufficient fluids and a balanced diet to enhance breast-feeding.
- Suggest to the patient applying a warm, wet towel to the affected breast or taking a warm shower to relax and improve breast-feeding.

Common characteristics
- Red, swollen, warm, and tender breasts
- Nipple cracks or fissures
- Enlarged axillary lymph nodes

Complications
- Abscess

Assessment

History
- Fever
- Malaise
- Flulike symptoms
- Tenderness

Physical findings
- Nipple abrasion or fissure
- Enlarged axillary lymph nodes
- Involved breast red, edematous, warm, and hard

Test results
Laboratory
- Cultures of expressed milk confirming generalized mastitis
- Cultures of breast skin confirming localized mastitis

Treatment

General
- Warm soaks
- Avoidance of tight bras and clothing
- Continuation of breast-feeding in both breasts to prevent engorgement, with proper infant sucking and changing of feeding positions to drain the milk

Medication
- Broad-spectrum antibiotics
- Analgesics

Surgery
- Breast abscess incision and drainage

Nursing considerations

Key outcomes
The patient will:
- express feelings of increased comfort
- exhibit no signs or symptoms of infection
- resume breast-feeding without further complications
- maintain skin integrity.

Nursing interventions
- Give prescribed drugs.
- Provide warm soaks.
- Use meticulous hand-washing technique.
- Provide meticulous skin care.

Monitoring
○ Signs and symptoms of infection
○ Abscess development
○ Breast engorgement
○ Skin integrity
○ Breast-feeding

Patient teaching

Be sure to cover:
○ the disorder, diagnosis, and treatment
○ prescribed antibiotic therapy and potential adverse reactions
○ reassurance that breast-feeding won't harm the infant because he's the source of the infection
○ offering the infant the unaffected breast first to promote complete emptying and prevent clogged ducts
○ need to stop breast-feeding with abscessed breast
○ use of a breast pump until abscess heals
○ continuation of breast-feeding on the unaffected side
○ prevention of mastitis (see *Preventing mastitis*)

Discharge planning
○ Refer the patient to a lactation specialist, if indicated.

Melanoma, malignant

Overview

Description
○ Neoplasm that arises from melanocytes
○ Potentially the most lethal of the skin cancers
○ Common sites are head and neck in men, legs in women, and backs of people exposed to excessive sunlight
○ Four types:
　– superficial spreading melanoma — most common type; usually develops between ages 40 and 50
　– nodular melanoma — grows vertically, invades the dermis, and metastasizes early; usually develops between ages 40 and 50
　– acral-lentiginous melanoma — occurs on the palms and soles and under the tongue; most common among Hispanics, Asians, and Blacks
　– lentigo maligna melanoma — relatively rare; most benign, slowest growing, and least aggressive of the four types; most commonly occurs in areas heavily exposed to the sun; arises from a lentigo maligna on an exposed skin surface; usually occurs between ages 60 and 70

Pathophysiology
○ Melanomas arise as a result of malignant degeneration of melanocytes located either along the basal layer of the epidermis or in a benign melanocytic nevus.
○ Up to 70% of malignant melanomas arise from a preexisting nevus.
○ Malignant melanoma spreads through the lymphatic and vascular systems and metastasizes to the regional lymph nodes, skin, liver, lungs, and central nervous system.
○ Malignant melanoma follows an unpredictable course; recurrence and metastasis may not appear for more than 5 years after resection of the primary lesion.

Causes
○ Ultraviolet rays from the sun damage the skin and can cause malignant melanoma.

Risk factors
○ Excessive exposure to sunlight
○ Skin type (blond or red hair, fair skin, and blue eyes; prone to sunburn; and Celtic or Scandinavian ancestry)
○ Hormonal factors (pregnancy)
○ Family history
○ Past history of melanoma
○ Preexisting pigmented mole or nevus

Incidence
○ Account for 1% to 2% of all malignant tumors
○ Slightly more common in women than in men
○ Unusual in children
○ Peak incidence between ages 50 and 70, but incidence in younger age groups increasing

Common characteristics
○ Sore that doesn't heal
○ Preexisting lesion or nevus that enlarges

Complications
○ Metastasis to the lungs, liver, or brain

Assessment

History
○ A sore that doesn't heal, a persistent lump or swelling, and changes in preexisting skin markings, such as moles, birthmarks, scars, freckles, or warts
○ Preexisting skin lesion or nevus that enlarges, changes color, becomes inflamed or sore, itches, ulcerates, bleeds, changes texture, or shows signs of surrounding pigment regression

Physical findings
○ Lesions on the ankles or the inside surfaces of the knees
○ Uniformly discolored nodule on knee or ankle
○ Small, elevated tumor nodules that may ulcerate and bleed
○ Palpable polypoid nodules that resemble the surface of a blackberry
○ Pigmented lesions on the palms and soles or under the nails
○ Long-standing lesion that has ulcerated
○ Flat nodule with smaller nodules scattered over the surface

Test results
Laboratory
○ Complete blood count with differential showing anemia
○ Elevated erythrocyte sedimentation rate
○ Abnormal platelet count if metastasis
○ Abnormal liver function studies if metastasis
Imaging
○ Chest X-rays assist in staging.
Diagnostic procedures
○ Excisional biopsy and full-depth punch biopsy with histologic examination can show tumor thickness and disease stage.

Treatment

General
○ Close long-term follow-up care to detect metastasis and recurrences
○ Radiation therapy (usually for metastatic disease)
○ Well-balanced diet
○ Avoidance of sun exposure

Medication

○ Chemotherapy
○ Biotherapy
○ Immunotherapy
○ Immunostimulants

Surgery

○ Surgical resection to remove tumor and 3- to 5-cm margin
○ Regional lymphadenectomy

Nursing considerations

Key outcomes

The patient will:
○ have no further weight loss
○ express positive feelings about self
○ demonstrate effective coping mechanisms
○ experience healing of wound without signs of infection
○ express feelings of increased comfort.

Nursing interventions

○ Encourage verbalization and provide support.
○ Provide appropriate wound care.
○ Give prescribed drugs.
○ Provide a high-protein, high-calorie diet.

Monitoring

○ Complications of treatment
○ Pain control
○ Wound site
○ Postoperative complications

Patient teaching

Be sure to cover:
○ the disorder, diagnosis, and treatment
○ preoperative and postoperative care
○ need for close follow-up care to detect recurrences early
○ signs and symptoms of recurrence
○ detrimental effects of overexposure to solar radiation and benefits of regular use of a sunblock or a sunscreen and protective clothing.

Discharge planning

○ Refer the patient to available resources and support services.

Ménière's disease

Overview

Description

- Inner ear disease that results from a labyrinthine dysfunction
- Causes severe vertigo, sensorineural hearing loss, and tinnitus
- Usually, only one ear involved
- After multiple attacks over several years, possibly incapacitating residual tinnitus and hearing loss
- Also known as *endolymphatic hydrops*

Pathophysiology

- Ménière's disease may result from overproduction or decreased absorption of endolymph—the fluid contained in the labyrinth of the ear.
- Accumulated endolymph dilates the semicircular canals, utricle, and saccule and causes degeneration of the vestibular and cochlear hair cells.
- Overstimulation of the vestibular branch of cranial nerve VIII impairs postural reflexes and stimulates the vomiting reflex. (See *Normal vestibular function.*)
- Perception of sound is impaired as a result of this excessive cranial nerve stimulation, and injury to sensory receptors for hearing may affect auditory acuity.

Causes

- Unknown, but may be associated with:
  - family history
  - immune disorder
  - migraine headaches
  - middle ear infection
  - head trauma
  - autonomic nervous system dysfunction
  - premenstrual edema

 Alert

In some women, premenstrual edema may precipitate outbreaks of Ménière's disease.

Normal vestibular function

The three semicircular canals and the vestibule of the inner ear are responsible for equilibrium and balance. Each of the semicircular canals lies at a 90° angle to the others. Head movement in one direction causes the endolymph inside each semicircular canal to move in the opposite direction and causes vestibular otoliths (crystals of calcium salts) to shift in their gel medium. This movement stimulates hair cells, sending electrical impulses to the brain through the vestibular portion of cranial nerve VIII. Together, these organs help detect the body's present position as well as any change in its direction or motion.

Incidence

- Usually affects adults between ages 30 and 60; rare in children
- Slightly more common in men than in women

Common characteristics

- Sudden severe spinning, whirling vertigo, lasting from 10 minutes to several hours
- Tinnitus
- Hearing impairment
- Feeling of fullness or blockage in the affected ear preceding an attack
- Severe nausea, vomiting, sweating, and pallor during an acute attack
- Nystagmus
- Loss of balance and falling to the affected side

Complications

- Continued tinnitus
- Hearing loss
- Injury

Assessment

History

- Vertigo
- Nausea
- Tinnitus
- Falls

Physical findings

- Inability to maintain upright posture
- Unsteady gait
- Diplopia
- Hypotension

Test results

Imaging
- Computed tomography scan and magnetic resonance imaging to rule out acoustic neuroma as a cause of symptoms

Diagnostic procedures
- Audiometric testing showing a sensorineural hearing loss and loss of discrimination and recruitment
- Electronystagmography showing normal or reduced vestibular response on the affected side
- Cold caloric testing showing impairment of oculovestibular reflex
- Electrocochleography showing increased ratio of summating potential to action potential
- Brain stem evoked response audiometry test to rule out acoustic neuroma, brain tumor, and vascular lesions in the brain stem

Other

- Patient history

Treatment

General

- Lying down to minimize head movement, and avoiding sudden movements and glaring lights to reduce dizziness (during an attack)

Medication

- Promethazine (Phenergan) or prochlorperazine (Compazine)
- Atropine
- Dimenhydrinate (Dramamine)
- Central nervous system depressants, such as lorazepam (Ativan) or diazepam (Valium) during an acute attack
- Antihistamines, such as meclizine (Antivert) or diphenhydramine (Benadryl)

For long-term management

- Diuretics
- Betahistine dihydrochloride
- Vasodilators
- Sodium restriction
- Antihistamines or mild sedatives
- Systemic streptomycin (chemical ablation)

Surgery

- Endolymphatic drainage and shunt procedures
- Vestibular nerve resection
- Labyrinthectomy
- Cochlear implantation

Nursing considerations

Key outcomes

The patient will:

- express feelings of increased comfort
- remain safe from injury
- maintain adequate fluid balance
- seek appropriate support to assist with coping.

Nursing interventions

- Maintain a safe environment; provide assistance when necessary.
- Give prescribed drugs.

Monitoring

- Intake and output
- Frequency of attacks
- Response to treatment

Patient teaching

Be sure to cover:

- avoidance of reading and exposure to glaring lights to reduce dizziness
- avoidance of sudden position changes and any tasks that vertigo makes hazardous.

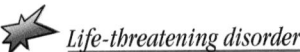 *Life-threatening disorder*

Meningitis

Overview

Description

- Inflammation of brain and spinal cord meninges
- May affect all three meningeal membranes (dura mater, arachnoid membrane, and pia mater)
- Usually follows onset of respiratory symptoms
- Sudden onset, causing serious illness within 24 hours
- Prognosis good; complications rare
- Bacterial meningitis: acute infection in the subarachnoid space

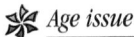 **Age issue**

Prognosis is poor for infants and elderly people.

Pathophysiology

- Inflammation of pia-arachnoid and subarachnoid space progresses to congestion of adjacent tissues.
- Nerve cells are destroyed.
- Intracranial pressure (ICP) increases because of exudates.
- Results can include:
  - engorged blood vessels
  - disrupted blood supply
  - edema of the brain tissue
  - thrombosis
  - rupture
  - acute hydrocephalus.

Causes

- Bacterial infection, usually from *Neisseria meningitidis* and *Streptococcus pneumoniae* (Before the 1990s, *Haemophilus influenzae* type b [Hib] was the leading cause of bacterial meningitis. However, new vaccines have reduced its occurrence in children.)
- Viruses
- Protozoa
- Fungi
- Secondary to another bacterial infection such as pneumonia
- May follow skull fracture, penetrating head wound, lumbar puncture, or ventricular shunting procedures

Incidence

- Infants, children, and elderly people are at highest risk
- An increasing threat to college students

Common characteristics

- Nuchal rigidity
- Headache
- Fever
- Meningismus, typically with signs of cerebral dysfunction
- Seizures

Complications

- Visual impairment; optic neuritis
- Cranial nerve palsies; deafness
- Paresis or paralysis
- Endocarditis
- Coma
- Vasculitis
- Cerebral infarction
- Seizures

Assessment

History

- Headache
- Fever
- Nausea, vomiting
- Weakness
- Myalgia
- Photophobia
- Confusion, delirium
- Seizures

Physical findings

- Meningismus
- Rigors
- Profuse sweating
- Kernig's and Brudzinski's signs (elicited in only 50% of adults)
- Declining level of consciousness (LOC)
- Cranial nerve palsies
- Rash (with meningococcemia)
- Focal neurologic deficits such as visual field defects
- Signs of increased ICP (in later stages)

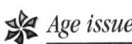 **Age issue**

Meningismus and fever are commonly absent in neonates and the only clinical clues may be nonspecific, such as refusal to feed, high-pitched cry, and irritability.

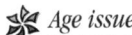 **Age issue**

Elderly patients may exhibit an insidious onset, exhibiting lethargy and variable signs of meningismus and no fever.

Test results

Laboratory
○ White blood cell count showing leukocytosis
○ Positive blood cultures in bacterial meningitis, depending on the pathogen

Imaging
○ Chest X-rays may reveal a coexisting pneumonia.
○ Neuroimaging techniques, such as computed tomography scanning and magnetic resonance imaging, may detect complications and a parameningeal source of infection.

Diagnostic procedures
○ Lumbar puncture and cerebrospinal fluid analysis shows:
  – increased opening pressure
  – neutrophilic pleocytosis
  – elevated protein
  – hypoglycorrhachia
  – positive Gram stain
  – positive culture.

Treatment

General
○ Hypothermia
○ Fluid therapy
○ Pain control
○ Bed rest (in acute phase)

Medication
○ I.V. antibiotics
○ Oral antibiotics
○ Antiarrhythmics
○ Osmotic diuretics
○ Anticonvulsants
○ Aspirin or acetaminophen

Nursing considerations

Key outcomes
The patient will:
○ maintain adequate ventilation
○ have normal temperature
○ express feelings of increased comfort and pain relief
○ maintain normal fluid volume
○ have intact skin.

Nursing interventions
○ Follow standard precautions.
○ Maintain respiratory isolation for first 24 hours (with meningococcal meningitis).
○ Give prescribed oxygen.
○ Position the patient in proper body alignment.
○ Encourage active range-of-motion (ROM) exercises when appropriate.
○ Provide passive ROM exercises when appropriate.
○ Maintain adequate nutrition.
○ Give prescribed laxatives or stool softeners.
○ Provide meticulous skin and mouth care.
○ Give prescribed drugs.

Monitoring
○ Neurologic status
○ Vital signs
○ Signs and symptoms of cranial nerve involvement
○ Signs and symptoms of increased ICP
○ LOC
○ Seizures
○ Respiratory status
○ Arterial blood gas results
○ Fluid balance
○ Response to medications
○ Complications

Patient teaching

Be sure to cover:
○ the disorder, diagnosis, and treatment
○ contagion risks for close contacts
○ medication regimen
○ adverse drug effects
○ signs and symptoms of meningitis
○ polysaccharide meningococcal vaccine, pneumococcal vaccine, and Hib vaccine.

Metabolic syndrome

Overview

Description

- A cluster of symptoms triggered by insulin resistance: abdominal fat; obesity; high blood pressure; and high levels of blood glucose, triglycerides, and cholesterol
- Increased risk of diabetes, heart disease, and stroke
- Often unrecognized
- Also known as *syndrome X, insulin resistance syndrome, dysmetabolic syndrome,* and *multiple metabolic syndrome*

Pathophysiology

- The body breaks food down into basic components, one of which is glucose.
- Glucose provides energy for cellular activity.
- Excess glucose is stored in cells for future use. It's guided into storage cells by insulin, which is secreted by the pancreas.
- In those with metabolic syndrome, glucose doesn't respond to insulin's attempt to guide it into storage cells. This is called insulin resistance.
- To overcome this resistance, the pancreas produces excess insulin, which causes damage to arterial lining.
- Excessive insulin secretion also promotes fat storage deposits and prevents fat breakdown.
- This series of events can lead to diabetes, blood clots, and coronary events.

Causes

- Genetic predisposition
- Acquired

Risk factors

- Obesity
- Improper diet
- Insufficient physical activity
- Aging
- Hyperinsulinemia/impaired glucose tolerance
- Previous heart attack

Incidence

- Affects an estimated 47 million Americans
- Most common in Mexican Americans (highest rate at 32%)
- In Black and Mexican American persons, women more susceptible than men; otherwise, men and women equally affected

Common characteristics

- Waist size: more than 40″ (101.6 cm) in men; more than 35″ (88.9 cm) in women (see *Why abdominal obesity is dangerous*)
- Lethargy, especially after eating

Complications

- Coronary artery disease
- Diabetes
- Hyperlipidemia
- Premature death

Assessment

History

- Familial history
- Hypertension
- High low-density lipoproteins (LDL) and triglyceride levels
- Low high-density lipoproteins (HDL) levels
- Abdominal obesity
- Sedentary lifestyle
- Poor diet

Physical findings

- Abdominal obesity

Test results

Laboratory
- High blood glucose levels
- High LDL and triglyceride levels
- Low HDL levels
- Hyperinsulinemia
- Elevated serum uric acid

Other
- Blood pressure greater than 130/85 mm/Hg

Treatment

General

- Weight-reduction program
- Low alcohol intake
- Low-cholesterol diet
- Diet high in complex carbohydrates (grains, beans, vegetables, fruit) and low in refined carbohydrates (soda, table sugar, high fructose corn syrup)
- Daily physical activity of at least 20 minutes

Medication

- Oral antidiabetic agents
- Antihypertensives
- Statins

Nursing considerations

Key outcomes

The patient will:
- maintain a healthy weight
- increase his level of activity
- consume a proper diet.

Why abdominal obesity is dangerous

People with excess weight around the waist have a greater risk of developing metabolic syndrome than people with excess weight around the hips. That's because intra-abdominal fat tends to be more resistant to insulin than fat in other areas of the body. Insulin resistance increases the release of free fatty acid into the portal system, leading to increased apolipoprotein B, increased low-density lipoprotein (LDL), decreased high-density lipoprotein (HDL), and increased triglyceride levels. As a result, the risk of cardiovascular disease increases.

Nursing interventions

○ Promote lifestyle changes and give appropriate support.

Monitoring

○ Blood pressure
○ Ordered laboratory tests

Patient teaching

Be sure to cover:
○ the disorder, diagnosis, and treatment
○ principles of healthy diet
○ relationship of diet, inactivity, and obesity to metabolic syndrome
○ benefits of increased physical activity
○ prescribed medication, administration, and possible adverse reactions.

Methicillin-resistant *Staphylococcus aureus*

Overview

Description

○ A mutation of a very common bacterium easily spread by direct person-to-person contact
○ Also known as *MRSA*

Pathophysiology

○ 90% of *Staphylococcus aureus* isolates or strains are penicillin-resistant, and about 27% of all *S. aureus* isolates are resistant to methicillin, a penicillin derivative. These strains may also resist cephalosporins, aminoglycosides, erythromycin, tetracycline, and clindamycin.
○ When natural defense systems break down (after invasive procedures, trauma, or chemotherapy), the usually benign bacteria can invade tissue, proliferate, and cause infection.
○ The most frequent colonization site is the anterior nares (40% of adults and most children become transient nasal carriers). The groin, armpits, and intestines are less common colonization sites.

Causes

○ Methicillin-resistant *S. aureus* that enters a health care facility through an infected or colonized patient (symptom-free carrier of the bacteria) or colonized health care worker
○ Transmitted mainly by health care workers' hands

Risk factors

○ Immunosuppression
○ Prolonged facility stays
○ Extended therapy with multiple or broad-spectrum antibiotics
○ Proximity to others colonized or infected with methicillin-resistant *S. aureus*

Incidence

○ Endemic in nursing homes, long-term care facilities, and community facilities

Common characteristics

○ Dependent upon body system affected

Complications

○ Sepsis
○ Death

Assessment

History

○ Possible risk factors for methicillin-resistant *S. aureus*
○ Carrier patient commonly asymptomatic

Physical findings

○ In symptomatic patients, signs and symptoms related to the primary diagnosis (respiratory, cardiac, or other major system symptoms)

Test results

Laboratory
○ Cultures from suspicious wounds, skin, urine, or blood showing methicillin-resistant *S. aureus*

Treatment

General

○ Transmission precautions: contact isolation for wound, skin, and urine infection; respiratory isolation for sputum infection
○ No treatment needed for patient with colonization only
○ High-protein diet
○ Rest periods, as needed

Medication

○ Vancomycin and imipenem

Nursing considerations

Key outcomes

The patient will:
○ maintain collateral circulation
○ attain hemodynamic stability
○ maintain adequate cardiac output
○ remain afebrile
○ have an adequate fluid volume.

Nursing interventions

○ Provide emotional support to the patient and family members.
○ Consider grouping infected patients together and having the same nursing staff care for them.
○ Use proper hand-washing technique.
○ Use contact precautions and standard precautions.

Monitoring

○ Vital signs
○ Culture results
○ Response to treatment
○ Adverse drug reactions
○ Complications

Patient teaching

Be sure to cover:
- ○ the disorder, diagnosis, and treatment
- ○ difference between methicillin-resistant *S. aureus* infection and colonization
- ○ prevention of methicillin-resistant *S. aureus* spread
- ○ proper hand-washing technique
- ○ need for family and friends to wear protective garb (and to dispose of it properly) when they visit the patient
- ○ medication administration, dosage, and possible adverse effects
- ○ need to take antibiotics for the full prescription period, even if the patient begins to feel better.

Discharge planning
- ○ Refer the patient to an infectious disease specialist, if indicated.

Mitral stenosis

Overview

Description

○ Narrowing of the mitral valve orifice, which is normally 3 to 6 cm
○ Mild mitral stenosis: valve orifice of 2 cm
○ Severe mitral stenosis: valve orifice of 1 cm
○ Also called *MS*

Pathophysiology

○ Valve leaflets become diffusely thickened by fibrosis and calcification.
○ The mitral commissures and the chordae tendinae fuse and shorten, the valvular cusps become rigid, and the valve's apex becomes narrowed.
○ This obstructs blood flow from the left atrium to the left ventricle, resulting in incomplete emptying.
○ Left atrial volume and pressure increase, and the atrial chamber dilates.
○ Increased resistance to blood flow causes pulmonary hypertension, right ventricular hypertrophy and, eventually, right-sided heart failure and reduced cardiac output.

Causes

○ Rheumatic fever
○ Congenital anomalies
○ Atrial myxoma
○ Endocarditis
○ Adverse effects of fenfluramine and phentermine (Fen-phen) diet drug combination

Incidence

○ Two-thirds of all MS patients female
○ Occurs in approximately 40% of patients with rheumatic heart disease

Common characteristics

○ Gradual decline in exercise tolerance
○ Dyspnea on exertion
○ Shortness of breath
○ Chest pain, palpitations

Identifying the murmur of mitral stenosis

A low, rumbling crescendo-decrescendo murmur in the mitral valve area characterizes mitral stenosis.

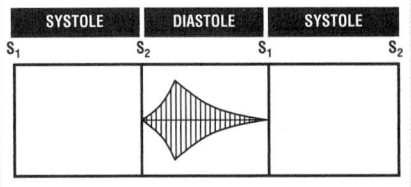

SYSTOLE	DIASTOLE	SYSTOLE
S_1	S_2	S_1	S_2

Complications

○ Cardiac arrhythmias, especially atrial fibrillation
○ Thromboembolism

Assessment

History

Mild mitral stenosis
○ Asymptomatic
Moderate to severe mitral stenosis
○ Gradual decline in exercise tolerance
○ Dyspnea on exertion; shortness of breath
○ Paroxysmal nocturnal dyspnea
○ Orthopnea
○ Weakness
○ Fatigue
○ Palpitations
○ Cough

Physical findings

○ Hemoptysis
○ Peripheral and facial cyanosis
○ Malar rash
○ Jugular vein distention
○ Ascites
○ Peripheral edema
○ Hepatomegaly
○ A loud S_1 or opening snap
○ A diastolic murmur at the apex (see *Identifying the murmur of mitral stenosis*)
○ Crackles over lung fields
○ Right ventricular lift
○ Resting tachycardia; irregularly irregular heart rhythm

Test results

Imaging
○ Chest X-rays show left atrial and ventricular enlargement (in severe mitral stenosis), straightening of the left border of the cardiac silhouette, enlarged pulmonary arteries, dilation of the upper lobe pulmonary veins, and mitral valve calcification.
○ Echocardiography discloses thickened mitral valve leaflets and left atrial enlargement.
Diagnostic procedures
○ Cardiac catheterization shows a diastolic pressure gradient across the valve, elevated pulmonary artery wedge pressure (greater than 15 mm Hg), and pulmonary artery pressure in the left atrium with severe pulmonary hypertension.
○ Electrocardiography reveals left atrial enlargement, right ventricular hypertrophy, right axis deviation, and (in 40% to 50% of cases) atrial fibrillation.

Treatment

General

- Synchronized electrical cardioversion to correct atrial fibrillation
- Sodium-restricted diet
- Activity, as tolerated

Medication

- Digoxin
- Diuretics
- Oxygen
- Beta-adrenergic blockers
- Calcium channel blockers
- Anticoagulants
- Infective endocarditis antibiotic prophylaxis
- Nitrates

Surgery

- Commissurotomy or valve replacement
- Percutaneous balloon valvuloplasty

Nursing considerations

Key outcomes

The patient will:
- carry out activities of daily living without weakness or fatigue
- maintain hemodynamic stability and adequate cardiac output
- have no complications from fluid excess
- exhibit adequate coping mechanisms.

Nursing interventions

- Check for hypersensitivity reaction to antibiotics.
- If the patient needs bed rest, stress its importance.
- Provide a bedside commode.
- Allow the patient to express concerns over her inability to meet responsibilities because of activity restrictions.
- Place the patient in an upright position to relieve dyspnea, if needed.
- Provide a low-sodium diet.

Monitoring

- Vital signs and hemodynamics
- Intake and output
- Signs and symptoms of heart failure and pulmonary edema
- Signs and symptoms of thromboembolism
- Adverse drug reactions
- Cardiac arrhythmias
- Postoperatively: hypotension, arrhythmias, and thrombus formation

Patient teaching

Be sure to cover:
- the disorder, diagnosis, and treatment
- need to plan for periodic rest in daily routine
- how to take the pulse
- dietary restrictions
- prescribed medications and potential adverse effects
- signs and symptoms to report
- importance of consistent follow-up care
- when to notify the physician
- use of prophylactic antibiotics for procedures.

Mitral valve insufficiency

Overview

Description

- Valvular disease of the mitral valve that allows the backflow of blood from the left ventricle to the left atrium
- May be acute (sudden volume overload of the left ventricle), chronic compensated (left ventricle compensates and left ventricular enlargement occurs), or chronic decompensated (left ventricle unable to sustain forward cardiac output)
- Also known as *mitral regurgitation*

Pathophysiology

- Blood from the left ventricle flows back into the left atrium during systole, causing the atrium to enlarge to accommodate the backflow.
- As a result, the left ventricle dilates to accommodate the increased volume of blood from the atrium and to compensate for diminishing cardiac output.
- Ventricular hypertrophy and increased end-diastolic pressure result in increased pulmonary artery pressure, eventually leading to left- and right-sided heart failure.

Causes

- Trauma
- Rheumatic fever
- Systemic lupus erythematosus
- Scleroderma
- Hypertrophic cardiomyopathy
- Infective endocarditis
- Mitral valve prolapse
- Myocardial infarction
- Severe left-sided heart failure
- Ruptured chordae tendineae
- Associated with congenital anomalies such as transposition of the great arteries

---

Identifying the murmur of mitral valve insufficiency

A high-pitched, rumbling pansystolic murmur that radiates from the mitral area to the left axillary line characterizes mitral valve insufficiency.

SYSTOLE	DIASTOLE	SYSTOLE	
S_1	S_2	S_1	S_2

Incidence

- Can occur at any age
- Affects both sexes equally

Common characteristics

- Dyspnea
- Peripheral edema
- Tachycardia

Complications

- Heart failure
- Pulmonary edema
- Thromboembolism
- Endocarditis
- Arrhythmias

Assessment

History

- Causal occurrence
- Orthopnea
- Dyspnea
- Fatigue
- Angina
- Palpitations

Physical findings

- Tachycardia
- Crackles in the lungs
- Hepatomegaly (right-sided failure)
- Holosystolic murmur at the apex (see *Identifying the murmur of mitral valve insufficiency*)
- Possible split S_2
- S_3

Test results

Imaging
- Chest X-ray reveals left atrial and ventricular enlargement and pulmonary congestion.
- Echocardiography shows abnormal valve leaflet motion and left atrial enlargement.

Diagnostic procedures
- Cardiac catheterization reveals mitral insufficiency with increased left ventricular end-diastolic volume and pressure, increased atrial pressure and pulmonary artery wedge pressure, and decreased cardiac output.
- Electrocardiogram may show left atrial and ventricular hypertrophy, sinus tachycardia, or atrial fibrillation.

Treatment

General

- Treat underlying cause appropriately
- Low-sodium diet
- Activity, as tolerated

Medication

○ Diuretics
○ Inotropic agents
○ Angiotensin-converting enzyme inhibitors
○ Oxygen
○ Anticoagulants
○ Prophylactic antibiotics before and after surgery or dental care to prevent endocarditis
○ Beta-adrenergic blockers or digoxin to slow the ventricular rate in atrial fibrillation or atrial flutter

Surgery

○ Annuloplasty or valvuloplasty to reconstruct or repair the valve
○ Valve replacement with a prosthetic valve

Nursing considerations

Key outcomes

The patient will:
○ carry out activities of daily living without weakness or fatigue
○ maintain hemodynamic stability
○ maintain adequate ventilation.

Nursing interventions

○ Give prescribed oxygen.
○ Watch for signs of heart failure or pulmonary edema.

Monitoring

○ Vital signs and pulse oximetry
○ Cardiac rhythm
○ Pulmonary artery catheter readings
○ Intake and output
○ Adverse effects of drug therapy

Patient teaching

Be sure to cover:
○ the disorder, diagnosis, and treatment
○ dietary restrictions and medication.

Mitral valve prolapse

Overview

Description

○ Portion of the mitral valve (MV) prolapses into the left atrium during ventricular contraction (systole)

Pathophysiology

○ Myxomatous degeneration of MV leaflets with redundant tissue leads to prolapse of the MV into the left atrium during systole.
○ In some patients, this results in leakage of blood into the left atrium from the left ventricle.

Causes

○ Connective tissue disorders, such as systemic lupus erythematosus and Marfan syndrome
○ Congenital heart disease
○ Acquired heart disease, such as coronary artery disease and rheumatic heart disease

Incidence

○ More prevalent in females than males
○ Usually detected in young adulthood
○ Affects 2.5% to 5% of the general population

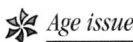 *Age issue*

Mitral valve prolapse is most common in women ages 20 to 40.

Common characteristics

○ Palpitations
○ Atypical chest pain

Complications

○ Arrhythmias
○ Infective endocarditis
○ Mitral insufficiency from chordal rupture
○ Mitral regurgitation

Assessment

History

○ Usually asymptomatic
○ Possible fatigue, syncope, palpitations, chest pain, or dyspnea on exertion

Physical findings

○ Orthostatic hypotension
○ Mid-to-late systolic click and late systolic murmur

Test results

Imaging
○ Echocardiography may reveal mitral valve prolapse (MVP) with or without mitral insufficiency.
Diagnostic procedures
○ Electrocardiography (ECG) is usually normal but may reveal atrial or ventricular arrhythmia.
○ Signal-averaged ECG may show ventricular and supraventricular arrhythmias.
○ Holter monitor worn for 24 hours may show an arrhythmia.

Treatment

General

○ Usually requires no treatment; only regular monitoring
○ Decreased caffeine intake
○ Fluid intake to maintain hydration

Medication

○ Antibiotic prophylaxis
○ Beta-adrenergic blockers
○ Anticoagulants
○ Antiarrhythmics

Nursing considerations

Key outcomes

The patient will:
○ carry out activities of daily living without fatigue or decreased energy
○ maintain adequate cardiac output, without arrhythmias
○ exhibit adequate coping mechanisms.

Nursing interventions

○ Provide reassurance and comfort if the patient experiences anxiety.
○ If fatigue is a concern, plan rest periods.
○ Discuss the patient's drug therapy including dosage, adverse reactions, and when to notify the physician if a problem arises.
○ Discuss the importance of adequate hydration.

Monitoring

○ Vital signs
○ Blood pressure while lying, sitting, and standing
○ Heart sounds
○ Signs and symptoms of mitral insufficiency
○ Serial echocardiograms
○ ECG for arrhythmias

Patient teaching

Be sure to cover:
○ the disorder, diagnosis, and treatment
○ need to perform the most important activities of the day when energy levels are highest
○ need for antibiotic prophylaxis therapy before dental or surgical procedures as indicated (not all patients with MVP require antibiotic prophylaxis)
○ avoidance of foods and beverages high in caffeine.

Discharge planning

○ If the patient is being discharged with a Holter monitor, make sure she understands the importance of documenting her activities throughout the monitoring process.
○ Refer the patient to an MVP support group.

Multiple myeloma

Overview

Description

○ Disseminated neoplasm of marrow plasma cells
○ Prognosis usually poor because by the time it's diagnosed, it has already infiltrated the vertebrae, pelvis, skull, ribs, clavicles, and sternum (without treatment, leads to vertebral collapse; within 3 months of diagnosis, 52% of patients die; within 2 years, 90% die)
○ With early diagnosis and treatment, life often prolonged by 3 to 5 years
○ Also called malignant *plasmacytoma, plasma cell myeloma,* and *myelomatosis*

Pathophysiology

○ Infiltration of the bone produces osteolytic lesions throughout the skeleton.
○ In late stages, the malignant plasma cells infiltrate into the lymph nodes, liver, spleen, and kidneys.

Causes

○ Exact cause unknown

Risk factors

○ Genetic factors
○ Occupational exposure to radiation

Incidence

○ Most common in men older than age 40.

Common characteristics

○ History of neoplastic fractures
○ Joint and back pain

Complications

○ Infections (such as pneumonia)
○ Pyelonephritis, renal calculi, and renal failure
○ Hematologic imbalance
○ Fractures
○ Hypercalcemia
○ Hyperuricemia
○ Dehydration

Assessment

History

○ History of neoplastic fractures
○ Severe, constant back pain, which may increase with exercise
○ Arthritic symptoms
○ Peripheral paresthesia
○ Progressive weakness
○ History of pneumonia
○ Pain on movement or weight bearing, especially in the thoracic and lumbar vertebrae

Physical findings

○ Noticeable thoracic deformities and reduction in body height of 5″ (12.7 cm)

Test results

Laboratory
○ Complete blood count shows moderate or severe anemia; the differential may show 40% to 50% lymphocytes but seldom more than 3% plasma cells; Rouleau formation, often the first clue, is seen on differential smear and results from elevation of the erythrocyte sedimentation rate.
○ Urine studies may show protein urea, Bence Jones protein, and hypercalciuria; absence of Bence Jones protein doesn't rule out multiple myeloma, but its presence almost invariably confirms the disease.
○ Serum electrophoresis shows an elevated globulin spike that's electrophoretically and immunologically abnormal.

Imaging
○ X-rays during the early stages may reveal only diffuse osteoporosis. Eventually, they show the characteristic lesions of multiple myeloma: multiple, sharply circumscribed osteolytic, or punched out lesions, particularly on the skull, pelvis, and spine.

Diagnostic procedures
○ Bone marrow aspiration reveals myelomatous cells and abnormal number of immature plasma cells (10% to 95% instead of the normal 3% to 5%).

Treatment

General

○ Adjuvant local radiation
○ Dialysis (if renal complications develop)
○ Plasmapheresis to remove the M protein from the blood and return the cells to the patient (temporary effect)
○ Peripheral blood stem cell transplantation
○ Well-balanced diet
○ Activity, as tolerated

Medication

○ Bisphosphonates
○ Analgesics
○ Chemotherapeutic agents
○ Possible use of thalidomide
○ Immunotherapy

Surgery

○ Laminectomy if the patient develops vertebral compression

Nursing considerations

Key outcomes

The patient will:
○ express feelings regarding illness
○ maintain adequate ventilation

- express feelings of increased comfort and decreased pain
- demonstrate effective coping skills.

Nursing interventions

- Encourage fluid intake (3 to 4 qt [3 to 4 L] daily).
- Give prescribed drugs.

After surgery

- Encourage mobilization.

Monitoring

- Complications of treatment
- Signs and symptoms of severe anemia and fractures
- Proper positioning (alignment)
- Pain control

Patient teaching

Be sure to cover:
- the disorder, diagnosis, and treatment
- importance of deep breathing and changing position every 2 hours after surgery
- appropriate dress for weather conditions (because the patient may be sensitive to cold)
- avoidance of crowds and people with infections
- medication administration, dosage, and possible adverse effects.

Discharge planning

- Refer the patient to available resources and support services.

Multiple sclerosis

Overview

Description

○ Progressive demyelination of white matter of brain and spinal cord
○ Characterized by exacerbations and remissions
○ May progress rapidly, causing death within months
○ Prognosis varies (70% of patients with multiple sclerosis lead active lives with prolonged remissions)
○ Also known as *MS*

Pathophysiology

○ Sporadic patches of demyelination occur in the central nervous system, resulting in widespread and varied neurologic dysfunction.

Causes

○ Exact cause unknown
○ Slow-acting viral infection
○ An autoimmune response of the nervous system
○ Allergic response
○ Events that precede the onset:
  – emotional stress
  – overwork
  – fatigue
  – pregnancy
  – acute respiratory tract infections
○ Genetic factors possibly also involved

Risk factors

○ Trauma
○ Anoxia
○ Toxins
○ Nutritional deficiencies
○ Vascular lesions
○ Anorexia nervosa

Incidence

○ Highest in women
○ Highest among people in northern urban areas
○ Highest in higher socioeconomic groups
○ Low incidence in Japan
○ Family history increases incidence
○ Increased incidence with living in a cold, damp climate
○ Major cause of chronic disability in young adults ages 20 to 40

Common characteristics

○ Dependent on the extent and site of myelin destruction
○ Sensory impairment
○ Muscle dysfunction
○ Bladder and bowel disturbances
○ Speech problems
○ Fatigue

Complications

○ Injuries from falls
○ Urinary tract infections
○ Constipation
○ Contractures
○ Pressure ulcers
○ Pneumonia
○ Depression

Assessment

History

○ Symptoms related to extent and site of myelin destruction, extent of remyelination, and adequacy of subsequent restored synaptic transmission
○ Symptoms possibly transient or last for hours or weeks
○ Symptoms unpredictable and difficult to describe
○ Visual problems and sensory impairment (the first signs)
○ Blurred vision or diplopia
○ Urinary problems
○ Emotional lability
○ Dysphagia
○ Bowel disturbances (involuntary evacuation or constipation)
○ Fatigue (typically the most disabling symptom)

Physical findings

○ Poor articulation
○ Muscle weakness of the involved area
○ Spasticity; hyperreflexia
○ Intention tremor
○ Gait ataxia
○ Paralysis, ranging from monoplegia to quadriplegia
○ Nystagmus; scotoma
○ Optic neuritis
○ Ophthalmoplegia

Test results

○ Years of testing and observation may be required for diagnosis.
Laboratory
○ Cerebrospinal fluid analysis showing mononuclear cell pleocytosis, an elevation in the level of total immunoglobulin (Ig) G, and presence of oligoclonal Ig
Imaging
○ Magnetic resonance imaging is the most sensitive method of detecting multiple sclerosis focal lesions.
Other
○ EEG abnormalities occur in one-third of patients with MS.
○ Evoked potential studies show slowed conduction of nerve impulses.

Treatment

General

○ Symptomatic treatment for acute exacerbations and related signs and symptoms
○ High fluid diet and fiber intake in case of constipation
○ Frequent rest periods

Medication

○ I.V. steroids followed by oral steroids
○ Immunosuppressants
○ Antimetabolites
○ Alkylating drugs
○ Biological response modifiers

Nursing considerations

Key outcomes

The patient will:
○ perform activities of daily living
○ remain free from infection
○ maintain joint mobility and range of motion
○ express feelings of increased energy and decreased fatigue
○ develop regular bowel and bladder habits
○ use available support systems and coping mechanisms.

Nursing interventions

○ Provide emotional and psychological support.
○ Assist with physical therapy program.
○ Provide adequate rest periods.
○ Promote emotional stability.
○ Keep the bedpan or urinal readily available because the need to void is immediate.
○ Provide bowel and bladder training, if indicated.
○ Give prescribed drugs.

Monitoring

○ Response to medications
○ Adverse drug reactions
○ Sensory impairment
○ Muscle dysfunction
○ Energy level
○ Signs and symptoms of infection
○ Speech
○ Elimination patterns
○ Vision changes
○ Laboratory results

Patient teaching

Be sure to cover:
○ disease process (see *Describing multiple sclerosis*)
○ medication and adverse effects
○ avoidance of stress, infections, and fatigue

Describing multiple sclerosis

Various terms are used to describe multiple sclerosis (MS).
○ *Elapsing-remitting:* clear relapses (or acute attacks or exacerbations) with full recovery and lasting disability. Between attacks, the disease doesn't worsen.
○ *Primary progressive:* steadily progressing or worsening with minor recovery or plateaus. This form is uncommon and may involve different brain and spinal cord damage from other forms.
○ *Secondary progressive:* beginning as a pattern of clear-cut relapses and recovery but becoming steadily progressive and worsening between acute attacks.
○ *Progressive-relapsing:* steadily progressing from the onset but also has clear, acute attacks. This form is rare. In addition, differential diagnosis must rule out spinal cord compression, foramen magnum tumor (which may mimic the exacerbations and remissions of MS), multiple small strokes, syphilis or another infection, thyroid disease, and chronic fatigue syndrome.

○ maintaining independence
○ avoiding exposure to bacterial and viral infections
○ nutritional management
○ adequate fluid intake and regular urination.

Discharge planning

○ Refer the patient to the National Multiple Sclerosis Society.
○ Refer the patient to physical and occupational rehabilitation programs, as indicated.

Mumps

Overview

Description

○ An acute inflammation of one or both parotid glands, and sometimes the sublingual or submaxillary glands
○ Also called *infectious* or *epidemic parotitisan*

Pathophysiology

○ Virus replication occurs in the epithelium of the upper respiratory tract, leading to viremia.
○ Infection of the central nervous system (CNS) or glandular tissues (or both) occurs, resulting in perivascular and interstitial mononuclear cell infiltrates with edema.
○ Necrosis of acinar and epithelial duct cells occurs in the salivary glands and germinal epithelium of the seminiferous tubules.

Causes

○ A paramyxovirus found in the saliva of an infected person
○ Transmitted by droplets or by direct contact with the saliva of an infected person

Incidence

○ Seldom occurs in infants younger than age 1 because of passive immunity from maternal antibodies
○ About 50% of cases in young adults; remainder in young children or immunocompromised adults
○ Peak incidence during late winter and early spring

Common characteristics

○ Usually begins with prodromal symptoms that last for 24 hours
○ Myalgia, anorexia, malaise, headache, an earache aggravated by chewing, and pain when drinking sour or acidic liquids; may have a fever of 101° to 104° F (38.3° to 40° C)

Complications

○ Epididymoorchitis
○ Meningoencephalitis
○ Sterility
○ Pancreatitis
○ Transient sensorineural hearing loss
○ Arthritis
○ Nephritis
○ Spontaneous abortion (with contact during the first trimester)

Assessment

History

○ Inadequate immunization and exposure to someone with mumps within the preceding 2 to 3 weeks

○ Myalgia, headache
○ Malaise, fever
○ Earache aggravated by chewing

Physical findings

○ Swelling and tenderness of the parotid glands
○ Simultaneous or subsequent swelling of one or more other salivary glands (see *Parotid inflammation in mumps*)

Test results

○ Glandular swelling confirms the diagnosis.
Laboratory
○ Serologic testing showing mumps antibodies.

Treatment

General

○ Rest
○ Cold compresses for swollen glands
○ Use of athletic supporter if testicles are tender
○ Liquid to mechanical soft diet until able to swallow
○ Increased fluid intake
○ Bed rest until fever resolves
○ Rest periods when fatigued

Medication

○ Analgesics
○ Antipyretics

Nursing considerations

Key outcomes

The patient will:
○ remain afebrile
○ express feelings of increased comfort and decreased pain
○ maintain adequate fluid volume
○ achieve adequate nutritional intake.

Nursing interventions

○ Apply warm or cool compresses to the neck area to relieve pain.
○ Give prescribed drugs.
○ Provide scrotal support, if needed.
○ Report all cases of mumps to local public health authorities.
○ Disinfect articles soiled with nose and throat secretions.

Monitoring

○ Response to treatment
○ Signs of CNS involvement
○ Auditory acuity
○ Complications

The mumps virus (paramyxovirus) attacks the parotid glands—the main salivary glands. Inflammation causes characteristic swelling and discomfort with eating, drinking, swallowing, and talking.

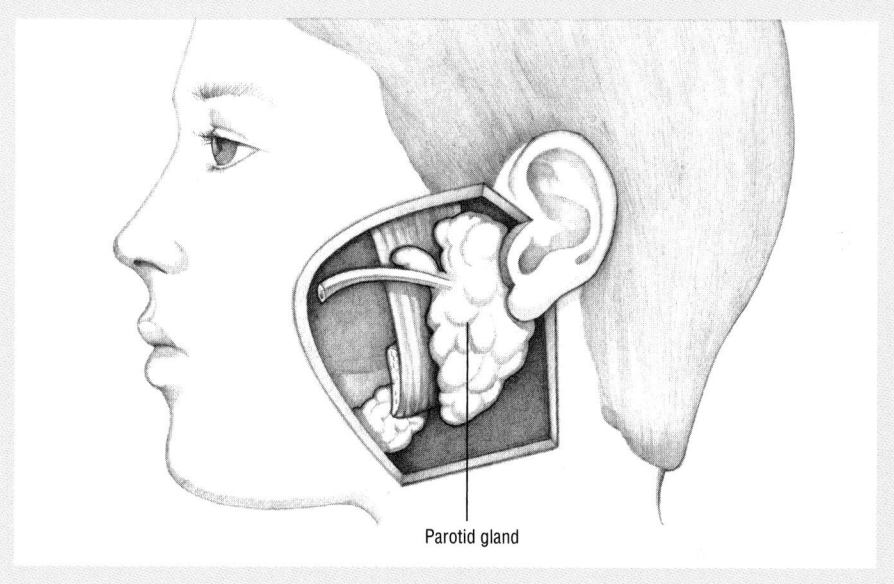

Parotid gland

Patient teaching

Be sure to cover:
- the disorder, diagnosis, and treatment
- need to stay away from school or work from days 12 through 25 after exposure
- importance of having children immunized with live attenuated mumps vaccine at age 15 months or older, if applicable
- if epididymoorchitis occurs, reassurance that it won't cause impotence and sterility (occurs only with bilateral orchitis)
- need for bed rest during febrile period
- need to avoid spicy, irritating foods, and those that require much chewing; advise a soft, bland diet
- need for family members to follow respiratory isolation precautions until symptoms subside.

Discharge planning

- Refer the patient to a urologist for orchitis, if indicated.

Muscular dystrophy

Overview

Description

- Hereditary disorder characterized by progressive symmetrical wasting of skeletal muscles
- No neural or sensory defects
- Four main types are Duchenne's (pseudohypertrophic), Becker's (benign pseudohypertrophic), Landouzy-Dejerine (facioscapulohumeral) dystrophy, and Erb's (limb-girdle) dystrophy
- Duchenne's begins during early childhood, death occurs within 10 to 15 years

Pathophysiology

- Muscle fibers necrotize and regenerate in various states.
- Regeneration slows and degeneration dominates.
- Fat and connective tissue replace muscle fibers.
- Weakness results.

Causes

- Various genetic mechanisms (band Xp 21)
- Duchenne's and Becker's X-linked recessive
- Landouzy-Dejerine autosomal dominant
- Erb's usually autosomal recessive

Incidence

- Duchenne's and Becker's affect males almost exclusively.
- Landouzy-Dejerine and Erb's affect both sexes about equally.

Common characteristics

- Waddling gait
- Toe walking
- Lumbar lordosis
- Frequent falls
- Dyspnea
- Dysphagia

Complications

- Crippling disability
- Contractures
- Pneumonia
- Arrhythmias
- Cardiac hypertrophy
- Dysphagia

Assessment

History

- Evidence of genetic transmission
- Progressive muscle weakness

Duchenne's
- Onset insidious
- Onset between ages 3 and 5
- Pelvic muscle weakness
- Interferes with child's ability to run, climb, and walk

Becker's
- Onset after age 5
- Symptoms the same as Duchenne's, but slower progression

Landouzy-Dejerine
- Onset before age 10
- Weakness of eye, face, and shoulder muscles
- Inability to raise arms over head
- Inability to close eyes
- Inability to pucker lips or whistle
- Abnormal facial movements
- Absence of facial movements when laughing or crying
- Pelvic muscles weaken as disease progresses

Erb's
- Symptoms the same as in Landouzy-Dejerine but slower progression
- Less of a disability than in Landouzy-Dejerine
- Onset between ages 6 and 10
- Muscle weakness of upper arm and pelvic muscles

Physical findings

Duchenne's and Becker's
- Wide stance and waddling gait
- Gowers' sign when rising from a sitting or supine position
- Muscle hypertrophy and atrophy
- Calves enlarged because of fat infiltration into the muscle
- Posture changes
- Lordosis and a protuberant abdomen
- Scapular "'winging'" or flaring when raising arms
- Contractures
- Tachypnea and shortness of breath

Landouzy-Dejerine
- Pendulous lower lip
- Possible disappearance of nasolabial fold
- Diffuse facial flattening leading to a masklike expression
- Inability to suckle (infants)
- Scapulae with a winglike appearance; inability to raise arms above head

Erb's
- Effects of muscle weakness apparent
- Muscle wasting
- Winging of the scapulae
- Lordosis with abdominal protrusion
- Waddling gait
- Poor balance
- Inability to raise the arms

Test results

Laboratory
- Elevated urine creatinine, serum creatine kinase, lactate dehydrogenase, alanine aminotransferase, and aspartate aminotransferase

Diagnostic procedures
○ Muscle biopsy result confirms the diagnosis.
○ Immunologic and biological results facilitate prenatal and postnatal diagnosis.
○ Electromyography shows abnormal muscle movements.
○ Amniocentesis detects sex of fetus for high-risk family.

Other
○ Genetic testing may be used to detect the gene defect that leads to muscular dystrophy in some families.

Treatment

General
○ No known treatment to stop progression
○ Orthopedic appliances
○ Low-calorie, high-protein, high-fiber diet
○ Tube feedings, as needed
○ Exercise, as tolerated
○ Physical therapy

Medication
○ Stool softeners
○ Possible steroids

Surgery
○ Surgery to correct contractures
○ Spinal fusion

Nursing considerations

Key outcomes
The patient will:
○ perform activities of daily living without muscle fatigue or intolerance
○ maintain muscle strength, joint mobility, and range of motion
○ show no evidence of complications
○ maintain respiratory rate within 5 breaths/minute of baseline.

Nursing interventions
○ Encourage coughing and deep-breathing exercises.
○ Take steps to prevent muscle atrophy.
○ Use splints, braces, grab bars, and overhead slings.
○ Use a footboard or high-topped shoes and a foot cradle.
○ Provide a low-calorie, high-protein, high-fiber diet.

Monitoring
○ Intake and output
○ Respiratory status
○ Joint mobility
○ Muscle weakness
○ Complications

Patient teaching

Be sure to cover:
○ the disorder, diagnosis, and treatment
○ maintenance of peer relationships
○ how to maintain mobility and independence
○ possible complications and prevention
○ signs and symptoms of respiratory tract infections
○ need for a low-calorie, high-protein, high-fiber diet
○ need to avoid long periods of bed rest and inactivity.

Discharge planning
○ Refer the patient for sexual counseling, if indicated.
○ Refer the patient for physical therapy, vocational rehabilitation, social services, and financial assistance.
○ Refer the patient to the Muscular Dystrophy Association.
○ Refer the patient for genetic counseling.

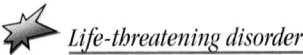
Life-threatening disorder

Myasthenia gravis

Overview

Description
- An acquired autoimmune disorder characterized by abnormal fatigability of striated (skeletal) muscles
- Sporadic but progressive weakness
- Muscle weakness exacerbated by exercise and repetitive movement
- Initial symptoms related to cranial nerves
- With respiratory system involvement, may be life-threatening
- Spontaneous remissions in about 25% of patients

Pathophysiology
- Blood cells and thymus gland produce antibodies that block, destroy, or weaken neuroreceptors (which transmit nerve impulses).
- The result is failure in transmission of nerve impulses at the neuromuscular junction.

Causes
- Autoimmune disorder associated with the thymus gland
- Accompanies other immune and thyroid disorders

Incidence
- Occurs at any age
- Three times more common in women than men
- Highest in women ages 18 to 25
- Highest in men ages 50 to 60
- Transient myasthenia in about 20% of infants born to myasthenic mothers

Common characteristics
- Weak eye closure; ptosis
- Diplopia
- Skeletal muscle weakness; paralysis

Complications
- Respiratory distress
- Pneumonia
- Aspiration

Assessment

History
- Varying assessment findings
- Progressive muscle weakness
- Extreme muscle weakness and fatigue (cardinal symptoms)
- Ptosis and diplopia (the most common sign and symptom)
- Difficulty chewing and swallowing
- Jaw hanging open (especially when tired)
- Head bobbing
- Symptoms milder on awakening; worsen as the day progresses
- Short rest periods that temporarily restore muscle function
- Symptoms that become more intense during menses, after emotional stress, after prolonged exposure to sunlight or cold, and with infections

Physical findings
- Sleepy, masklike expression
- Drooping jaw
- Ptosis
- Decreased breath sounds
- Decreased tidal volume
- Respiratory distress and myasthenic crisis

Test results
Imaging
- Chest X-rays or computed tomography scan shows thymoma.
Other
- Positive Tensilon test shows temporary improved muscle function and confirms the diagnosis.
- Electrodiagnostic testing shows a rapid reduction of more than 10% in the amplitude of evoked responses.

Treatment

General
- Plasmapheresis
- Emergency airway and ventilation management
- Diet, as tolerated
- Activity, as tolerated (Exercise may exacerbate symptoms; planned rest periods may retard symptoms.)

Medication
- Anticholinesterase drugs
- Corticosteroids
- I.V. immune globulin

Surgery
- Thymectomy

Nursing considerations

Key outcomes
The patient will:
- maintain a patent airway and adequate ventilation
- maintain respiratory rate within 5 breaths/minute of baseline
- perform activities of daily living
- maintain range of motion and joint mobility
- express positive feelings about self.

Nursing interventions
- Provide psychological support.

○ Provide frequent rest periods.
○ Maintain nutritional management program.
○ Maintain social activity.
○ Give prescribed drugs.

Monitoring

○ Neurologic and respiratory function
○ Response to medications

 Alert

Monitor patient for signs of impending myasthenic crisis, including increased muscle weakness, respiratory distress, and difficulty talking or chewing.

Patient teaching

Be sure to cover:
○ the disorder, diagnosis, and treatment
○ surgery (preoperative and postoperative teaching)
○ energy conservation techniques
○ medication and adverse drug effects
○ avoidance of strenuous exercise, stress, infection, needless exposure to the sun or cold weather
○ nutritional management program
○ swallowing therapy program.

Discharge planning

○ Refer the patient to the Myasthenia Gravis Foundation.

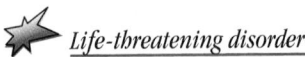 *Life-threatening disorder*

Myocardial infarction

Overview

Description

- Reduced blood flow through one or more coronary arteries causing myocardial ischemia and necrosis
- Infarction site depends on the vessels involved
- Also called *MI* and *heart attack*

Pathophysiology

- One or more coronary arteries become occluded.
- If coronary occlusion causes ischemia lasting longer than 30 to 45 minutes, irreversible myocardial cell damage and muscle death occur.
- Every MI has a central area of necrosis surrounded by an area of hypoxic injury. This injured tissue is potentially viable and may be salvaged if circulation is restored, or it may progress to necrosis.

Causes

- Atherosclerosis
- Thrombosis
- Platelet aggregation
- Coronary artery stenosis or spasm

Risk factors

- Increased age (40 to 70)
- Diabetes mellitus
- Elevated serum triglyceride, low-density lipoprotein, and cholesterol levels, and decreased serum high-density lipoprotein levels
- Excessive intake of saturated fats, carbohydrates, or salt
- Hypertension
- Obesity
- Positive family history of coronary artery disease (CAD)
- Sedentary lifestyle
- Smoking
- Stress or a type A personality
- Use of drugs, such as amphetamines or cocaine

Incidence

- Men more susceptible than premenopausal women
- Increasing among women who smoke and take hormonal contraceptives
- In postmenopausal women, similar to incidence in men

Common characteristics

- Substernal chest pain or pressure with radiation in men
- Shoulder or jaw pain
- Dyspnea
- Atypical symptoms such as nausea in women

Complications

- Arrhythmias
- Cardiogenic shock
- Heart failure causing pulmonary edema
- Pericarditis
- Rupture of the atrial or ventricular septum, ventricular wall
- Ventricular aneurysm
- Cerebral or pulmonary emboli
- Extensions of the original infarction
- Mitral insufficiency

Assessment

History

- Possible CAD with increasing anginal frequency, severity, or duration
- Cardinal symptom of MI: persistent, crushing substernal pain or pressure possibly radiating to the left arm, jaw, neck, and shoulder blades, and possibly persisting for 12 or more hours
- In elderly patient or one with diabetes, pain possibly absent; in others, pain possibly mild and confused with indigestion
- A feeling of impending doom, fatigue, nausea, vomiting, and shortness of breath
- Sudden death (may be the first and only indication of MI)

Physical findings

- Extreme anxiety and restlessness
- Dyspnea
- Diaphoresis
- Tachycardia
- Hypertension
- Bradycardia and hypotension, in inferior MI
- An S_4, an S_3, and paradoxical splitting of S_2 with ventricular dysfunction
- Systolic murmur of mitral insufficiency
- Pericardial friction rub with transmural MI or pericarditis
- Low-grade fever during the next few days

Test results

Laboratory

- Elevated serum creatine kinase (CK) level, especially the CK-MB isoenzyme, the cardiac muscle fraction of CK
- Elevated serum lactate dehydrogenase (LD) level; higher LD_1 isoenzyme (found in cardiac tissue) than LD_2 (in serum)
- Elevated white blood cell count usually appearing on the second day and lasting 1 week
- Detection of myoglobin (the hemoprotein found in cardiac and skeletal muscle) that's released with muscle damage as soon as 2 hours after MI
- Elevated troponin I, a structural protein found in cardiac muscle, only in cardiac muscle damage; more specific than the CK-MB level (Troponin levels in-

crease within 4 to 6 hours of myocardial injury and may remain elevated for 5 to 11 days.)

Imaging
- Nuclear medicine scans, using I.V. technetium 99m pertechnetate, can identify acutely damaged muscle by picking up accumulations of radioactive nucleotide, which appear as a "hot spot" on the film. Myocardial perfusion imaging with thallium 201 reveals a "cold spot" in most patients during the first few hours after a transmural MI.
- Echocardiography shows ventricular wall dyskinesia with a transmural MI and helps to evaluate the ejection fraction.

Diagnostic procedures
- Serial 12-lead electrocardiography (ECG) readings may be normal or inconclusive during the first few hours after an MI. Characteristic abnormalities include serial ST-segment depression in subendocardial MI and ST-segment elevation and Q waves, representing scarring and necrosis, in transmural MI.
- Pulmonary artery catheterization may be performed to detect left- or right-sided heart failure and to monitor response to treatment.

Treatment

General
- For arrhythmias, a pacemaker or electrical cardioversion
- Intra-aortic balloon pump for cardiogenic shock
- Low-fat, low-cholesterol diet
- Calorie restriction, if indicated
- Bed rest with bedside commode
- Gradual increase in activity, as tolerated

Medication
- I.V. thrombolytic therapy started within 3 hours of the onset of symptoms
- Aspirin
- Antiarrhythmics, antianginals
- Calcium channel blockers
- Heparin I.V.
- Morphine I.V.
- Inotropic drugs
- Beta-adrenergic blockers
- Angiotensin-converting inhibitors
- Stool softeners
- Oxygen

Surgery
- Surgical revascularization
- Percutaneous revascularization

Nursing considerations

Key outcomes
The patient will:
- maintain adequate cardiac output
- maintain hemodynamic stability
- develop no arrhythmia
- develop no complications of fluid volume excess
- express feelings of increased comfort and decreased pain
- exhibit adequate coping skills.

Nursing interventions
- Assess pain and give prescribed analgesics. Record the severity, location, type, and duration of pain. Avoid I.M. injections.
- Check the patient's blood pressure before and after giving nitroglycerin.
- During episodes of chest pain, obtain ECG.
- Organize patient care and activities to provide periods of uninterrupted rest.
- Provide a low-cholesterol, low-sodium diet with caffeine-free beverages.
- Allow the patient to use a bedside commode.
- Assist with range-of-motion exercises.
- Provide emotional support, and help to reduce stress and anxiety.
- If the patient has undergone percutaneous transluminal coronary angioplasty, sheath care is necessary. Watch for bleeding. Keep the leg with the sheath insertion site immobile. Maintain strict bed rest. Check peripheral pulses in the affected leg frequently.

Monitoring
- Serial ECGs
- Vital signs and heart and breath sounds

 Alert

Watch for crackles, cough, tachypnea, and edema, which may indicate impending left-sided heart failure.

- Daily weight; intake and output
- Cardiac enzyme levels; coagulation studies
- Cardiac rhythm for reperfusion arrhythmias (treat according to facility protocol)

Patient teaching

Be sure to cover:
- procedures (answering questions for the patient and family members)
- medication dosages, adverse reactions, and signs of toxicity to watch for and report
- dietary restrictions
- progressive resumption of sexual activity
- appropriate responses to new or recurrent symptoms
- typical or atypical chest pain to report.

Discharge planning
- Refer the patient to a cardiac rehabilitation program.
- Refer the patient to a smoking-cessation program, if needed.
- Refer the patient to a weight-reduction program, if needed.

Myocarditis

Overview

Description

- Focal or diffuse inflammation of the myocardium typically uncomplicated and self-limiting
- May be acute or chronic
- Recovery usually spontaneous and without residual defects

Pathophysiology

- An infectious organism triggers an autoimmune, cellular, and humoral reaction.
- Inflammation may lead to hypertrophy, fibrosis, and inflammatory changes of the myocardium and conduction system.
- Heart muscle weakens and contractility is reduced.

Causes

- Viruses
- Bacteria
- Hypersensitive immune reactions such as acute rheumatic fever
- Radiation therapy
- Chronic alcoholism
- Parasitic infections
- Helminthic infections such as trichinosis

Incidence

- Can occur at any age

Common characteristics

- Mild, continuous chest soreness or pressure

Complications

- Left-sided heart failure
- Cardiomyopathy
- Chronic valvulitis (when it results from rheumatic fever)
- Arrhythmias
- Thromboembolism

Assessment

History

- Possible recent upper respiratory tract infection with fever, viral pharyngitis, or tonsillitis
- Nonspecific symptoms, such as fatigue, dyspnea, palpitations, persistent tachycardia, and persistent fever
- Mild, continuous pressure or soreness in the chest

Physical findings

- S_3 and S_4 gallops, muffled S_1
- Pericardial friction rub

Test results

Laboratory

- Elevated cardiac enzyme levels, including creatine kinase (CK), CK-MB, aspartate aminotransferase, and lactate dehydrogenase
- Elevated white blood cell count and erythrocyte sedimentation rate
- Elevated antibody titers, such as antistreptolysin-O titer in rheumatic fever
- Cultures of stool, throat, pharyngeal washings, or other body fluids showing the causative bacteria or virus

Diagnostic procedures

- Endomyocardial biopsy can be used to confirm a myocarditis diagnosis.
- Electrocardiography typically shows diffuse ST-segment and T-wave abnormalities as in pericarditis, conduction defects (prolonged PR interval), and ventricular and supraventricular ectopic arrhythmias.

Treatment

General

- For patient with signs and symptoms of heart failure, hospitalization until stabilized
- Oxygen therapy, if indicated
- Avoidance of alcohol
- Low-sodium diet
- Modified bed rest
- Activity, as tolerated

Medication

- Anti-infectives
- Antiarrhythmics
- Anticoagulants
- Anti-inflammatory agents
- Angiotensin-converting enzyme inhibitors
- Diuretics
- Inotropic agents

Surgery

- Pacemaker implantation
- Ventricular assist device
- Heart transplantation

Nursing considerations

Key outcomes

The patient will:
- carry out activities of daily living without weakness or fatigue
- maintain hemodynamic stability and adequate cardiac output without arrhythmia
- maintain adequate ventilation.

Nursing interventions

- Stress the importance of bed rest. Provide a bedside commode.

○ Allow the patient to express his concerns about the effects of activity restrictions on his responsibilities and routines.
○ Give prescribed oxygen.
○ Give prescribed parenteral anti-infectives and other drugs.

Monitoring

○ Vital signs
○ Cardiovascular status
○ Intake and output
○ Signs and symptoms of heart failure
○ For digoxin toxicity
○ Cardiac rhythm
○ Arterial blood gas levels
○ Daily weight
○ Response to treatment

Patient teaching

Be sure to cover:
○ the disorder, diagnosis, and treatment
○ prescribed medications and potential adverse reactions
○ prevention of myocarditis
○ signs and symptoms of heart failure
○ for a patient taking cardiac glycosides at home, how to check the pulse for 1 full minute before taking the dose, and the need to withhold the dose and notify the physician if the heart rate falls below the predetermined rate (usually 60 beats/minute)
○ when to notify the physician.

Near drowning

Overview

Description

○ Victim survives physiologic effects of submersion
○ Primary problems: hypoxemia and acidosis
○ "Dry" near drowning: fluid not aspirated; respiratory obstruction or asphyxia
○ "Wet" near drowning: fluid aspirated; asphyxia or secondary changes from fluid aspiration
○ "Secondary" near drowning: recurrence of respiratory distress

Pathophysiology

○ Immersion stimulates hyperventilation.
○ Voluntary apnea occurs.
○ Laryngospasm develops.
○ Hypoxemia develops and can lead to brain damage and cardiac arrest.

Causes

○ Inability to swim
○ Panic
○ Boating accident
○ Sudden acute illness
○ Blow to the head while in the water
○ Venomous stings from aquatic animals
○ Excessive alcohol consumption before swimming
○ Decompression sickness from deep-water diving
○ Dangerous water conditions
○ Suicide attempt

Incidence

○ Most common cause of injury and death in children ages 1 month to 14 years
○ Incidence greater in males

Common characteristics

○ Altered vital signs
○ Dyspnea
○ Hypoxia
○ Altered level of consciousness
○ Cardiopulmonary arrest

Complications

○ Neurologic impairment
○ Seizure disorder
○ Pulmonary edema
○ Renal damage
○ Bacterial aspiration
○ Pulmonary complications
○ Cardiac complications

Assessment

History

○ Victim found in water

Physical findings

○ Fever or hypothermia
○ Rapid, slow, or absent pulse
○ Shallow, gasping, or absent respirations
○ Altered level of consciousness
○ Seizures
○ Cyanosis or pink, frothy sputum or both
○ Abdominal distention
○ Crackles, rhonchi, wheezing, or apnea
○ Tachycardia
○ Irregular heartbeat

Test results

Laboratory
○ Arterial blood gas (ABG) level showing degree of hypoxia, intrapulmonary shunt, and acid-base balance
○ Imbalanced electrolyte levels
○ Complete blood count showing hemolysis
○ Blood urea nitrogen and creatinine levels revealing impaired renal function
○ Urinalysis showing signs of impaired renal function
Imaging
○ Cervical spine X-ray may show evidence of fracture.
○ Serial chest X-rays may show pulmonary edema.
Other
○ Electrocardiogram may show myocardial ischemia or infarct or cardiac arrhythmias.

Treatment

General

○ Stabilize neck
○ Establish airway and provide ventilation
○ Correct abnormal laboratory values
○ Warming measures, if hypothermic
○ Nothing by mouth until swallowing ability has returned
○ Activity based on extent of injury and success of resuscitation

Medication

○ Bronchodilators
○ Cardiac drug therapy if appropriate

Nursing considerations

Key outcomes

The patient will:
○ maintain adequate cardiac output
○ maintain adequate ventilation
○ have a patent airway at all times
○ maintain a normal body temperature
○ develop effective coping mechanisms.

Nursing interventions

○ Perform cardiopulmonary resuscitation as indicated.
○ Perform active external rewarming and passive re-warming measures for mild hypothermia (93.2° to 96.8° F [34° to 36° C]); for active external rewarming of truncal areas only and passive rewarming measures for moderate hypothermia (86° F [30° C] to 93.2° F) for active internal rewarming measures for severe hypothermia (less than 86° F).
○ Protect the cervical spine.
○ Give prescribed drugs.
○ Provide emotional support.

Monitoring

○ Electrolyte and ABG measurement results
○ Cardiac rhythm
○ Vital signs
○ Neurologic status
○ Respiratory status
○ Core body temperature
○ Psychological state

Patient teaching

Be sure to cover:
○ the injury, diagnosis, and treatment
○ the need to avoid using alcohol or drugs before swimming
○ water safety measures (such as the "buddy system").

Discharge planning

○ Recommend a water safety course given by the Red Cross, YMCA, or YWCA.
○ Refer the patient or family for psychological counseling if appropriate.
○ Refer the patient or family to resource and support services.

Necrotizing fasciitis

Overview

Description

○ A progressive, rapidly spreading inflammatory infection of the deep fascia
○ Mortality rate: 70% to 80%
○ Most commonly called *flesh-eating bacteria*
○ Also called *hemolytic streptococcal gangrene, acute dermal gangrene, suppurative fasciitis,* and *synergistic necrotizing cellulitis*

Pathophysiology

○ Infecting bacteria enter the host through a local tissue injury or a breach in a mucous membrane barrier.
○ Organisms proliferate in an environment of tissue hypoxia caused by trauma, recent surgery, or a medical condition that compromises the patient.
○ Necrosis of the surrounding tissue results, accelerating the disease process by creating a favorable environment for organisms.
○ The fascia and fat tissues are destroyed, with secondary necrosis of subcutaneous tissue.

Causes

○ Group A beta-hemolytic *Streptococcus* (GAS) and *Staphylococcus aureus,* alone or together, are the most common primary infecting bacteria. (More than 80 types of the causative bacteria, *Streptococcus pyogenes,* makes epidemiology of GAS infections complex.)

Incidence

○ Three times more likely in men than women
○ Rarely occurs in children except in countries with poor hygiene practices
○ Mean age is 38 to 44
○ Increased risk for elderly or immunocompromised patients and those with chronic illnesses or using steroids

Common characteristics

○ Pain out of proportion to the size of the wound or injury
○ Rapid deterioration in overall clinical status

Complications

○ Renal failure
○ Septic shock
○ Scarring with cosmetic deformities
○ Myositis
○ Myonecrosis
○ Amputation

Assessment

History

○ Associated risk factors
○ Pain
○ Tissue injury

Physical findings

○ Rapidly progressing erythema at the site of insult
○ Fluid-filled blisters and bullae (indicate rapid progression of the necrotizing process)
○ By days 4 and 5, large areas of gangrenous skin
○ By days 7 to 10, extensive necrosis of the subcutaneous tissue
○ Fever
○ Sepsis
○ Hypovolemia
○ Hypotension
○ Respiratory insufficiency
○ Deterioration in level of consciousness
○ Signs of sepsis

Test results

Laboratory

○ Tissue biopsy showing infiltration of the deep dermis, fascia, and muscular planes with bacteria and polymorphonuclear cells, and necrosis of fatty and muscular tissue
○ Cultures of microorganisms from the periphery of the spreading infection or from deeper tissues during surgical debridement identifying the causative organism
○ Gram stain and culture of biopsied tissue identifying the causative organism

Imaging

○ Radiographic studies may pinpoint the presence of subcutaneous gases.
○ Computed tomography scans may show the anatomic site of involvement by locating necrosis.
○ Magnetic resonance imaging shows areas of necrosis and areas that require surgical debridement.

Treatment

General

○ Wound care
○ Hyperbaric oxygen therapy
○ High-protein, high-calorie diet
○ Increased fluid intake
○ Bed rest until treatment effective

Medication

○ Antimicrobials
○ Analgesics

Surgery

○ Immediate surgical debridement, fasciectomy, or amputation

Nursing considerations

Key outcomes

The patient will:
○ maintain collateral circulation
○ attain hemodynamic stability
○ maintain adequate cardiac output
○ remain afebrile
○ maintain adequate fluid volume.

Nursing interventions

○ Give prescribed drugs.
○ Provide supportive care and supplemental oxygen, as appropriate.
○ Provide emotional support.

Monitoring

○ Signs and symptoms of complications
○ Vital signs
○ Mental status
○ Wound status
○ Pain control

Patient teaching

Be sure to cover:
○ the disorder, diagnosis, and treatment
○ importance of strict sterile technique and proper hand-washing technique for wound care
○ drug administration, dosage, and possible adverse effects
○ importance of recognizing and reporting signs and symptoms of complications.

Discharge planning

○ Refer the patient for follow-up with an infectious disease specialist and surgeon, as indicated.
○ Refer the patient to physical rehabilitation, if indicated.
○ For education and support, refer the patient to organizations such as the National Necrotizing Fasciitis Foundation.

Nephrotic syndrome

Overview

Description

○ Kidney disorder characterized by marked protein-uria, hypoalbuminemia, hyperlipidemia, increased coagulation, and edema
○ Results from a glomerular defect that affects perme-ability, indicating renal damage
○ Prognosis highly variable, depending on underlying cause
○ Some forms possibly progressing to end-stage renal failure

Pathophysiology

○ Glomerular protein permeability increases.
○ Urinary excretion of protein, especially albumin, increases.
○ Hypoalbuminemia develops and causes decreased colloidal oncotic pressure.
○ Leakage of fluid into interstitial spaces leads to acute, generalized edema.
○ Vascular volume loss leads to increased blood vis-cosity and coagulation disorders.
○ The renin-angiotensin system is triggered, causing tubular reabsorption of sodium and water and con-tributing to edema.

Causes

○ Primary (idiopathic) glomerulonephritis (about 75% of cases)
○ Lipid nephrosis (main cause in children younger than age 8)
○ Membranous glomerulonephritis (most common lesion in adult idiopathic nephrotic syndrome)
○ Focal glomerulosclerosis (can develop spontaneous-ly at any age, occur after kidney transplantation, or result from heroin injection; develops in about 10% of childhood cases and up to 20% of adult cases)
○ Membranoproliferative glomerulonephritis (may fol-low infection, particularly streptococcal infection; occurs primarily in children and young adults)
○ Metabolic diseases
○ Collagen-vascular disorders
○ Circulatory diseases
○ Certain neoplastic diseases such as multiple myeloma

Risk factors

○ Nephrotoxins
○ Infection
○ Allergic reactions
○ Pregnancy
○ Hereditary nephritis
○ Chronic analgesic abuse

Incidence

○ In children, 1 in 50,000 new cases per year
○ In adults, 1 or 2 in 50,000 new cases per year
○ In children, peak incidence between ages 2 and 3
○ Slightly more common in males than in females

Common characteristics

○ Fluid retention
○ Anorexia
○ Hypertension
○ Decreased urine output

Complications

○ Malnutrition
○ Infection
○ Coagulation disorders
○ Thromboembolic vascular occlusion
○ Accelerated atherosclerosis
○ Acute renal failure

Assessment

History

○ Lethargy
○ Depression
○ Anorexia
○ Underlying cause
○ Presence of risk factor
○ Decreased urination

Physical findings

○ Periorbital edema
○ Mild to severe dependent edema
○ Orthostatic hypotension
○ Ascites
○ Swollen external genitalia
○ Signs of pleural effusion
○ Pallor

Test results

Laboratory

○ Urinalysis revealing an increased number of hyaline, granular, waxy, fatty casts and oval fat bodies; consis-tent, heavy proteinuria (levels over 3.5 mg/dl for 24 hours) strongly suggesting nephrotic syndrome
○ Increased serum cholesterol, serum phospholipids, serum triglycerides, and decreased serum albumin levels

Diagnostic procedures

○ Renal biopsy allows histologic identification of the lesion.

Treatment

General

○ Correction of the underlying cause if possible
○ Diet consisting of 0.6 g of protein per kilogram of body weight
○ Restricted sodium intake
○ Frequent rest periods

Medication

- Diuretics
- Antibiotics for infection
- Glucocorticoids
- Possible alkylating agents
- Possible cytotoxic agents

Nursing considerations

Key outcomes

The patient will:
- avoid or have minimal complications
- maintain fluid balance
- identify risk factors that worsen tissue perfusion, and modify lifestyle appropriately
- maintain hemodynamic stability.

Nursing interventions

- Offer the patient reassurance and support, especially during the acute phase, when severe edema changes body image.
- Provide information regarding dietary restrictions and fluid restriction.

Monitoring

- Urine for protein
- Intake and output
- Daily weight
- Plasma albumin and transferrin levels
- Edema

Patient teaching

Be sure to cover:
- the disorder, diagnosis, and treatments
- signs of infection that should be reported
- adherence to diet
- drug administration, dosage, and possible adverse effects.

Discharge planning

- Refer the patient to resource and support services.

Neural tube defects

Overview

Description
- ○ Birth defects that involve the spine or skull
- ○ Result from neural tube's failure to close approximately 28 days after conception
- ○ Different forms include spina bifida (50% of cases), anencephaly (40%), and encephalocele (10%)

Pathophysiology
- ○ Spina bifida occulta, the least severe neural tube defect (NTD), is characterized by incomplete closure of one or more vertebrae without protrusion of the spinal cord or meninges. More severe forms have incomplete closure of one or more vertebrae, causing protrusion of the spinal contents in an external sac or cystic lesion (spina bifida cystica). (See *Types of spinal cord defects*.)
- ○ In encephalocele, a saclike portion of the meninges and brain protrudes through a defective opening in the skull. Usually it occurs in the occipital area, but it may also occur in the parietal, nasopharyngeal, or frontal area.
- ○ In anencephaly, the closure defect occurs at the cranial end of the neuroaxis and, as a result, part or the entire top of the skull is missing, severely damaging the brain. Portions of the brain stem and spinal cord may also be missing. This condition is fatal.

Causes
- ○ Exposure to a teratogen
- ○ Part of a multiple malformation syndrome such as trisomy 18 or 13 syndrome
- ○ A combination of genetic and environmental factors; possibly a lack of folic acid in the mother's diet

Incidence
- ○ Spina bifida occulta most common NTD
- ○ At least twice the incidence in North Carolina and South Carolina than in the rest of the United States
- ○ More common in Whites than in Blacks

Common characteristics
- ○ Some degree of neurological dysfunction

Complications
- ○ Paralysis below the level of the defect
- ○ Infection such as meningitis
- ○ Hydrocephalus
- ○ Death

Assessment

History
- ○ Maternal history revealing factors that cause defect

Physical findings
Spina bifida
- ○ Possibly a depression or dimple, tuft of hair, soft fatty deposit, port wine nevi, or a combination of these abnormalities on the skin over the spinal area
- ○ Saclike protrusion over the spinal cord
- ○ Flaccid or spastic paralysis
Encephalocele
- ○ Saclike protrusion through a defective opening in the skull
- ○ Paralysis
Anencephaly
- ○ Part or entire top of skull missing

Test results
Laboratory
- ○ Elevated maternal alpha-fetoprotein, amniotic fluid alpha-fetoprotein, and amniotic fluid acetylcholinesterase levels indicate further testing is needed.
- ○ Fetal karyotype detects chromosomal abnormalities (present in 5% to 7% of NTDs).
- ○ Maternal serum AFP screening in combination with other serum markers, such as human chorionic gonadotropin (hCG), free beta-hCG, or unconjugated estriol (for patients with a lower risk of NTDs and those who will be younger than age 34½ at the time of delivery) estimates a fetus' risk of NTD as well as possible increased risk for perinatal complications, such as premature rupture of the membranes, abruptio placentae, or fetal death.
Imaging
- ○ Ultrasound (when increased risk of open NTD exists, based on family history or abnormal serum screening results; not conclusive for open NTDs or ventral wall defects)
- ○ Spinal X-rays reveal spina bifida occulta
- ○ Myelography differentiates spina bifida occulta from other spinal abnormalities, especially spinal cord tumors
- ○ Skull X-rays, cephalic measurements, and computed tomography (CT) scan demonstrate associated hydrocephalus
- ○ X-rays show a basilar bony skull defect (CT scan and ultrasonography further define the defect [with encephalocele])
Other
- ○ Transillumination of the protruding sac distinguishes between myelomeningocele (typically doesn't transilluminate) and meningocele (typically transilluminates).

There are three major types of spinal cord defects. Spina bifida occulta is characterized by a depression or raised area and a tuft of hair over the defect. In myelomeningocele, an external sac contains meninges, cerebrospinal fluid, and a portion of the spinal cord or nerve roots. In meningocele, an external sac contains only meninges and cerebrospinal fluid.

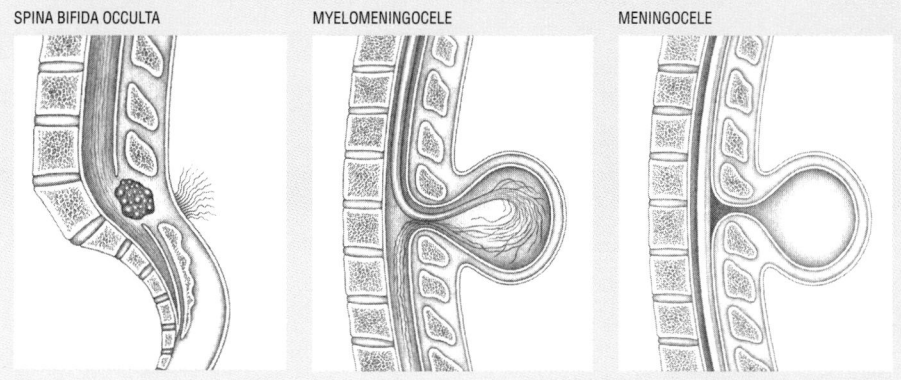

SPINA BIFIDA OCCULTA   MYELOMENINGOCELE   MENINGOCELE

Treatment

General

○ Symptomatic according to neurological effects of defect
○ Assessment of growth and development throughout lifetime
○ Diet, as tolerated
○ Physical therapy

Medication

○ Antibiotics, as indicated

Surgery

○ Surgical closure of the protruding sac
○ Shunt to relieve associated hydrocephalus
○ Surgery during infancy to place protruding tissues back in the skull, excise the sac, and correct associated craniofacial abnormalities (encephalocele)

Nursing considerations

Key outcomes

The patient will:
○ maintain intact skin integrity
○ maintain joint mobility and range of motion
○ attain appropriate growth and development for age.

Nursing interventions

○ Provide psychological support.

Before surgery
○ Clean the defect gently with sterile saline solution or other solutions, as ordered.
○ Handle the infant carefully, and don't apply pressure to the defect.
○ Provide adequate time for parent-child bonding, if possible.

After surgery
○ Change the dressing regularly, as ordered, and check and report any signs of drainage, wound rupture, and infection.
○ Place the infant prone to protect and assess the site.
○ If leg casts have been applied, watch for signs that the child is outgrowing the cast. Regularly check distal pulses to ensure adequate circulation.

Monitoring

Before surgery
○ Neurologic status
○ Feeding ability
○ Nutritional status

After surgery
○ Signs of infection
○ Signs of increased intracranial pressure
○ Intake and output
○ Vital signs

Patient teaching

Be sure to cover:
○ the disorder, diagnosis, and treatment
○ how to prevent contractures, pressure ulcers, and urinary tract infections.

Discharge planning

○ When an NTD has been diagnosed prenatally, refer the prospective parents to a genetic counselor
○ Refer the family for psychological and support services

Neurogenic bladder

Overview

Description
- All types of bladder dysfunction caused by an interruption of normal bladder innervation by the nervous system
- Can be hyperreflexic (hypertonic, spastic, or automatic) or flaccid (hypotonic, atonic, or autonomous)
- Also known as *neuromuscular dysfunction of the lower urinary tract, neurologic bladder dysfunction,* and *neuropathic bladder*

Pathophysiology
- An upper motor neuron lesion (at or above T12) causes spastic neurogenic bladder, with spontaneous contractions of detrusor muscles, increased intravesical voiding pressure, bladder wall hypertrophy with trabeculation, and urinary sphincter spasms.
- A lower motor neuron lesion (at or below S2 to S4) affects the spinal reflex that controls micturition. The result is a flaccid neurogenic bladder with decreased intravesical pressure, and increased bladder capacity, residual urine retention, and poor detrusor contraction. The bladder may not empty spontaneously.
- Interruption of the efferent nerves at the cortical level results in loss of voluntary control. Higher centers also control micturition, and voiding may be incomplete. Sensory neuron interruption leads to dribbling and overflow incontinence. (See *Types of neurogenic bladder.*)

Causes
- Cerebral disorders
- Spinal cord disease
- Trauma
- Metabolic disturbances
- Acute infectious diseases
- Heavy metal toxicity
- Chronic alcoholism
- Collagen diseases
- Vascular diseases
- Herpes zoster
- Sacral agenesis (absence of a completely formed sacrum)

Incidence
- Based on type of neurogenic bladder disorder

Common characteristics
- Some degree of incontinence
- Changes in initiation or interruption of micturition
- Inability to completely empty the bladder

Complications
- Incontinence
- Residual urine retention
- Urinary tract infections (UTIs)
- Calculus formation
- Renal failure

Assessment

History
- Frequent UTIs
- Hyperactive autonomic reflexes (autonomic dysreflexia) when the bladder is distended and the lesion is at upper thoracic or cervical level
- Involuntary or frequent, scant urination without a feeling of bladder fullness
- Overflow incontinence and diminished anal sphincter tone, due to flaccid neurogenic bladder

Physical findings
- Severe hypertension, bradycardia, and vasodilation (blotchy skin) above the level of the lesion
- Piloerection and profuse sweating above the level of the lesion
- Spontaneous spasms (caused by voiding) of the arms and legs
- Increased anal sphincter tone
- Greatly distended bladder without feeling of bladder fullness, due to sensory impairment

Test results
Imaging
- Retrograde urethrography shows strictures and diverticula.

Diagnostic procedures
- Voiding cystourethrography evaluates bladder neck function, vesicoureteral reflux, and continence.
- Urodynamic studies evaluate how urine is stored in the bladder, how well the bladder empties urine, and urine's movement out of the bladder during voiding.
- Urine flow study (uroflow) shows diminished or impaired urine flow.
- Cystometry evaluates bladder nerve supply, detrusor muscle tone, and intravesical pressures during bladder filling and contraction.
- Urethral pressure profile determines urethral function with respect to the urethra's length and outlet pressure resistance.
- Sphincter electromyelography correlates neuromuscular function of the external sphincter with bladder muscle function during bladder filling and contraction; it also evaluates how well the bladder and urinary sphincter muscles work together.
- Videourodynamic studies correlate visual documentation of bladder function with pressure studies.

Treatment

General
- Absorbent products
- Urethral occlusive devices
- Catheterization of the bladder

Types of neurogenic bladder

Neural lesion	Type	Cause
Upper motor	Uninhibited	• Lack of voluntary control in infancy • Multiple sclerosis
	Reflex or automatic	• Spinal cord transaction • Cord tumors • Multiple sclerosis
Lower motor	Autonomous	• Sacral cord trauma • Tumors • Herniated disk • Abdominal surgery with transection of pelvic parasympathetic nerves
	Motor paralysis	• Lesions at levels S2, S3, S4 • Poliomyelitis • Trauma • Tumors
	Sensory paralysis	• Posterior lumbar nerve roots • Diabetes mellitus • Tabes dorsalis

○ Avoidance of dietary stimulants, such as spicy foods, citrus fruits, and chocolate
○ Avoidance of excessive fluid intake
○ Avoidance of caffeinated and carbonated products
○ Pelvic muscle exercises
○ Bladder training program

Medication

○ Anticholinergics
○ Alpha-adrenergic stimulators
○ Antispasmodics

Surgery

○ External sphincterotomy, urethral dilation, urinary diversion, or transurethral resection of the bladder neck to correct structural impairment
○ Possible implantation of an artificial urinary sphincter if permanent incontinence follows surgery

Nursing considerations

Key outcomes

The patient will:
○ regain normal voiding habits
○ express positive feelings regarding self-image
○ demonstrate effective coping mechanisms
○ follow bladder training program, as indicated.

Nursing interventions

○ Catheterize the patient, as appropriate.
○ Provide emotional support, as appropriate.

Monitoring

○ Intake and output
○ Signs of infection

Patient teaching

Be sure to cover:
○ the disorder, diagnosis, and treatment
○ dietary adjustments
○ pelvic exercises
○ bladder evacuation techniques.

Nocardiosis

Overview

Description

○ Acute, subacute, or chronic bacterial infection caused by a weakly gram-positive species of the genus *Nocardia* — usually *Nocardia asteroides*

Pathophysiology

○ *Nocardia* are aerobic gram-positive bacteria with branching filaments resembling fungi.
○ Normally found in soil, these organisms cause occasional sporadic disease in humans and animals throughout the world.
○ Their incubation period is unknown but probably lasts several weeks.
○ The usual mode of transmission is inhalation of organisms suspended in dust. Transmission by direct inoculation through puncture wounds or abrasions is less common.

Causes

○ Inhalation or inoculation of *Nocardia* bacteria

Risk factors

○ Immunocompromised state
○ Alcoholism
○ Pulmonary alveolar proteinosis
○ Male gender

Incidence

○ About 500 to 1,000 cases annually in the United States
○ More common in men (3:1), especially those with a compromised immune system
○ In patients with brain infection, mortality exceeds 80%; in other forms, mortality is 50%

Common characteristics

Cutaneous infection
○ Cellulitis
○ Erythematous nodule at site of inoculation
Pulmonary infection
○ Cough that produces thick, tenacious, purulent, mucopurulent and, possibly, blood-tinged sputum
○ Fever
Disseminated infection
○ Confusion and disorientation
○ Dizziness and nausea
○ Headache
○ Seizures

Complications

○ Pleurisy
○ Intrapleural effusions
○ Empyema
○ Tracheitis
○ Bronchitis
○ Pericarditis
○ Endocarditis
○ Peritonitis
○ Mediastinitis
○ Septic arthritis
○ Keratoconjunctivitis
○ Purulent meningitis
○ Seizures

Assessment

History

○ Immunocompromising condition
○ Chills
○ Night sweats
○ Anorexia
○ Malaise
○ Weight loss
○ Dyspnea
○ Pleural pain
○ Puncture wound or abrasion

Physical findings

○ Fever
○ Cellulitis
○ Productive cough
○ Subcutaneous abscesses that lack induration
○ Crackles

Test results

Laboratory
○ Culture of causative organism from site of infection
Imaging
○ Chest X-rays vary and may show fluffy or interstitial infiltrates, nodules, or abscesses.
Diagnostic procedures
○ Biopsy of lung or other tissue
○ In brain infection with meningitis, lumbar puncture showing nonspecific changes such as increased opening pressure; cerebrospinal fluid showing increased white blood cell and protein levels and decreased glucose levels compared to serum glucose

Treatment

General

○ Diet, as tolerated
○ Activity, as tolerated (during acute phase, bed rest)
○ Safety measures

Medication

○ Antimicrobial therapy for at least 6 to 12 months
○ Combination drug therapy (sulfonamide, ceftriaxone) and amikacin
○ Antipyretics

Surgery

○ Drainage of abscesses and excision of necrotic tissue

Nursing considerations

Key outcomes

The patient will:
- show no signs of infection
- maintain adequate ventilation
- demonstrate effective coping mechanisms
- cough effectively
- have normal breath sounds.

Nursing interventions

- Encourage coughing and deep-breathing exercises.
- Provide psychological support.
- Give prescribed antibiotics.
- Provide adequate nourishment.
- Give tepid sponge bath to reduce fever.
- Perform chest physiotherapy.
- Assist with range-of-motion exercises.

Monitoring

- Vital signs
- Respiratory status
- Sputum production and character
- Compliance with treatment
- Allergic reaction to antibiotics

Patient teaching

Be sure to cover:
- the disorder, diagnosis, and treatment
- need for long-term antibiotic therapy
- signs of worsening infection.
- allergic reaction to antibiotics

Discharge planning

- Encourage follow-up care, as indicated.

Obesity

Overview

Description

- An excess of body fat, generally 20% above ideal body weight
- Body mass index (BMI) of 30 or greater (see *BMI measurements*)
- Second-leading cause of preventable deaths

Pathophysiology

- Fat cells increase in size in response to dietary intake.
- When the cells can no longer expand, they increase in number.
- With weight loss, the size of the fat cells decreases, but the number of cells doesn't.

Causes

- Excessive caloric intake combined with inadequate energy expenditure
- Theories to explain obesity include:
  - hypothalamic dysfunction of hunger and satiety centers
  - genetic predisposition
  - abnormal absorption of nutrients
  - impaired action of GI and growth hormones and of hormonal regulators such as insulin
  - socioeconomic status
  - environmental factors
  - psychological factors.

Incidence

- More than 50% of U.S. residents are overweight.
- Obesity affects one in five children.

Common characteristics

- BMI of 30 or greater

Complications

- Respiratory difficulties
- Hypertension
- Cardiovascular disease
- Diabetes mellitus
- Renal disease
- Gallbladder disease
- Psychosocial difficulties
- Premature death

Assessment

History

- Increasing weight
- Complications of obesity

Physical findings

- BMI of 30 or greater

Test results

Other

- Comparison of height and weight to a standard table
- Measurement of the thickness of subcutaneous fat folds with calipers to approximate total body fat (see *Taking anthropometric arm measurements*)
- BMI calculation

Treatment

General

- Hypnosis and behavior modification techniques
- Psychological counseling
- Reduction in daily caloric intake
- Increase in daily activity level

Surgery

- Vertical banded gastroplasty
- Gastric bypass

Nursing considerations

Key outcomes

The patient will:
- reduce BMI to normal level
- safely reduce weight
- demonstrate effective coping mechanisms to deal with long-term compliance.

Nursing interventions

- Obtain an accurate diet history to identify the patient's eating patterns and the importance of food to his lifestyle.
- Promote increased physical activity as appropriate.

Monitoring

- Diet
- Intake and output
- Vital signs
- Weight and BMI

BMI measurements

Use these steps to calculate body mass index (BMI):
- Multiply weight in pounds by 705.
- Divide this number by height in inches.
- Then divide this by height in inches again.
- Compare results to these standards:
  - 18.5 to 24.9: normal
  - 25.0 to 29.9: overweight
  - 30 to 39.9: obese
  - 40 or greater: morbidly obese.

Follow these steps to determine triceps skinfold thickness, midarm circumference, and midarm muscle circumference.

Triceps skinfold thickness
○ Find the midpoint circumference of the arm by placing the tape measure halfway between the axilla and the elbow. Grasp the patient's skin with your thumb and forefinger, about ⅜" (1 cm) above the midpoint, as shown below.
○ Place calipers at the midpoint, and squeeze for 3 seconds.
○ Record the measurement to the nearest millimeter.
○ Take two more readings, and use the average.

Midarm circumference and midarm muscle circumference
○ At the midpoint, measure the midarm circumference, as shown below. Record the measurement in centimeters.
○ Calculate the midarm muscle circumference by multiplying the triceps skinfold thickness — measured in millimeters — by 3.14.
○ Subtract this number from the midarm circumference.

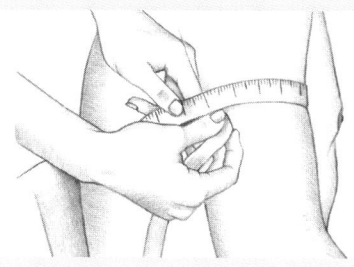

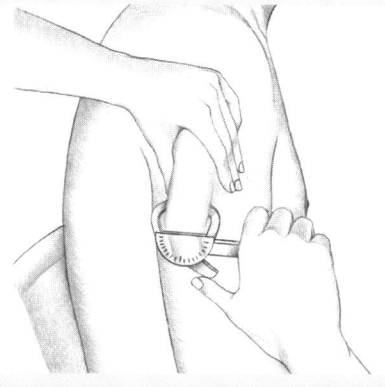

Recording the measurements
Record all three measurements as a percentage of the standard measurements (see table below), using this formula:

$$\frac{\text{Actual measurement}}{\text{Standard measurement}} \times 100\%$$

Remember, a measurement less than 90% of the standard indicates caloric deprivation. A measurement over 90% indicates adequate or more-than-adequate energy reserves.

Measurement	*Standard*	*90%*
Triceps skinfold thickness	Men: 12.5 mm Women: 16.5 mm	Men: 11.3 mm Women: 14.9 mm
Midarm circumference	Men: 29.3 cm Women: 28.5 cm	Men: 26.4 cm Women: 25.7 cm
Midarm muscle circumference	Men: 25.3 cm Women: 23.3 cm	Men: 22. 8 cm Women: 20.9 cm

Patient teaching

Be sure to cover:
○ need for long-term maintenance after desired weight is achieved
○ dietary guidelines
○ safe weight loss practices.

Discharge planning
○ Refer the patient to a weight-reduction program.

Obsessive-compulsive disorder

Overview

Description

○ Obsessive thoughts and compulsive behaviors that impair everyday functioning
○ May be simple or complex and ritualized
○ Also known as *OCD*

Pathophysiology

○ This anatomic-physiologic disturbance is thought to involve an alteration in the frontal-subcortical neural circuitry of the brain.

Causes

○ Decrease in caudate nucleus volume

Risk factors

○ Coexisting mental disorder
○ Tic disorders

Incidence

○ Affects 1 in 50 U.S. residents
○ Can occur at any age
○ More common in males and first-born children

Common characteristics

○ Repetitive behaviors and activities for more than 1 hour per day.
○ Activities alleviate anxiety triggered by a core fear.

Complications

○ Impairment of occupational and social functioning
○ Endangerment of health and safety

Assessment

History

○ Presence of obsessive thoughts, words, or mental images that persistently and involuntarily invade the consciousness
○ Moderate to severe impairment of social and occupational functioning
○ Patient usually rigid and conscientious, with great aspirations
○ Patient takes responsibility seriously and finds decision-making difficult
○ Patient lacks creativity and the ability to find alternate solutions to problems

Physical findings

○ Formal, reserved manner
○ Patient is accurate and complete, carefully qualifying statements and anticipating every move and gesture of person to whom he speaks

○ Affect is flat and unemotional, except for controlled anxiety
○ Self-awareness is intellectual, without accompanying emotion or feeling

DSM-IV-TR criteria

Diagnosis is confirmed when the patient meets these criteria:

Obsessions

○ Patient experiences recurrent and persistent ideas, thoughts, impulses, or images as intrusive and senseless.
○ Patient attempts to ignore or suppress such thoughts or impulses or to neutralize them with some other thought or action.
○ Patient recognizes that the obsessions are products of his mind, not externally imposed.
○ Patient's obsession is unrelated to another Axis I disorder.

Compulsions

○ Patient performs repetitive, purposeful, and intentional behaviors in response to an obsession or according to certain rules or in a stereotypical manner.
○ Behavior is intended to neutralize or prevent discomfort or some dreaded event or situation, but the behavior isn't connected in a realistic way with intended outcome, or is clearly excessive.
○ Patient recognizes that the behavior is excessive or unreasonable.

Treatment

General

○ Behavioral therapy
○ Increasing exposure to stressful situations
○ Keeping a diary of daily stressors
○ Substituting new activities for compulsive behavior

Medication

○ Selective serotonin-reuptake inhibitors

Nursing considerations

Key outcomes

The patient will:

○ reduce the amount of time spent each day on obsessing and ritualizing
○ produce no harmful effects from ritualistic behavior
○ express feelings of anxiety as they occur
○ cope with stress without excessive obsessive-compulsive behavior.

Nursing interventions

○ Provide an accepting, patient atmosphere.
○ Allow time for ritualistic behavior (unless it's dangerous) until distraction occurs.
○ Provide for basic needs.
○ Make reasonable demands and set reasonable limits; make the patient's purpose clear.

- Explore patterns leading to the behavior or recurring problems.
- Encourage active diversional resources.
- Assist with individualized problem-solving.
- Identify insight and improved behavior.

Monitoring

- Behavioral changes
- Disturbing topics of conversation
- Effective interventions
- Effects of pharmacologic therapy

Patient teaching

Be sure to cover:
- the disorder, diagnosis, and treatment
- how to identify progress
- importance of realistic expectations of self and others
- stress relief by channeling emotional energy
- relaxation and breathing techniques.

Discharge planning

- Refer the patient to social services and support services.

Osgood-Schlatter disease

Overview

Description

- Partial separation of the epiphysis of the tibial tubercle from the tibial shaft, leading to tendinitis
- Affects one or both knees
- Also known as *osteochondrosis*

Pathophysiology

- Bone growth is faster than soft tissue growth
- Muscle tendon tightness occurs across the joint
- Flexibility is decreased
- Mechanical inefficiency of the extensor mechanism follows incomplete separation of the epiphysis from the shaft.
- Tendinitis of the knee results.

Causes

- Traumatic avulsion of the proximal tibial tuberosity at the patellar tendon insertion
- Locally deficient blood supply
- Genetic factors
- Exercise

Risk factors

- Male gender
- Age 11 to 18 years
- Rapid skeletal growth
- Repetitive jumping sports

Incidence

- Most common in active adolescent boys after undergoing a rapid growth spurt

Common characteristics

- Frequent fractures
- Pain at inferior aspect of patella

Complications

- Irregular growth of the proximal tibial epiphysis
- Partial avascular necrosis of the proximal tibial epiphysis
- Chronic pain
- Patellar tendon avulsion

Assessment

History

- Intermittent aching, pain, swelling, and tenderness below the kneecap
- Pain that worsens from running, jumping, squatting, and ascending or descending stairs
- Symptoms relieved with rest
- Precipitating trauma

Physical findings

- Soft-tissue swelling
- Localized heat and tenderness
- Decreased flexibility and restriction in the hamstrings, triceps surae, and quadriceps muscle
- Pain at 30-degree flexion with tibia starting at 90 degrees in internal rotation
- Palpable firm mass

Test results

Imaging

- X-rays show epiphyseal closings, soft tissue swelling, and bone fragmentation
- Bone scan may reveal increased uptake in the area of the tibial tuberosity

Treatment

General

- Ice application for 20 minutes every 2 to 4 hours
- Reinforced elastic knee support, plaster cast, or splint
- Reduction of sports activities or exercise
- Avoidance of exercises that demand quadriceps contraction
- In severe cases, immobilization for 6 to 8 weeks
- Rehabilitation exercises

Medication

- Nonsteroidal anti-inflammatory drugs
- Analgesics

Surgery

- Removal or fixation of the epiphysis

Nursing considerations

Key outcomes

The patient will:

- express feelings of increased comfort and decreased pain
- maintain joint mobility and range of motion
- perform activities of daily living
- exhibit developmental milestones
- express positive feelings about self.

Nursing interventions

- Give prescribed analgesics and assess response.
- Ensure proper application of knee support or splint.
- Provide the patient with crutches if needed.
- Promote and allow adequate time for self-care.
- Encourage verbalization and provide support.

Monitoring

- Limitation of movement
- Muscle atrophy
- After surgery: circulation, sensation, and pain
- Excessive bleeding

Patient teaching

Be sure to cover:
- ❍ the disorder, diagnosis, and treatment
- ❍ prescribed exercise program
- ❍ use of crutches if needed
- ❍ protection of the injured knee.
- ❍ avoidance of activities that requires deep knee bending for 2 to 4 months

Discharge planning

- ❍ Refer the patient for occupational and physical therapy as appropriate.

Osteoarthritis

Overview

Description

○ Chronic degeneration of joint cartilage
○ Most common form of arthritis
○ Disability from minor limitation to near immobility
○ Most commonly affects the hips and knees
○ Varying progression rates

Pathophysiology

○ Deterioration of the joint cartilage occurs.
○ Reactive new bone forms at the margins and sub-chondral areas.
○ Breakdown of chondrocytes occurs.
○ Cartilage flakes irritate synovial lining.
○ The cartilage lining becomes fibrotic.
○ Joint movement is limited.
○ Synovial fluid leaks into bone defects, causing cysts.

Causes

○ Advancing age
○ Hereditary, possibly
○ Secondary osteoarthritis
○ Traumatic injury
○ Congenital abnormality
○ Endocrine disorders such as diabetes mellitus
○ Metabolic disorders such as chondrocalcinosis

Incidence

○ Occurs equally in both sexes
○ Occurs after age 40

Common characteristics

○ Deep, aching joint pain
○ Stiffness, especially in morning and after exercise
○ Crepitus of the joint during motion
○ Heberden's nodes (bony enlargements of distal inter-phalangeal joints)
○ Altered gait
○ Decreased range of motion (ROM)
○ Localized headaches

Complications

○ Flexion contractures
○ Subluxation
○ Deformity
○ Ankylosis
○ Bony cysts
○ Gross bony overgrowth
○ Central cord syndrome
○ Nerve root compression
○ Cauda equina syndrome

Assessment

History

○ Predisposing traumatic injury
○ Deep, aching joint pain
○ Pain after exercise or weight bearing
○ Pain possibly relieved by rest
○ Stiffness in morning and after exercise
○ Aching during changes in weather
○ "Grating" feeling when the joint moves
○ Limited movement

Physical findings

○ Contractures
○ Joint swelling
○ Muscle atrophy
○ Deformity of the involved areas
○ Gait abnormalities
○ Hard nodes that may be red, swollen, and tender on the distal and proximal interphalangeal joints (see *Signs of osteoarthritis*)
○ Loss of finger dexterity
○ Muscle spasms, limited movement, and joint instability

Test results

Laboratory
○ Synovial fluid analysis ruling out inflammatory arthritis
Imaging
○ X-rays of the affected joint may show a narrowing of the joint space or margin, cystlike bony deposits in the joint space and margins, sclerosis of the sub-chondral space, joint deformity or articular damage, bony growths at weight-bearing areas, and possible joint fusion.
○ Radionuclide bone scan may be used to rule out in-flammatory arthritis by showing normal uptake of the radionuclide.
○ Magnetic resonance imaging shows affected joint, adjacent bones, and disease progression.
Diagnostic procedures
○ Neuromuscular tests may show reduced muscle strength.
Other
○ Arthroscopy shows internal joint structures and identifies soft-tissue swelling.

Treatment

General

○ Relieve pain
○ Improve mobility
○ Minimize disability
○ Activity, as tolerated
○ Physical therapy
○ Assistive mobility devices

Heberden's nodes appear on the dorsolateral aspect of the distal interphalangeal joints. These bony and cartilaginous enlargements are usually hard and painless. They typically occur in middle-aged and elderly patients with osteoarthritis.

Bouchard's nodes are similar to Heberden's nodes but are less common and appear on the proximal interphalangeal joints.

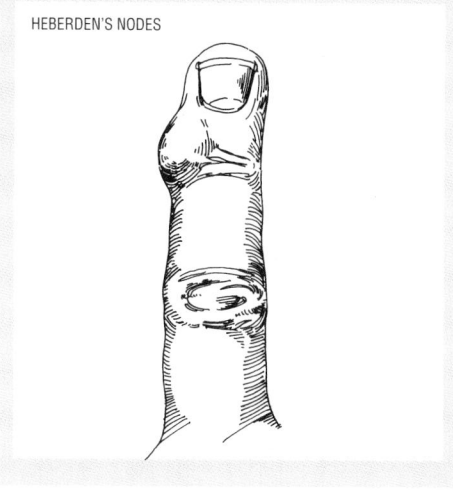

HEBERDEN'S NODES

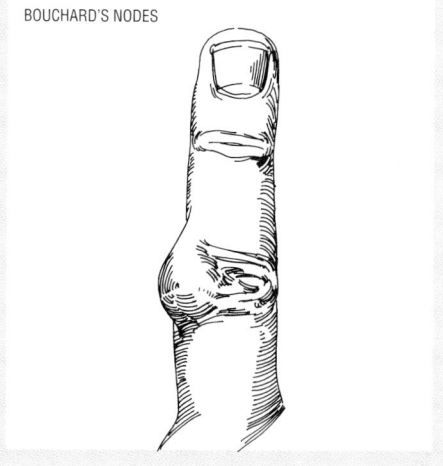

BOUCHARD'S NODES

Medication

○ Analgesics

Surgery

○ Arthroplasty (partial or total)
○ Arthrodesis
○ Osteoplasty
○ Osteotomy

Nursing considerations

Key outcomes

The patient will:
○ express feelings of increased comfort and decreased pain
○ maintain joint mobility and ROM
○ perform activities of daily living within confines of the disease
○ achieve the highest level of mobility
○ express positive feelings about self.

Nursing interventions

○ Allow adequate time for self-care.
○ Adjust pain medications to allow maximum rest.
○ Identify techniques that promote rest and relaxation.
○ Give prescribed anti-inflammatories.
○ For affected hand joints, use hot soaks and paraffin dips.
○ For affected lumbosacral spinal joints, provide a firm mattress.
○ For affected cervical spinal joints, apply a cervical collar.

○ For an affected hip, apply moist heat pads and give antispasmodics.
○ For an affected knee, help with ROM exercises.
○ Apply elastic supports or braces.
○ Check crutches, cane, braces, or walker for proper fit.

Monitoring

○ Pain pattern
○ Response to analgesics
○ ROM

Patient teaching

Be sure to cover:
○ the disorder, diagnosis, and treatment
○ need for adequate rest during the day, after exertion, and at night
○ energy conservation methods
○ need to take medications exactly as prescribed
○ adverse reactions to drugs
○ wearing support shoes that fit well and repairing worn heels
○ installation of safety devices at home
○ ROM exercises, performing them as gently as possible
○ need to maintain proper body weight
○ use of crutches or other orthopedic devices.

Discharge planning

○ Refer the patient to occupational or physical therapist as indicated.

Osteogenesis imperfecta

○ Cord compression
○ Cerebral hemorrhage caused by birth trauma

Overview

Description

○ Genetic disease in which bones are thin, poorly developed, and fracture easily
○ Expression varies, depending on whether the defect is carried as a trait or is clinically obvious
○ Also called *little bone disease*

Pathophysiology

○ The pathogenesis begins when mutations in the genes change the structure of collagen.
○ Possible mutations in other genes may cause variations in the assembly and maintenance of bone and other connective tissues.
○ Collectively or alone, these mutated genes lead to pathologic fractures and impaired healing.

Causes

○ Genetic disease, typically autosomal dominant (characterized by a defect in the synthesis of connective tissue)
○ Autosomal recessive carriage of gene defects producing osteogenesis imperfecta in homozygotes (osteoporosis in some)

Incidence

○ Autosomal dominant disorder occurs in about 1 in 30,000 live births.
○ Affects males and females equally

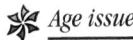 *Age issue*

Age of onset of symptoms ranges from in utero to infancy.

Common characteristics

○ Frequent fractures caused by falls as toddler begins to walk; poor healing
○ Short stature due to multiple fractures caused by minor physical stress
○ Deformed cranial structure and limbs due to multiple fractures
○ Thin skin and bluish sclera of the eyes; thin collagen fibers of the sclera allowing the choroid layer to be seen
○ Abnormal tooth and enamel development due to improper deposition of dentin
○ Middle ear deafness

Complications

○ Deafness
○ Stillbirth or death within the first year of life (autosomal-recessive disorder)
○ Hyperplastic callus formation
○ Repeated respiratory infections

Assessment

History

○ Fractures early in life
○ Hearing loss
○ Easy bruising

Physical findings

○ Blue sclerae, showing that mutation is expressed in more than one connective tissue
○ Short trunk
○ Hearing loss
○ Fractures
○ Kyphoscoliosis

Test results

Laboratory
○ Elevated serum alkaline phosphatase levels (during periods of rapid bone formation and cellular injury)
○ Skin culture showing reduced quantity of fibroblasts
Imaging
○ Echocardiography, possibly showing mitral insufficiency or floppy mitral valves
○ Prenatal ultrasound (during second trimester) reveals bowing of long bones, fractures, limb shortening, and decreased skull echogenicity
○ Skull, long bone, and pelvis X-rays reveal thin bones, fractures with deformities, beaded ribs, and osteopenia

Treatment

General

○ Prevention of fractures
○ Nutritious, well-balanced diet
○ Safety during periods of activity
○ Physical therapy

Medication

○ Antibiotics (when infection occurs)

Surgery

○ Internal fixation of fractures to ensure stabilization and prevent deformities
○ Spinal fusion for scoliosis

Nursing considerations

Key outcomes

The patient (and his family) will:
○ follow safety measures to prevent fractures
○ understand the disorder and its treatment
○ demonstrate effective coping mechanisms.

Nursing interventions
○ Ensure a safe environment.
○ Encourage activities based on ability.
○ Provide psychological support.

Monitoring
○ Environment
○ Bone condition

Patient teaching

Be sure to cover:
○ safe handling of infant
○ how to recognize fractures and correctly splint them
○ how to protect the child during diapering, dressing, and other activities of daily living
○ encouraging interests that don't require strenuous physical activity
○ the importance of good nutrition to heal bones and promote growth
○ use of shock-absorbing footwear
○ importance of not letting infants younger than age 1 year sit upright

Discharge planning
○ Refer the child and his parents for genetic counseling to assess the recurrence risk.
○ Instruct the parents to provide their child with a medical identification jewelry.

Osteomalacia and rickets

Overview

Description
- Vitamin D deficiency that doesn't allow bone to calcify normally
- Also called *rickets* in infants and young children; *osteomalacia* in adults
- Prognosis good with treatment
- Possible disappearance of bone deformities in adults; usually persist in children

Pathophysiology
- Vitamin D regulates the absorption of calcium ions from the intestine.
- When vitamin D is lacking, falling serum calcium concentration stimulates synthesis and secretion of parathyroid hormone.
- This causes the release of calcium from bone, decreasing renal calcium excretion and increasing renal phosphate excretion.
- When the concentration of phosphate in the bone decreases, osteoid may be produced but mineralization can't proceed normally.
- This causes large quantities of osteoid to accumulate, coating the trabeculae and linings of the haversian canals and areas beneath the periosteum.
- When bone matrix mineralization is delayed or inadequate, bone is disorganized in structure and lacks density. The result is gross deformity of both spongy and compact bone.

Causes
- Inadequate dietary intake of vitamin D
- Malabsorption of vitamin D
- Inadequate exposure to sunlight
- Inherited impairment of renal tubular reabsorption of phosphate (from vitamin D insensitivity) in vitamin D–resistant rickets (refractory rickets, familial hypophosphatemia)
- Conditions reducing the absorption of fat-soluble vitamin D
- Hepatic or renal disease
- Malfunctioning parathyroid gland contributing to calcium deficiency and interfering with vitamin D activation in the kidneys

Incidence
- Rare in the United States
- Does appear occasionally in breast-fed infants who don't receive a vitamin D supplement or in infants fed a formula with a nonfortified milk base
- Occurs in overcrowded, urban areas where smog limits sunlight penetration

 Alert

Incidence of rickets is highest in children with darkly pigmented skin who, because of their pigmentation, absorb less sunlight.

Common characteristics
- May be asymptomatic until a fracture occurs
- Leg and lower back pain due to vertebral collapse
- Bowed legs
- Knock knees
- Rachitic rosary (beading of ends of ribs)
- Enlarged wrists and ankles
- Pigeon breast (protruding ribs and sternum)
- Delayed closing of fontanels
- Softening skull
- Bulging forehead
- Poorly developed muscles (pot belly)
- Difficulty walking and climbing stairs
- Kyphoscoliosis

Complications
- Spontaneous multiple fractures
- Tetany in infants
- Bone deformities

Assessment

History
- Poor diet
- Leg and lower back pain

Physical findings
- Bowed legs
- Knock knees
- Rachitic rosary (beading of ends of ribs)
- Enlarged wrists and ankles
- Pigeon breast (protruding ribs and sternum)
- Bulging forehead
- Poorly developed muscles (pot belly)
- Kyphoscoliosis

Test results
Laboratory
- Serum calcium concentration less than 7.5 mg/dl
- Serum inorganic phosphorus concentration less than 3 mg/dl
- Serum citrate level less than 2.5 mg/dl
- Alkaline phosphatase level less than 4 Bodansky units/dl

Imaging
- X-rays showing characteristic bone deformities and abnormalities such as Looser's transformation zones (radiolucent bands perpendicular to the surface of the bones indicating reduced bone ossification confirm the diagnosis)

Treatment

General

○ Sufficient sun exposure
○ Diet high in vitamin D (fortified milk, fish liver oils, herring, liver, and egg yolks)
○ Treatment of bone deformities or fractures

Medication

○ Massive oral doses of vitamin D or cod liver oil
○ For rickets refractory to vitamin D, or in rickets accompanied by hepatic or renal disease, 25-hydroxycholecalciferol, 1,25-dihydroxycholecalciferol, or a synthetic-analogue of active vitamin D

Surgery

○ Possible surgical intervention for intestinal disease
○ Appropriate repair of bone fractures

Nursing considerations

Key outcomes

The patient will:
○ have increased vitamin D intake
○ remain free of fractures
○ express understanding of the disorder and its treatment.

Nursing interventions

○ Obtain a dietary history to assess the patient's vitamin D intake.

Monitoring

○ Dietary intake
○ Bone integrity

Patient teaching

Be sure to cover:
○ symptoms of vitamin D toxicity (headache, nausea, constipation and, after prolonged use, renal calculi).

Discharge planning

○ If the patient's vitamin D deficiency appears to be linked to adverse socioeconomic conditions, refer him to an appropriate community agency.

Osteomyelitis

Overview

Description
- Pyogenic bone infection
- Chronic or acute
- Good prognosis for acute form (with prompt treatment)
- Poor prognosis for chronic form

Pathophysiology
- Organisms settle in a hematoma or weakened area and spread directly to bone.
- Pus is produced and pressure builds within the rigid medullary cavity.
- Pus is forced through the haversian canals.
- Subperiosteal abscess forms.
- Bone is deprived of its blood supply.
- Necrosis results and new bone formation is stimulated.
- Dead bone detaches and exits through an abscess or the sinuses.
- Osteomyelitis becomes chronic.

Causes
- Minor traumatic injury
- Acute infection originating elsewhere in the body
- *Staphylococcus aureus*
- *Streptococcus pyogenes*
- *Pseudomonas aeruginosa*
- *Escherichia coli*
- *Proteus vulgaris*
- Fungi or viruses

Incidence
- Incidence of both types declining, except in drug abusers

 Age issue

The acute form affects rapidly growing children, especially boys.

Common characteristics
- Sudden pain in affected bone
- Tenderness, heat, swelling
- Restricted movement
- Chronic infection

Complications
- Chronic infection
- Skeletal deformities
- Joint deformities
- Disturbed bone growth in children
- Differing leg lengths
- Impaired mobility

Assessment

History
- Previous injury, surgery, or primary infection
- Sudden, severe pain in the affected bone
- Pain unrelieved by rest and worse with motion
- Related chills, nausea, and malaise
- Refusal to use the affected area

Physical findings
- Tachycardia and fever
- Swelling and restricted movement over the infection site
- Tenderness and warmth over the infection site
- Persistent pus drainage from an old pocket in a sinus tract

Test results
Laboratory
- White blood cell count showing leukocytosis
- Increased erythrocyte sedimentation rate
- Blood culture identifying pathogen

Imaging
- X-rays may show bone involvement.
- Bone scans may detect early infection.
- Computed tomography scan and magnetic resonance imaging can show extent of infection.

Treatment

General
- Decrease internal bone pressure
- Prevent bone necrosis
- Hyperbaric oxygen therapy
- Free tissue transfers
- I.V. fluids, as needed
- High-protein diet rich in vitamin C
- Bed rest
- Immobilization of involved bone and joint with a cast or traction

Medication
- I.V. antibiotics
- Analgesics
- Intracavitary instillation of antibiotics for open wounds

Surgery
- Surgical drainage
- Local muscle flaps
- Sequestrectomy
- Amputation for chronic and unrelieved symptoms

Nursing considerations

Key outcomes
The patient will:
- experience increased comfort and decreased pain

- maintain joint mobility and range of motion
- exhibit adequate fluid volume
- exhibit adequate tissue perfusion and pulses distally
- perform activities of daily living.

Nursing interventions

- Control infection.
- Protect the bone from injury.
- Provide emotional support.
- Promote and allow adequate time for self-care.
- Promote activities that promote rest and relaxation.
- Use strict sterile technique.
- With skeletal traction, cover the pin insertion points with small, dry dressings.
- Provide firm pillows.
- Provide thorough skin care.
- Provide complete cast care.
- Give prescribed analgesics.

Monitoring

- Vital signs
- Wound appearance and healing
- Pain control
- Drainage and suctioning equipment
- Sudden malpositioning of the limb

Patient teaching

Be sure to cover:
- the disorder, diagnosis, and treatment
- drug administration, dosage, and possible adverse effects
- techniques for promoting rest and relaxation
- wound site care
- signs of recurring infection
- importance of follow-up examinations.

Discharge planning

- Refer the patient for occupational therapy, as appropriate.

Osteoporosis

Overview

Description

- Loss of calcium and phosphate from bones causing increased vulnerability to fractures
- Primary or secondary to underlying disease
- Types of primary osteoporosis: postmenopausal osteoporosis (type I) and age-associated osteoporosis (type II)
- Secondary osteoporosis: caused by an identifiable agent or disease

Pathophysiology

- The rate of bone resorption accelerates as the rate of bone formation decelerates.
- Decreased bone mass results and bones become porous and brittle.

Causes

- Exact cause unknown
- Prolonged therapy with steroids or heparin
- Bone immobilization
- Alcoholism
- Malnutrition
- Rheumatoid arthritis
- Liver disease
- Malabsorption
- Scurvy
- Lactose intolerance
- Hyperthyroidism
- Osteogenesis imperfecta
- Sudeck's atrophy (localized in hands and feet, with recurring attacks)

Risk factors

- Mild, prolonged negative calcium balance
- Declining gonadal adrenal function
- Faulty protein metabolism (caused by estrogen deficiency)
- Sedentary lifestyle

Incidence

- Idiopathic affects children and adults
- Type I (or postmenopausal): affects women ages 51 to 75
- Type II (or senile): most common between ages 70 and 85

Common characteristics

- Sudden pain associated with bending or lifting
- Back pain (if vertebral collapse occurs)
- Increasing deformity
- Kyphosis
- Loss of height
- Decreased exercise tolerance
- Spontaneous wedge fractures

Complications

- Bone fractures (vertebrae, femoral neck, and distal radius)

Assessment

History

- Postmenopausal patient
- Condition known to cause secondary osteoporosis
- Snapping sound or sudden pain in lower back when bending down to lift something
- Possible slow development of pain (over several years)
- With vertebral collapse, backache and pain radiating around the trunk
- Pain aggravated by movement or jarring

Physical findings

- Humped back
- Markedly aged appearance
- Loss of height
- Muscle spasm
- Decreased spinal movement with flexion more limited than extension

Test results

Laboratory
- Normal serum calcium, phosphorus, and alkaline levels
- Elevated parathyroid hormone level

Imaging
- X-ray studies show characteristic degeneration in the lower thoracolumbar vertebrae.
- Computed tomography scan assesses spinal bone loss.
- Bone scans show injured or diseased areas.

Diagnostic procedures
- Bone biopsy shows thin, porous, but otherwise normal bone.

Other
- Dual or single photon absorptiometry (measurement of bone mass) shows loss of bone mass.

Treatment

General

- Control bone loss
- Prevent additional fractures
- Control pain
- Reduction and immobilization of fractures
- Diet rich in vitamin D, calcium, and protein
- Physical therapy program of gentle exercise and activity
- Supportive devices

Medication

- Estrogen
- Sodium fluoride
- Calcium and vitamin D supplements

○ Calcitonin

Surgery

○ Open reduction and internal fixation for femur fractures

Nursing considerations

Key outcomes

The patient will:
○ maintain joint mobility and range of motion (ROM)
○ experience increased comfort and decreased pain
○ demonstrate measures to prevent injury
○ perform activities of daily living.

Nursing interventions

○ Encourage careful positioning, ambulation, and prescribed exercises.
○ Promote self-care while allowing adequate time.
○ Encourage mild exercise.
○ Assist with walking.
○ Perform passive ROM exercises.
○ Promote physical therapy sessions.
○ Use safety precautions.
○ Give prescribed analgesia.
○ Apply heat.

Monitoring

○ Skin for redness, warmth, and new pain sites
○ Response to analgesia
○ Nutritional status
○ Height
○ Exercise tolerance
○ Joint mobility

Patient teaching

Be sure to cover:
○ the disorder, diagnosis, and treatment
○ drug administration, dosage, and possible adverse effects
○ performing monthly breast self-examination while on estrogen therapy
○ need to report vaginal bleeding promptly
○ need to report new pain sites immediately
○ sleeping on a firm mattress
○ avoiding excessive bed rest
○ use of back brace, if appropriate
○ proper body mechanics
○ home safety devices
○ diet rich in calcium.

Discharge planning

○ Refer the patient for physical and occupational therapy, as appropriate.

Otitis externa

Overview

Description

○ Acute or chronic inflammation of the external ear canal
○ With treatment, usually subsides within 7 days
○ May become chronic and tends to recur
○ If severe and chronic, may reflect underlying diabetes mellitus, hypothyroidism, or nephritis
○ Also known as *external otitis* and *swimmer's ear*

Pathophysiology

○ External ear canal inflammation results from invasion by infecting organisms.

Causes

○ Traumatic injury or excessive moisture that predisposes canal to infection
○ Bacteria (common) and fungi (less common)
○ Occasionally, dermatologic conditions, such as seborrhea or psoriasis

Risk factors

○ Swimming in contaminated water
○ Cleaning ear canal with cotton-tipped applicator, bobby pin, finger, or other object
○ Exposure to dust, hair-care products, or other irritants
○ Regular use of earphones, earplugs, or earmuffs
○ Chronic drainage from a perforated tympanic membrane

Incidence

○ Most common during summer, but can occur any time of the year

Common characteristics

○ Swollen, inflamed ear canal
○ Mild to severe itching or pain aggravated by jaw motion, clenching the teeth, opening the mouth, or chewing

Complications

○ Complete closure of the ear canal
○ Significant hearing loss
○ Otitis media
○ Cellulitis
○ Abscesses
○ Disfigurement of the pinna
○ Lymphadenopathy
○ Osteitis
○ Septicemia
○ Stenosis

Assessment

History

○ Repeated exposure to ear trauma, water, use of earphones, or allergic response to hair spray, dye, or other hair-care products
○ Mild to severe ear itching or pain aggravated by jaw motion, clenching the teeth, opening the mouth, or chewing
○ Fungal otitis externa possibly asymptomatic

Physical findings

○ Swollen, inflamed ear canal
○ Ear discharge that may be foul-smelling and yellow to green in color
○ Thick red epithelium in canal with chronic otitis externa
○ Increased pain or itching on palpation or manipulation

Test results

Laboratory
○ Microscopic examination showing the causative organism
Diagnostic procedures
○ Audiometric testing may reveal a partial hearing loss.
○ Otoscopy reveals a swollen external ear canal, periauricular lymphadenopathy and, occasionally, regional cellulitis.

Treatment

General

○ Cleaning of debris from canal under direct visualization
○ With mild, chronic otitis externa, use of specially fitted earplugs for showering or swimming

Medication

○ Analgesics
○ Antibiotic drops
○ Oral antibiotics if lymphadenopathy is present, or if external ear is swollen

Surgery

○ Excision and abscess drainage

Nursing considerations

Key outcomes

The patient will:
○ show no signs or symptoms of infection
○ express feelings of increased comfort
○ express understanding of the disorder and treatment
○ regain hearing function or develop other ways to communicate.

- To prevent recurrence, tell the patient to avoid potential irritants, such as hair-care products and earrings.
- Advise the patient to use lamb's wool earplugs coated with petroleum jelly to keep water out of the ears when showering or shampooing.
- Inform the parents of a young child that modeling clay makes a tight seal and can be used to prevent water from getting into the external canal.
- Tell the patient to wear earplugs or to keep his head above water when swimming and to instill two or three drops of 3% boric acid solution in 70% alcohol into the ear before and after swimming to toughen the skin of the external ear canal.
- Warn against cleaning the ears with cotton-tipped applicators or other objects.

Nursing interventions

- Clean and dry the ear gently and thoroughly.
- Use wet soaks on infected skin.
- Give prescribed drugs.

With hearing loss

- Encourage discussion of concerns.
- Reassure the patient that hearing loss from an external ear infection is temporary.
- Face the patient when speaking.
- Enunciate words clearly, slowly, and in a normal tone.
- Allow adequate time to grasp what was said.
- Provide a pencil and paper to aid communication.
- Alert staff to the communication problem.

Monitoring

- Vital signs, especially temperature
- Auditory acuity
- Type and amount of aural drainage
- Response to treatment
- Complications

Patient teaching

Be sure to cover:

- the disorder, diagnosis, and treatment
- proper hand washing and daily ear cleaning
- administration of ear drops, ointment, and ear wash
- antibiotics, as prescribed
- recognizing and reporting adverse reactions
- preventing recurrence. (See *Preventing otitis externa.*)

Otitis media

Overview

Description
- Inflammation of the middle ear associated with fluid accumulation
- Acute, chronic, suppurative, or secretory

Pathophysiology
- Differs with otitis media type

Suppurative form
- Nasopharyngeal flora reflux through the eustachian tube and colonize the middle ear.
- Respiratory tract infections, allergic reactions, and position changes allow reflux of nasopharyngeal flora through the eustachian tube and colonization in the middle ear.

Secretory form
- Obstruction of the eustachian tube promotes transudation of sterile serous fluid from blood vessels in the middle ear membrane.

Causes
- Suppurative otitis media: bacterial infection with pneumococci, group A beta-hemolytic streptococci, staphylococci, and gram-negative bacteria
- Chronic suppurative otitis media: inadequate treatment of acute otitis episodes or infection by resistant strains of bacteria
- Secretory otitis media: viral infection, allergy, or barotrauma
- Chronic secretory otitis media: adenoidal tissue overgrowth, edema, chronic sinus infection, or inadequate treatment of acute suppurative otitis media

Incidence
- Most common in infants and children

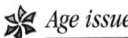 *Age issue*

Acute otitis media is an emergency in an immunocompromised child.

- Peaks between ages 6 and 24 months
- Subsides after age 3 years
- Most common during winter months

Common characteristics
- Severe, deep, throbbing ear pain
- Mild to high fever

Complications
- Spontaneous rupture of the tympanic membrane
- Persistent perforation
- Chronic otitis media
- Mastoiditis
- Meningitis
- Cholesteatomas
- Abscesses, septicemia
- Lymphadenopathy, leukocytosis
- Permanent hearing loss and tympanosclerosis
- Vertigo

Assessment

History
- Upper respiratory tract infection
- Allergies
- Severe, deep, throbbing ear pain
- Dizziness
- Nausea, vomiting

Acute secretory otitis media
- Sensation of fullness in the ear
- Popping, crackling, or clicking sounds on swallowing or moving the jaw
- Describes hearing an echo when speaking

Tympanic membrane rupture
- Pain that suddenly stops
- Recent air travel or scuba diving

Physical findings
- Sneezing and coughing with upper respiratory tract infection
- Mild to high fever
- Painless, purulent discharge in chronic suppurative otitis media
- Obscured or distorted bony landmarks of the tympanic membrane in acute suppurative otitis media
- Tympanic membrane retraction in acute secretory otitis media
- Clear or amber fluid behind the tympanic membrane
- Blue-black tympanic membrane with hemorrhage into the middle ear
- Pulsating discharge with tympanic perforation
- Conductive hearing loss (varies with the size and type of tympanic membrane perforation and ossicular destruction)

Chronic otitis media
- Thickening and scarring of tympanic membrane
- Decreased or absent tympanic membrane mobility
- Cholesteatoma

Test results
Laboratory
- Culture and sensitivity tests of exudate show the causative organism.
- Complete blood count shows leukocytosis.

Imaging
- Radiographic studies demonstrate mastoid involvement.

Diagnostic procedures
- Tympanometry detects hearing loss and evaluates the condition of the middle ear.
- Audiometry shows degree of hearing loss.
- Pneumatic otoscopy may show decreased tympanic membrane mobility.

Alert

In adults, unilateral serous otitis media should always be evaluated for a nasopharyngeal-obstructing lesion such as carcinoma.

Treatment

General

○ In acute secretory otitis media, Valsalva's maneuver several times per day (may be the only treatment required)
○ Concomitant treatment of the underlying cause
○ Elimination of eustachian tube obstruction

Medication

○ Antibiotic therapy
○ Aspirin or acetaminophen
○ Analgesics
○ Sedatives (small children)
○ Nasopharyngeal decongestant therapy

Surgery

○ Myringotomy and aspiration of middle ear fluid, followed by insertion of a polyethylene tube into the tympanic membrane
○ Myringoplasty
○ Tympanoplasty
○ Mastoidectomy
○ Cholesteatoma excision
○ Stapedectomy for otosclerosis

Nursing considerations

Key outcomes

The patient will:
○ express feelings of increased comfort
○ exhibit no signs or symptoms of infection
○ verbalize understanding of the disorder and treatment regimen
○ regain hearing loss or develop compensatory mechanisms
○ experience no injury or harm.

Nursing interventions

○ Answer all questions.
○ Encourage discussion of concerns about hearing loss.
With hearing loss
○ Offer reassurance, when appropriate, that hearing loss caused by serious otitis media is temporary.
○ Provide clear, concise explanations.
○ Face the patient when speaking and enunciate clearly and slowly.
○ Allow time for the patient to grasp what was said.
○ Provide a pencil and paper.
○ Alert the staff to the patient's communication problem.

Preventing otitis media

For a patient recovering from otitis media at home, instruct the patient or his family to follow these guidelines to help prevent a recurrence:
○ Teach the patient how to recognize upper respiratory tract infections, and encourage early treatment of them.
○ Instruct parents not to feed an infant in a supine position and not to put him to bed with a bottle. Explain that doing so could cause reflux of nasopharyngeal flora.
○ If appropriate, teach the patient to promote eustachian tube patency by performing Valsalva's maneuver several times per day, especially during airplane travel.
○ After tympanoplasty, advise the patient not to blow his nose or get his ear wet when bathing.
○ Explain adverse reactions to the prescribed medication, emphasizing those that require immediate medical attention.

After myringotomy
○ Wash hands before and after ear care.
○ Maintain drainage flow.
○ Place sterile cotton loosely in the external ear to absorb drainage and prevent infection. Change the cotton when damp. Avoid placing cotton or plugs deep in ear canal.
○ Give prescribed analgesics.
○ Give antiemetics after tympanoplasty and reinforce dressings.

Monitoring

○ Pain level
○ Excessive bleeding or discharge
○ Auditory acuity
○ Response to treatment
○ Complications

 Alert

Watch for and immediately report pain and fever due to acute secretory otitis media.

Patient teaching

Be sure to cover:
○ proper instillation of ointment, drops, and ear wash, as ordered
○ drug administration, dosage, and possible adverse effects
○ importance of taking antibiotics
○ adequate fluid intake
○ correct instillation of nasopharyngeal decongestants
○ use of fitted earplugs for swimming after myringotomy and tympanostomy tube insertion
○ notification of the physician if tube falls out and for ear pain, fever, or pus-filled discharge
○ preventing recurrence. (See *Preventing otitis media.*)

Otosclerosis

Overview

Description

- Bone disease that occurs only in the middle ear and results in an overgrowth of abnormal bone, usually involving the stapes bone
- Most common cause of conductive hearing loss
- With surgery, prognosis good
- Also known as *hardening of the ear* and *otospongiosis*

Pathophysiology

- Normal bone of otic capsule is gradually replaced with highly vascular spongy bone.
- Spongy bone immobilizes the footplate of the normally mobile stapes.
- Conduction of vibrations from the tympanic membrane to the cochlea is disrupted, and conductive hearing loss results.
- If the inner ear is involved, sensorineural hearing loss may develop.

Causes

- Genetic factor transmitted as an autosomal dominant trait
- Pregnancy (may trigger the onset)

Incidence

- Occurs in at least 10% of whites
- Twice as common in women as in men
- Usually occurs between ages 15 and 50

Common characteristics

- Slow, progressive hearing loss in one ear, with progression to both ears, without middle ear infection
- Tinnitus

Complications

- Bilateral conductive hearing loss
- Taste disturbance

Assessment

History

- Family history of hearing loss (excluding presbycusis)
- Tinnitus
- Ability to hear a conversation better in a noisy environment than in a quiet one (paracusis of Willis)
- Vertigo, especially after bending over

Physical findings

- Tympanic membrane appears normal
- Schwartze's sign (faint pink blush throughout the tympanic membrane from vascularity of active otosclerotic bone)

Test results

Diagnostic procedures

- Rinne test result shows bone-conducted tone is heard longer than air-conducted tone.
- Weber's test result shows that sound lateralizes to the more damaged ear.
- Audiometric testing reveals hearing loss.

Treatment

General

- Hearing aids
- Avoidance of activities that provoke dizziness

Medication

- Antibiotics
- Sodium fluoride (may prevent further worsening of hearing)

Surgery

- Stapedectomy
- Prosthesis insertion to restore partial or total hearing
- Fenestration
- Stapes mobilization

Nursing considerations

Key outcomes

The patient will:
- show no evidence of infection
- experience no injury or harm
- express needs and feelings
- regain hearing or develop alternative ways of communicating
- express understanding of illness and treatment.

Nursing interventions

- Encourage discussion of concerns about hearing loss.
- Offer reassurance with hearing loss, when appropriate.
- Give clear, concise explanations.
- Face the patient when speaking.
- Enunciate clearly and slowly, in a normal tone.
- Allow adequate time to grasp what was said.
- Provide a pencil and paper to aid communication.
- Alert the staff to communication problem.

After surgery

- Position as ordered.
- Assist with ambulation when indicated.
- Give prescribed drugs for pain.
- Reassure the patient that taste disturbance is common and usually subsides in a few weeks.

Monitoring

- For vertigo
- Response to medication
- Hearing loss

Alert

Watch for and report postoperative facial drooping, which may indicate swelling of or around the facial nerve.

Patient teaching

Be sure to cover:
- ○ the disorder, diagnosis, and treatment
- ○ preoperative and postoperative teaching, if indicated
- ○ slow movement to prevent vertigo
- ○ drug administration, dosage, and possible adverse effects
- ○ importance of protecting ears against the cold
- ○ need to avoid activities that provoke dizziness
- ○ avoidance of anyone with upper respiratory tract infection
- ○ changing external ear dressing and incision care
- ○ completion of prescribed drug regimen
- ○ need for follow-up care
- ○ how hearing may be masked by packing, dressing, and postoperative edema
- ○ why hearing may not be noticeably improved for 1 to 4 weeks after surgery
- ○ avoidance of loud noises and sudden pressure changes until healing is complete
- ○ avoidance of blowing nose for at least 1 week to prevent contaminated air and bacteria from entering the eustachian tube
- ○ avoidance of sudden movements
- ○ avoidance of wetting head in shower or swimming for about 6 weeks
- ○ avoidance of getting water in the ear for an additional 4 weeks
- ○ prevention of constipation and avoidance of straining while defecating.

Ovarian cancer

Overview

Description

- ○ Malignancy arising from the ovary; a rapidly progressing cancer that's difficult to diagnose
- ○ Prognosis varying with histologic type and stage
- ○ 90% primary epithelial tumors
- ○ Stromal and germ cell tumors also important tumor types

Pathophysiology

- ○ Ovarian cancer spreads rapidly intraperitoneally by local extension or surface seeding and, occasionally, through the lymphatics and the bloodstream.
- ○ Metastasis to the ovary can occur from breast, colon, gastric, and pancreatic cancers.

Causes

- ○ Exact cause unknown

Risk factors

- ○ Infertility problems or nulliparity
- ○ Celibacy
- ○ Exposure to asbestos and talc
- ○ History of breast or uterine cancer
- ○ Family history of ovarian cancer
- ○ Diets high in saturated fat

Incidence

- ○ After lung, breast, and colon cancer, primary ovarian cancer is the most common cause of cancer death among women in the United States (about 40% survive for 5 years)
- ○ More common after age 50
- ○ Women in industrialized nations at greater risk
- ○ Metastatic ovarian cancer is more common than cancer at any other site in women with previously treated breast cancer.

Common characteristics

- ○ Initially no signs
- ○ Weight loss
- ○ Abdominal pain

Complications

- ○ Fluid and electrolyte imbalance
- ○ Leg edema
- ○ Ascites
- ○ Intestinal obstruction
- ○ Profound cachexia
- ○ Recurrent malignant effusions

Assessment

History

- ○ Lack of obvious signs, or signs and symptoms that vary with tumor size and extent of metastasis (disease usually metastasized before diagnosis is made)
- ○ In later stages: urinary frequency, constipation, pelvic discomfort, distention, weight loss, abdominal pain

Physical findings

- ○ Gaunt appearance
- ○ Grossly distended abdomen accompanied by ascites
- ○ Palpable abdominal mass with rocky hardness or rubbery or cystlike quality

Test results

Laboratory
- ○ Laboratory tumor marker studies (such as ovarian carcinoma antigen, carcinoembryonic antigen, and human chorionic gonadotropin) showing abnormalities that may indicate complications

Imaging
- ○ Abdominal ultrasonography, computed tomography scan, or X-rays delineate tumor size.

Diagnostic procedures
- ○ Aspiration of ascitic fluid can reveal atypical cells.

Other
- ○ Exploratory laparotomy, including lymph node evaluation and tumor resection, is required for accurate diagnosis and staging.

Treatment

General

- ○ Radiation therapy (not commonly used because it causes myelosuppression, which limits effectiveness of chemotherapy)
- ○ Radioisotopes as adjuvant therapy
- ○ High-protein diet
- ○ Small, frequent meals

Medication

- ○ Chemotherapy after surgery
- ○ Immunotherapy (under investigation)
- ○ Hormone replacement therapy in prepubertal girls who had bilateral salpingo-oophorectomy

Surgery

- ○ Total abdominal hysterectomy and bilateral salpingo-oophorectomy with tumor resection
- ○ Omentectomy, appendectomy, lymph node palpation with probable lymphadenectomy, tissue biopsies, and peritoneal washings
- ○ Resection of involved ovary
- ○ Biopsies of omentum and uninvolved ovary
- ○ Peritoneal washings for cytologic examination of pelvic fluid

Nursing considerations

Key outcomes

The patient will:
- show no further evidence of weight loss
- express feelings about the potential loss
- express feelings of increased comfort and decreased pain
- establish effective coping mechanisms.

Nursing interventions

- Encourage verbalization and provide support.
- Give prescribed drugs.
- Provide abdominal support, and be alert for abdominal distention.
- Encourage coughing and deep breathing.

Monitoring

- Vital signs
- Intake and output
- Wound site
- Pain control
- Effects of medication
- Hydration and nutrition status

Patient teaching

Be sure to cover:
- the disorder, diagnosis, and treatment
- dietary needs
- relaxation techniques
- importance of preventing infection, emphasizing proper hand-washing technique
- drug administration, dosage, and possible adverse effects.

Discharge planning

- Refer the patient to resource and support services.

Ovarian cysts

Overview

Description

- Non-neoplastic sacs on an ovary that contain fluid or semisolid material
- Usually small and nonsymptomatic
- May be single or multiple (polycystic ovarian disease)
- Include follicular cysts, theca-lutein cysts, and corpus luteum cysts
- Can develop any time between puberty and menopause, including during pregnancy
- Excellent prognosis for non-neoplastic ovarian cysts (The risk for ovarian malignancy is not increased with a functional (physiologic) ovarian cyst.)

Pathophysiology

- Follicular cysts are generally very small and arise from follicles that overdistend, either because they haven't ruptured or have ruptured and resealed before their fluid was reabsorbed. (See *Follicular cyst*.)
- Luteal cysts develop if a mature corpus luteum persists abnormally and continues to secrete progesterone. They consist of blood or fluid that accumulates in the cavity of the corpus luteum and are typically more symptomatic than follicular cysts.
- When luteal cysts persist into menopause, they secrete excessive amounts of estrogen in response to the hypersecretion of follicle-stimulating hormone and luteinizing hormone that normally occurs during menopause.

Follicular cyst

A common type of ovarian cyst, a follicular cyst is usually semitransparent and overdistended, with watery fluid visible through its thin walls.

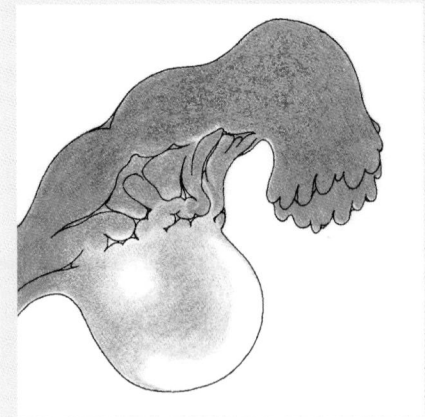

Causes

- Granulosa-lutein cysts (excessive accumulation of blood during menstruation)
- Theca-lutein cysts
- Hydatidiform mole
- Choriocarcinoma
- Hormone therapy

Incidence

- Can occur at any age, but occur more frequently in women of reproductive age

Common characteristics

- Possibly no symptoms (small ovarian cysts such as follicular cysts)
- Mild pelvic discomfort, lower back pain, dyspareunia, or abnormal uterine bleeding, secondary to a disturbed ovulatory pattern (large or multiple cysts)
- Acute abdominal pain similar to that of appendicitis (ovarian cysts with torsion)
- Unilateral pelvic discomfort (from granulosa-lutein cysts appearing early in pregnancy and growing as large as 2″ to 2½″ [5 to 6 cm] in diameter)
- Delayed menses, followed by prolonged or irregular bleeding (granulosa-lutein cysts in nonpregnant women)

Complications

- Torsion or rupture of cyst
- Infertility
- Amenorrhea
- Secondary dysmenorrhea
- Oligomenorrhea

Assessment

History

- Mild pelvic discomfort
- Lower back pain
- Dyspareunia
- Irregular bleeding

Physical findings

- Abdominal tenderness
- Abdominal distention
- Rigid abdomen
- Enlarged ovaries

Test results

Laboratory
- Elevated human chorionic gonadotropin (HCG) titer (theca-lutein cyst)
- Slightly elevated urine 17-ketosteroids (polycystic ovarian disease)

Imaging
- Ultrasound reveals cyst.

Other
- Laparoscopy (usually for another condition) reveals cyst.

Treatment

General

○ Follicular cysts: no treatment because cysts commonly disappear spontaneously within one to two menstrual cycles (excision of persistent cysts to rule out malignancy)
○ Theca-lutein cysts: discontinuation of HCG or clomiphene citrate therapy
○ Ruptured cysts: culdocentesis to drain intraperitoneal fluid
○ Activity, as tolerated

Medication

○ Hormonal contraceptives
○ Gonadotropin-releasing hormonal agonists
○ Analgesics

Surgery

○ Laparoscopy or exploratory laparotomy with possible ovarian cystectomy or oophorectomy for persistent or suspicious ovarian cyst

Nursing considerations

Nursing interventions

○ Provide emotional support.
After surgery
○ Encourage early ambulation.

Monitoring

○ Signs of rupture
○ Vital signs
○ Vaginal bleeding

Patient teaching

Be sure to cover:
○ the disorder, diagnosis, and treatment
○ importance of follow-up care
○ need to report increased menstrual bleeding
○ need to report abdominal mass.

Paget's disease

Overview

Description

- Bone disorder that causes an irregular bone formation
- Affects one or several skeletal areas (spine, pelvis, femur, and skull)
- Slow and progressive
- Causes malignant bone changes in about 5% of patients
- Can be fatal, particularly when associated with heart failure, bone sarcoma, or giant cell tumors
- Also known as *osteitis deformans*

 Alert

Paget's disease of the breast, a form of breast cancer, is a different disorder than Paget's disease. (See Paget's disease of the breast.*)*

Pathophysiology

- In the initial phase (osteoclastic phase) excessive bone resorption occurs.
- The second phase (osteoblastic phase) involves excessive abnormal bone formation.
- Affected bones enlarge and soften.
- New bone structure is chaotic, fragile, and weak.

Causes

- Exact cause unknown
- Theory: slow or dormant viral infection (possibly mumps)

Incidence

- More common after age 40
- More common in men

Common characteristics

- Severe, persistent pain
- Pain worsened by weight-bearing activities
- Cranial enlargement
- Barrel-shaped chest
- Kyphosis
- Asymmetric bowing of the tibia and femur
- Waddling gait

Paget's disease of the breast

Often misdiagnosed as a dermatologic problem, this rare type of breast cancer appears as a red, scaly crust on the nipple, causing itchiness and burning. Biopsy confirms the diagnosis. Treatment should be started to prevent spread of malignancy to the lymph nodes and other parts of the body.

- Pathologic fractures
- Muscle weakness

Complications

- Fractures
- Paraplegia
- Blindness and hearing loss with tinnitus and vertigo
- Osteoarthritis
- Sarcoma
- Hypertension
- Renal calculi
- Hypercalcemia
- Gout
- Heart failure

Assessment

History

- Severe, persistent pain
- Impaired mobility
- Pain that worsens with weight bearing
- Increased hat size
- Headaches

Physical findings

- Cranial enlargement over frontal and occipital areas
- Kyphosis
- Barrel-shaped chest
- Asymmetrical bowing of the tibia and femur
- Warmth and tenderness over affected sites

Test results

Laboratory
- Red blood cell count showing anemia
- Elevated serum alkaline phosphatase level
- Elevated 24-hour urine hydroxyproline level

Imaging
- X-ray studies show bone expansion and increased bone density.
- Bone scans clearly show early pagetic lesions.

Diagnostic procedures
- Bone biopsy shows a characteristic mosaic pattern of bone tissue.

Treatment

General

- Heat therapy
- Massage
- Well-balanced diet
- Activity, as tolerated
- Pacing of activities
- Use of assistive devices

Medication

- Calcitonin
- Nonsteroidal anti-inflammatory drugs
- Biphosphonates

○ Calcium supplements
○ Vitamin D

Surgery

○ Reduction of pathologic fractures
○ Correction of secondary deformities
○ Relief of neurologic impairment

Nursing considerations

Key outcomes

The patient will:
○ express feelings of increased comfort and decreased pain
○ perform activities of daily living to the extent possible
○ maintain adequate skin integrity
○ demonstrate measures to prevent self-injury
○ maintain joint mobility and range of motion.

Nursing interventions

○ Take measures to prevent pressure ulcers.
○ Instruct the patient with footdrop to wear high-topped sneakers or use a footboard.

Monitoring

○ Pain level, response to analgesic therapy
○ New areas of pain
○ New movement restrictions
○ Sensory and motor disturbances
○ Serum calcium and alkaline phosphatase levels
○ Intake and output

Patient teaching

Be sure to cover:
○ the disorder, diagnosis, and treatment
○ pacing of activities
○ use of assistive devices
○ exercise program
○ use of a firm mattress or a bed board
○ home safety measures
○ how to take prescribed drugs
○ adverse reactions to report.

Discharge planning

○ Refer the patient to community resource and support sources, as appropriate.
○ Refer the patient to physical and occupational therapy.

Pancreatic cancer

Overview

Description

○ Proliferation of cancer cells in the pancreas
○ Fifth most lethal type of carcinoma
○ Poor prognosis (most patients die within 1 year of diagnosis)

Pathophysiology

○ Pancreatic cancer is almost always adenocarcinoma.
○ Nearly two-thirds of tumors appear in the head of the pancreas; islet cell tumors are rare.
○ Two main tissue types form fibrotic nodes. Cylinder cells arise in ducts and degenerate into cysts; large, fatty, granular cells arise in parenchyma.
○ A high-fat or excessive protein diet induces chronic hyperplasia of the pancreas, with increased cell turnover.

Causes

○ Possible link to inhalation or absorption of carcinogens (such as cigarette smoke, excessive fat and protein, food additives, and industrial chemicals), which the pancreas then excretes

Risk factors

○ Chronic pancreatitis
○ Diabetes
○ Chronic alcohol abuse
○ Smoking
○ Occupational exposure to chemicals
○ High-fat diet

Incidence

○ Three to four times more common in smokers than nonsmokers
○ Highest in black men ages 35 to 70
○ Highest in Israel, United States, Sweden, and Canada; lowest in Switzerland, Belgium, and Italy

Common characteristics

○ Intermittent epigastric pain
○ Weight loss
○ Anorexia, nausea, and vomiting
○ Jaundice

Complications

○ Nutrient malabsorption
○ Type 1 diabetes
○ Liver and GI problems
○ Mental status changes
○ Hemorrhage
○ Pulmonary congestion

Assessment

History

○ Colicky, dull, or vague intermittent epigastric pain, which may radiate to the right upper quadrant or dorsolumbar area; unrelated to posture or activity and aggravated by meals
○ Anorexia, nausea, and vomiting
○ Rapid, profound weight loss

Physical findings

○ Jaundice
○ Large, palpable, well-defined mass in the subumbilical or left hypochondrial region
○ Abdominal bruit or pulsation

Test results

Laboratory
○ Absence of pancreatic enzymes
○ Increased serum bilirubin
○ Possible increase in serum lipase and amylase levels
○ Prolonged thrombin time
○ Elevated levels of aspartate aminotransferase and alanine aminotransferase (if liver cell necrosis present)
○ Markedly elevated alkaline phosphatase level (in biliary obstruction)
○ Measurable serum insulin (if islet cell tumor present)
○ Hypoglycemia or hyperglycemia
○ Elevation in specific tumor markers for pancreatic cancer, including carcinoembryonic antigen, pancreatic oncofetal antigen, alpha-fetoprotein, and serum immunoreactive elastase I
○ Conjugated equine estrogen plasma level
Imaging
○ Barium swallow, retroperitoneal insufflation, cholangiography, and scintigraphy locate the neoplasm and detect changes in the duodenum or stomach.
○ Ultrasonography and computed tomography scans identify masses.
○ Magnetic resonance imaging scan discloses tumor location and size.
○ Angiography reveals tumor vascularity.
○ Endoscopic retrograde cholangiopancreatography allows tumor visualization and specimen biopsy.
Diagnostic procedures
○ Percutaneous fine-needle aspiration biopsy may detect tumor cells.
○ Laparotomy with biopsy allows definitive diagnosis.

Treatment

General

○ Mainly palliative
○ May involve radiation therapy as adjunct to fluorouracil chemotherapy
○ Well-balanced diet, as tolerated
○ Small, frequent meals

○ Postoperative avoidance of lifting and contact sports
○ After recovery, no activity restrictions

Medication

○ Chemotherapy
○ Antibiotics
○ Anticholinergics
○ Antacids
○ Diuretics
○ Insulin
○ Analgesics
○ Pancreatic enzymes

Surgery

○ Total pancreatectomy
○ Cholecystojejunostomy, choledochoduodenostomy, and choledochojejunostomy
○ Gastrojejunostomy
○ Whipple's operation or radical pancreatoduodenectomy

Nursing considerations

Key outcomes

The patient will:
○ maintain an adequate weight
○ maintain normal fluid volume status
○ maintain skin integrity
○ verbalize increased comfort and pain relief
○ avoid injury.

Nursing interventions

○ Give prescribed drugs and blood transfusions.
○ Provide small, frequent meals.
○ Ensure adequate rest and sleep.
○ Assist with range-of-motion and isometric exercises, as appropriate.
○ Perform scrupulous skin care.
○ Apply antiembolism stockings.
○ Encourage verbalization and provide emotional support.

Monitoring

○ Fluid balance and nutrition
○ Abdominal girth, metabolic state, and daily weight
○ Blood glucose levels
○ Complete blood count
○ Pain control
○ Bleeding

Patient teaching

Be sure to cover:
○ the disorder, diagnosis, and treatment
○ end-of-life issues
○ drug administration, dosage, and possible adverse effects
○ expected postoperative care

○ information about diabetes, including signs and symptoms of hypoglycemia and hyperglycemia
○ adverse effects of radiation therapy and chemotherapy.

Discharge planning

○ Refer the patient to community resource and support services
○ Refer the patient to hospice care, if indicated.
○ Refer the patient to the American Cancer Society.

Pancreatitis

Overview

Description

- Inflammation of the pancreas
- Occurs in acute and chronic forms; acute form has 10% mortality
- Irreversible tissue damage with chronic form, which tends to progress to significant pancreatic function loss
- Can be idiopathic but sometimes associated with biliary tract disease, alcoholism, trauma, and certain drugs

Pathophysiology

- Enzymes normally excreted into the duodenum by the pancreas are activated in the pancreas or its ducts and start to autodigest pancreatic tissue.
- Consequent inflammation causes intense pain, third spacing of large fluid volumes, pancreatic fat necrosis with consumption of serum calcium and, occasionally, hemorrhage.

Causes

- Biliary tract disease
- Alcoholism
- Abnormal organ structure
- Metabolic or endocrine disorders
- Pancreatic cysts or tumors
- Penetrating peptic ulcers
- Penetrating trauma
- Viral or bacterial infection

Risk factors

- Use of glucocorticoids, sulfonamides, thiazides, and hormonal contraceptives
- Renal failure and kidney transplantation
- Endoscopic retrograde cholangiopancreatography (ERCP)
- Heredity
- Emotional or neurogenic factors

Incidence

- Acute form: 2 of every 10,000 people
- Chronic form: 2 of every 25,000 people
- Affects more men than women
- Affects Blacks four times more than Whites

Common characteristics

- Intense epigastric pain
- History of predisposing factors
- Foul-smelling foamy stools

Complications

- Diabetes mellitus
- Massive hemorrhage
- Diabetic acidosis
- Shock and coma
- Acute respiratory distress syndrome
- Atelectasis and pleural effusion
- Pneumonia
- Paralytic ileus
- GI bleeding
- Pancreatic abscess and cancer
- Pseudocysts

Assessment

History

- Intense epigastric pain centered close to the umbilicus and radiating to the back, between the 10th thoracic and 6th lumbar vertebrae
- Pain aggravated by fatty foods, alcohol consumption, or recumbent position
- Weight loss with nausea and vomiting
- Predisposing factor

Physical findings

- Hypotension
- Tachycardia
- Fever
- Dyspnea, orthopnea
- Generalized jaundice
- Cullen's sign (bluish periumbilical discoloration)
- Turner's sign (bluish flank discoloration)
- Steatorrhea (with chronic pancreatitis)
- Abdominal tenderness, rigidity, and guarding

Test results

Laboratory

- Elevated serum amylase and lipase levels
- Elevated white blood cell count
- Elevated serum bilirubin level
- Transient hyperglycemia and glycosuria
- Increased urinary amylase level
- In chronic pancreatitis: elevations in serum alkaline phosphatase, amylase, and bilirubin levels; transient elevation in serum glucose level; and elevated lipid and trypsin level in stool

Imaging

- Abdominal and chest X-rays differentiate pancreatitis from other diseases that cause similar symptoms; they also detect pleural effusions.
- Computed tomography scans and ultrasonography show increased pancreatic diameter, pancreatic cysts, and pseudocysts.

Diagnostic procedures

- ERCP shows pancreatic anatomy, identifies ductal system abnormalities, and differentiates pancreatitis from other disorders.

Treatment

General

- Emergency treatment of shock, as needed; vigorous I.V. replacement of fluid, electrolytes, and proteins
- Blood transfusions (for hemorrhage)

- Nasogastric suctioning
- Nothing by mouth
- Once crisis starts to resolve, oral low-fat, low-protein feedings implemented gradually
- Alcohol and caffeine abstention
- Activity, as tolerated

Medication

- Analgesics
- Antacids
- Histamine antagonists
- Antibiotics
- Anticholinergics
- Total parenteral nutrition
- Pancreatic enzymes
- Insulin
- Albumin

Surgery

- Not indicated in acute pancreatitis unless complications occur
- For chronic pancreatitis: sphincterotomy
- Pancreaticojejunostomy

Nursing considerations

Key outcomes

The patient will:
- maintain normal fluid volume
- maintain a patent airway
- verbalize feelings of increased comfort
- avoid complications
- maintain skin integrity
- initiate lifestyle changes.

Nursing interventions

- Give prescribed drugs and I.V. therapy.
- Encourage the patient to express his feelings.
- Provide emotional support.

Monitoring

- Vital signs
- Nasogastric tube function and drainage
- Respiratory status
- Acid-base balance
- Serum glucose level
- Fluid and electrolyte balance
- Daily weight
- Pain control
- Nutritional status and metabolic requirements

Patient teaching

Be sure to cover:
- the disorder, diagnosis, and treatment
- identification and avoidance of acute pancreatitis triggers
- dietary needs

- drug administration, dosage, and possible adverse effects.

Discharge planning

- Refer the patient to community resource and support services, as needed.

Panic disorder

Overview

Description

○ Anxiety in its most severe form, characterized by recurrent episodes of intense apprehension, terror, and impending doom
○ May be associated with specific situations or tasks
○ Commonly exists concurrently with agoraphobia
○ May be triggered by severe separation anxiety experienced during early childhood
○ Can persist for years without treatment, with alternating exacerbations and remissions

Pathophysiology

○ Increased sensitivity to adrenergic central nervous system discharges, with hypersensitivity of presynaptic alpha-2 receptors

Causes

○ Combination of physiologic and psychological factors
○ Hereditary
○ Temporal lobe dysfunction
○ May develop as a persistent pattern of maladaptive behavior acquired by learning
○ Alterations in brain biochemistry, especially in norepinephrine, serotonin, and gamma-aminobutyric acid activity, may be contributing factors
○ Possibly related to stressful events or unconscious conflicts that occur early in childhood

Incidence

○ Men and women affected equally
○ Panic disorder with agoraphobia about twice as common in women than in men
○ Typical onset in late adolescence or early adulthood, commonly in response to a sudden loss

Common characteristics

○ Repeated episodes of unexpected apprehension, fear, and intense discomfort that may last for minutes or hours and leave the patient shaken, fearful, and exhausted
○ Attacks that occur several times a week, sometimes daily
○ Hyperventilation
○ Tachycardia
○ Trembling
○ Profuse sweating
○ Digestive disturbances
○ Chest pain

Complications

○ Psychoactive substance use disorder

Assessment

History

○ Repeated episodes of unexpected apprehension or fear

Physical findings

○ During a panic attack:
  – trembling
  – digestive disturbances
  – hyperventilation
  – tachycardia
  – profuse sweating.

DSM-IV-TR criteria

Diagnosis of panic disorder is confirmed when the patient meets the following criteria:
○ recurrent, unexpected panic attacks with at least one of the attacks having been followed by 1 month (or more) of one (or more) of the following:
  – persistent concern about having additional attacks
  – worry about the attack's implications or consequences
  – significant change in behavior related to the attack
  – agoraphobia
○ attacks not due to the direct physiologic effects of a substance or a general medical condition
○ attacks not better accounted for by another mental disorder, such as social phobia, specific phobia, obsessive-compulsive disorder, posttraumatic stress disorder, or separation anxiety.

Test results

Laboratory
○ Urine and serum toxicology tests may reveal the presence of psychoactive substances that can precipitate panic attacks, including barbiturates, caffeine, and amphetamines.
Other
○ Various tests may be ordered to rule out an organic basis for the symptoms.

Treatment

General

○ Behavioral therapy
○ Supportive psychotherapy

Medication

○ Antianxiety agents
○ Antidepressants

Nursing considerations

Key outcomes

The patient will:
○ experience reduced anxiety by identifying internal precipitating situation

○ identify current stressors
○ set limits and compromises on behavior when ready
○ develop effective coping mechanisms.

Nursing interventions

○ Stay with the patient until the attack subsides.
○ Speak in short, simple sentences and slowly give one direction at a time. Avoid giving lengthy explanations and asking too many questions.
○ Give prescribed drugs.

Monitoring

○ Response to therapy
○ Vital signs during an attack

Patient teaching

Be sure to cover:
○ relaxation techniques such as focusing on slow, deep breathing
○ drug administration, dosage, and possible adverse effects.

Discharge planning

○ Encourage the patient and his family to use community resources such as the Anxiety Disorders Association of America.

Parkinson's disease

Overview

Description

- Brain disorder causing progressive deterioration, with muscle rigidity, akinesia, and involuntary tremors
- Usual cause of death: aspiration pneumonia
- One of the most common crippling diseases in the United States

Pathophysiology

- Dopaminergic neurons degenerate, causing loss of available dopamine.
- Dopamine deficiency prevents affected brain cells from performing their normal inhibitory function.
- Excess excitatory acetylcholine occurs at synapses.
- Nondopaminergic receptors are also involved.
- Motor neurons are depressed. (See *Understanding Parkinson's disease.*)

Causes

- Usually unknown
- Exposure to such toxins as manganese dust and carbon monoxide
- Type A encephalitis
- Drug-induced (Haldol, methyldopa, reserpine)

Incidence

- More common in men than women
- Occurs in middle age or later
- Rare in blacks

Common characteristics

- Muscle rigidity
- Tremor
- Resistance to passive muscle stretching
- Akinesia
- High-pitched, monotonous voice
- Drooling
- Loss of posture control
- Dysarthria
- Excessive sweating
- Decreased GI motility
- Orthostatic hypotension
- Oily skin
- Eyes fixed upward

Understanding Parkinson's disease

New research on the pathogenesis of Parkinson's disease focuses on damage to the substantia nigra from oxidative stress. Oxidative stress is believed to:
- alter the brain's iron content
- impair mitochondrial function
- alter antioxidant and protective systems
- reduce glutathione
- damage lipids, proteins, and deoxyribonucleic acid.

Complications

- Injury from falls
- Food aspiration
- Urinary tract infections
- Skin breakdown

Assessment

History

- Muscle rigidity
- Akinesia
- Insidious (unilateral pill-roll) tremor, which increases during stress or anxiety and decreases with purposeful movement and sleep
- Dysphagia
- Fatigue with activities of daily living (ADLs)
- Muscle cramps of legs, neck, and trunk
- Oily skin
- Increased perspiration
- Insomnia
- Mood changes
- Dysarthria

Physical findings

- High-pitched, monotonous voice
- Drooling
- Masklike facial expression
- Difficulty walking
- Lack of parallel motion in gait
- Loss of posture control with walking
- Oculogyric crises (eyes fixed upward, with involuntary tonic movements)
- Muscle rigidity causing resistance to passive muscle stretching
- Difficulty pivoting
- Loss of balance

Test results

Imaging
- Computed tomography scan or magnetic resonance rules out other disorders such as intracranial tumors.

Treatment

General

- Small, frequent meals
- High-bulk foods
- Physical therapy and occupational therapy
- Assistive devices to aid ambulation

Medication

- Dopamine replacement drugs
- Anticholinergics
- Antihistamines
- Antiviral agents
- Enzyme-inhibiting agents
- Tricyclic antidepressants

Surgery

○ Used when drug therapy fails
○ Stereotaxic neurosurgery
○ Destruction of ventrolateral nucleus of thalamus

Nursing considerations

Key outcomes

The patient will:
○ perform ADLs
○ avoid injury
○ maintain adequate caloric intake
○ express positive feelings about himself
○ develop adequate coping behaviors
○ seek support resources.

Nursing interventions

○ Take measures to prevent aspiration.
○ Protect the patient from injury.
○ Stress the importance of rest periods between activities.
○ Ensure adequate nutrition.
○ Provide frequent warm baths and massage.
○ Encourage the patient to enroll in a physical therapy program.
○ Provide emotional and psychological support.
○ Encourage the patient to be independent.
○ Assist with ambulation and range-of-motion exercises

Monitoring

○ Vital signs
○ Intake and output
○ Drug therapy
○ Adverse reactions to medications
○ Postoperatively: signs of hemorrhage and increased intracranial pressure
○ Swallowing

Patient teaching

Be sure to cover:
○ the disorder, diagnosis, and treatment
○ drug administration, dosage, and possible adverse effects
○ measures to prevent pressure ulcers and contractures
○ household safety measures
○ importance of daily bathing
○ methods to improve communication
○ swallowing therapy regimen (aspiration precautions).

Discharge planning

○ Refer the patient for occupational and physical rehabilitation, as indicated.

Patent ductus arteriosus

Overview

Description

- Heart condition in which the lumen of the ductus (fetal blood vessel that connects the pulmonary artery to the descending aorta) remains open after birth
- Initially may produce no clinical effects, but in time can precipitate pulmonary vascular disease, causing symptoms to appear by age 40
- Good prognosis if the shunt is small or surgical repair is effective; otherwise, may advance to intractable heart failure, which may be fatal

Pathophysiology

- The lumen of the ductus remains open after birth and creates a left-to-right shunt of blood from the aorta to the pulmonary artery, resulting in recirculation of arterial blood through the lungs.
- Prevalent in premature infants, probably as a result of abnormalities in oxygenation or the relaxant action of prostaglandin E, which prevents ductal spasm and contracture necessary for closure

Causes

- Prematurity
- Rubella syndrome
- Associated with other congenital defects, such as coarctation of the aorta, ventricular septal defect, and pulmonary and aortic stenoses

Incidence

- Twice as common in females than in males
- The most common congenital heart defect found in adults

Common characteristics

Infants
- Respiratory distress
- Signs and symptoms of heart failure
- Heightened susceptibility to respiratory tract infections
- Slow motor development
- Failure to thrive

Adults
- Pulmonary vascular disease
- Fatigability and dyspnea on exertion

Complications

- Chronic pulmonary hypertension
- Intractable left-sided heart failure
- Respiratory distress

Assessment

History

- Prematurity
- Rubella
- Difficulty breathing

Physical findings

- Gibson murmur during systole and diastole
- Thrill at the left sternal border
- Prominent left ventricular impulse
- Bounding peripheral arterial pulses (Corrigan's pulse)
- Widened pulse pressure

Test results

Imaging
- Chest X-rays may show increased pulmonary vascular markings, prominent pulmonary arteries, and enlargement of the left ventricle and aorta.
- Echocardiography detects and helps estimate the size of a patent ductus arteriosus (PDA). It also reveals an enlarged left atrium and left ventricle or right ventricular hypertrophy from pulmonary vascular disease.

Diagnostic procedures
- ECG may be normal or may indicate left atrial or ventricular hypertrophy and, in pulmonary vascular disease, biventricular hypertrophy.
- Cardiac catheterization shows pulmonary arterial oxygen content higher than right ventricular content because of the influx of aortic blood.

Treatment

General

- No immediate treatment (if asymptomatic)
- Fluid restriction
- Activity, as tolerated

Medication

- Diuretics
- Cardiac glycosides
- Antibiotics (preoperatively)

Surgery

- Ligation of the ductus

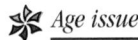 *Age issue*

If symptoms are mild, surgical correction is usually delayed until at least age 1. Before surgery, children with PDA require antibiotics to protect against infective endocarditis.

- Cardiac catheterization to deposit a plug in the ductus to stop shunting or for administration of indomethacin I.V. (a prostaglandin inhibitor that is an alternative to surgery in premature infants) to induce ductus spasm and closure

Nursing considerations

Key outcomes

The patient will:
○ maintain adequate ventilation
○ maintain hemodynamic stability
○ remain free from signs and symptoms of infection
○ utilize support groups to help cope effectively.

Nursing interventions

○ Give prescribed drugs.
○ Provide emotional support to the patient and her family.

Monitoring

○ Respiratory status
○ Vital signs
○ Cardiac rhythm
○ Intake and output

Patient teaching

Be sure to cover:
○ activity restrictions based on the child's tolerance and energy levels
○ importance of informing any physician who treats the child about his history of surgery for PDA — even if the child is being treated for an unrelated medical problem.

Discharge planning

○ Stress the need for regular medical follow-up examinations.

Pediculosis

Overview

Description

- Infestation of human parasitic lice, which feed exclusively on human blood and lay eggs (nits) on body hairs or clothing fibers; after nits hatch, lice must feed within 24 hours or die (see *Types of lice*)
- Pediculosis capitis (head lice): confined to scalp and, occasionally, eyebrows, eyelashes, and beard
- Pediculosis corporis (body lice): found next to skin in clothing seams; move to the host only to feed on blood
- Pediculosis pubis (crab lice): found primarily in pubic hairs; may extend to eyebrows, eyelashes, and axillary or body hair

Pathophysiology

- Lice crawl and attach superficially to the epidermis and hair. One female louse deposits approximately 60 to 150 nits to hair shafts. Nits survive by ingesting blood from the human host.
- A louse bite injects a toxin into the skin. Mild irritation and a purpuric spot result.
- Repeated bites cause sensitization to the toxin, leading to more serious inflammation. In severe cases, sensitization causes wheals or a rash on the trunk.
- Scratching may result in secondary bacterial infection.

Causes

Pediculosis capitis
- *Pediculus humanus* var. *capitis, P. humanus* var. *corporis*
- Spreads through shared clothing, hats, combs, and hairbrushes

Pediculosis corporis
- *P. humanus* var. *corporis*
- Spreads through shared clothing and bedding, especially with environmental overcrowding, prolonged wearing of same clothing, or poor personal hygiene

Pediculosis pubis
- *Phthirus pubis*
- Spreads through sexual intercourse or contact with clothing, bedding, or towels harboring lice

Incidence

Pediculosis capitis
- More common in children

Pediculosis pubis
- More common in adults

Common characteristics

- Nits
- Pruritus
- Skin excoriation

Complications

- Skin excoriation
- Secondary bacterial infections
- Hyperpigmentation or residual scarring

Assessment

History

- Exposure to causative organism
- Headache
- Fever
- Malaise
- Pruritus
- Cutaneous changes

Physical findings

Pediculosis capitis
- Visible lice
- Skin excoriation on the scalp and neck
- Matted, lusterless hair (in severe cases)
- Occipital and cervical lymphadenopathy
- Oval, gray-white nits visible on hair shafts

Pediculosis corporis
- Red papules or macules, usually on the shoulders, trunk, or buttocks
- Excoriations from scratching
- Nits on clothing seams

Pediculosis pubis
- Visible brownish-gray lice
- Erythematous papules
- Small macules on the thighs, buttocks, or lower abdomen
- Coarse, grainy-feeling, white-gray nits attached to pubic hairs

Test results

Diagnostic procedures
- Direct inspection with hand lens showing visible lice or nits
- Wood's light examination showing fluorescence of live nits (dead nits don't fluoresce)

Treatment

General

- Use of fine-toothed comb dipped in vinegar
- Hair-washing with ordinary shampoo
- Laundering of potentially contaminated clothing and bed linen
- Bathing with soap and water
- Petroleum jelly applied to eyebrows or eyelashes

Medication

Pediculosis capitis
- Permethrin or pyrethrins

Pediculosis corporis
- Pediculicide cream (for severe infestation)

Pediculosis pubis
- Pediculicide shampoo

Types of lice

Head louse
Pediculus humanus var. capitis (head louse) resembles P. humanus var. corporis (body louse).

Body louse
Pediculus humanus var. corporis (body louse) has a long abdomen, and its legs are all about the same length.

Pubic louse
Phthirus pubis (pubic, or crab, louse) is slightly translucent. Its first set of legs is shorter than its second and third sets.

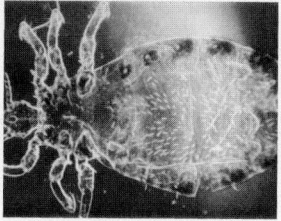 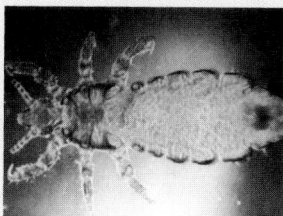 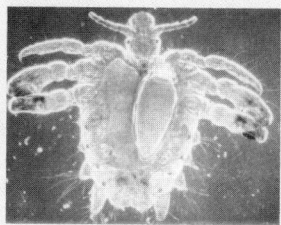

Nursing considerations

Key outcomes

The patient will:
○ exhibit resolution of the infestation
○ report feelings of increased comfort
○ demonstrate understanding of the treatment regimen
○ verbalize feelings about changed body image.

Nursing interventions

○ Give prescribed drugs.
○ Use personal protective equipment when administering delousing treatment.
○ Notify the school if infestation occurs in a child.
○ Encourage the patient to express feelings about the infestation.

Monitoring

○ Adverse reactions to insecticide treatment
○ Complications
○ Response to treatment

Patient teaching

Be sure to cover:
○ how to inspect for lice, eggs, and lesions
○ how to decontaminate infestation sources
○ how to apply insecticidal agents
○ removal of nits and lice
○ importance of not sharing personal articles
○ adverse reactions to treatment, including when to notify the physician
○ notification and treatment of sexual contacts within previous 30 days.

Pelvic inflammatory disease

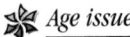
Overview

Description

○ Umbrella term that refers to any acute, subacute, recurrent, or chronic infection of the oviducts and ovaries, with adjacent tissue involvement
○ Includes inflammation of the cervix (cervicitis), uterus (endometritis), fallopian tubes (salpingitis), and ovaries (oophoritis)
○ Possible extension of the inflammation to connective tissue lying between the broad ligaments (parametritis)
○ Commonly called *PID*

Pathophysiology

○ Various conditions, procedures, or instrumentation can alter or destroy the cervical mucus, which normally serves as a protective barrier.
○ As a result, bacteria enter the uterine cavity, causing inflammation of various structures.

Causes

○ Aerobic or anaerobic organisms (commonly, overgrowth of one or more of the bacterial species found in the cervical mucus)
○ Sexually transmitted infections (*Neisseria gonorrhoeae* and *Chlamydia trachomatis*)
○ Septicemia
○ Infected drainage from a chronically infected fallopian tube
○ Ruptured appendix
○ Diverticulitis of the sigmoid colon
○ Pelvic abscess
○ Use of intrauterine device

Risk factors

○ Multiple sex partners
○ Conditions or procedures that alter or destroy cervical mucus
○ Procedures that risk transfer of contaminated cervical mucus into the endometrial cavity by an instrument
○ Infection during or after pregnancy
○ Cigarette smoking
○ Multiparity
○ Douching
○ Intercourse during menses
○ Therapeutic abortion

Incidence

○ Primarily affects women ages 16 to 40

Common characteristics

○ Profuse, purulent vaginal discharge
○ Lower abdominal pain
○ Vaginal bleeding

Complications

○ Septicemia (potentially fatal)
○ Pulmonary embolism
○ Infertility
○ Peritonitis
○ Shock
○ Death
○ Ectopic pregnancy

Assessment

History

○ Profuse, purulent vaginal discharge
○ Low-grade fever
○ Malaise
○ Lower abdominal pain
○ Vaginal bleeding

Physical findings

○ Pain with cervical movement or adnexal palpation
○ Vaginal discharge
○ Unilaterally or bilaterally tender adnexal mass

Test results

Laboratory
○ Culture and sensitivity and Gram stain of endocervix or cul-de-sac secretions showing the causative agent
○ Urethral and rectal secretions showing the causative agent
○ Elevated C-reactive protein level

Imaging
○ Transvaginal ultrasonography may show the presence of thickened, fluid-filled fallopian tubes.
○ Computed tomography scan may show complex tubo-ovarian abscesses and is useful in diagnosing PID.
○ Magnetic resonance imaging provides images of soft tissue; useful not only for establishing the diagnosis of PID but also for detecting other processes responsible for symptoms.

Diagnostic procedures
○ Culdocentesis obtains peritoneal fluid or pus for culture and sensitivity testing.
○ Diagnostic laparoscopy identifies cul-de-sac fluid, tubal distention, and masses in pelvic abscess.

Treatment

General
○ Frequent perineal care if vaginal discharge occurs
○ Bed rest

Medication
○ Antibiotics
○ Analgesics
○ I.V. fluids, as needed

Surgery
○ Drainage of pelvic abscess

 Alert

A ruptured pelvic abscess is a life-threatening condition. The patient may need a total abdominal hysterectomy with bilateral salpingo-oophorectomy.

Nursing considerations

Key outcomes
The patient will:
○ express feelings of increased comfort
○ remain free from signs or symptoms of infection
○ exhibit stable vital signs
○ maintain fluid balance
○ express feelings about having PID.

Nursing interventions
○ Give prescribed antibiotics and analgesics.
○ Provide frequent perineal care.
○ Use meticulous hand-washing technique.
○ Encourage the patient to discuss her feelings, and offer emotional support.
○ Help the patient develop effective coping strategies.
○ Assess discharge.

Monitoring
○ Vital signs
○ Fluid intake and output
○ Signs and symptoms of dehydration

 Alert

Watch for and report abdominal rigidity and distention. These signs may indicate development of peritonitis.

Patient teaching

Be sure to cover:
○ the disorder, diagnosis, and treatment
○ ways to prevent a recurrence
○ importance of avoiding multiple sexual partners

○ need for the patient's sexual partner to be examined and, if necessary, treated for infection
○ condom use
○ causes of PID, such as dyspareunia and sexual activity
○ signs and symptoms of infection after a minor gynecologic procedure.

 Alert

Tell the patient to immediately report fever, increased vaginal discharge, or pain — especially after a minor gynecologic procedure.

○ avoidance of douching or intercourse for at least 7 days after a minor gynecologic procedure.

Discharge planning
○ Refer the patient to infertility counseling, if indicated.
○ Refer the patient to a smoking-cessation program, if indicated.

Peptic ulcer

Overview

Description
- Circumscribed lesion in the mucosal membrane of the lower esophagus, stomach, duodenum, or jejunum
- Occurs in two major forms: duodenal ulcer and gastric ulcer (both forms chronic)
- Duodenal ulcers: represent about 80% of peptic ulcers; affect the proximal part of the small intestine and follow a chronic course characterized by remissions and exacerbations (about 5% to 10% of patients with duodenal ulcers develop complications that necessitate surgery)

Pathophysiology
- *Helicobacter pylori* releases a toxin that promotes mucosal inflammation and ulceration.
- In a peptic ulcer resulting from *H. pylori,* acid isn't the dominant cause of bacterial infection but contributes to the consequences.
- Ulceration stems from inhibition of prostaglandin synthesis, increased gastric acid and pepsin secretion, reduced gastric mucosal blood flow, or decreased cytoprotective mucus production.

Causes
- *H. pylori*
- Use of nonsteroidal anti-inflammatory drugs (NSAIDs) or glucocorticoids
- Pathologic hypersecretory states

Risk factors
- Type A blood (for gastric ulcer)
- Type O blood (for duodenal ulcer)
- Other genetic factors
- Exposure to irritants
- Cigarette smoking
- Trauma
- Psychogenic factors
- Normal aging

Incidence
- Gastric ulcers: most common in middle-aged and elderly men, especially those who are poor and undernourished; prevalence higher in chronic users of aspirin or alcohol
- Duodenal ulcers: most common in men ages 20 to 50

Common characteristics
- Left epigastric or abdominal pain with exacerbations and remissions
- History of predisposing factor

Complications
- GI hemorrhage
- Abdominal or intestinal infarction
- Ulcer penetration into attached structures

Assessment

History
- Periods of symptom exacerbation and remission, with remissions lasting longer than exacerbations
- History of predisposing factor
- Left epigastric pain described as heartburn or indigestion, accompanied by feeling of fullness or distention

Gastric ulcer
- Recent weight or appetite loss
- Nausea or vomiting
- Pain triggered or worsened by eating

Duodenal ulcer
- Pain relieved by eating; may occur 1½ to 3 hours after food intake
- Pain that awakens the patient from sleep
- Weight gain

Physical findings
- Pallor
- Epigastric tenderness
- Hyperactive bowel sounds

Test results
Laboratory
- Complete blood count showing anemia
- Occult blood in stools
- Venous blood sample showing *H. pylori* antibodies
- Elevated white blood cell count
- Low levels of exhaled carbon 13 (^{13}C) in urea breath test
- Fasting serum gastrin level (rules out Zollinger-Ellison syndrome)

Imaging
- Barium swallow or upper GI and small-bowel series may reveal the ulcer.
- Upper GI tract X-rays reveal mucosal abnormalities.

Diagnostic procedures
- Upper GI endoscopy or esophagogastroduodenoscopy confirm the ulcer and permit cytologic studies and biopsy to rule out *H. pylori* or cancer.
- Gastric secretory studies show hyperchlorhydria.

Treatment

General
- Symptomatic
- Iced saline lavage, possibly containing norepinephrine
- Laser or cautery during endoscopy
- Stress reduction
- Smoking cessation
- Avoidance of dietary irritants
- Nothing by mouth if GI bleeding evident

Medication

For H. pylori
○ Amoxicillin, biaxin, and prilosec

For gastric or duodenal ulcer
○ Proton pump inhibitors
○ Antacids
○ Histamine-receptor antagonists or gastric acid pump inhibitor
○ Coating agents (for duodenal ulcer)
○ Antisecretory agents if ulcer resulted from NSAID use, when NSAIDs must be continued
○ Sedatives and tranquilizers (for gastric ulcer)
○ Anticholinergics (for duodenal ulcers; usually contraindicated in gastric ulcers)
○ Prostaglandin analogs

Surgery
○ Indicated for perforation, lack of response to conservative treatment, suspected cancer, or other complications
○ Type varies with ulcer location and extent; major operations: bilateral vagotomy, pyloroplasty, and gastrectomy

Nursing considerations

Key outcomes
The patient will:
○ maintain adequate fluid volume
○ express feelings of increased comfort
○ verbalize an understanding of the illness
○ comply with the treatment regimen.

Nursing interventions
○ Give prescribed drugs.
○ Provide six small meals or small hourly meals, as ordered.
○ Offer emotional support.

Monitoring
○ Medication effects
○ Vital signs
○ Signs and symptoms of bleeding
○ Pain control

If patient had surgery
○ Nasogastric tube function and drainage
○ Bowel function
○ Fluid and nutritional status
○ Wound site
○ Signs and symptoms of metabolic alkalosis or perforation

Patient teaching

Be sure to cover:
○ the disorder, diagnosis, and treatment
○ drug administration, dosage, and possible adverse effects

○ warnings against avoid over-the-counter medications, especially aspirin, aspirin-containing products, and NSAIDS, unless the physician approves
○ warnings against caffeine and alcohol intake during exacerbations
○ appropriate lifestyle changes
○ dietary modifications.

Discharge planning
○ Refer the patient to a smoking-cessation program, if indicated.

Perforated eardrum

Overview

Description
- Rupture of the tympanic membrane
- May cause hearing loss
- Typically heals spontaneously

Pathophysiology
- Pressure on the tympanic membrane causes a traumatic opening that allows release of pressure.
- The rupture may be central or marginal.
- The hole exposes the middle and inner ear to damage or infection.

Causes
- Bacterial infection (acute or chronic suppurative otitis media)
- Trauma
- Puncture
- Skull fracture
- Burns
- Excessive change in pressure

Incidence
- More common in children

Common characteristics
- Ear pain
- Ear discharge
- Vertigo (may be transient)
- Tinnitus
- Hearing loss
- Fever or chills
- Nausea or vomiting

Complications
- Mastoiditis
- Meningitis
- Permanent hearing loss

Assessment

History
- Mild or severe ear trauma
- Recent airline flight during an upper respiratory infection
- Sudden onset of severe earache and bleeding from ear
- Hearing loss
- Tinnitus
- Vertigo

Physical findings
- Signs of hearing loss
- Outer ear drainage
- Perforated tympanic membrane seen on otoscopic examination

Test results
Laboratory
- Ear drainage culture identifies causative organism or determines if an infection caused the rupture

Imaging
- Skull and temporal lobe X-rays may reveal an associated fracture, especially when a bad fall caused the eardrum rupture.

Diagnostic procedures
- Audiometric testing evaluates middle ear function.

Treatment

General
- May heal spontaneously
- No dietary restrictions unless nausea occurs; in that case, clear liquids until nausea passes
- Safety precautions if the patient has vertigo

Medication
- Analgesics (acetaminophen)
- Antibiotics if perforation resulted from infection

Surgery
- Myringoplasty
- Tympanoplasty

Nursing considerations

Key outcomes
The patient (or parents) will:
- express an understanding of hearing changes
- demonstrate appropriate use of pain relief methods
- express an understanding of the potential causes of ear injury
- remain free from infection.

Nursing interventions
- Give prescribed drugs.
- Insert a sterile wick.
- When talking, face the patient and speak distinctly and slowly.

Monitoring
- Hearing ability
- Ear drainage
- Safety
- Signs of complications

Patient teaching

Be sure to cover:

○ the disorder, diagnosis, and treatment
○ warnings against irrigating the ear or cleaning the middle ear canal with a cotton-tipped applicator
○ importance of avoiding swimming or use of ear plugs
○ care during hair washing
○ the need to complete the course of antibiotic therapy as prescribed.
○ use of safety equipment in the workplace and at home to prevent injury to the ear.

Pericarditis

Overview

Description

- Inflammation of the pericardium—the fibroserous sac that envelops, supports, and protects the heart
- Occurs in acute and chronic forms
- Acute form: can be fibrinous or effusive; characterized by serous, purulent, or hemorrhagic exudate
- Chronic form: characterized by dense fibrous pericardial thickening
- Chronic form called *constrictive pericarditis*

Pathophysiology

- Pericardial tissue is damaged by bacteria or another substance that releases chemical mediators of inflammation into surrounding tissue.
- Friction occurs as the inflamed layers rub against each other.
- Chemical mediators dilate blood vessels and increase vessel permeability.
- Vessel walls leak fluids and proteins, causing extracellular edema.

Causes

- Bacterial, fungal, or viral infection (in infectious pericarditis)
- Neoplasms (primary or metastatic)
- High-dose chest radiation
- Uremia
- Hypersensitivity or autoimmune disease
- Drugs, such as hydralazine or procainamide
- Idiopathic factors
- Myocardial infarction (MI)
- Chest trauma
- Aortic aneurysm with pericardial leakage
- Myxedema with cholesterol deposits in pericardium
- Radiation
- Rheumatologic conditions
- Tuberculosis

Incidence

- Affects males more than females
- Most common in men ages 20 to 50

Common characteristics

- Pericardial friction rub
- Chest pain

Complications

- Pericardial effusion
- Cardiac tamponade

Assessment

History

- Predisposing factor
- Sharp, sudden pain, usually starting over the sternum and radiating to the neck, shoulders, back, and arms
- Pleuritic pain, increasing with deep inspiration and decreasing when the patient sits up and leans forward
- Dyspnea
- Chest pain (may mimic MI pain)

Physical findings

- Pericardial friction rub
- Diminished apical impulse
- Fluid retention, ascites, hepatomegaly (resembling those of chronic right-sided heart failure)
- With pericardial effusion: tachycardia
- With cardiac tamponade: pallor, clammy skin, hypotension, pulsus paradoxus, jugular vein distention, and dyspnea

Test results

Laboratory
- Elevated white blood cell count (especially in infectious pericarditis)
- Elevated erythrocyte sedimentation rate
- Slightly elevated serum creatine kinase-MB levels (with associated myocarditis)
- Pericardial fluid culture; may identify a causative organism in bacterial or fungal pericarditis
- Elevated blood urea nitrogen in uremia
- Elevated antistreptolysin-O titers; may indicate rheumatic fever
- Positive reaction in purified protein derivative skin test; indicates tuberculosis

Imaging
- Echocardiography showing an echo-free space between the ventricular wall and the pericardium indicates pericardial effusion
- High-resolution computed tomography and magnetic resonance imaging reveals pericardial thickness.

Diagnostic procedures
- Electrocardiography shows initial ST-segment elevation across the precordium.

Treatment

General

- Management of rheumatic fever, uremia, tuberculosis, or other underlying disorder
- Dietary restrictions based on underlying disorder
- Bed rest as long as fever and pain persist

Medication

- Nonsteroidal anti-inflammatory drugs
- Corticosteroids
- Antibiotics

Surgery

○ Surgical drainage
○ Pericardiocentesis
○ Partial pericardectomy (for recurrent pericarditis)
○ Total pericardectomy (for constrictive pericarditis)

Nursing considerations

Key outcomes

The patient will:
○ maintain hemodynamic stability and adequate cardiac output
○ avoid arrhythmias
○ maintain adequate ventilation
○ verbalize feelings of increased comfort and decreased pain.

Nursing interventions

○ Give prescribed analgesics and oxygen.
○ Give prescribed antibiotics on time.
○ Stress the importance of bed rest. Provide a bedside commode.
○ Place the patient upright to relieve dyspnea and chest pain.

 Alert

Keep a pericardiocentesis set readily available whenever you suspect pericardial effusion.

○ Encourage the patient to express concerns about the effects of activity restrictions on responsibilities and routines.
○ Review the patient's allergy history.
○ Provide appropriate postoperative care.

Monitoring

○ Vital signs
○ Heart rhythm
○ Heart sounds
○ Hemodynamic values

Patient teaching

Be sure to cover:
○ the disorder, diagnosis, and treatments
○ how to perform deep-breathing and coughing exercises
○ the need to resume daily activities slowly and to schedule rest periods in daily routine, as instructed by the physician.

Peritonitis

Overview

Description

- Inflammation of the peritoneum; may extend throughout the peritoneum or localize as an abscess
- Commonly decreases intestinal motility and causes intestinal distention with gas
- Fatal in 10% of cases, with bowel obstruction the usual cause of death
- Can be acute or chronic

Pathophysiology

- Bacteria invade the peritoneum after inflammation and perforation of the GI tract.
- Fluid containing protein and electrolytes accumulates in the peritoneal cavity; normally transparent, the peritoneum becomes opaque, red, inflamed, and edematous.
- Infection may localize as an abscess rather than disseminate as a generalized infection.

Causes

- GI tract perforation (from appendicitis, diverticulitis, peptic ulcer, or ulcerative colitis)
- Bacterial or chemical inflammation
- Ruptured ectopic pregnancy

Incidence

- More common in men

Common characteristics

- Abdominal pain
- Fever
- Rebound tenderness

Complications

- Abscess
- Septicemia
- Respiratory compromise
- Bowel obstruction
- Shock

Assessment

History

Early phase
- Vague, generalized abdominal pain
- If localized: pain over a specific area (usually the inflammation site)
- If generalized: diffuse pain over the abdomen

With progression
- Increasingly severe and constant abdominal pain that increases with movement and respirations
- Possible referral of pain to shoulder or thoracic area
- Anorexia, nausea, and vomiting
- Inability to pass stools and flatus
- Hiccups

Physical findings

- Fever
- Tachycardia
- Hypotension
- Shallow breathing
- Signs of dehydration
- Positive bowel sounds (early); absent bowel sounds (later)
- Abdominal rigidity
- General abdominal tenderness
- Rebound tenderness
- Typical patient positioning: lying very still with knees flexed

Test results

Laboratory
- Complete blood count showing leukocytosis

Imaging
- Abdominal X-rays show edematous and gaseous distention of the small and large bowel. With perforation of a visceral organ, X-rays show air in the abdominal cavity.
- Chest X-rays may reveal elevation of the diaphragm.
- Computed tomography reveals fluid and inflammation.

Diagnostic procedures
- Paracentesis shows the exudate's nature and permits bacterial culture testing.

Treatment

General

- I.V. fluids
- Nasogastric (NG) intubation
- Nothing by mouth until bowel function returns
- Gradual increase in diet
- Parenteral nutrition, if necessary
- Bed rest until condition improves
- Semi-Fowler's position
- Avoidance of lifting for at least 6 weeks postoperatively

Medication

- Antibiotics, based on infecting organism
- Electrolyte replacement
- Analgesics

Surgery

- Treatment of choice; procedure varies with the cause of peritonitis

Nursing considerations

Key outcomes

The patient will:
- regain normal vital signs
- express feelings of increased comfort

○ maintain normal fluid volume
○ show no signs or symptoms of infection.

Nursing interventions

○ Give prescribed drugs.
○ Encourage early postoperative ambulation.
○ Encourage the patient to express his feelings.
○ Provide emotional support.

Monitoring

○ Fluid and nutritional status
○ Pain control
○ Vital signs
○ NG tube function and drainage
○ Bowel function
○ Wound site
○ Signs and symptoms of dehiscence

 Alert

*Watch for signs and symptoms of abscess forma-
tion, including persistent abdominal tenderness
and fever.*

Patient teaching

Be sure to cover:
○ the disorder, diagnosis, and treatment
○ preoperatively, coughing and deep-breathing techniques
○ postoperative care procedures
○ signs and symptoms of infection
○ proper wound care
○ drug administration, dosage, and possible adverse
effects
○ dietary and activity limitations (depending on type of
surgery).

...us respiratory infection
...ses an irritating cough that becomes
... and ends in a high-pitched, inspiratory

a 6- to 8-week course that includes three
...к stages with varying symptoms
called *whooping cough*

...ophysiology

The infecting organism adheres to ciliated epithelial cells and multiplies.
○ The resulting local mucosal damage induces paroxysmal coughing, which enhances disease transmission.
○ Various toxins produced during the infection impair local defenses and cause local tissue damage. Toxins may cause direct central nervous system injury.

Causes

○ Nonmotile, gram-negative coccobacillus *B. pertussis;* occasionally, *B. parapertussis* or *B. bronchiseptica* (see *Bordetella pertussis*)
○ Typically transmitted by direct inhalation of contaminated droplets from someone in the acute disease stage
○ Spreads indirectly through soiled linen and other articles contaminated by respiratory secretions

Bordetella pertussis

This microscopic enlargement shows *Bordetella pertussis*, the nonmotile, gram-negative coccobacillus that commonly causes whooping cough. After entering the tracheobronchial tree, pertussis causes mucus to become increasingly tenacious. The classic 6-week course of whooping cough follows.

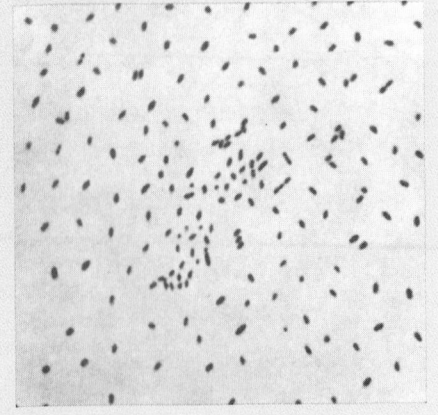

Incidence

○ 50% of cases seen in underimmunized children younger than age 1
○ Commonly occurs in schools, nursing homes, and residential facilities
○ Epidemics occurring every 3 to 5 years without seasonal variation

Common characteristics

Catarrhal (first) stage
○ Hacking nocturnal cough
○ Anorexia
○ Sneezing, lacrimation, and rhinorrhea
Paroxysmal (second) stage
○ Spasmodic, recurrent coughing (usually at night) with tenacious mucus; cough typically ends in a loud, crowing, inspiratory whoop
○ Vomiting if the patient chokes on mucus
Convalescent (third) stage
○ Gradual subsidence of paroxysmal coughing and vomiting

Complications

○ Increased venous pressure
○ Anterior eye chamber hemorrhage
○ Detached retina and blindness
○ Rectal prolapse
○ Inguinal or umbilical hernia
○ Encephalopathy, seizures
○ Atelectasis, pneumonitis, or pneumonia
○ In infants: apnea, anoxia
○ Otitis media
○ Pneumonia

Assessment

History

○ Possible lack of immunization coupled with exposure to pertussis during previous 3 weeks

Physical findings

○ Low or normal body temperature
○ Mild conjunctivitis
○ Listlessness
○ Engorged neck veins
○ Epistaxis during paroxysmal coughing
○ Exhaustion and cyanosis after coughing spell
○ Diminished breath sounds, upper airway wheezing

Test results

Laboratory
○ White blood cell count and differential showing lymphocytosis
○ *B. pertussis* found in nasopharyngeal swabs and sputum culture in early disease stages
○ Direct immunofluorescence showing antigen

Treatment

General

- ○ For infants and elderly patients: hospitalization with vigorous supportive therapy and fluid and electrolyte replacement
- ○ Oxygen therapy, as warranted
- ○ Adequate nutrition with small, frequent meals
- ○ Increased fluid intake
- ○ Rest periods when fatigued

Medication

- ○ Antitussives
- ○ Antibiotics

Nursing considerations

Key outcomes

The patient will:
- ○ remain free from adventitious breath sounds
- ○ maintain a patent airway
- ○ regain normal arterial blood gas levels
- ○ show no evidence of pathogens in cultures.

Nursing interventions

- ○ Maintain respiratory isolation (mask only) for 5 to 7 days after antibiotic therapy begins.
- ○ Provide oxygen and moist air, as ordered; if needed, assist respiration.
- ○ Suction secretions, as necessary. Elevate the head of the bed to ease breathing.
- ○ Create a quiet environment to decrease coughing stimulation.
- ○ Assess for complications caused by excessive coughing.
- ○ Provide emotional support to the patient and parents, as appropriate.
- ○ Report pertussis cases to local public health authorities.

Monitoring

- ○ Respiratory status
- ○ Acid-base balance
- ○ Fluid and electrolyte balance

Patient teaching

Be sure to cover (with the patient or parents, as appropriate):
- ○ the disease process and medical procedures
- ○ need for the patient's close contacts to get medical care
- ○ when to notify the physician

- ○ importance of immunization and vaccination the need to notify the physician of adverse r to the vaccine.

Discharge planning

- ○ Refer the patient to a pulmonologist for follow-care, as indicated.

...c inflammation of the pharynx
..., throat disorder
...ides in 3 to 10 days unless complications

...ysiology

...ar damage caused by a virus or bacteria causes
...nflammatory response.
...yperemia and fluid exudation result.

...auses

○ Viral or bacterial infection
○ Beta-hemolytic streptococci (15% to 20% of acute pharyngitis cases)
○ Mononucleosis
In children
○ Streptococcal bacteria infections
Gonococcal pharyngitis
○ Release of a toxin produced by *Corynebacterium diphtheria*
Fungal pharyngitis
○ Prolonged antibiotic use (in immunosuppressed patients)

Incidence

Widespread among adults who:
○ live or work in dusty or dry environments
○ use their voices excessively
○ use tobacco or alcohol habitually
○ suffer from chronic sinusitis, persistent coughs, or allergies

Common characteristics

○ Sore throat
○ Pharyngeal edema

Complications

○ Otitis media
○ Sinusitis
○ Mastoiditis
○ Rheumatic fever
○ Nephritis

Assessment

History

○ Sore throat
○ Slight difficulty swallowing (swallowing saliva more painful than swallowing food)
○ Sensation of a lump in the throat
○ Constant, aggravating urge to swallow
○ Headache
○ Muscle and joint pain

Physical findings

○ Mild fever
○ Fiery red appearance of the posterior pharyngeal wall
○ Swollen, exudate-flecked tonsils
○ Lymphoid follicles
Bacterial pharyngitis
○ Acutely inflamed throat, with patches of white and yellow follicles
○ Strawberry-red tongue
○ Enlarged, tender cervical lymph nodes

Test results

Laboratory
○ Throat culture identifying the causative organism
○ Rapid strep test showing group A beta-hemolytic streptococcal infection
○ White blood cell count and differential showing atypical lymphocytes
Imaging
○ Computed tomography scans identify abscesses.

Treatment

General

○ Warm saline gargles
○ Hospitalization for dehydration
○ Elimination of the underlying cause
○ Adequate humidification
○ Adequate fluid intake
○ Avoidance of citrus juices
○ Bed rest while febrile

Medication

○ Anesthetic throat lozenges
○ Analgesics, as needed
○ Antibiotics
○ Antifungal agents (for fungal pharyngitis)
○ Equine antitoxins (for diphtherial pharyngitis)

Surgery

○ Abscess drainage

Nursing considerations

Key outcomes

The patient will:
○ maintain intact mucous membranes
○ maintain normal fluid volume
○ express feelings of increased comfort
○ achieve adequate daily calorie intake.

Nursing interventions

○ Give prescribed drugs.
○ Obtain throat cultures, as ordered.
○ Instruct the patient to use warm saline gargles.
○ Encourage adequate oral fluid intake.
○ Perform meticulous mouth care.
○ Maintain a restful environment.

Monitoring
○ Intake and output
○ Signs and symptoms of dehydration

 Alert

Examine the patient's skin twice per day for rashes caused by drug sensitivity or rashes that could indicate a communicable disease.

Patient teaching

Be sure to cover:
○ the disorder, diagnosis, and treatment
○ importance of completing prescribed antibiotic therapy
○ drug administration, dosage, and possible adverse effects
○ preventive measures
○ avoidance of excessive exposure to air conditioning
○ smoking cessation
○ ways to minimize environmental sources of throat irritation
○ importance of throat cultures for all family members if the patient has a streptococcal infection.

Discharge planning
○ Refer the patient to a smoking-cessation program, if indicated.

Pheochromocytoma

Overview

Description

- Catecholamine-producing tumor, typically benign; usually derived from adrenal medullary cells
- Most common cause of adrenal medullary hypersecretion
- Usually produces norepinephrine; large tumors secrete both epinephrine and norepinephrine
- Potentially fatal, but with treatment carries a good prognosis
- Also known as *chromaffin tumor*

Pathophysiology

- Pheochromocytoma causes excessive catecholamine production from autonomous tumor functioning.
- The tumor stems from a chromaffin cell tumor of the adrenal medulla or sympathetic ganglia (more commonly in the right adrenal gland than in the left).
- Extra-adrenal pheochromocytomas may occur in the abdomen, thorax, urinary bladder, and neck and in association with the 9th and 10th cranial nerves.

Causes

- May be inherited as an autosomal dominant trait

Incidence

- Rare; seen in about 0.5% of newly diagnosed hypertensive patients
- Seen in all races
- Affects both sexes equally
- Typically familial
- Most common in patients ages 30 to 50

Common characteristics

- Paroxysmal or sustained hypertension
- Hypertensive crises triggered by conditions that displace the abdominal contents or by use of opiates, histamine, glucagon, or corticotropin
- Headache
- Flushing
- Diaphoresis
- Tachycardia
- Retinal changes

Complications

- Stroke
- Retinopathy
- Irreversible kidney damage
- Acute pulmonary edema
- Cholelithiasis
- Cardiac arrhythmias
- Heart failure

Alert

Pheochromocytoma may occur during pregnancy when uterine pressure on the tumor causes more frequent hypertensive crises. These crises carry a high risk for spontaneous abortion and can be fatal for both the mother and fetus.

Assessment

History

- Unpredictable episodes of hypertensive crisis
- Paroxysmal symptoms suggesting a seizure disorder or anxiety attack
- Hypertension that responds poorly to conventional treatment
- Hypotension or shock after surgery or diagnostic procedures

During paroxysms or crises
- Throbbing headache
- Palpitations
- Visual blurring
- Nausea and vomiting
- Severe diaphoresis
- Feelings of impending doom
- Precordial or abdominal pain
- Moderate weight loss
- Dizziness or light-headedness when moving to an upright position

Physical findings

During paroxysms or crises
- Hypertension
- Tachypnea
- Pallor or flushing
- Profuse sweating
- Tremor
- Seizures
- Tachycardia

Test results

Laboratory
- Increased levels of vanillylmandelic acid and metanephrine in 24-hour urine specimen
- Total plasma catecholamine levels 10 to 50 times higher than normal on direct assay

Imaging
- Computed tomography (CT) scan or magnetic resonance imaging of adrenal glands may show intra-adrenal lesions.
- CT scan, chest X-rays, or abdominal aortography may reveal extra-adrenal pheochromocytoma.

Treatment

General

- High-protein diet with adequate calories
- Rest during acute attacks

Medication

- Alpha-adrenergic blockers
- Catecholamine-synthesis antagonists
- Beta-adrenergic blockers
- Calcium channel blockers
- I.V. phentolamine or nitroprusside during paroxysms or crises

 Alert

Because severe and occasionally fatal paroxysms have been induced by opiates, histamine, and other drugs, all medications should be considered carefully and administered cautiously in patients with known or suspected pheochromocytoma.

Surgery

- Removal of pheochromocytoma

Nursing considerations

Key outcomes

The patient will:
- maintain stable vital signs
- maintain fluid balance
- maintain normal cardiac output
- express feelings of increased comfort
- avoid complications.

Nursing interventions

- Take orthostatic blood pressures.
- Give prescribed drugs.
- Ensure the reliability of urine catecholamine measurements.
- Provide comfort measures.
- Consult a dietitian, as needed.
- Tell the patient to report symptoms of an acute attack.
- Encourage the patient to express his feelings.
- Help the patient develop effective coping strategies.

After adrenalectomy

 Alert

Be aware that postoperative hypertension is common because the stress of surgery and adrenal gland manipulation stimulate catecholamine secretion.

Monitoring

- Vital signs, especially blood pressure
- Serum glucose level
- Daily weight
- Neurologic status
- Renal function
- Cardiovascular status
- Adverse reactions to medications

After adrenalectomy
- Vital signs
- Bowel sounds
- Wound dressings
- Incision
- Signs and symptoms of hemorrhage
- Pain

Patient teaching

Be sure to cover:
- the disorder, diagnosis, and treatment
- drug administration, dosage, and possible adverse effects
- when to notify the physician
- way to prevent paroxysmal attacks
- signs and symptoms of adrenal insufficiency
- importance of wearing medical identification jewelry
- how to monitor his own blood pressure.

Discharge planning

- Refer family members for genetic counseling if autosomal dominant transmission of pheochromocytoma is suspected.

Pituitary tumors

Overview

Description

- Nonmalignant intracranial tumor; accounts for 10% of all intracranial neoplasms
- Most common tumor tissue types: chromophobe adenoma (90%), basophil adenoma, and eosinophil adenoma
- Most common site: anterior pituitary (adenohypophysis)
- Considered a neoplastic condition because of the tumor's invasive growth
- Carries a fair to good prognosis, depending on how far the tumor spreads beyond the sella turcica

Pathophysiology

- As a pituitary adenoma grows, it replaces normal glandular tissue and enlarges the sella turcica (which houses it).
- Chromophobe adenoma may be associated with production of corticotropin, melanocyte-stimulating hormone, growth hormone, and prolactin.
- Basophil adenoma may be associated with excess corticotropin production and, consequently, Cushing's syndrome.
- Eosinophil adenoma may be associated with excessive growth hormone.

Causes

- Unknown

Risk factors

- Autosomal dominant trait

Incidence

- Affects adults of both sexes between ages 30 and 50
- Twice more common in females than in males

Common characteristics

- Headache, visual changes, double vision, and drooping eyelids
- Nipple discharge
- Gynecomastia
- Menses cessation
- Decreased libido, male impotence
- Cold intolerance
- Nausea, vomiting, and constipation
- Personality changes
- Skin changes
- Hair loss
- Fatigue
- Seizures
- Hypotension

Complications

- Endocrine abnormalities throughout the body, unless lost hormones are replaced
- Diabetes insipidus from tumor compression of the hypothalamus

Assessment

History

- Neurologic and endocrine abnormalities
- Personality changes or dementia
- Amenorrhea
- Decreased libido
- Impotence
- Lethargy, weakness, increased fatigability
- Sensitivity to cold
- Constipation
- Seizures
- With cranial nerve involvement: diplopia and dizziness

Physical findings

- Rhinorrhea
- Head tilting during physical examination
- Skin changes
- Strabismus

Test results

Laboratory
- Increased protein level in cerebrospinal fluid

Imaging
- Skull X-rays with tomography may show an enlarged sella turcica or erosion of its floor; if growth hormone secretion predominates, X-rays show enlargement of the paranasal sinuses and mandible, thickened cranial bones, and separated teeth.
- Carotid angiography may identify displacement of the anterior cerebral and internal carotid arteries from tumor enlargement and may rule out intracerebral aneurysm.
- Computed tomography scan may confirm an adenoma and accurately depict its size.
- Magnetic resonance imaging scan differentiates healthy, benign, and malignant tissues and blood vessels.

Treatment

General

- Radiation therapy used for small, nonsecretory tumors confined to the sella turcica or for patients considered poor surgical risks
- Individualized diet according to tumor manifestations; possible sodium or caloric restriction
- In initial postoperative period, avoidance of coughing, sneezing, bending, and other movements that may increase intracranial pressure (ICP) or cause cerebrospinal fluid leakage

Medication

○ Corticosteroids or thyroid or sex hormones
○ Electrolyte replacement
○ Insulin
○ Bromocriptine (a dopamine agent)

Surgery

○ Transfrontal removal of a large tumor impinging on the optic apparatus
○ Transsphenoidal resection for a smaller tumor confined to the pituitary fossa
○ Cryohypophysectomy

Nursing considerations

Key outcomes

The patient will:
○ remain free from injury
○ express positive feelings about himself
○ report an increased sense of well-being
○ exhibit increased energy
○ participate in care and prescribed therapies (along with family members).

Nursing interventions

○ Give prescribed drugs.
○ Maintain patient safety.
○ Provide rest periods to avoid fatigue.
○ Establish a supportive, trusting relationship with the patient.

Monitoring

After supratentorial or transsphenoidal hypophysectomy
○ Proper positioning (head of the bed elevated 30 degrees)
○ Intake and output
○ Signs and symptoms of infection
○ Blood glucose level
After craniotomy
○ Vital signs
○ Neurologic status
○ Signs and symptoms of increased ICP

Patient teaching

Be sure to cover:
○ the disorder, diagnosis, and treatment
○ preoperative instructions on surgery, treatments, and postoperative course
○ avoidance of coughing, sneezing, and bending
○ importance of immediately reporting persistent postnasal drip or constant swallowing.

Discharge planning

○ Encourage the patient to wear medical identification that indicates his medical condition and its proper treatment.

Placenta previa

Overview

Description

- Placental implantation in the lower uterine segment, encroaching on the internal cervical os
- Common cause of bleeding during the second half of pregnancy (Among patients who develop placenta previa during the second trimester, less than 15% have persistent previa at term.)
- Carries good maternal prognosis if hemorrhage can be controlled
- Usually necessitates pregnancy termination if bleeding is heavy
- Fetal prognosis dependent on gestational age and amount of blood lost; risk for death greatly reduced by frequent monitoring and prompt management

Pathophysiology

- The placenta covers all or part of the internal cervical os. (See *Three types of placenta previa.*)

Causes

- Unknown

Factors that may affect the site of placental attachment to the uterine wall
- Defective vascularization of the decidua
- Multiple pregnancy
- Previous uterine surgery
- Multiparity
- Advanced maternal age
- Endometriosis
- Smoking

Incidence

- About 1 in every 200 pregnancies
- More common in multigravidas than primigravidas
- Occurs more commonly after age 35

Common characteristics

- Painless, bright red, vaginal bleeding
- Vaginal bleeding after 20th week of pregnancy

Complications

- Anemia
- Hemorrhage
- Disseminated intravascular coagulation
- Shock
- Renal damage
- Cerebral ischemia
- Maternal or fetal death

Assessment

History

- Onset of painless, bright red, vaginal bleeding after 20th week of pregnancy
- Vaginal bleeding before labor onset, typically episodic and stopping spontaneously
- May be asymptomatic

Physical findings

- Soft, nontender uterus
- Fetal malpresentation
- Minimal descent of fetal presenting part
- Good fetal heart tones

Test results

Laboratory
- Decreased maternal hemoglobin level

Imaging
- Transvaginal ultrasound scanning determines placental position.

Diagnostic procedures
- Pelvic examination confirms diagnosis.

 Alert

Pelvic examination isn't commonly performed because it increases maternal bleeding and can dislodge more of the placenta.

Treatment

General

- Control of blood loss, blood replacement
- Delivery of viable neonate
- Prevention of coagulation disorders
- With premature fetus, careful observation to give fetus more time to mature
- With complete placenta previa, hospitalization
- Possible vaginal delivery if bleeding is minimal and placenta previa is marginal or when labor is rapid

 Alert

Because of possible fetal blood loss through the placenta, a pediatric team should be on hand during delivery to immediately assess and treat neonatal shock, blood loss, and hypoxia.

- Nothing by mouth initially, then as guided by clinical status
- Bed rest

Medication

- I.V. fluids, using large-bore catheter

The degree of placenta previa depends largely on the extent of cervical dilation at the time of examination because the dilating cervix gradually uncovers the placenta, as shown below.

Marginal placenta previa
If the placenta covers just a fraction of the internal cervical os, the patient has marginal, or low-lying, placenta previa.

Partial placenta previa
The patient has the partial, or incomplete, form of the disorder if the placenta caps a larger part of the internal os.

Total placenta previa
If the placenta covers all of the internal os, the patient has total, complete, or central placenta previa.

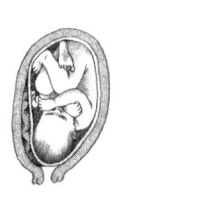
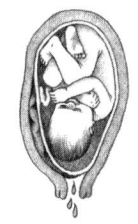
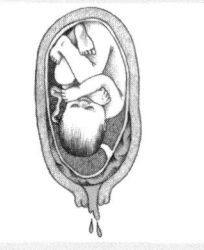

Surgery

○ Immediate cesarean delivery in case of severe hemorrhage or as soon as fetus is sufficiently mature

Nursing considerations

Key outcomes

The patient will:
○ maintain stable vital signs
○ maintain normal fluid volume
○ express feelings of increased comfort
○ verbalize her feelings about her condition
○ use available support systems to aid coping.

Nursing interventions

○ Obtain blood specimens for complete blood count and blood type and cross match.
○ Initiate external electronic fetal monitoring.
○ Give prescribed I.V. fluids and blood products.
○ If the patient is Rh-negative, give Rho(D) immune globulin (RhoGAM) after every bleeding episode, as ordered.
○ Offer emotional support during labor.
○ Provide information about labor progress and the condition of the fetus.
○ Encourage the patient to express her feelings.
○ Help the patient develop effective coping strategies.

Monitoring

○ Vital signs
○ Vaginal bleeding, including character of blood loss
○ Central venous pressure
○ Intake and output
○ Fetal heart tones
○ Signs and symptoms of hemorrhage and shock

Patient teaching

Be sure to cover:
○ the disorder, diagnosis, and treatment
○ signs and symptoms of placenta previa
○ possibility of emergency cesarean delivery
○ possibility of the birth of a premature neonate
○ possibility of neonatal death
○ postpartum physical and emotional changes to expect.

Discharge planning

○ Refer the patient for professional counseling if necessary.

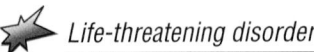 *Life-threatening disorder*

Plague

Overview

Description

- Acute, febrile, zoonotic infection caused by the gram-negative, nonsporulating bacillus *Yersinia pestis*
- Usually transmitted to humans through the bite of a flea from an infected rodent host, such as a rat or squirrel; occasional transmission from handling infected animals or their tissues (see *Bubonic plague carrier*)
- Potential bioterrorism and biological warfare agent

Forms of plague
- *Bubonic:* most common form; causes swollen and sometimes suppurating, lymph glands (buboes)
- *Septicemic:* rapid, severe systemic form
- *Pneumonic:* can be primary or secondary to the other two forms; highly contagious, with secondary spread a serious concern (Primary pneumonic plague is an acutely fulminant form causing acute prostration, respiratory distress, and death, possibly within 2 to 3 days after onset. Secondary pneumonic plague is transmitted by contaminated respiratory droplets.)
- Without treatment, 60% mortality in bubonic plague and nearly 100% in septicemic and pneumonic plague; with treatment, 18% mortality

Pathophysiology

- *Y. pestis* is one of the most invasive bacterium known; mechanisms by which it causes disease aren't fully understood.
- Once inoculated through the skin or mucous membranes, *Y. pestis* usually invades cutaneous lymphatic vessels and regional lymph nodes; direct bloodstream inoculation may also occur.
- Organisms probably are phagocytized by mononuclear phagocytes without being destroyed and are then disseminated to distant sites in the body.
- Plague can involve almost any organ and usually results in massive and widespread tissue destruction, especially if left untreated.

Causes

- *Y. pestis*

Incidence

- Becoming more prevalent in the United States
- Most common between May and September; in hunters who skin wild animals, between October and February
- Affects both sexes equally

Common characteristics
- Fever
- Chills
- Weakness
- Headache

Bubonic plague
- Characteristic buboes
- History of exposure to rodents

Complications
- Peritoneal or pleural effusions
- Septicemia
- Fulminant pneumonia
- Pericarditis
- Seizures
- Diffuse interstitial myocarditis
- Multifocal hepatic necrosis
- Diffuse hemorrhagic splenic necrosis
- Respiratory failure
- Cardiovascular collapse
- Disseminated intravascular coagulation
- Meningitis
- Death

Assessment

History

Milder form of bubonic plague
- History of exposure to rodents
- Malaise
- Fever
- Excruciatingly painful bubo

Severe form of bubonic plague
- Sudden fever of 103° to 106° F (39.4° to 41.1° C)
- Chills, myalgia, and headache
- Restlessness, disorientation
- Abdominal pain, nausea, and vomiting
- Constipation followed by bloody diarrhea

Physical findings

Milder form of bubonic plague
- Fever
- Pain or tenderness in regional lymph nodes
- Painful, inflamed, and possibly suppurative buboes (usually in the axillary, cervical, or inguinal areas)
- Necrotization of hemorrhagic areas
- Moribund state within hours after onset

Bubonic plague
- Fever
- Prostration
- Restlessness, disorientation, delirium
- Toxemia
- Staggering gait
- Skin mottling, petechiae
- Circulatory collapse
- Coma

Test results

Laboratory

○ *Y. pestis* found in capsular antigen testing, Wayson stain, or fluorescent antibody stain
○ White blood cell count above 20,000/μl, with increased polymorphonuclear leukocytes and hemoagglutination reaction
○ *Y. pestis* present in culture and Gram stain of skin-lesion needle aspirate or lymph node aspirate, blood, or sputum

Imaging

○ Chest X-rays show fulminating pneumonia in pneumonic plague.

Treatment

General

○ Supportive management to control fever, shock, and seizures and maintain fluid balance
○ Warm, moist compresses on buboes
○ Diet, as tolerated
○ Tube feedings or total parenteral nutrition, if required
○ Supplemental I.V. fluids
○ Bed rest during the acute phase

Medication

○ Antibiotics
○ Oxygen
○ Corticosteroids
○ Benzodiazepines
○ Anticonvulsants
○ Antipyretics

Surgery

○ Incision and drainage of necrotic buboes

Nursing considerations

Key outcomes

The patient will:
○ maintain acceptable tissue perfusion and cellular oxygenation
○ maintain effective ventilation
○ maintain fluid balance
○ verbalize feelings of fear and anxiety
○ demonstrate effective coping mechanisms.

Nursing interventions

○ Give drugs, I.V. fluids, and oxygen, as prescribed and needed.
○ If pneumonic plague, use standard and droplet precautions.
○ Provide adequate nutrition.
○ Maintain a patent airway and adequate oxygenation.
○ Apply warm, moist compresses to buboes.
○ Provide meticulous skin care.
○ Prevent further injury to necrotic tissue areas.

Bubonic plague carrier

Bubonic plague is usually transmitted to humans through the bite of an infected flea (*Xenopsylla cheopis*), shown here.

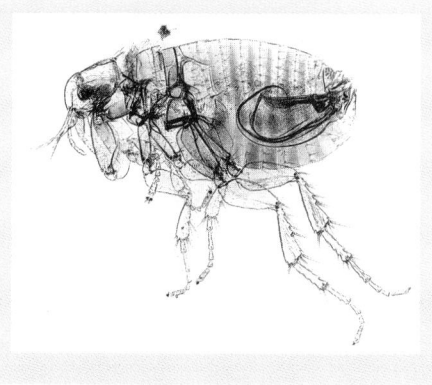

○ Institute seizure precautions.
○ Report suspected plague cases to local public health department.

Monitoring

○ Vital signs
○ Intake and output
○ Skin integrity
○ Pulmonary status
○ Cardiovascular status
○ Nutritional status
○ Seizures
○ Complications
○ Abnormal bleeding
○ Mentation

Patient teaching

Be sure to cover:
○ the disorder, diagnosis, and treatment
○ drug administration, dosage, and possible adverse effects
○ isolation procedures
○ personal protective measures
○ avoidance of contact with sick or dead wild animals and the need to wear gloves when handling animal carcasses
○ importance of insect and rodent population control
○ use of repellents, insecticides, and protective clothing when at risk for exposure to rodents' fleas
○ elimination of rodent food and habitats
○ insecticide control of fleas.

Pleural effusion and empyema

Overview

Description

○ Fluid accumulation in the pleural space; the fluid may be extracellular, pus (empyema), blood (hemothorax), chyle (chylothorax), or bilious
○ Effusion classified as transudative or exudative

Pathophysiology

○ Typically, fluid and other blood components migrate through the walls of intact capillaries bordering the pleura.
○ In *transudative* effusion, fluid is watery and diffuses out of the capillaries if hydrostatic pressure increases or capillary oncotic pressure decreases.
○ In *exudative* effusion, inflammatory processes increase capillary permeability. Exudative effusion is less watery and contains high concentrations of white blood cells and plasma proteins.
○ Empyema occurs when pulmonary lymphatics become blocked, leading to outpouring of contaminated lymphatic fluid into the pleural space.

Causes

Transudative pleural effusion
○ Cardiovascular disease
○ Hepatic disease
○ Renal disease
○ Hypoproteinemia
Exudative pleural effusion
○ Pleural infection
○ Pleural inflammation
○ Pleural malignancy
Empyema
○ Pulmonary infection
○ Lung abscess
○ Infected wound
○ Intra-abdominal infection
○ Thoracic surgery

Incidence

○ Can occur at any age
○ Affects both sexes equally

Common characteristics

○ Shortness of breath
○ Chest pain
○ Malaise
○ Nonproductive cough

Complications

○ Atelectasis
○ Infection
○ Hypoxemia

Assessment

History

○ Underlying pulmonary disease
○ Shortness of breath
○ Chest pain
○ Malaise

Physical findings

○ Fever
○ Trachea deviated away from the affected side
○ Dullness and decreased tactile fremitus over the effusion
○ Diminished or absent breath sounds
○ Pleural friction rub
○ Bronchial breath sounds
○ In empyema, foul-smelling sputum

Test results

Laboratory
PLEURAL FLUID ANALYSIS FINDINGS
○ In transudative effusion: specific gravity below 1.015; less than 3 g/dl of protein
○ In exudative effusion: 0.5 or higher ratio of protein in pleural fluid to protein in serum; lactate dehydrogenase (LDH) level of 200 IU or higher; 0.6 or higher ratio of LDH in pleural fluid to LDH in serum
○ In empyema: microorganisms, increased white blood cell count, decreased glucose level
○ In esophageal rupture or pancreatitis: pleural fluid amylase levels exceeding serum amylase levels
Imaging
○ Chest X-rays may show pleural effusions; lateral decubitus films may show loculated pleural effusions or small pleural effusions not visible on standard chest X-rays.
○ Computed tomography scan of the thorax shows small pleural effusions.
Diagnostic procedures
○ Thoracentesis obtains pleural fluid specimens for analysis
Other
○ Tuberculin skin test may be positive for tuberculosis.
○ Pleural biopsy may be positive for carcinoma.

Treatment

General

○ Thoracentesis to remove fluid
○ Possible chest tube insertion
○ Possible chemical pleurodesis
○ High-calorie diet
○ Activity, as tolerated

Medication

○ Antibiotics
○ Oxygen

Surgery

○ Removal of thick coating over lung (decortication)

Nursing considerations

Key outcomes

The patient will:
○ maintain adequate ventilation
○ remain free from signs and symptoms of infection
○ consume the specified number of calories daily
○ express an understanding of the illness
○ demonstrate effective coping mechanisms.

Nursing interventions

○ Give prescribed drugs and oxygen.
○ Assist during thoracentesis.
○ Encourage the patient to use incentive spirometry.
○ Encourage deep-breathing exercises.
○ Provide meticulous chest tube care.
○ Ensure chest tube patency.
○ Keep petroleum gauze at the bedside.

Monitoring

○ Vital signs
○ Intake and output
○ Respiratory status
○ Pulse oximetry
○ Signs and symptoms of pneumothorax
○ Chest tube drainage

Patient teaching

Be sure to cover:
○ the disorder, diagnosis, and treatment
○ drug administration, dosage, and possible adverse effects
○ how thoracentesis is performed
○ chest tube insertion and drainage
○ signs and symptoms of infection
○ signs and symptoms of pleural fluid reaccumulation
○ when to notify the physician.

Discharge planning

○ Provide a home health referral for follow-up care.
○ Refer the patient to a smoking-cessation program, if indicated.

Pleurisy

Overview

Description
○ Inflammation of the visceral and parietal pleurae that line the inside of the thoracic cage and envelop the lungs
○ Also called *pleuritis*

Pathophysiology
○ The pleurae become swollen and congested.
○ As a result, pleural fluid transport is hampered, and friction between the pleural surfaces increases.

Causes
○ Pneumonia
○ Tuberculosis
○ Viruses
○ Systemic lupus erythematosus
○ Rheumatoid arthritis
○ Uremia
○ Dressler's syndrome
○ Cancer
○ Pulmonary infarction
○ Chest trauma
○ Pathologic rib fractures
○ Pneumothorax
○ Sickle cell disease
○ Radiation therapy
○ Human immunodeficiency virus
○ Certain drugs, such as methotrexate or penicillin

Incidence
○ Affects both sexes equally

Common characteristics
○ Sudden dull, aching, burning, or sharp pain that worsens on inspiration
○ Limited movement on the affected side during breathing
○ Shortness of breath

Complications
○ Adhesions
○ Pleural effusion
○ Chronic pain or shortness of breath

Assessment

History
○ Sudden dull, aching, burning, or sharp pain that worsens on inspiration
○ Predisposing factor
○ Cough
○ Shortness of breath
○ Fever

Physical findings
○ Characteristic late-inspiration and early-expiration pleural friction rub
○ Coarse vibration on palpation of the affected area

Test results
Imaging
○ Chest X-rays show absence of pneumonia.
Diagnostic procedures
○ Electrocardiography shows absence of ischemic heart disease.

Treatment

General
○ Symptomatic
○ Possible intercostal nerve block
○ Diet, as tolerated
○ Bed rest

Medication
○ Anti-inflammatory agents
○ Analgesics

Surgery
○ Thoracentesis

Nursing considerations

Key outcomes
The patient will:
○ maintain a patent airway
○ maintain adequate ventilation
○ express feelings of increased comfort and relief of pain
○ demonstrate energy conservation techniques
○ demonstrate effective coping strategies.

Nursing interventions
○ Give prescribed drugs.
○ Encourage deep breathing and coughing.
○ Encourage the patient to use incentive spirometry.
○ Assist the patient in splinting the affected side.
○ Position the patient in high Fowler's position.
○ Plan care to allow frequent rest periods.
○ Assist with passive range-of-motion (ROM) exercises.
○ Encourage active ROM exercises.
○ Provide comfort measures.
○ Assist with thoracentesis.
○ Encourage verbalization and provide emotional support.

Monitoring
○ Vital signs
○ Intake and output
○ Response to treatment
○ Pain control
○ Complications

○ Breath sounds
○ Respiratory status

Patient teaching

Be sure to cover:
○ the disorder, diagnosis, and treatment
○ drug administration, dosage, and possible adverse effects
○ how to perform splinting and deep-breathing exercises
○ importance of regular rest periods
○ signs and symptoms of possible complications
○ when to notify the physician.

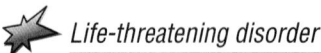

Pneumocystis carinii pneumonia

Overview

Description

○ Communicable, opportunistic lung infection frequently associated with human immunodeficiency virus (HIV)
○ A leading cause of opportunistic infection and death among patients with acquired immunodeficiency syndrome (AIDS) in industrialized countries

Pathophysiology

○ The infecting organism invades the lungs bilaterally, multiplies extracellularly, and fills alveoli with organisms and exudate.
○ As a result, gas exchange is impaired.
○ Alveoli hypertrophy and thicken, eventually leading to extensive consolidation.

Causes

○ *P. carinii;* spreads mainly through the air (although part of the normal flora in most healthy people, this organism becomes an aggressive pathogen in immunocompromised patients)
○ Possible role of B-cell function defects

Incidence

○ Most common in premature or malnourished infants, children with primary immunodeficiency disease, patients receiving immunosuppressive therapy, and those with HIV/AIDS

Common characteristics

○ Insidious onset, with increasing shortness of breath and nonproductive cough
○ Hypoxemia and hypercapnia (may not cause significant clinical symptoms)

Complications

○ Disseminated infection
○ Pulmonary insufficiency and death

Assessment

History

○ Immunodepression, as from HIV infection, leukemia, lymphoma, or organ transplantation

Physical findings

○ Low-grade, intermittent fever
○ Tachypnea
○ Dyspnea
○ Accessory muscle use for breathing
○ Cyanosis (with acute illness)
○ Dullness on percussion (with consolidation)
○ Crackles
○ Decreased breath sounds

Test results

Laboratory
○ *P. carinii* found on histologic sputum specimen studies
○ Hypoxia, increased A-a gradient on arterial blood gas (ABG) values
Imaging
○ Chest X-rays may show slowly progressing, fluffy infiltrates, occasional nodular lesions, or spontaneous pneumothorax.
○ Gallium scan may show increased uptake over the lungs.
Diagnostic procedures
○ Fiber-optic bronchoscopy
○ Transbronchial biopsy
○ Open lung biopsy

Treatment

General

○ Oxygen therapy
○ Mechanical ventilation
○ High-calorie, high-protein diet
○ Nutritional supplements, as needed
○ Small, frequent meals
○ Increased fluid intake
○ Rest periods when fatigued

Medication

○ Co-trimoxazole (may be given prophylactically to AIDS and other high-risk patients)
○ Pentamidine

Nursing considerations

Key outcomes

The patient will:
○ maintain normal vital signs
○ maintain adequate fluid volume
○ maintain normal breath sounds
○ regain normal ABG values
○ demonstrate correct bronchial hygiene techniques
○ verbalize fears, feelings, and concerns.

Nursing interventions

○ Implement standard precautions.
○ Give prescribed drugs and oxygen.
○ Encourage ambulation, deep-breathing exercises, and use of incentive spirometry.
○ Provide adequate rest periods.
○ Encourage the patient to express fears, feelings, and concerns.
○ Provide emotional support.

Monitoring
○ Respiratory status
○ ABG values
○ Fluid and electrolyte status

Patient teaching

Be sure to cover:
○ the disorder, diagnosis, and treatment
○ drug administration, dosage, and possible adverse
  effects
○ energy conservation techniques
○ prevention (for HIV-infected patients and other immunocompromised individuals)
○ home oxygen therapy, if indicated.

Discharge planning
○ Refer the patient to a pulmonologist or an infectious
  diseases specialist for follow-up care, as needed.
○ If the patient has AIDS or HIV, provide information
  about resources and support organizations.

Pneumonia

Overview

Description

○ Acute infection of the lung parenchyma that impairs gas exchange
○ May be classified by etiology, location, or type

Pathophysiology

○ A gel-like substance forms as microorganisms and phagocytic cells break down.
○ This substance consolidates within the lower airway structure.
○ Inflammation involves the alveoli, alveolar ducts, and interstitial spaces surrounding the alveolar walls.
○ In lobar pneumonia, inflammation starts in one area and may extend to the entire lobe. In bronchopneumonia, it starts simultaneously in several areas, producing patchy, diffuse consolidation. In atypical pneumonia, inflammation is confined to the alveolar ducts and interstitial spaces.

Causes

Bacterial and viral pneumonia
○ Chronic illness and debilitation
○ Cancer
○ Abdominal and thoracic surgery
○ Atelectasis
○ Bacterial or viral respiratory infections
○ Chronic respiratory disease
○ Influenza
○ Smoking
○ Malnutrition
○ Alcoholism
○ Sickle cell disease
○ Tracheostomy
○ Exposure to noxious gases
○ Aspiration
○ Immunosuppressive therapy
○ Endotracheal intubation or mechanical ventilation
Aspiration pneumonia
○ Caustic substance entering airway

Risk factors

○ Advanced age
○ Debilitation
○ Nasogastric (NG) tube feedings
○ Impaired gag reflex
○ Poor oral hygiene
○ Decreased level of consciousness

Incidence

○ Affects both sexes and all ages
○ More than four million cases annually in the United States

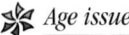 *Age issue*

Incidence and mortality are highest in elderly patients.

Common characteristics

○ Pleuritic chest pain
○ Cough
○ Excessive sputum production
○ Chills

Complications

○ Septic shock
○ Hypoxemia
○ Respiratory failure
○ Empyema
○ Bacteremia
○ Endocarditis
○ Pericarditis
○ Meningitis
○ Lung abscess
○ Pleural effusion

Assessment

History

Bacterial pneumonia
○ Sudden onset of:
  – Pleuritic chest pain
  – Cough
  – Purulent sputum production
  – Chills
Viral pneumonia
○ Nonproductive cough
○ Constitutional symptoms
○ Fever
Aspiration pneumonia
○ Fever
○ Weight loss
○ Malaise

Physical findings

○ Fever
○ Sputum production
○ Dullness over the affected area
○ Crackles, wheezing, or rhonchi
○ Decreased breath sounds
○ Decreased fremitus
○ Tachypnea
○ Use of accessory muscles

Test results

Laboratory
○ Complete blood count showing leukocytosis
○ Positive blood cultures for causative organism
○ Arterial blood gas (ABG) values showing hypoxemia
○ Fungal or acid-fast bacilli cultures identifying the etiologic agent

- Assay for legionella soluble antigen in urine detecting presence of antigen
- Sputum culture, Gram stain, and smear revealing the infecting organism

Imaging
- Chest X-rays generally show patchy or lobar infiltrates.

Diagnostic procedures
- Bronchoscopy or transtracheal aspiration specimens identify the etiologic agent.

Other
- Pulse oximetry may reveal decreased oxygen saturation.

Treatment

General
- Mechanical ventilation (positive end-expiratory pressure) for respiratory failure
- High-calorie, high-protein diet
- Adequate fluids
- Bed rest initially; progress as tolerated

Medication
- Antibiotics
- Humidified oxygen
- Antitussives
- Analgesics
- Bronchodilators

Surgery
- Drainage of parapneumonic pleural effusion or lung abscess

Nursing considerations

Key outcomes
The patient will:
- maintain adequate ventilation
- maintain fluid balance
- maintain adequate caloric intake
- express feelings of increased comfort
- demonstrate effective coping strategies.

Nursing interventions
- Give prescribed drugs.
- Give prescribed I.V. fluids and electrolyte replacement.
- Maintain a patent airway and adequate oxygenation.
- Give prescribed supplemental oxygen. Give oxygen cautiously if the patient has chronic lung disease.
- Suction the patient, as needed.
- Obtain sputum specimens, as needed.
- Provide a high-calorie, high-protein diet of soft foods.
- Give supplemental oral feedings, NG tube feedings, or parenteral nutrition, if needed.
- Take steps to prevent aspiration during NG feedings.
- Dispose of secretions properly.

Preventing pneumonia

- Urge bedridden and postoperative patients to perform deep-breathing and coughing exercises frequently. Position these patients properly to promote full aeration and secretion drainage.
- Advise the patient to avoid using antibiotics indiscriminately for minor infections. Doing so could produce upper airway colonization with antibiotic-resistant bacteria. If pneumonia develops, the causative organisms may require treatment with more toxic antibiotics.
- Encourage the high-risk patient to ask the physician about an annual influenza vaccination and pneumococcal pneumonia vaccination. A single dose of pneumococcal vaccine is recommended for most patients age 54 and older; certain patients may need one booster dose after 5 years.
- Discuss ways to avoid spreading the infection to others. Remind the patient to sneeze and cough into tissues and to dispose of tissues in a waxed or plastic bag. Advise the patient to wash his hands thoroughly after handling contaminated tissues.

- Provide a quiet, calm environment with frequent rest periods.
- Include the patient in care decisions whenever possible.

Monitoring
- Vital signs
- Intake and output
- Daily weight
- Sputum production
- Respiratory status
- Breath sounds
- Pulse oximetry
- ABG values

Patient teaching

Be sure to cover:
- the disorder, diagnosis, and treatment
- drug administration, dosage, and possible adverse effects
- need for adequate fluid intake
- importance of adequate rest
- deep-breathing and coughing exercises
- adequate fluid intake
- chest physiotherapy
- avoidance of irritants that stimulate secretions
- when to notify the physician
- home oxygen therapy, if required
- ways to prevent pneumonia. (See *Preventing pneumonia*.)

Discharge planning
- Refer the patient to a smoking-cessation program, if indicated.

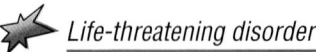 *Life-threatening disorder*

Pneumothorax

Overview

Description
○ Accumulation of air or gas between the parietal and visceral pleurae, leading to lung collapse
○ Degree of lung collapse determined by amount of trapped air or gas
○ Most common pneumothorax types: open, closed, and tension

Pathophysiology
○ Air accumulates and separates the visceral and parietal pleurae.
○ Negative pressure is eliminated, affecting elastic recoil forces.
○ The lung recoils and collapses toward the hilus.
○ In open pneumothorax, atmospheric air flows directly into the pleural cavity, collapsing the lung on the affected side.
○ In closed pneumothorax, air enters the pleural space from within the lung, increasing pleural pressure and preventing lung expansion.
○ In tension pneumothorax, air in the pleural space is under higher pressure than air in the adjacent lung. Air enters the pleural space from a pleural rupture only on inspiration. This air pressure exceeds barometric pressure, causing compression atelectasis. Increased pressure may displace the heart and great vessels and cause mediastinal shift.

Causes
Open pneumothorax
○ Penetrating chest injury
○ Central venous catheter insertion
○ Chest surgery
○ Transbronchial biopsy
○ Thoracentesis
○ Percutaneous lung biopsy
Closed pneumothorax
○ Blunt chest trauma
○ Rib fracture
○ Clavicle fracture
○ Congenital bleb rupture
○ Emphysematous bullae rupture
○ Barotrauma
○ Erosive tubercular or cancerous lesions
○ Interstitial lung disease
Tension pneumothorax
○ Penetrating chest wound
○ Lung or airway puncture from positive-pressure ventilation
○ Mechanical ventilation after chest injury
○ High positive end-expiratory pressures, causing rupture of alveolar blebs

○ Chest tube occlusion or malfunction

Incidence
○ Occurs in 9,000 U.S. residents annually

Common characteristics
○ Sudden, sharp, pleuritic pain
○ Pain exacerbated by chest movement
○ Shortness of breath

Complications
○ Fatal pulmonary and circulatory impairment

Assessment

History
○ Possibly asymptomatic (with small pneumothorax)
○ Sudden, sharp, pleuritic pain
○ Pain that worsens with chest movement, breathing, and coughing
○ Shortness of breath

Physical findings
○ Asymmetrical chest wall movement
○ Overexpansion and rigidity on the affected side
○ Possible cyanosis
○ Subcutaneous emphysema
○ Hyperresonance on the affected side
○ Decreased or absent breath sounds on the affected side
○ Decreased tactile fremitus over the affected side
Tension pneumothorax
○ Distended jugular veins
○ Pallor
○ Anxiety
○ Tracheal deviation away from the affected side
○ Weak, rapid pulse
○ Hypotension
○ Tachypnea
○ Cyanosis

Test results
Laboratory
○ Arterial blood gas analysis possibly showing hypoxemia
Imaging
○ Chest X-rays may show air in the pleural space and, possibly, a mediastinal shift.
Other
○ Pulse oximetry may show decreased oxygen saturation.

Treatment

General
○ Conservative treatment of spontaneous pneumothorax with no signs of increased pleural pressure, less than 30% lung collapse, and no obvious physiologic compromise

- Diet, as tolerated
- Bed rest
- Chest tube insertion
- Needle thoracostomy

Medication

- Oxygen
- Analgesics

Surgery

- Thoracotomy, pleurectomy for recurring spontaneous pneumothorax
- Repair of traumatic pneumothorax
- Doxycycline or talc installation into pleural space

Nursing considerations

Key outcomes

The patient will:
- maintain adequate ventilation
- remain free from signs and symptoms of infection
- express feelings of increased comfort
- demonstrate effective coping strategies.

Nursing interventions

- Give prescribed drugs.
- Assist with chest tube insertion.

 Alert

If the chest tube dislodges, immediately place a petroleum gauze dressing over the opening.

- Provide comfort measures.
- Encourage deep-breathing and coughing exercises.
- Offer reassurance, as appropriate.
- Include the patient and family members in care decisions whenever possible.

Monitoring

- Vital signs
- Intake and output
- Respiratory status
- Breath sounds
- Chest tube system
- Complications
- Pneumothorax recurrence

 Alert

Watch for signs and symptoms of tension pneumothorax, which can be fatal. These include anxiety, hypotension, tachycardia, tachypnea, and cyanosis.

Patient teaching

Be sure to cover:
- the disorder, diagnosis, and treatment
- drug administration, dosage, and possible adverse effects
- chest tube insertion
- deep-breathing exercises
- signs and symptoms of recurrent spontaneous pneumothorax and when to notify the physician.

Discharge planning

- Refer the patient to a smoking-cessation program, if appropriate.

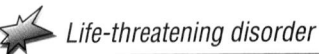

Life-threatening disorder

Poisoning

Overview

Description

- Contact with a harmful substance by inhalation, ingestion, injection, or skin contact
- Prognosis varies with the amount of poison absorbed, its toxicity, and the time lapse between poisoning and treatment

Pathophysiology

- Varies with the type of poison.

Causes

- Accidental ingestion of medication
- Improper cooking, canning, or storage of food
- Suicide attempt
- Homicide attempt

Risk factors

- Employment in chemical plant
- Inappropriate storage of medications or chemicals
- Inappropriate labeling

Incidence

- Affects 1 million people annually; fatal in about 800 cases
- Fourth most common cause of death in children

Common characteristics

- Hypotension
- Altered neurologic status
- Changes in skin temperature and color
- Cardiopulmonary arrest

Complications

- Cardiac arrhythmias
- Seizures
- Neurogenic shock
- Cardiovascular collapse
- Coma and death

Assessment

History

- Poison exposure
- Drug overdose

Physical findings

- Vary with type of poison. May include:
  - central nervous system depression or excitability
  - respiratory depression
  - cardiovascular depression
  - cardiovascular excitation

- cardiac arrhythmias
- acute renal failure
- liver failure.

Test results

Laboratory

- Increased or decreased lactate level
- Increased serum calcium
- Increased serum magnesium
- Toxicology studies showing poison levels in the patient's mouth, vomitus, urine, feces, or blood or on the patient's hands or clothing
- Arterial blood gas values identifying hypoxemia or metabolic derangements
- Imbalanced serum electrolyte levels such as hypokalemia; possibly showing anion-gap metabolic acidosis

Imaging

- Chest X-rays may show pulmonary infiltrates or edema in inhalation poisoning; may show aspiration pneumonia in petroleum distillate inhalation.
- Abdominal X-rays may show the presence of iron pills or other radiopaque substances.

Diagnostic procedures

- Electrocardiogram may show arrhythmias or QRS- and QT-interval prolongation.

Treatment

General

- Emergency resuscitation, as needed
- Recommendations of local poison control center
- Symptomatic care
- Airway and ventilation maintenance
- Oxygen administration
- Nothing by mouth until the episode resolves
- Safety measures

Medication

- Specific antidote, if available
- Activated charcoal, if appropriate

Nursing considerations

Key outcomes

The patient will:
- maintain adequate ventilation
- maintain a patent airway
- maintain orientation to time, place, and person
- express feelings of increased comfort and pain relief
- identify factors that increase the risk for injury.

Nursing interventions

- Perform cardiopulmonary resuscitation, if needed.
- Induce emesis, if recommended.
- Perform gastric lavage and administer a cathartic, as ordered.
- Provide supplemental oxygen as ordered and needed.

○ Send vomitus and aspirate for analysis.
○ In severe poisoning, provide peritoneal dialysis or hemodialysis.

Monitoring

○ Vital signs
○ Level of consciousness
○ Respiratory status
○ Suicidal ideations, if indicated

Patient teaching

Be sure to cover:
○ importance of reading all labels before taking medications
○ proper medication and chemical storage
○ dangers of taking medications prescribed for someone else
○ dangers of transferring medications or chemicals from their original container
○ dangers of telling children that medication is "candy"
○ importance of keeping ipecac syrup available at home
○ use of childproof caps on medication containers.

Discharge teaching

○ Refer the patient for psychological counseling in case of suicide attempt.
○ Refer the patient to the proper authorities in case of deliberate poisoning.

Poliomyelitis

Overview

Description

- An acute communicable disease caused by the polio virus
- Ranges in severity from inapparent infection to fatal paralytic illness (mortality 5% to 10%)
- Prognosis excellent if central nervous system (CNS) is spared
- Also called *polio* or *infantile paralysis*

Pathophysiology

- The poliovirus has three antigenically distinct serotypes (types I, II, and III) that cause poliomyelitis.
- The incubation period ranges from 5 to 35 days (7 to 14 days on average).
- The virus usually enters the body through the alimentary tract, multiplies in the oropharynx and lower intestinal tract, and then spreads to regional lymph nodes and the blood.
- Factors that increase the risk of paralysis include pregnancy; old age; localized trauma, such as a recent tonsillectomy, tooth extraction, or inoculation; and unusual physical exertion at or just before the clinical onset of poliomyelitis.

Causes

- Contraction of the virus from direct contact with infected oropharyngeal secretions or feces

Incidence

- Minor polio outbreaks, usually among nonimmunized groups
- Onset during the summer and fall
- Mostly occurs in people over age 15
- Adults and girls at greater risk for infection; boys, for paralysis

Common characteristics

Abortive infection
- Slight fever
- Malaise
- Headache
- Sore throat
- Inflamed pharynx
- Vomiting

Major poliomyelitis
NONPARALYTIC
- Moderate fever
- Headache
- Vomiting
- Lethargy
- Irritability
- Pains in neck, back, arms, legs, and abdomen
- Muscle tenderness, weakness, and spasms in the extensors of the neck and back and sometimes in the hamstring and other muscles

PARALYTIC
- Symptoms similar to those of nonparalytic poliomyelitis
- Asymmetrical weakness of various muscles
- Loss of superficial and deep reflexes
- Paresthesia
- Hypersensitivity to touch
- Urine retention
- Constipation
- Abdominal distention

BULBAR PARALYTIC
- Respiratory paralysis
- Symptoms of encephalitis
- Facial weakness
- Diplopia
- Dysphasia
- Difficulty chewing
- Inability to swallow or expel saliva
- Regurgitation of food through the nasal passages
- Dyspnea

Complications

- Hypertension
- Urinary tract infection
- Urolithiasis
- Atelectasis
- Pneumonia
- Myocarditis
- Cor pulmonale
- Skeletal and soft-tissue deformities
- Paralytic ileus

Assessment

History

- Exposure to polio virus
- Fever

Physical findings

- Muscle weakness
- Resistance to neck flexion (nonparalytic and paralytic poliomyelitis)
- Patient "tripods" (extend his arms behind him for support) when sitting up
- Patient's head falls back when supine and shoulders are elevated (Hoyne's sign)
- Unable to raise legs 90 degrees when in a supine position
- Kernig's and Brudzinski's signs (paralytic poliomyelitis)

Test results

Laboratory
- Polio virus isolated from throat washings early in the disease, from stools throughout the disease, and from cerebrospinal fluid cultures in CNS infection.

- ○ Convalescent serum antibody titers are four times greater than acute titers.
- ○ Tests to rule out coxsackievirus and echovirus infections must be performed.

Treatment

General

- ○ Supportive
- ○ Moist heat applications
- ○ Well-balanced diet
- ○ Activity, as tolerated
- ○ Physical therapy
- ○ Assistive devices

Medication

- ○ Analgesics
- ○ Antipyretics

Nursing considerations

Key outcomes

The patient will:
- ○ report feelings of increased comfort
- ○ maintain adequate ventilation
- ○ demonstrate effective coping mechanisms
- ○ utilize available support systems.

Nursing interventions

- ○ Provide emotional support.
- ○ Provide good skin care, reposition the patient often, and keep the bed dry.
- ○ Maintain contact isolation.

Monitoring

- ○ Signs of paralysis
- ○ Respiratory status
- ○ Vital signs
- ○ Nutritional status

Patient teaching

Be sure to cover:
- ○ physical therapy
- ○ avoiding complications of limited mobility
- ○ proper hand-washing and contact isolation techniques.

Discharge planning

- ○ Refer the patient to support services, as appropriate.

Polycystic kidney disease

Overview

Description

- Growth of multiple, bilateral, grapelike clusters of fluid-filled cysts in the kidneys
- May progress slowly even after renal insufficiency symptoms appear
- Has two distinct forms: *infantile* form, which causes stillbirth or early neonatal death; and *adult* form, which has insidious onset but usually becomes obvious between ages 30 and 50
- Usually fatal within 4 years of uremic symptom onset, unless dialysis begins
- Carries a widely varying prognosis in adults
- Also known as *PKD*

Pathophysiology

- Cysts enlarge the kidneys, compressing and eventually replacing functioning renal tissue.
- Renal deterioration results; deterioration is more gradual in adults than in infants.
- The condition progresses relentlessly to fatal uremia.

Causes

- Familial
- Infantile form inherited as an autosomal recessive trait
- Adult form inherited as an autosomal dominant trait

Risk factors

- If one parent has autosomal dominant PKD, there's a 50% chance that the disease will pass to a child
- In autosomal recessive PKD, parents who don't have the disease can have a child with the disease if both parents carry the abnormal gene and both pass the gene to their child (one in four chance).

Incidence

- Affects both sexes equally
- Infantile form: 1 in 6,000 to 40,000 infants
- Adult form: 1 in 50 to 1,000 adults

Common characteristics

- Enlarged kidneys
- Signs and symptoms of renal failure
- Abdominal or flank pain
- Hypertension
- Nocturia

Complications

- Hepatic failure
- Renal failure
- Respiratory failure
- Heart failure
- Recurrent hematuria
- Life-threatening retroperitoneal bleeding
- Proteinuria

Assessment

History

Adult polycystic disease

- Family history
- Polyuria
- Urinary tract infections
- Headaches
- Pain in back or flank area
- Gross hematuria
- Abdominal pain, usually worsened on exertion and eased by lying down

Physical findings

Infantile form

- Pronounced epicanthal folds
- Pointed nose
- Small chin
- Floppy, low-set ears (Potter facies)
- Huge, bilateral, symmetrical flank masses that are tense and can't be transilluminated
- Signs of respiratory distress, heart failure and, eventually, uremia and renal failure
- Signs of portal hypertension (bleeding varices)

Adult form

- Hypertension
- Signs of an enlarging kidney mass
- Grossly enlarged kidneys (in advanced stages)

Test results

Laboratory

- Urinalysis possibly showing hematuria or bacteria or protein
- Creatinine clearance test results possibly showing renal insufficiency or failure
- Possibly sodium loss or retention

Imaging

- Excretory or retrograde urography reveals enlarged kidneys, with pelvic elongation, flattening of the calyces, and indentations caused by cysts. In a neonate, excretory urography shows poor excretion of contrast medium.
- Ultrasonography, tomography, and radioisotopic scans show kidney enlargement and cysts.
- Tomography, computed tomography scan, and magnetic resonance imaging show multiple areas of cystic damage.

Treatment

General

- Monitoring of renal function
- Dialysis
- Low-protein and, possibly, low-sodium diet
- Fluid restriction (in renal failure)
- Avoidance of contact sports

Medication

○ Analgesics
○ Antibiotics for urinary tract infection
○ Antihypertensive agents for hypertension

Surgery

○ Kidney transplantation
○ Surgical drainage for cystic abscess or retroperitoneal bleeding

Nursing considerations

Key outcomes

The patient will:
○ maintain fluid balance
○ maintain urine specific gravity within designated limits
○ maintain hemodynamic stability
○ report feelings of increased comfort
○ identify risk factors that worsen decreased tissue perfusion, and modify lifestyle appropriately.

Nursing interventions

○ Give prescribed drugs.
○ Provide supportive care to minimize symptoms.
○ Individualize patient care accordingly.

Monitoring

○ Urine (for blood, cloudiness, calculi, and granules)
○ Intake and output
○ Electrolytes
○ Vital signs
○ Access site for dialysis

Patient teaching

Be sure to cover:
○ the disorder, diagnosis, and treatment
○ drug administration, dosage, and possible adverse effects
○ follow-up with the physician for severe or recurring headaches
○ signs and symptoms of urinary tract infection and prompt notification of the physician
○ importance of blood pressure control
○ possible need for dialysis or transplantation.

Discharge planning

○ Refer a young adult patient or the parents of an infant with polycystic kidney disease for genetic counseling.

Polycystic ovarian syndrome

Overview

Description

○ Metabolic disorder characterized by multiple ovarian cysts
○ Prognosis good for ovulation and fertility with appropriate treatment

Pathophysiology

○ A general feature of all anovulation syndromes is a lack of pulsatile release of gonadotropin-releasing hormone.
○ Initial ovarian follicle development is normal.
○ Many small follicles begin to accumulate because there's no selection of a dominant follicle.
○ These follicles may respond abnormally to the hormonal stimulation, causing an abnormal pattern of estrogen secretion during the menstrual cycle.
○ Endocrine abnormalities may be the cause of polycystic ovarian syndrome or cystic abnormalities; muscle and adipose tissue are resistant to the effects of insulin, and lipid metabolism is abnormal.

Causes

○ Exact cause unknown, but theories include:
  – abnormal enzyme activity triggering excess androgen secretion
  – endocrine abnormalities.

Incidence

○ Polycystic ovarian syndrome occurs in 6% to 10% of women in the United States; 50% to 80% of these women are obese.
○ Among women who seek treatment for infertility, more than 75% have some degree of polycystic ovarian syndrome, usually manifested by anovulation alone.
○ Women of reproductive age are affected.

Common characteristics

○ Mild pelvic discomfort
○ Lower back pain
○ Dyspareunia
○ Abnormal uterine bleeding secondary to disturbed ovulatory pattern
○ Hirsutism
○ Acne
○ Male-pattern hair loss
○ Infertility
○ Obesity
○ Impaired glucose tolerance (by age 40)

Complications

○ Malignancy
○ Increased risk for cardiovascular disease and type 2 diabetes mellitus
○ Secondary amenorrhea
○ Oligomenorrhea
○ Infertility
○ Addison's disease
○ Ovarian atrophy

Assessment

History

○ Diabetes
○ Mild pelvic discomfort
○ Lower back pain
○ Dyspareunia
○ Abnormal uterine bleeding secondary to disturbed ovulatory pattern

Physical findings

○ Obesity
○ Hirsutism
○ Acne
○ Male-pattern hair loss
○ Hyperpigmentation of the skin

Test results

Laboratory
○ Slightly elevated urinary 17-ketosteroid levels
○ Anovulation
○ Unopposed estrogen action during menstrual cycle (due to anovulation)
○ Elevated ratio of luteinizing hormone to follicle-stimulating hormone (usually 3:1 or greater)
○ Elevated testosterone and androstenedione levels
Imaging
○ Ultrasound permits visualization of the ovary.
Surgery
○ Surgery may confirm ovarian cysts.
Other
○ History and physical examination
○ Direct visualization by laparoscopy

Treatment

General

○ Lifestyle modifications
○ Weight-loss diet
○ Daily exercise program
○ Hair removal

Medication

○ Clomiphene
○ Medroxyprogesterone
○ Low-dose hormonal contraceptives

- Metformin
- Antiandrogens (for hirsutism)

Surgery

- Ovarian wedge resection
- Laparoscopic surgery to create focal areas of damage in the ovarian cortex and stoma

Nursing considerations

Key outcomes

The patient will:
- report feelings of increased comfort
- express understanding of condition and treatment
- demonstrate effective coping mechanisms.

Nursing interventions

- Postoperatively, encourage frequent movement in bed and early ambulation.
- Provide emotional support.
- Encourage weight reduction, if appropriate.
- Provide guidelines for exercise program.

Monitoring

Preoperatively
- Signs of cyst rupture

Postoperatively
- Vital signs
- Signs of infection

Patient teaching

Be sure to cover:
- the disorder, diagnosis, and treatment
- diabetic diet, if appropriate
- low-calorie diet
- importance of regular follow-up care.

Discharge planning

- Refer the patient to a reproductive endocrinologist.
- Refer the patient to supportive services as appropriate.

Polycythemia, secondary

Overview

Description

- Excessive production of circulating red blood cells (RBCs) due to hypoxia, tumor, or disease
- Also called *reactive polycythemia*

Pathophysiology

- May result from increased production of the hormone erythropoietin
- Bone marrow is stimulated to produce RBCs (increased production of erythropoietin possibly an inappropriate pathologic response to renal, central nervous system, or endocrine disorders or to certain neoplasms)
- Compensatory response to several conditions, such as:
  - hypoxemia
  - hemoglobin abnormalities
  - heart failure
  - right-to-left shunting of blood in the heart
  - central or peripheral alveolar hypoventilation
  - low oxygen content at high altitudes
- May be an inappropriate (pathologic) response to:
  - renal disease
  - central nervous system disease
  - neoplasms
  - endocrine disorders

Causes

- Increased production of erythropoietin
- Conditions that cause prolonged tissue hypoxia, such as shock or compression of major blood vessels
- Recessive genetic trait

Incidence

- Occurs in 2 of every 100,000 people living at or near sea level
- Greater incidence among those living at high altitude

Common characteristics

- Ruddy, cyanotic skin
- Emphysema
- Hypoxemia without hepatomegaly or hypertension (in the hypoxic patient)
- Clubbing of the fingers (when underlying cause is cardiovascular)

Complications

- Hemorrhage
- Thromboembolism secondary to hemoconcentration

Assessment

History

- Emphysema
- Headaches
- Lethargy

Physical findings

- Clubbed fingers
- Ruddy skin
- Cyanosis
- Splenomegaly
- Shortness of breath
- Hypoxemia

Test results

Laboratory
- Increased RBC mass
- Elevated hematocrit and hemoglobin level
- Elevated mean corpuscular volume and mean corpuscular hemoglobin level
- Elevated urinary erythropoietin count
- Elevated blood histamine level
- Normal to low arterial oxygen saturation level

Diagnostic procedures
- Bone marrow biopsy reveals hyperplasia confined to the erythroid series

Treatment

General

- Correction of underlying disease or environmental condition
- Phlebotomy
- Plasmapheresis
- Smoking cessation
- Low-sodium diet
- Activity, as tolerated

Medication

- Analgesics
- Low-flow oxygen therapy

Nursing considerations

Key outcomes

The patient will:
- maintain adequate gas exchange
- express understanding of condition and treatment
- report feelings of increased comfort
- maintain normal fluid balance
- remain free from signs of infection.

Nursing interventions

- Promote optimal activity.
- Before and after phlebotomy, check the patient's blood pressure with him lying down. After the proce-

dure, have the patient drink approximately 24 oz (710 ml) of water or juice. To prevent syncope, have him sit up for about 5 minutes before walking.
○ Encourage verbalization and provide support.
○ Give prescribed drugs.

Monitoring

○ Signs of thrombosis
○ Respiratory status
○ Vital signs

Patient teaching

Be sure to cover:
○ the disorder, diagnosis, and treatment
○ symptoms of recurring polycythemia and the importance of reporting them promptly
○ the importance of regular blood studies (every 2 to 3 months), even after the disease is controlled
○ the need for relocation if altitude is a contributing factor
○ dietary restrictions
○ using an electric razor
○ maintaining a safe environment
○ alternating rest periods and activity.

Discharge planning

○ Refer the patient to social services as appropriate.

Polycythemia vera

Overview

Description

○ Chronic, myeloproliferative disorder of increased red blood cell (RBC) mass, leukocytosis, thrombocytosis, and increased hemoglobin concentration

○ Also called *primary polycythemia, erythema, polycythemia rubra vera, splenomegalic polycythemia,* and *Vaquez-Osler disease*

Pathophysiology

○ Uncontrolled and rapid cellular reproduction and maturation cause proliferation or hyperplasia of all bone marrow cells.

○ Increased RBC mass makes the blood abnormally viscous and inhibits blood flow to the microcirculation.

○ Diminished blood flow and thrombocytosis set the stage for intravascular thrombosis.

Causes

○ Hyperplasia of all bone marrow cells (panmyelosis)

Incidence

○ Onset usually between ages 40 and 60

○ Most common among Jewish men

○ Rare in children and blacks

Common characteristics

○ Joint pain

○ Hypertension

Complications

○ Hemorrhage

○ Vascular thromboses

○ Uric acid calculi

○ Myelofibrosis

○ Acute leukemia

Assessment

History

○ Vague feeling of fullness in the head or rushing in the ears

○ Tinnitus

○ Headache

○ Dizziness, vertigo

○ Epistaxis

○ Night sweats

○ Epigastric and joint pain

○ Vision alterations, such as scotomas, double vision, and blurred vision

○ Pruritus

○ Abdominal fullness

Physical findings

○ Congestion of the conjunctiva, retina, and retinal veins

○ Oral mucous membrane congestion

○ Hypertension

○ Ruddy cyanosis

○ Ecchymosis

○ Hepatosplenomegaly

Test results

Laboratory

○ Increased uric acid level

○ Increased RBC mass and normal arterial oxygen saturation confirming diagnosis with splenomegaly or two of the following:

　－ Platelet count above 400,000/μl (thrombocytopenia)

　－ White blood cell count above 10,000/μl in adults

　－ Elevated leukocyte alkaline phosphatase level

　－ Elevated serum vitamin B_{12} levels or unbound B_{12}-binding capacity

Diagnostic procedures

○ Bone marrow biopsy shows panmyelosis.

Treatment

General

○ Phlebotomy

○ Pheresis

Medication

○ Myelosuppressive agents

○ Radioactive phosphorus

○ Chemotherapy

Nursing considerations

Key outcomes

The patient will:

○ maintain strong peripheral pulses

○ maintain normal skin color and temperature

○ remain free from evidence of infection

○ express feelings of increased comfort and decreased pain.

Nursing interventions

○ Keep the patient active and ambulatory.

○ If bed rest is necessary, implement a daily program of active and passive range-of-motion exercises.

○ Encourage additional fluid intake.

○ If the patient has symptomatic splenomegaly, suggest or provide small, frequent meals followed by a rest period.

○ If the patient has pruritus, give prescribed drugs.

○ Encourage the patient to express concerns about the disease and its treatment.

Report acute abdominal pain immediately. It may signal splenic infarction, renal calculus formation, or abdominal organ thrombosis.

During and after phlebotomy
○ Make sure the patient is lying down comfortably. Stay alert for tachycardia, clamminess, and complaints of vertigo. If these effects occur, the procedure should be stopped.
○ Immediately after phlebotomy, have the patient sit up for about 5 minutes before letting him walk. Give 24 oz (710 ml) of juice or water.

During myelosuppressive chemotherapy
○ If nausea and vomiting occur, begin antiemetic therapy and adjust the patient's diet.
○ During treatment with radioactive phosphorus, obtain a blood sample for complete blood cell (CBC) count and platelet count before starting treatment. (Personnel who administer radioactive phosphorus should take radiation precautions to prevent contamination.)
○ Have the patient lie down during I.V. administration and for 15 to 20 minutes afterward.

Monitoring
○ Vital signs
○ Adverse reactions to drugs
○ CBC and platelet count before and during therapy
○ Complications
○ Signs and symptoms of impending stroke
○ Hypertension
○ Signs and symptoms of heart failure
○ Signs and symptoms of bleeding

Patient teaching

Be sure to cover:
○ the disorder, diagnosis, and treatment
○ importance of staying as active as possible
○ use of an electric razor to prevent accidental cuts
○ ways to minimize falls and contusions at home
○ avoidance of high altitudes
○ common bleeding sites, if the patient has thrombocytopenia
○ importance of reporting abnormal bleeding promptly
○ phlebotomy procedure (if scheduled) and its effects
○ symptoms of iron deficiency to report
○ possible adverse reactions to myelosuppressive therapy
○ instructions on infection prevention for an outpatient who develops leukopenia (including avoiding crowds and watching for infection symptoms)
○ radioactive phosphorus administration procedure (if scheduled) and the possible need for repeated phlebotomies
○ dental care
○ use of gloves when outdoors if temperature is below 50° F (9.9° C).

Polyps, intestinal

Overview

Description
- A small, tumorlike growth that projects from a mucous membrane surface
- May develop in the colon or rectum, where they protrude into the GI tract

Pathophysiology
- Masses of tissue resulting from unrestrained cell growth in the upper epithelium rise above the mucosal membrane and protrude into the GI tract.
- They may be described by their appearance:
  - pedunculated: attached by a stalk to the intestinal wall
  - sessile: attached to the intestinal wall with a broad base and no stalk.
- Polyps are classified according to tissue type:
  - adenomatous polyps, such as tubular adenoma, tubulovillous adenoma, and villous adenoma
  - nonadenomatous polyps, such as hyperplastic polyps, inflammatory polyps, and juvenile polyps.
- Most polyps are benign. However, villous and familial polyps show a marked inclination to become malignant.

 Alert

Familial polyposis is commonly linked to rectosigmoid adenocarcinoma.

Causes
- Unknown

Risk factors
- Heredity
- Age
- High-fat, low-fiber diet

Incidence
- Villous adenomas most prevalent in men older than age 55
- Common polypoid adenomas most prevalent in white women between ages 45 and 60
- Incidence in both sexes increased after age 70
- Juvenile polyps most common in children younger than age 10

Common characteristics
- Rectal bleeding
- Painful defecation
- Changes in bowel habits

Complications
- Anemia
- Bowel obstruction
- Rectal bleeding
- Intussusception
- Colorectal cancer (villous adenomas and familial polyps)
- Electrolyte imbalance

Assessment

History
- Diarrhea
- Bloody stools
- Painful defecation
- Changes in bowel habits

Physical findings
- Polyp felt during digital rectal examination

Test results
Laboratory
- Occult blood in the stools
- Low hemoglobin level
- Low hematocrit level (with anemia)
- Serum electrolyte imbalances (with villous adenomas)

Imaging
- Barium enema identifies polyps that are located high in the colon.

Diagnostic procedures
- Sigmoidoscopy, colonoscopy, and rectal biopsy identify polyps.

Treatment

General
- Activity, as tolerated
- Diet, as tolerated

Medication
- Analgesics

Surgery
- Polypectomy, commonly by fulguration (destruction by high-frequency electricity) during endoscopy
- Abdominoperineal resection, low anterior resection, ileostomy, colostomy
- Biopsy
- Snare removal during colonoscopy

Nursing considerations

Key outcomes
The patient will:
- return to normal bowel habits
- express increased comfort
- maintain electrolyte balance.

Nursing interventions
- Observe the amount and character of stools.

- Prepare the patient with precancerous or familial lesions for abdominoperineal resection.
- Provide emotional support.

Monitoring

- Electrolyte levels
- Rectal bleeding
- Vital signs
- Intake and output

After surgery
- Signs of bleeding
- Wound condition

Patient teaching

Be sure to cover:
- the disorder, diagnosis, and treatment
- wound care, if appropriate
- enterostomal therapy and care.

Discharge planning

- If the patient has benign polyps, stress the need for routine follow-up studies to check for new polypoid growth.

Porphyrias

Overview

Description

- Umbrella term for a group of metabolic disorders that affect the biosynthesis of heme (a hemoglobin component), resulting in excessive porphyrin production
- Classified by the site of excessive porphyrin production as erythropoietic, hepatic, or erythrohepatic porphyria

Pathophysiology

- Various metabolic disorders affect heme biosynthesis.
- This leads to excessive production and excretion of porphyrins or their precursors.

Causes

- Inherited as an autosomal dominant trait, except Günther's disease (inherited as an autosomal recessive trait) and toxic-acquired porphyria (which results from lead ingestion or exposure)

Incidence

- More common in Whites than Blacks or Asians

Common characteristics

- Neuropsychiatric, dermatologic, and abdominal symptoms

Precipitating factors
- Certain medications
- Hormonal changes
- Infection
- Malnutrition

Complications

- With hepatic porphyria: neurologic and hepatic dysfunction
- With acute intermittent porphyria: flaccid paralysis, respiratory paralysis, and death
- With erythropoietic porphyria: hemolytic anemia

Assessment

History

- Mild or severe abdominal pain
- Photosensitivity
- Paresthesia
- Neuritic pain

Physical findings

- Wide variation, depending on the type of porphyria
- Psychosis
- Seizures
- Skin lesions
- Darkening of urine left in the light or air
- Neurologic signs of wristdrop or footdrop
- Muscle weakness
- Fever (with an acute attack)
- Splenomegaly (if hemolytic anemia is present)
- Wheezing and dyspnea (with acute intermittent porphyria)

Test results

Laboratory
- Urine aminolevulinic acid in the ion-exchange chromatography test
- In acute intermittent porphyria: urine porphobilinogen (as shown by the Watson-Schwartz test), leukocytosis, elevated bilirubin and alkaline phosphatase levels, and hyponatremia
- In variegate porphyria: protoporphyrin and coproporphyrin in stools
- In hereditary coproporphyria: abundant coproporphyrin in stools and, to a lesser extent, in urine
- In porphyria cutanea tarda: increased uroporphyrin excretion, with varying amounts of fecal porphyrins
- In Günther's disease: urine porphyrins
- In erythropoietic protoporphyria: protoporphyrin in red blood cells
- In toxic acquired porphyria: urine lead level of 0.2 mg/L or higher
- In porphyria cutanea tarda: increased serum iron levels

Treatment

- High-carbohydrate diet
- Fluid restriction
- Avoidance of direct sun exposure

Medication

- Beta-caotene supplements
- Chlorpromazine I.V.
- Analgesics
- Hemin
- Sunscreen preparations

Surgery

- In hemolytic anemia: splenectomy

Nursing considerations

Key outcomes

The patient will:
- maintain adequate ventilation
- maintain intact skin integrity
- avoid complications
- regain normal bowel movements
- express feelings of increased comfort.

Nursing interventions

- Check the patient's history for use of medications that can trigger an acute attack. (See *Drugs that aggravate porphyria.*)

- Give prescribed drugs.
- Perform passive and active range-of-motion exercises.
- Encourage the patient to express feelings and concerns about the disease.
- Provide emotional support.

Monitoring

- Respiratory status
- GI motility
- Vital signs
- Response to treatment

Patient teaching

Be sure to cover:
- the disorder, diagnosis, and treatment
- avoidance of excessive sun exposure
- importance of wearing medical identification
- lead sources (if the patient has toxic-acquired porphyria)
- precipitating factors, including crash diets, fasting, and use of alcohol, estrogens, and barbiturates
- stress-management techniques
- ways to prevent infection
- value of a high-carbohydrate diet.

Discharge planning

- For toxic-acquired porphyria, refer the patient and family to resources that can help identify lead sources in the home.

Posttraumatic stress disorder

Overview

Description

- Development of psychological symptoms, such as intense fear and feelings of hopelessness and loss of control, after exposure to extreme trauma
- Can be acute, chronic, or delayed

Pathophysiology

- The alpha$_2$-adrenergic receptor response that inhibits stress-induced release of norepinephrine is impaired.
- Progressive behavioral sensitization results, with generalization to stimulus cues from the original trauma.
- Consequently, responses of increased sympathetic activity occur.

Causes

- An event that the patient views as traumatic (typically an event outside the range of usual human experience)

Risk factors

- History of psychopathology
- Neurotic and extroverted characteristics
- History of child abuse or neglect

Incidence

- Affects 30% of trauma victims
- Occurs in up to 15% of U.S. residents at some time in their lives
- More common in women than men

Common characteristics

- Detachment and loss of emotional response
- Feelings of depersonalization
- Inability to recall specific aspects of the traumatic event
- Flashbacks within dreams or thoughts when cues to the event occur
- Nightmares of the traumatic event

Complications

- Increased risk for other anxiety, mood, and substance-related disorders
- Substance abuse
- Feelings of detachment or estrangement, which may damage interpersonal relationships

Assessment

History

- Difficulty falling or staying asleep
- Aggressive outbursts on awakening
- Panic attacks
- Phobic avoidance of situations that arouse memories of the traumatic event
- Early life experiences, interpersonal factors, military experiences, or other incidents that suggest the traumatic event
- Symptoms that began immediately or soon after the trauma (although in some cases, symptoms don't develop until months or years later)
- Pangs of painful emotions and unwelcome thoughts
- Traumatic re-experiencing of the traumatic event
- Chronic anxiety
- Rage and survivor guilt
- Use of violence to solve problems
- Depression and suicidal thoughts
- Fantasies of retaliation

Physical findings

- Emotional numbing (diminished or constricted response)
- Memory impairment
- Difficulty concentrating
- Signs of substance abuse
- Physiologic reactivity on exposure to internal or external cues that symbolize or resemble an aspect of the traumatic event

DSM-IV-TR criteria

Diagnosis is confirmed when the patient meets the following criteria:

- Exposure to a traumatic event that included both of the following:
  - actual or threatened death or serious injury or threat to the physical integrity of self or others
  - a response of intense fear, helplessness, or horror.
- Persistent reexperiencing of this traumatic event in at least one of these ways:
  - recurrent and intrusive distressing recollections of the event
  - recurrent distressing dreams of the event
  - flashbacks of the event
  - intense psychological distress at exposure to events
  - physiologic reactivity on exposure to events.
- Persistent avoidance of stimuli associated with the trauma, or numbing of general responsiveness not present before the trauma, as indicated by at least three of these criteria:
  - efforts to avoid thoughts or feelings associated with the traumatic event
  - efforts to avoid activities or situations that arouse recollections of the traumatic event
  - inability to recall an important aspect of the event
  - sharply decreased interest in significant activities
  - feeling of detachment or estrangement from others
  - restricted range of effect
  - sense of a foreshortened future.
- Persistent symptoms of increased arousal (not previously present) as indicated by two or more of these criteria:
  - difficulty falling or staying asleep

- irritability or outbursts of anger
- difficulty concentrating
- hypervigilance
- exaggerated startle response.

The disturbance must have lasted at least 1 month and must cause significant distress or impairment of social, occupational, or other important areas of functioning.

Treatment

General

○ Supportive or expressive psychotherapy
○ Behavior therapies
○ Support groups
○ Rehabilitation programs in physical, social, and occupational areas
○ Treatment of alcohol or drug abuse, as needed
○ Active avoidance of stimuli that trigger memories of the traumatic event

Medication

○ Benzodiazepines (short-term use)
○ Tricyclic antidepressants
○ Monoamine oxidase inhibitors
○ Selective serotonin-reuptake inhibitors
○ Sedating antidepressants
○ Anticonvulsants

Nursing considerations

Key outcomes

The patient will:
○ express feelings and fears related to the traumatic event
○ use available support systems
○ use effective coping mechanisms
○ maintain or reestablish adaptive social interactions with family members.

Nursing interventions

○ Encourage the patient to express feelings of grief, mourning, and anger.
○ Practice crisis intervention techniques, as needed.
○ Assume a positive, consistent, honest, and nonjudgmental attitude.
○ Help the patient evaluate behavior.

Monitoring

○ Response to drug therapy

Patient teaching

Be sure to cover:
○ the disorder, diagnosis, and treatment
○ healing process

○ importance of identifying and avoiding cues that worsen symptoms
○ problem-solving skills
○ relaxation and breathing techniques
○ drug administration, dosage, and possible adverse effects.

Discharge planning

○ Refer the patient to support services.
○ Refer the patient for psychotherapy.
○ Refer the patient to physical, social, and occupational rehabilitation programs, as indicated.
○ Refer the patient to drug treatment programs, as appropriate.

Precocious puberty

Overview

Description

○ Early sexual maturity
○ True precocious puberty: early maturation of the hypothalamic-pituitary-gonadal axis, development of secondary sex characteristics, gonadal development, and spermatogenesis
○ Pseudoprecocious puberty: development of secondary sex characteristics without gonadal development

Pathophysiology

○ In males, results from pituitary or hypothalamic intracranial lesions that cause excessive secretion of gonadotropin
○ In females, results from early development and activation of the endocrine glands without corresponding abnormality

Causes

In males
TRUE PRECOCIOUS PUBERTY
○ Idiopathic
○ Genetically transmitted as a dominant gene
PSEUDOPRECOCIOUS PUBERTY
○ Testicular tumors
○ Congenital adrenogenital syndrome
In females
TRUE PRECOCIOUS PUBERTY
○ Idiopathic
○ Central nervous system (CNS) disorders
PSEUDOPRECOCIOUS PUBERTY
○ Ovarian and adrenocortical tumors
○ Estrogen or androgen ingestion
○ Increased end-organ sensitivity to low levels of circulating sex hormones

Incidence

○ Five times more common in females than in males

Common characteristics

In males
○ Early bone development; initial growth spurt
○ Early muscle development
○ Stunted adult stature
○ Adult hair pattern
○ Penile growth
○ Bilateral enlarged testes

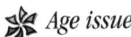 *Age issue*

Males as young as 7 with true precocious puberty have fathered children.

In females
○ Rapid growth spurt
○ Breast development at early age
○ Pubic hair
○ Early menarche

Complications

○ Testicular tumor (males)
○ Ovarian or adrenal malignancy (females)

Assessment

History

○ Rapid growth spurt
○ Early muscle development (males)
○ Early menarche (females)

Physical findings

○ Enlarged penis or testicles (males)
○ Enlarged breasts (females)
○ Pubic hair

Test results

Laboratory
IN MALES WITH TRUE PRECOCIOUS PUBERTY
○ Elevated plasma testosterone levels
○ Ejaculate showing live spermatozoa
○ Elevated levels of luteinizing and follicle-stimulating hormones and corticotropins
IN MALES WITH PSEUDOPRECOCIOUS PUBERTY
○ Chromosomal karyotype analysis showing abnormal pattern of autosomes and sex chromosomes
○ Elevated levels of 24-hour urinary 17-ketosteroids and other steroids
IN FEMALES WITH PSEUDOPRECOCIOUS PUBERTY
○ Vaginal smear showing estrogen secretion
○ Urinary tests for gonadotropic activity and excretion of 17-ketosteroids
○ Elevated levels of luteinizing and follicle-stimulating hormones
Imaging
○ X-rays of the hands, wrists, knees, and hips determines bone age and possibly premature epiphyseal closure.
○ Ultrasound verifies suspected abdominal lesion.
○ X-rays possibly show CNS tumors.

Treatment

General

○ Aimed at underlying cause
○ Supportive psychological counseling

Medication

○ Medroxyprogesterone (females)

Surgery

○ Removal of ovarian or adrenal tumors
○ Removal of thyroid gland

Nursing considerations

Key outcomes

The patient will:
○ express understanding of condition and treatment
○ demonstrate effective coping mechanisms
○ avoid complications.

Nursing interventions

○ Provide emotional support.

Monitoring

○ Complications

Patient teaching

Be sure to cover:
○ the disorder, diagnosis, and treatment
○ drug administration, dosage, and possible adverse effects
○ the need to continue social and emotional support.

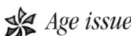
Pregnancy-induced hypertension

Overview

Description

○ High blood pressure, most often occurring after the 20th week of gestation in a nulliparous woman
○ Carries a high risk for fetal mortality because of the increased incidence of premature delivery
○ Among the most common causes of maternal death in developed countries (especially when complications occur)
○ Nonconvulsive form (also called *preeclampsia*) occurring after the 20th week of gestation; may be mild or severe
○ Convulsive form (also called *eclampsia*) occurring between the 24th week of gestation and the end of the first postpartum week

Pathophysiology

○ Generalized arteriolar vasoconstriction is thought to cause decreased blood flow through the placenta and maternal organs.
○ This leads to intrauterine growth retardation or restriction, placental infarcts, and abruptio placentae.

Causes

○ Unknown
○ Contributing factors include:
 – Geographic, ethnic, racial, nutritional, immunologic, and familial factors
 – Preexisting vascular disease
 – Maternal age
 – Autolysis of placental infarcts
 – Autointoxication
 – Uremia
 – Maternal sensitization to total proteins
 – Pyelonephritis
 – Diabetes

✳ Age issue

Adolescents and primiparas older than age 35 are at higher risk for preeclampsia.

Risk factors

○ First-time pregnancy
○ Multiple fetuses
○ History of vascular disease

Incidence

○ Occurs in about 7% of pregnancies; more common in women from lower socioeconomic groups

○ Roughly 5% incidence of preeclampsia progressing to eclampsia

Common characteristics

○ Hypertension
○ Sudden weight gain
○ Irritability
○ Emotional tension

Complications

○ Abruptio placentae
○ HELLP syndrome: hemolysis, elevated liver enzyme levels, low platelet count
○ Coagulopathy
○ Stillbirth
○ Seizures
○ Coma
○ Premature labor
○ Renal failure
○ Maternal hepatic damage

Assessment

History

○ Sudden weight gain
○ Irritability
○ Emotional tension
○ Severe frontal headache
○ Blurred vision
○ Epigastric pain or heartburn

Physical findings

○ Preeclampsia: blood pressure of 160/110 mm Hg or higher
○ Eclampsia: systolic blood pressure of 180 or 200 mm Hg or higher
○ Generalized edema, especially of the face
○ Pitting edema of the legs and feet
○ Hyperreflexia
○ Oliguria
○ Vascular spasm, papilledema, retinal edema or detachment, and arteriovenous nicking or hemorrhage (seen on ophthalmoscopy)
○ Seizures

Test results

Laboratory
○ In preeclampsia: proteinuria of more than 300 mg/24 hours [1+]
○ In severe eclampsia: proteinuria of 5 g/24 hours [5+] or more
○ In HELLP syndrome: hemolysis, elevated liver enzymes and decreased platelet count
Imaging
○ Ultrasonography aids evaluation of fetal well-being.
Diagnostic procedures
○ Stress and nonstress tests and biophysical profiles help evaluate fetal well-being.

Treatment

General

- Measures to halt progression of the disorder and ensure fetal survival
- Prompt labor induction, especially if the patient is near term (advocated by some clinicians)
- Adequate nutrition
- Low-sodium diet, if indicated
- Limited caffeine
- Complete bed rest
- Left lateral lying position

Medication

- Antihypertensives
- Magnesium sulfate
- Oxytocin
- Oxygen

Surgery

- Possible cesarean delivery

Nursing considerations

Key outcomes

The patient will:
- maintain normal vital signs
- maintain adequate fluid volume
- avoid complications
- remain oriented to the environment.

Nursing interventions

- Give prescribed drugs.
- Elevate edematous arms or legs.
- Eliminate constricting hose, slippers, and bed linens.
- Assist with or insert an indwelling urinary catheter, if necessary.
- Provide a quiet, darkened room.
- Enforce absolute bed rest.
- Provide emotional support.
- Encourage the patient to express feelings.
- Help the patient develop effective coping strategies. (See *Emergency interventions for PIH.*)

Monitoring

- Vital signs
- Fetal heart rate
- Vision
- Edema
- Daily weight
- Intake and output
- Level of consciousness
- Deep tendon reflexes
- Headache unrelieved by medication
- Complications

Emergency interventions for PIH

When caring for a patient with pregnancy-induced hypertension (PIH), be prepared to perform the following interventions:

- Observe for signs of fetal distress by closely monitoring results of stress and nonstress tests.
- Keep emergency resuscitative equipment and anticonvulsants at hand in case of seizures and cardiac or respiratory arrest.
- Carefully monitor magnesium sulfate administration. Signs of drug toxicity include absence of patellar reflexes, flushing, muscle flaccidity, decreased urinary output, significant blood pressure drop (> 15 mm Hg), and a respiratory rate below 12 per minute. Keep calcium gluconate at the bedside to counteract the toxic effects of magnesium sulfate.
- Prepare for emergency cesarean delivery, if indicated. Alert the anesthesiologist and pediatrician.
- To protect the patient from injury, maintain seizure precautions. Don't leave an unstable patient unattended. Maintain a patent airway, and have supplemental oxygen readily available.

Patient teaching

Be sure to cover:
- the disorder, diagnosis, and treatment
- signs and symptoms of preeclampsia and eclampsia
- importance of bed rest in the left lateral position, as ordered
- adequate nutrition and a low-sodium diet
- good prenatal care
- control of preexisting hypertension
- early recognition and prompt treatment of preeclampsia
- likelihood that the neonate will be small for gestational age, with the probability that he'll do better than other premature babies of the same weight.

Discharge planning

- Refer the patient for professional counseling, as indicated.

Premenstrual syndrome

Overview

Description

- Group of somatic, behavioral, cognitive, and mood-related symptoms occurring 1 to 14 days before menses and usually subsiding with menses onset
- Causes effects that range from minimal discomfort to severe, disruptive symptoms
- Also known as *PMS* and *premenstrual dysphoric disorder (PMDD)*

Pathophysiology

- PMS may result from a progesterone deficiency during the luteal phase of the ovarian cycle.
- Hormone levels and patterns in women with PMS don't differ significantly from those in women who don't experience PMS.

Causes

- Physiologic, psychological, and sociocultural factors
- Possible progesterone deficiency in the luteal phase
- Possible serotonin or norepinephrine deficiency

Incidence

- Affects 30% of women in the United States.

Age issue

- Moderate to severe symptoms occur in 14% to 88% of adolescent girls
- Usually occurs between ages 25 and 45
- Affects women in their 40s most severely
- PMS resolves completely at menopause

Common characteristics

- Anxiety
- Irritability
- Depression
- Multiple somatic complaints

Complications

- Psychosocial problems
- Reduced self-esteem
- Depression
- Inability to function (in PMDD)

Assessment

History

- Behavioral changes
- Breast tenderness or swelling
- Abdominal tenderness or bloating
- Joint pain
- Headache
- Edema
- Diarrhea or constipation
- Exacerbations of skin, respiratory, or neurologic problems

Physical findings

- Possible edema

Test results

Laboratory
- Blood studies to rule out anemia, thyroid disease, or other hormonal imbalances

Other
- A daily symptom calendar aids diagnosis of PMS.
- Psychological evaluation may be used to rule out or detect an underlying psychiatric disorder.

Treatment

General

- Symptom relief
- Stress reduction
- Relaxation techniques
- Diet low in simple sugars, caffeine intake, animal fat, and sodium
- Increased calcium and complex carbohydrate intake
- Aerobic exercise

Medication

- Antidepressants
- Vitamins (such as B complex)
- Progestins
- Prostaglandin inhibitors
- Monophasic birth control pills
- Nonsteroidal anti-inflammatory drugs
- Pituitary-ovarian axis supplements
- Gonadotropin-releasing hormone agonists

Nursing considerations

Key outcomes

The patient will:
- identify effective and ineffective coping techniques
- use available support systems, such as family, friends, and groups, to develop and maintain effective coping skills
- express feelings of increased comfort
- express positive feelings about herself.

Nursing interventions

- Encourage adequate fluid intake.
- Provide comfort measures.
- Offer emotional support and reassurance.
- Encourage the patient to express feelings.
- Help the patient develop effective coping strategies.
- Instruct the patient to chart symptoms daily for two cycles.

Monitoring

- Response to treatment
- Coping skills

Patient teaching

Be sure to cover:
○ the disorder, diagnosis, and treatment
○ physiologic basis of PMS
○ beneficial lifestyle changes
○ relaxation and stress-reduction techniques
○ dietary management.

Discharge planning

○ Refer the patient to a self-help group for women with PMS.
○ Refer the patient for psychological counseling, as indicated.
○ Refer the patient to a dietitian, as needed.

Pressure ulcers

Overview

Description

○ Localized areas of ischemic tissue caused by pressure, shearing, or friction
○ Most common over bony prominences, especially the sacrum, ischial tuberosities, greater trochanter, heels, malleoli, and elbows
○ May be superficial, caused by localized skin irritation (with subsequent surface maceration), or deep, arising in underlying tissue (Deep lesions may go undetected until they penetrate the skin.)
○ Also called *decubitus ulcers, pressure sores,* or *bedsores*

Pathophysiology

○ Impaired skin capillary pressure results in local tissue anoxia.
○ Anoxia leads to edema and multiple capillary thromboses.
○ An inflammatory reaction results in ulceration and necrosis of ischemic cells.

Causes

○ Local tissue compression
○ Shearing force
○ Friction

Risk factors

○ Poor nutrition
○ Diabetes mellitus
○ Immobility or paralysis
○ Cardiovascular disorders
○ Advanced age
○ Incontinence
○ Obesity
○ Edema
○ Anemia
○ Poor hygiene
○ Exposure to chemicals
○ Steroids

Incidence

○ Affect roughly 10% of hospitalized patients and 20% to 40% of patients in long-term care facilities

Common characteristics

○ Vary with the ulcer stage (see *Four stages of pressure ulcers*)

Complications

○ Secondary bacterial infection
○ Septicemia
○ Gangrene

Assessment

History

○ One or more risk factors

Physical findings

○ Shiny, erythematous superficial lesion (early)
○ Small blisters or erosions with progression of superficial erythema
○ Possible necrosis and ulceration with deeper erosions and ulcerations
○ Malodorous, purulent discharge (suggesting secondary bacterial infection)
○ Black eschar around and over the lesion

Test results

Laboratory
○ Infecting organism identified by wound culture and sensitivity testing of exudate
○ Decreased total serum protein
Other
○ Diagnosis typically made from inspection

Treatment

General

○ Measures to prevent pressure ulcers
○ Relief of pressure on the affected area
○ Meticulous skin care
○ Devices such as pads, mattresses, and special beds
○ Moist wound therapy dressings
○ Whirlpool baths
○ Diet high in protein, iron, and vitamin C (unless contraindicated)
○ Activity, as tolerated
○ Active and passive range-of-motion (ROM) exercises
○ Frequent turning and repositioning

Medication

○ Enzymatic ointments
○ Healing ointments
○ Antibiotics, if indicated

Surgery

○ Debridement of necrotic tissue
○ Skin grafting (in severe cases)

Nursing considerations

Key outcomes

The patient will:
○ exhibit improved or healed lesions or wounds
○ maintain adequate daily caloric intake
○ maintain joint mobility and ROM
○ avoid infection and other complications.

To protect the patient from pressure ulcer complications, learn to recognize the four stages of ulcer formation.

Stage I
The skin is red and intact and doesn't blanche with external pressure. (A black person's skin may look purple.) The skin feels warm and firm. Usually, the sore reverses after pressure is removed.

Stage III
A hole develops that oozes foul-smelling yellow or green fluid. The ulcer extends into the muscle and may develop a black, leathery crust, or eschar, at its edges and eventually, at the center. Undermining may or may not be present. The ulcer isn't painful, but healing may take months.

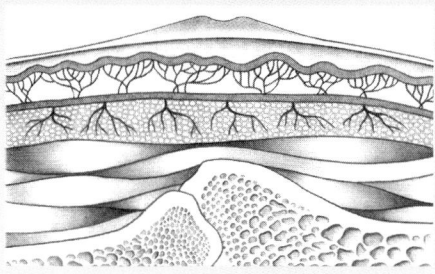

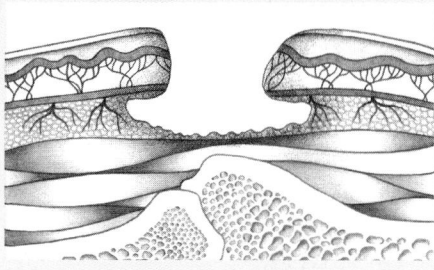

Stage II
Skin breaks appear and discoloration may occur. Penetrating to the subcutaneous fat layer, the sore is painful and visibly swollen. The ulcer may be characterized as an abrasion, blister, or shallow crater. If pressure is removed, the sore may heal within 1 to 2 weeks.

Stage IV
The ulcer destroys tissue from the skin to the bone and becomes necrotic. Findings include foul drainage and deep tunnels that extend from the ulcer. The ulcer may take months or even a year to heal.

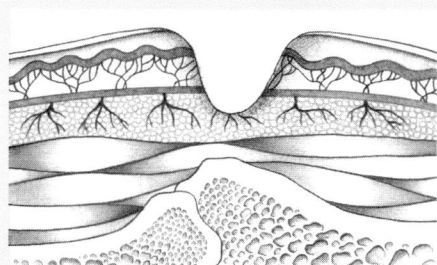

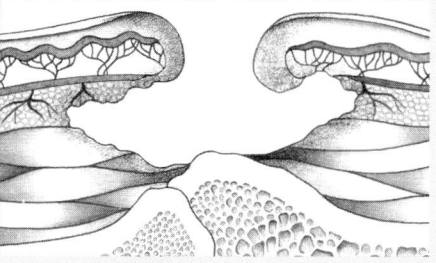

Nursing interventions
○ Give prescribed drugs.
○ Apply dressings appropriate for the ulcer stage.
○ Encourage adequate food and fluid intake.
○ Reposition the bedridden patient at least every 2 hours.
○ Elevate the head of the bed 30 degrees or less.
○ Perform passive ROM exercises.
○ Encourage active ROM exercises, if possible.
○ Use pressure-relief aids on the bed.
○ Provide meticulous skin care.

Monitoring
○ Changes in skin color, turgor, temperature, sensation, and drainage
○ Change in the ulcer stage
○ Laboratory results
○ Complications
○ Response to treatment
○ Intake and output

Patient teaching

Be sure to cover:
○ the disorder, diagnosis, and treatment
○ techniques for changing positions
○ active and passive ROM exercises
○ avoidance of skin-damaging agents
○ debridement procedures
○ skin graft surgery, if required
○ signs and stages of healing
○ importance of a well-balanced diet and adequate fluid intake
○ drug administration, dosage, and possible adverse effects
○ importance of notifying the physician immediately of signs and symptoms of infection.

Discharge planning
○ Refer the patient to a wound care specialist, if indicated.

Proctitis

Overview

Description
- An acute or chronic inflammation of the rectal mucosa
- Good prognosis unless massive bleeding occurs

Pathophysiology
- Mucosal cell loss occurs along with acute inflammation of the lamina propria, eosinophilic crypt abscess, and endothelial edema of the arterioles
- Rectal tissue ischemia occurs
- Mucosal friability, ulcers, bleeding, and fistulas result

Causes
- Crohn's disease
- Amebiasis
- Immunodeficiency disorders
- *Neisseria gonorrhoeae*
- *Chlamydia trachomatis*
- Herpes simplex virus 1 and 2
- Syphilis
- Radiation therapy
- Papillomavirus
- Ischemia
- Toxins
- Vasculitis

Risk factors
- High-risk sexual practices
- Homosexuality
- Autoimmune disorders

Incidence
- Occurs in 5% to 20% of patients receiving radiation therapy
- More common in Jewish people
- More common in males than females
- Occurs predominantly in adults

Common characteristics
- Tenesmus
- Constipation
- Feeling of rectal fullness
- Left-sided abdominal

Complications
- Ulcerations
- Crypt abscesses
- Bleeding
- Fissures
- Fistulas
- Ulcerative colitis

Assessment

History
- Tenesmus
- Abdominal cramping
- Loose stool with or without abdominal pain
- Pruritus
- Rectal and anal pain

Physical findings
- Bloody or mucoid stools
- Superficial ulcers
- Mucosal erythema
- Painless chancres
- Mucosal friability

Test results
Laboratory
- Complete blood count evaluates blood loss
- C-reactive protein may be elevated
- Rectal swab identifies gonorrhea or chlamydia
- Venereal disease research laboratory test diagnosis syphilis
- Culture of vesicular fluid identifies herpes simplex virus

Diagnostic procedures
- In acute proctitis, sigmoidoscopy shows edematous, bright-red, or pink rectal mucosa that's thick, shiny, friable and, possibly, ulcerated.
- In chronic proctitis, sigmoidoscopy shows thickened mucosa, loss of vascular pattern, and stricture of the rectal lumen.
- Biopsy rules out carcinoma.

Treatment

General
- Elimination of the underlying cause
- Increased fluids
- Activity as tolerated
- Sitz baths

Medication
- Enemas
- Steroid (hydrocortisone) suppositories
- Tranquilizers
- Antibiotics (based on cause)
- Antivirals

Surgery
- Diverting colostomy may be necessary.

Nursing considerations

Key outcomes

The patient will:
○ express feelings of increased comfort
○ understand the disease process and treatment regimen
○ exhibit adequate coping mechanisms.

Nursing interventions

○ Offer emotional support.
○ Give prescribed drugs.

Monitoring

○ Response to treatment
○ Rectal bleeding
○ Amount and character of stools

Patient teaching

Be sure to cover:
○ the disorder, diagnosis, and treatment
○ importance of watching for and reporting bleeding and other persistent symptoms.

Discharge planning

○ Refer the patient to a colorectal surgeon, if appropriate.

Prostatic cancer

Overview

Description

○ Proliferation of cancer cells that usually take the form of adenocarcinomas and typically originate in the posterior prostate gland
○ May progress to widespread bone metastases and death
○ Is the leading cause of cancer death in men

Pathophysiology

○ Slow-growing prostatic cancer seldom causes signs and symptoms until it's well advanced.
○ Typically, when a primary prostatic lesion spreads beyond the prostate gland, it invades the prostatic capsule and spreads along ejaculatory ducts in the space between the seminal vesicles or perivesicular fascia.
○ Endocrine factors may play a role, leading re-searchers to suspect that androgens speed tumor growth.
○ Malignant prostatic tumors seldom result from the benign hyperplastic enlargement that commonly de-velops around the prostatic urethra in older men.

Causes

○ Unknown

Risk factors

○ Older than age 40
○ Infection
○ Vasectomy
○ Family history
○ Heavy metal exposure

Common characteristics

○ Urinary problems

Incidence

○ Most common among Blacks; least common among Asians
○ Incidence not affected by socioeconomic status or fertility
○ Most common neoplasm in men older than age 50

Complications

○ Spinal cord compression
○ Deep vein thrombosis
○ Pulmonary emboli
○ Myelophthisis
○ Death

Assessment

History

○ Symptoms rare in early stages
○ Later, urinary problems, such as difficulty initiating a urinary stream, dribbling, and urine retention

Physical findings

○ In early stages: nonraised, firm, nodular mass with a sharp edge
○ In advanced disease: edema of the scrotum or leg; a hard lump in the prostate region

Test results

Laboratory
○ Elevated serum prostate-specific antigen (PSA) level (may indicate cancer with or without metastases)
Imaging
○ Transrectal prostatic ultrasonography shows prostate size and presence of abnormal growths.
○ Bone scan and excretory urography determines the disease's extent.
○ Magnetic resonance imaging and computed tomography scan defines the extent of the tumor.
Other
○ Standard screening test: digital rectal examination and PSA test identify cancer (recommended yearly by the American Cancer Society for men older than age 40)

Treatment

General

○ Varies with cancer stage
○ Radiation therapy or internal beam radiation
○ Well-balanced diet

Medication

○ Hormonal therapy
○ Chemotherapy

Surgery

○ Prostatectomy
○ Orchiectomy
○ Radical prostatectomy
○ Transurethral resection of prostate
○ Cryosurgical ablation

Nursing considerations

Key outcomes

The patient will:
○ express feelings of increased comfort
○ discuss the disease's impact on self and family members
○ demonstrate effective coping mechanisms.

Nursing interventions

❍ Give prescribed drugs.
❍ Encourage the patient to express his feelings.
❍ Provide emotional support.

Monitoring

❍ Pain level
❍ Wound site
❍ Postoperative complications
❍ Medication effects

Patient teaching

Be sure to cover:
❍ the disorder, diagnosis, and treatment
❍ perineal exercises that decrease incontinence
❍ follow-up care
❍ drug administration, dosage, and possible adverse
effects.

Discharge planning

❍ Refer the patient to appropriate resources and support services.

Prostatitis

Overview

Description

- Inflammation of the prostate gland
- Occurs in acute, chronic, and several other forms

Acute prostatitis
- Easily recognized and treated

Chronic prostatitis
- Most common cause of recurrent urinary tract infection in men
- More difficult to recognize than acute prostatitis

Other prostatitis forms
- Granulomatous prostatitis (also called *tuberculous prostatitis*)
- Nonbacterial prostatitis
- Prostatodynia (painful prostate)

Pathophysiology

- Infectious organism spreads to the prostate gland by the hematogenous route, an ascending urethral infection, invasion of rectal bacteria via lymphatic vessels, or reflux of infected bladder urine into prostate ducts.
- Inflammation results.

Causes

- Bacterial prostatitis: *Escherichia coli* (80% of cases); *Klebsiella, Enterobacter, Proteus, Pseudomonas, Serratia, Streptococcus, Staphylococcus,* and diphtheroids (20% of cases)
- Chronic prostatitis: bacterial invasion from urethra
- Granulomatous prostatitis: miliary spread of *Mycobacterium tuberculosis*
- Nonbacterial prostatitis: *Mycoplasma, Ureaplasma, Chlamydia,* or *Trichomonas vaginalis,* or a virus
- Prostatodynia: unknown

Risk factors

- Invasive urethral procedures
- Infrequent or excessive sexual intercourse

Incidence

Chronic prostatitis
- Affects up to 35% of men older than age 50
- Seen in 5 of every 1,000 outpatient visits

Bacterial prostatitis
- Seen in 2 of every 10,000 outpatient visits

Nonbacterial prostatitis
- Seen in 5 of every 10,000 outpatient visits

Common characteristics

- Urinary frequency and urgency
- Fever

Complications

- Urinary tract infection
- Prostatic abscess
- Acute urinary retention
- Pyelonephritis
- Epididymitis

Assessment

History

- Sudden fever, chills
- Lower back pain
- Perineal fullness
- Arthralgia, myalgia
- Urinary urgency and frequency
- Dysuria, nocturia
- Transient erectile dysfunction

Chronic bacterial prostatitis
- May be asymptomatic
- Usually causes same urinary symptoms as the acute form, but to a lesser degree
- Hemospermia
- Persistent urethral discharge
- Painful ejaculation

Nonbacterial prostatitis
- Dysuria
- Mild perineal or lower back pain
- Frequent nocturia

Prostatodynia
- Perineal, lower back, or pelvic pain

Physical findings

- Cloudy urine
- Distended bladder
- Prostatic tenderness, induration, swelling, firmness, and warmth
- Crepitation (if prostatic calculi present)

Chronic bacterial prostatitis
- Stony, hard induration of the prostate

Test results

Laboratory
- Urine culture identifies infectious organism
- In nonbacterial prostatitis: inflammatory cells found in smears of prostatic secretion
- In prostatodynia: negative urine cultures and absence of inflammatory cells found in smears of prostatic secretions

Diagnostic procedures
- In granulomatous prostatitis: prostate tissue biopsy shows *M. tuberculosis.*
- Urodynamic evaluation reveals detrusor hyperreflexia and pelvic floor myalgia (from chronic spasms).

Other
- Rectal examination findings may suggest prostatitis.

Treatment

General

- Sitz baths
- Regular, protected sexual intercourse
- Prostatic massage
- Increased oral fluids
- Bed rest until the condition improves

After surgery
- Avoidance of lifting, strenuous exercise, and long automobile rides
- No sexual activity for several weeks after discharge

Medication

- Analgesics
- Antipyretics

Acute prostatitis
- Systemic antibiotic therapy

Chronic prostatitis
- Oral antibiotics

Granulomatous prostatitis
- Antitubercular drug combinations

Nonbacterial prostatitis
- Oral antibiotics
- Anticholinergics

Prostatodynia
- Muscle relaxants
- Alpha-adrenergic blocking agents

Surgery

- Transurethral resection of the prostate or total prostatectomy, if drug therapy unsuccessful

Nursing considerations

Key outcomes

The patient will:
- express feelings of increased comfort
- demonstrate skill in managing urinary elimination problems
- express his feelings about potential or actual changes in sexual function
- use available counseling, referrals, or support groups.

Nursing interventions

- Give prescribed drugs.
- Ensure bed rest and adequate hydration.
- Give sitz baths.
- Avoid rectal examinations.

Monitoring

After surgery
- Intake and output
- Catheter function and drainage
- Signs of infection
- Pain control

Patient teaching

Be sure to cover:
- the disorder, diagnosis, and treatment
- drug administration, dosage, and possible adverse effects
- importance of increased fluid intake
- benefits of regular sexual activity (with chronic prostatitis)
- prescribed activity limits
- importance of getting immediate medical attention for fever, inability to void, or bloody urine.

Pseudomembranous enterocolitis

Overview

Description

○ Acute inflammation and necrosis of the small and large intestines
○ Usually affects the mucosa but may extend into the submucosa and, rarely, into other layers
○ Marked by severe diarrhea
○ Can be fatal in 1 to 7 days from severe dehydration or from toxicity, peritonitis, or perforation

Pathophysiology

○ Associated with anibiotic use
○ Balance of normal intestinal flora is altered and over-growth of certain organisms occurs
○ Necrotic mucosa is replaced by a pseudomembrane filled with staphylococci, leukocytes, mucus, fibrin, and inflammatory cells.

Causes

○ Unknown
○ Possible role of *Clostridium difficile*

Risk factors

○ Antibiotic therapy
○ Recent abdominal surgery
○ Cancer chemotherapy
○ Compromised immune system
○ Advanced age
○ Bone-marrow transplantation
○ Intestinal ischemia
○ Uremia
○ Burns

Incidence

○ Affects both sexes equally
○ Most common in nursing home and hospital patients
○ Affects 6 of every 100,000 people treated with antibiotics

Common characteristics

○ Watery, green, foul-smelling diarrhea
○ Up to 30 stools per day

Complications

○ Severe dehydration
○ Electrolyte imbalance
○ Hemorrhage
○ Hypotension
○ Hypovolemia
○ Sepsis
○ Shock
○ Colonic perforation
○ Peritonitis
○ Toxic megacolon

Assessment

History

○ Current or recent antibiotic treatment
○ Sudden onset of copious, watery, or bloody diarrhea
○ Cramping abdominal pain
○ Low-grade fever
○ Nausea
○ Vomiting

Physical findings

○ Abdominal tenderness

Test results

Laboratory
○ Elevated white blood cell count
○ Hypoalbuminemia
○ Stool culture identifying *C. difficile*

Imaging
○ Abdominal X-ray reveals mucosal edema.
○ Computed tomography scan may show distention as well as diffuse and focal thickening of the colon wall.

Diagnostic procedures
○ Rectal biopsy through sigmoidoscopy confirms pseudomembranous enterocolitis.
○ Endoscopy reveals characteristic pseudomembranes.

Treatment

General

○ Discontinuation of offending antibiotics
○ Avoidance of opioids and antidiarrheals
○ Supportive treatment
○ I.V. fluids (if the condition is severe)
○ Nothing by mouth until bowel recovery occurs (if the condition is severe)
○ Bed rest until recovery begins
○ Enteric precautions

Medication

○ Oral metronidazole or oral vancomycin
○ Electrolyte replacement

Surgery

○ Diverting ileostomy or bowel resection (with perforation or toxic megacolon)
○ Early subtotal colectomy

Nursing considerations

Key outcomes

The patient will:
○ express feelings of increased comfort
○ maintain normal fluid volume
○ maintain stable vital signs
○ maintain adequate caloric intake
○ regain normal bowel function
○ regain normal laboratory values.

Nursing interventions

○ Give prescribed drugs and I.V. fluids.
○ Keep the patient as comfortable as possible.
○ Maintain precautions to prevent the infection from spreading to other patients.

Monitoring

○ Vital signs
○ Fluid and nutritional status
○ Skin integrity
○ Bowel function
○ Electrolytes

Patient teaching

Be sure to cover:
○ the disorder, diagnosis, and treatment
○ drug administration, dosage, and possible adverse effects
○ signs and symptoms of a recurrence
○ importance of cautioning future prescribers (if the disorder was antibiotic-related).

Psoriasis

Overview

Description

- Hereditary chronic skin disease marked by epidermal proliferation
- Causes lesions of erythematous papules and plaques covered with silvery scales (Lesions vary widely in severity and distribution.)
- Involves recurring remissions and exacerbations
- Exacerbations unpredictable, but usually controllable with therapy

Pathophysiology

- Psoriatic skin cells have a shortened maturation time as they migrate from the basal membrane to the surface or stratum corneum.
- As a result, the stratum corneum develops thick, scaly plaques (the cardinal manifestation of psoriasis).

Causes

- Genetic predisposition
- Possible autoimmune process
- Physical trauma
- Beta-hemolytic streptococci infection

Risk factors

- Pregnancy
- Endocrine changes
- Cold weather
- Emotional stress

Incidence

- Affects about 2% of the U.S. population
- Affects both sexes equally
- Can occur at any age
- More frequent among whites
- Two periods of onset: early (young adulthood) and late (middle adulthood)

Common characteristics

- Silvery scales on red plaques
- Pruritus
- Knee-elbow-scalp distribution

Complications

- Infection
- Altered self-image
- Social isolation
- Depression

Assessment

History

- Family history of psoriasis
- Risk factors

- Pruritus and burning
- Arthritic symptoms such as morning joint stiffness
- Remissions and exacerbations

Physical findings

- Erythematous, well-demarcated papules and plaques covered with silver scales, typically appearing on the scalp, chest, elbows, knees, back, and buttocks
- In mild psoriasis: plaques scattered over a small skin area
- In moderate psoriasis: plaques more numerous and larger (up to several centimeters in diameter)
- In severe psoriasis: plaques covering at least half the body
- Friable or adherent scales
- Fine bleeding points or Auspitz sign after attempts to remove scales
- Thin, erythematous guttate lesions, alone or with plaques, and with few scales (see *Identifying types of psoriasis*)
- Small indentations or pits, and yellow or brown discoloration of fingernails or toenails
- In severe cases, separation of nail from nail bed

Test results

Laboratory
- Elevated serum uric acid level
- In early-onset familial psoriasis: human leukocyte antigens Cw6, B13, and Bw-57

Diagnostic procedures
- Skin biopsy to help rule out other diseases

Treatment

General

- Depends on the psoriasis type, extent, and effect on the patient's quality of life
- Lesion management
- Lukewarm baths
- Ultraviolet B light or natural sunlight

Medication

- Topical corticosteroid creams and ointments
- Antihistamines
- Analgesics
- Nonsteroidal anti-inflammatory agents
- Occlusive ointment bases
- Urea or salicylic acid preparations
- Coal tar preparations
- Vitamin D analogs
- Emollients
- Kerolytic agents
- Methotrexate for severe, unresponsive psoriasis
- Potent retinoic acid derivative for resistant psoriasis
- Cyclosporine for severe, widespread psoriasis

Surgery

- Surgical nail removal to treat severely disfigured or damaged nails caused by psoriasis

Psoriasis occurs in various forms, ranging from one or two localized plaques that seldom require long-term medical attention to widespread lesions and crippling arthritis.

Erythrodermic psoriasis
This type is marked by extensive flushing all over the body, which may result in scaling. The rash may develop rapidly, signaling new psoriasis or gradually in chronic psoriasis. Sometimes the rash occurs as an adverse drug reaction.

Guttate psoriasis
This type typically affects children and young adults. Erupting in drop-sized plaques over the trunk, arms, legs and, sometimes, the scalp, this rash generalizes in several days. It's commonly associated with upper respiratory streptococcal infections.

Inverse psoriasis
Smooth, dry, bright red plaques characterize inverse psoriasis. Located in skin folds (armpits and groin, for example), the plaques fissure easily.

Psoriasis vulgaris
This psoriasis type is the most common. It begins with red, dotlike lesions that gradually enlarge and produce dry, silvery scales. The plaques usually appear symmetrically on the knees, elbows, extremities, genitalia, scalp, and nails.

Pustular psoriasis
This type features an eruption of local or extensive small, raised, pus-filled plaques. Possible triggers include emotional stress, sweating, infections, and adverse drug reactions.

Nursing considerations

Key outcomes

The patient will:
○ exhibit improved or healed lesions
○ report feelings of increased comfort
○ verbalize feelings about changed body image
○ demonstrate understanding of proper skin care
○ express an understanding of the condition and its treatment.

Nursing interventions

○ Give prescribed drugs.
○ Apply topical medications using a downward motion.
○ Encourage the patient to verbalize his feelings.
○ Provide emotional support.
○ Involve family members in the treatment regimen.

Monitoring

○ Response to treatment
○ Lipid profile results
○ Liver function tests
○ Renal function
○ Blood pressure
○ Signs and symptoms of hepatic or bone marrow toxicity

Patient teaching

Be sure to cover:
○ the disorder, diagnosis, and treatment
○ risk factors
○ incommunicability of psoriasis
○ likelihood of exacerbations and remissions
○ drug administration, dosage, and possible adverse effects
○ how to apply prescribed ointments, creams, and lotions

○ importance of avoiding scratching plaques
○ measures to relieve pruritus
○ importance of avoiding sun exposure
○ stress-reduction techniques
○ safety precautions
○ relationship between psoriasis and arthritis
○ when to notify the physician.

Discharge planning

○ Refer the patient to the National Psoriasis Foundation.

Ptosis

Overview

Description
○ Drooping of the upper eyelid
○ May be congenital or acquired, unilateral or bilateral, constant or intermittent
○ If severe, usually responds to treatment; if slight, may not require treatment
○ Also known as *blepharoptosis*

Pathophysiology
○ Dysfunction of one or both upper eyelid levator muscles

Causes
Congenital ptosis
○ Transmitted as an autosomal dominant trait
○ Results from a congenital anomaly in which the levator muscles of the eyelids fail to develop
Acquired ptosis
○ Advanced age (involutional ptosis, the most common form, usually seen in older patients following cataract surgery)
○ Mechanical factors that make the eyelid heavy
○ Myogenic factors
○ Neurogenic (paralytic) factors
○ Nutritional factors
○ Trauma
○ Ocular surgery

Incidence
○ Congenital ptosis occurs at birth
○ Acquired ptosis can occur at any age but mostly affects adults
○ Affects both sexes equally

Common characteristics
○ An infant with congenital ptosis has a smooth, flat upper eyelid, without the eyelid fold normally caused by the pull of the levator muscle; associated weakness of the superior rectus muscle isn't uncommon.
○ Ptosis due to oculomotor nerve damage produces a fixed, dilated pupil; divergent strabismus; and slight depression of the eyeball.

Complications
○ Disturbed vision
○ Amblyopia
○ Infection (after surgery)
○ Psychosocial effects

Assessment

History
○ History of causative factor
○ Family history
○ Trauma or ocular surgery

Physical findings
○ Abnormal eyelid
○ Drooping eyelid (see *Recognizing ptosis*)
○ Elevated eyebrow
○ Wrinkled forehead
○ Fixed, dilated pupil

Test results
Imaging
○ Digital subtraction angiography and magnetic resonance imaging (MRI) show aneurysm.
○ MRI reveals multiple sclerosis
Diagnostic procedures
○ Glucose tolerance test detects diabetes.
○ Tensilon test detects myasthenia gravis (in acquired ptosis with no history of trauma).
Other
○ Physical examination reveals upper lid retraction.
○ Examination with the Hertel exophthalmometer reveals the degree of proptosis.

Treatment

General
○ Treatment of underlying cause
○ Special glasses with an attached suspended crutch on the frames to elevate the eyelid
○ Eye protection with potentially dangerous activities

Medication
○ Topical antibiotic ointment (after surgery)

Surgery
○ Resection of the weak levator muscles

Nursing considerations

Key outcomes
The patient will:
○ avoid injury
○ demonstrate improvement in eyelid function
○ express understanding of the disorder and its treatment.

Nursing interventions
○ Provide a safe environment.
○ Apply ointment to the sutures as prescribed.

Monitoring
○ Signs of bleeding (after surgery)
○ Visual acuity

Recognizing ptosis

A drooping upper eyelid — typically apparent on visual examination — is the hallmark of ptosis. The disorder may affect one or both eyelids.

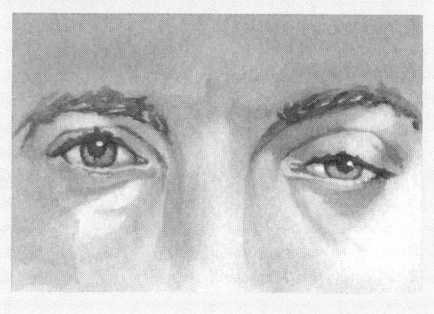

Patient teaching

Be sure to cover:
○ the need to report any postsurgery bleeding immediately
○ the need to prevent accidental trauma to the surgical site until healing is complete.

Discharge planning

○ Refer the patient to a neurologist if myasthenia gravis or multiple sclerosis is diagnosed.

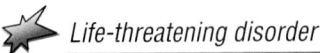 *Life-threatening disorder*

Pulmonary edema

Overview

Description

- ○ Accumulation of fluid in the extravascular spaces of the lung
- ○ Common complication of cardiovascular disorders
- ○ May be chronic or acute
- ○ Can become fatal rapidly

Pathophysiology

- ○ Pulmonary edema results from either increased pulmonary capillary hydrostatic pressure or decreased colloid osmotic pressure. Normally, the two pressures are in balance.
- ○ If pulmonary capillary hydrostatic pressure increases, the compromised left ventricle needs higher filling pressures to maintain adequate output; these pressures are transmitted to the left atrium, pulmonary veins, and pulmonary capillary bed. Fluids and solutes are then forced from the intravascular compartment into the lung interstitium. With fluid overloading the interstitium, some fluid floods peripheral alveoli and impairs gas exchange.
- ○ If colloid osmotic pressure decreases, the pulling force that contains intravascular fluids is lost, and nothing opposes the hydrostatic force. Fluid flows freely into the interstitium and alveoli, causing pulmonary edema.

Causes

- ○ Left-sided heart failure
- ○ Diastolic dysfunction
- ○ Valvular heart disease
- ○ Arrhythmias
- ○ Fluid overload
- ○ Acute myocardial ischemia and infarction
- ○ Barbiturate or opiate poisoning
- ○ Impaired pulmonary lymphatic drainage
- ○ Inhalation of irritating gases
- ○ Left atrial myxoma
- ○ Pneumonia
- ○ Pulmonary veno-occlusive disease

Incidence

- ○ More common in middle-aged and elderly people
- ○ Affects both sexes equally

Common characteristics

- ○ Persistent cough
- ○ Dyspnea on exertion
- ○ Orthopnea
- ○ Paroxysmal nocturnal dyspnea

Complications

- ○ Respiratory and metabolic acidosis
- ○ Cardiac or respiratory arrest
- ○ Death

Assessment

History

- ○ Predisposing factor
- ○ Persistent cough
- ○ Dyspnea on exertion
- ○ Paroxysmal nocturnal dyspnea
- ○ Orthopnea

Physical findings

- ○ Restlessness and anxiety
- ○ Rapid, labored breathing
- ○ Intense, productive cough
- ○ Frothy, bloody sputum
- ○ Mental status changes
- ○ Jugular vein distention
- ○ Sweaty, cold, clammy skin
- ○ Wheezing
- ○ Crackles
- ○ S_3
- ○ Tachycardia
- ○ Hypotension
- ○ Thready pulse
- ○ Peripheral edema
- ○ Hepatomegaly

Test results

Laboratory
- ○ Arterial blood gas (ABG) analysis showing hypoxemia, hypercapnia, or acidosis

Imaging
- ○ Chest X-rays show diffuse haziness of the lung fields, cardiomegaly, and pleural effusion.

Diagnostic procedures
- ○ Pulse oximetry may show decreased oxygen saturation.
- ○ Pulmonary artery catheterization may reveal increased pulmonary artery wedge pressures.
- ○ Electrocardiography may show valvular disease and left ventricular hypokinesis or akinesis.

Treatment

General

- ○ Fluid overload reduction
- ○ Improved gas exchange and myocardial function
- ○ Correction of underlying disease
- ○ Sodium-restricted diet
- ○ Fluid restriction
- ○ Activity, as tolerated

Medication

- ○ Supplemental oxygen
- ○ Diuretics

○ Antiarrhythmics
○ Morphine

 Alert

Be aware that morphine can further compromise respirations in a patient with respiratory distress. Keep resuscitation equipment at hand in case the patient stops breathing.

○ Preload-reducing agents
○ Afterload-reducing agents
○ Bronchodilators
○ Positive inotropic agents
○ Vasopressors

Surgery

○ Valve repair or replacement or myocardial revascularization if appropriate to correct the underlying cause

Nursing considerations

Key outcomes

The patient will:
○ maintain adequate ventilation
○ maintain fluid balance
○ maintain adequate cardiac output
○ verbalize decreased anxiety and fear
○ demonstrate adequate coping mechanisms.

Nursing interventions

○ Give prescribed drugs and oxygen.
○ Place the patient in high Fowler's position.
○ Restrict fluids and sodium intake.
○ Promote rest and relaxation.
○ Provide emotional support.

Monitoring

○ Vital signs
○ Intake and output
○ Daily weight
○ Respiratory status
○ Response to treatment
○ Complications
○ Heart rhythm
○ ABG values
○ Pulse oximetry values
○ Hemodynamic values

Patient teaching

Be sure to cover:
○ the disorder, diagnosis, and treatment
○ drug administration, dosage, and possible adverse effects
○ fluid and sodium restrictions
○ daily weight
○ signs and symptoms of fluid overload

○ energy conservation strategies
○ avoidance of alcohol
○ when to notify the physician.

Discharge planning

○ Refer the patient to a cardiac rehabilitation program, if indicated
○ Refer the patient to a smoking-cessation program, if indicated.

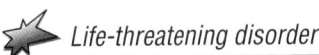

Pulmonary embolism

Overview

Description

- ○ Obstruction of the pulmonary arterial bed occurring when a mass (such as a dislodged thrombus) lodges in the main pulmonary artery or branch, partially or completely obstructing it
- ○ Most thrombi originate in deep veins of the leg
- ○ Can be asymptomatic, but sometimes causes rapid death from pulmonary infarction

Pathophysiology

- ○ Thrombus formation results from vascular wall damage, venous stasis, or blood hypercoagulability.
- ○ Trauma, clot dissolution, sudden muscle spasm, intravascular pressure changes, or peripheral blood flow changes can cause the thrombus to loosen or fragmentize.
- ○ The thrombus (now an embolus) floats to the heart's right side and enters the lung through the pulmonary artery. There, the embolus may dissolve, continue to fragmentize, or grow.
- ○ By occluding the pulmonary artery, the embolus prevents alveoli from producing enough surfactant to maintain alveolar integrity. Alveoli collapse and atelectasis develops.
- ○ If the embolus enlarges, it may occlude most or all of the pulmonary vessels and cause death.

Causes

- ○ Deep vein thrombosis
- ○ Pelvic, renal, and hepatic vein thrombosis
- ○ Right heart thrombus
- ○ Upper extremity thrombosis
- ○ Atrial fibrillation
- ○ Valvular heart disease
- ○ Rarely, other types of emboli, such as bone, air, fat, amniotic fluid, tumor cells, or a foreign body

Risk factors

- ○ Various disorders and treatments (See *Who's at risk for pulmonary embolism?*)

Incidence

- ○ 600,000 to 700,000 cases annually
- ○ Affects both sexes equally
- ○ More common with advancing age

Common characteristics

- ○ Shortness of breath for no apparent reason
- ○ Tachycardia
- ○ Anxiety
- ○ Pleuritic or anginal pain

Complications

- ○ Pulmonary infarction
- ○ Pulmonary hypertension
- ○ Embolic extension
- ○ Hepatic congestion and necrosis
- ○ Pulmonary abscess
- ○ Shock
- ○ Acute respiratory distress syndrome
- ○ Massive atelectasis
- ○ Right-sided heart failure
- ○ Ventilation-perfusion mismatch
- ○ Death

Assessment

History

- ○ Predisposing factor
- ○ Shortness of breath for no apparent reason
- ○ Pleuritic pain or angina

Physical findings

- ○ Tachycardia
- ○ Low-grade fever
- ○ Weak, rapid pulse
- ○ Hypotension
- ○ Productive cough, possibly with blood-tinged sputum
- ○ Warmth, tenderness, and edema of the lower leg
- ○ Restlessness
- ○ Transient pleural friction rub
- ○ Crackles
- ○ S_3 and S_4 with increased intensity of the pulmonic component of S_2
- ○ With a large embolus: cyanosis, syncope, distended neck veins

Test results

Laboratory
- ○ Arterial blood gas (ABG) values showing hypoxemia
- ○ Elevated D-dimer level

Imaging
- ○ Lung ventilation perfusion scan shows a ventilation-perfusion mismatch.
- ○ Pulmonary angiography shows a pulmonary vessel filling defect or an abrupt vessel ending and reveals the location and extent of pulmonary embolism.
- ○ Chest X-rays may show a small infiltrate or effusion.
- ○ Spiral chest computed tomography scan may show central pulmonary emboli.

Diagnostic procedures
- ○ Electrocardiography may reveal right axis deviation and right bundle-branch block; it also may show atrial fibrillation.

Treatment

General

- ○ Maintenance of adequate cardiovascular and pulmonary function
- ○ Mechanical ventilation, if indicated

Many disorders and treatments heighten the risk of pulmonary embolism. At particular risk are surgical patients. The anesthetic used during surgery can injure lung vessels, and surgery or prolonged bed rest can promote venous stasis, which compounds the risk.

Predisposing disorders
- Lung disorders, especially chronic types
- Cardiac disorders
- Infection
- Diabetes mellitus
- History of thromboembolism, thrombophlebitis, or vascular insufficiency
- Sickle cell disease
- Autoimmune hemolytic anemia
- Polycythemia
- Osteomyelitis
- Long-bone fracture
- Manipulation or disconnection of central lines

Venous stasis
- Prolonged bed rest or immobilization
- Obesity
- Older than age 40
- Burns
- Recent childbirth
- Orthopedic casts

Venous injury
- Surgery, particularly of the legs, pelvis, abdomen, or thorax
- Leg or pelvic fractures or injuries
- I.V. drug abuse
- I.V. therapy

Increased blood coagulability
- Cancer
- Use of high-estrogen hormonal contraceptives

- Possible fluid restriction
- Bed rest during the acute phase

Medication

- Oxygen therapy
- Thrombolytics
- Anticoagulation
- Corticosteroids (controversial)
- Diuretics
- Antiarrhythmics
- Vasopressors (for hypotension)
- Antibiotics (for septic embolus)

Surgery

- Vena caval interruption
- Vena caval filter placement
- Pulmonary embolectomy

Nursing considerations

Key outcomes

The patient will:
- maintain adequate ventilation
- maintain adequate cardiac output
- maintain a patent airway
- verbalize feelings of increased comfort
- demonstrate effective coping mechanisms.

Nursing interventions

- Give prescribed drugs.
- Avoid I.M. injections.
- Encourage active and passive range-of-motion exercises, unless contraindicated.
- Avoid massage of the lower legs.
- Apply antiembolism stockings.
- Provide adequate nutrition.

- Assist with ambulation as soon as the patient is stable.
- Encourage use of incentive spirometry.

Monitoring

- Vital signs
- Intake and output
- Respiratory status
- Pulse oximetry
- ABG values
- Signs of deep vein thrombosis
- Complications
- Coagulation study results
- Abnormal bleeding
- Stools for occult blood

Patient teaching

Be sure to cover:
- the disease, diagnosis, and treatment
- drug administration, dosage, and possible adverse effects
- ways to prevent deep vein thrombosis and pulmonary embolism
- signs and symptoms of abnormal bleeding
- prevention of abnormal bleeding
- how to monitor anticoagulant effects
- dietary sources of vitamin K
- when to notify the physician.

Discharge planning

- Refer the patient to a weight-management program, if indicated.

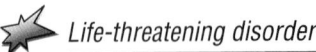

Pulmonary hypertension

Overview

Description

○ Pulmonary condition in which there's increased pressure in the pulmonary artery
○ Occurs in a primary form (rare) and a secondary form
○ In both forms, resting systolic pulmonary artery pressure (PAP) above 30 mm Hg and mean PAP above 20 mm Hg
○ Primary form also known as *PPH*

Pathophysiology

○ In primary pulmonary hypertension, the intimal lining of the pulmonary arteries thickens for no apparent reason. This narrows the artery and impairs distensibility, increasing vascular resistance.
○ Secondary pulmonary hypertension occurs from hypoxemia caused by conditions involving alveolar hypoventilation, vascular obstruction, or left-to-right shunting.

Causes

Primary pulmonary hypertension
○ Unknown
○ Possible hereditary factors
○ Possible altered autoimmune mechanisms
○ Associated with portal hypertension
Secondary pulmonary hypertension
○ Chronic obstructive pulmonary disease
○ Sarcoidosis
○ Diffuse interstitial pneumonia
○ Malignant metastases
○ Scleroderma
○ Use of some diet drugs
○ Obesity
○ Sleep apnea
○ Hypoventilation syndromes
○ Kyphoscoliosis
○ Pulmonary embolism
○ Vasculitis
○ Left atrial myxoma
○ Congenital cardiac defects
○ Mitral stenosis

Incidence

Primary pulmonary hypertension
○ Most common in women ages 20 to 40
○ More prevalent in people with collagen disease

Common characteristics

○ Dyspnea on exertion
○ Weakness, fatigue
○ Syncope

Complications

○ Cor pulmonale
○ Heart failure
○ Cardiac arrest
○ Death

Assessment

History

○ Shortness of breath with exertion
○ Weakness, fatigue
○ Pain during breathing
○ Near-syncope

Physical findings

○ Ascites
○ Jugular vein distention
○ Peripheral edema
○ Restlessness and agitation
○ Mental status changes
○ Decreased diaphragmatic excursion
○ Apical impulse displaced beyond mid-clavicular line
○ Right ventricular lift
○ Reduced carotid pulse
○ Hepatomegaly
○ Tachycardia
○ Systolic ejection murmur
○ Widely split S_2
○ S_3 and S_4
○ Hypotension
○ Decreased breath sounds
○ Tubular breath sounds

Test results

Laboratory
○ Arterial blood gas (ABG) values shows hypoxemia
Imaging
○ Ventilation-perfusion lung scan may show a ventilation-perfusion mismatch.
○ Pulmonary angiography may reveal filling defects in the pulmonary vasculature.
Diagnostic procedures
○ Electrocardiography may reveal right-axis deviation.
○ Pulmonary artery catheterization shows increased PAP, with systolic pressure above 30 mm Hg; increased pulmonary artery wedge pressure; decreased cardiac output; and decreased cardiac index.
○ Pulmonary function tests may show decreased flow rates and increased residual volume or reduced total lung capacity.
○ Echocardiography may show valvular heart disease or atrial myxoma.
Other
○ Lung biopsy may show tumor cells.

Treatment

General

○ Low-sodium diet
○ Fluid restriction (in right-sided heart failure)
○ Bed rest during acute phase

Medication

○ Oxygen therapy
○ Cardiac glycosides
○ Diuretics
○ Vasodilators
○ Calcium channel blockers
○ Bronchodilators
○ Beta-adrenergic blockers
○ Epoprostenol

Surgery

○ Heart-lung transplantation, if indicated

Nursing considerations

Key outcomes

The patient will:
○ maintain adequate ventilation
○ maintain adequate cardiac output
○ express an understanding of the disorder
○ demonstrate effective coping mechanisms.

Nursing interventions

○ Give prescribe drugs and oxygen.
○ Implement comfort measures.
○ Provide adequate rest periods.
○ Offer emotional support.

Monitoring

○ Vital signs
○ Intake and output
○ Daily weight
○ Respiratory status
○ Signs and symptoms of right-sided heart failure
○ Heart rhythm
○ ABG values
○ Hemodynamic values

Patient teaching

Be sure to cover:
○ the disorder, diagnosis, and treatment
○ drug administration, dosage, and possible adverse effects
○ dietary restrictions

○ frequent rest periods
○ signs and symptoms of right-sided heart failure
○ when to notify the physician.

Discharge planning

○ Refer the patient to a smoking-cessation program, if indicated.

Pulmonic insufficiency

Overview

Description

- Heart condition in which blood ejected into the pulmonary artery during systole flows back into the right ventricle during diastole
- Also called *pulmonary regurgitation*

Pathophysiology

- Pulmonic valve is incompetent.
- Incompetency is caused by:
  - dilation of the pulmonic valve ring
  - acquired alteration of pulmonic cusp morphology
  - congenital absence or malformation
- Blood flows back into the right ventricle from the pulmonary artery.
- Fluid overload occurs in the ventricle.
- Chronic backflow causes ventricular hypertrophy and right-sided heart failure.

Causes

- Pulmonary hypertension
- Infective endocarditis
- Tetralogy of Fallot
- Rheumatic heart disease
- Carcinoid heart disease
- Dilated cardiomyopathy

Incidence

- Variable age of occurrence
- Affects both males and females; frequency based on specific cause

Common characteristics

- Dyspnea on exertion
- Peripheral edema
- Tachycardia
- Fatigue

Complications

- Heart failure
- Pulmonary edema
- Thromboembolism
- Endocarditis
- Arrhythmias

Assessment

History

- Pulmonary hypertension
- Infective endocarditis
- Tetralogy of Fallot
- Rheumatic heart disease
- Carcinoid heart disease
- Orthopnea
- Dyspnea
- Fatigue
- Angina
- Palpitations

Physical findings

- Tachycardia
- Crackles in the lungs
- Hepatomegaly (right-sided failure)
- Jugular vein distention
- Palpable right ventricular systolic pulsation at left lower sternal border
- S_3 or S_4 at left mid-to-lower sternal border
- Hemoptysis

Test results

Imaging

- Chest X-rays reveal cardiomegaly, right-sided heart enlargement, and pulmonary hypertension.
- Echocardiography shows right ventricular hypertrophy and dilation.

Diagnostic procedures

- Electrocardiogram may show incomplete right bundle branch block and right axis deviation.
- Cardiac catheterization may determine underlying etiology.

Treatment

General

- Treatment of underlying cause
- Symptomatic treatment
- Low-sodium diet
- Activity, as tolerated

Medication

- Diuretics
- Inotropic agent
- Angiotensin-converting enzyme inhibitors
- Oxygen
- Prophylactic antibiotics before and after surgery or dental care to prevent endocarditis

Surgery

- Annuloplasty or valvuloplasty to reconstruct or repair the valve
- Valve replacement with a prosthetic valve

Nursing considerations

Key outcomes

The patient will:
- perform activities of daily living without weakness or fatigue
- maintain hemodynamic stability
- maintain adequate ventilation.

Nursing interventions

- Give prescribed oxygen.
- Watch for signs of heart failure or pulmonary edema.

Monitoring

○ Vital signs and pulse oximetry
○ Cardiac rhythm
○ Pulmonary artery catheter readings
○ Intake and output
○ Adverse effects of drug therapy

Patient teaching

Be sure to cover:
○ the disorder, diagnosis, and treatment
○ dietary restrictions
○ drug administration, dosage, and possible adverse
  effects.

Discharge planning

○ Encourage follow-up care with a cardiologist.

Pulmonic stenosis

Overview

Description
- Heart condition in which obstructed right ventricular outflow causes right-ventricular hypertrophy, eventually resulting in right-sided heart failure
- Also called *pulmonary regurgitation*

Pathophysiology
- Dynamic or fixed obstruction affects blood flow from the right ventricle to the pulmonary arteriole vasculature.
- Chronic obstruction may result in right-sided heart failure.

Causes
- Congenital defect
- Sinus of Valsalva aneurysm
- Aortic graft aneurysm
- Rheumatic heart disease
- Carcinoid heart disease

Incidence
- Affects females slightly more than males

Common characteristics
- Dyspnea on exertion
- Peripheral edema
- Cyanosis
- Tachycardia
- Fatigue

Complications
- Heart failure
- Pulmonary edema
- Thromboembolism
- Endocarditis
- Arrhythmias

Assessment

History
- Congenital defect
- Sinus of Valsalva aneurysm
- Aortic graft aneurysm
- Rheumatic heart disease
- Carcinoid heart disease
- Orthopnea
- Exertional dyspnea
- Fatigue
- Angina
- Palpitations

Physical findings
- Palpable impulse from the right ventricle along the left parasternal border
- Peripheral edema
- Split S_2
- Systolic ejection click
- Crackles in the lungs
- Hepatomegaly (right-sided failure)
- Jugular vein distention

Test results
Imaging
- Chest X-rays reveal prominence of the main, right, or left pulmonary arteries.
- Echocardiography shows thickening of the valves, characteristic doming of nondysplastic valves, and right ventricular hypertrophy.
- Cardiac ultrasound reveals thickening of valves, characteristic doming of nondysplastic valves, and right-ventricular hypertrophy.

Diagnostic procedures
- Electrocardiogram may show mild right axis deviation.

Treatment

General
- Treatment of underlying cause
- Low-sodium diet
- Avoidance of vigorous physical activity

Medication
- Diuretics
- Inotropic agents
- Angiotensin-converting enzyme inhibitors
- Oxygen
- Prophylactic antibiotics before and after surgery or dental care to prevent endocarditis

Surgery
- Balloon valvoplasty
- Pulmonary artery balloon angioplasty
- Valvotomy

Nursing considerations

Key outcomes
The patient will:
- perform activities of daily living without weakness or fatigue
- maintain hemodynamic stability
- maintain adequate ventilation
- state understanding of disorder and treatment.

Nursing interventions
- Give prescribed oxygen.
- Watch for signs of heart failure or pulmonary edema.
- Encourage verbalization and provide support.
- Give prescribed drugs.

Monitoring

○ Vital signs and pulse oximetry
○ Cardiac rhythm
○ Pulmonary artery catheter readings
○ Intake and output
○ Adverse effects of drug therapy

Patient teaching

Be sure to cover:
○ the disorder, diagnosis, and treatment
○ dietary restrictions
○ activity restrictions
○ drug administration, dosage, and possible adverse
effects.

Discharge planning

○ Encourage follow-up care with a cardiologist.

Q fever

Overview

Description
○ Acute systemic disease that affects people exposed to cattle, sheep, or goats
○ Rare human-to-human transmission; possible sexual transmission
○ May be acute or chronic

Pathophysiology
○ Coxiella burnetii is excreted in urine, milk, and feces of infected animals.
○ Once ingested, it proliferates in macrophages (in the acidic phagolysosome vacuole) and then gains access to the blood, producing a transient bacteremia.
○ It may invade many organs, most often the lungs and liver.
○ Inflammation occurs, manifested by granulomas in the liver, spleen, and bone marrow. These classic doughnut granulomas disappear with convalescence.

Causes
○ Coxiella burnetii

Incidence
○ Affects men more than women because men are more likely to be exposed to livestock
○ Most often affects people ages 25 to 40

Common characteristics
○ Self-limiting, febrile illness with headache, myalgia, chills
○ May have symptoms of pneumonia, hepatitis, or endocarditis (chronic)
○ May be asymptomatic

Complications
○ Chronic fatigue syndrome
○ Heart failure
○ Endocarditis (see *Treating Q fever endocarditis*)

Treating Q fever endocarditis

Chronic Q fever endocarditis often requires the use of multiple drugs to treat effectively. Two different drug treatment protocols have been evaluated:
○ doxycycline with quinolones, for at least 4 years
○ doxycycline with hydroxychloroquine, for 1½ to 3 years.
The second drug treatment protocol causes fewer relapses but requires routine eye examinations to detect accumulation of chloroquine.
  Some patients with *C. burnetii* endocarditis require surgery to remove damaged valves.

Assessment

History
○ Exposure to cattle, sheep, or goats
○ Headache
○ Mylagia
○ Chills, fever

Physical findings
○ Crackles (pneumonia)
○ Hepatomegaly and jaundice (hepatitis)
○ Heart murmur, signs of heart failure (endocarditis)

Test results
Laboratory
○ Patients with acute form may have an elevated white blood cell count, transient thrombocytopenia, and elevated transaminases and ALP.
○ CSF evaluation reveals lymphocytosis, elevated protein level, and normal glucose level.
○ Complement fixation reveals antephase II antibody titers of 40 or more (acute disease) and antiphase I antibody titers of 200 of more (chronic disease).
○ Microimmunofluorescence reveals immunoglobulin (Ig) G antiphase II antibody titers of 200 or more and IgM antephase II antibody titers of 50 or more (acute). (The presence of antephase I antibodies indicates chronic Q fever; the presence of IgG antephase I antibody titers of 800 or more is highly predictive of endocarditis.)
Imaging
○ Chest X-rays may show segmental or lobar opacities, multiple round opacities, and pleural effusion.
○ Echocardiogram may show pericardial effusion with pericarditis.
Diagnostic procedures
○ Electrocardiogram shows T-wave abnormalities with myocarditis and pericarditis.

Treatment

General
○ Symptomatic
○ Diet as tolerated
○ Activity as tolerated

Medication
○ Antibiotics
○ Antimalarial agents

Surgery
○ Possible valve replacement

Nursing considerations

Key outcomes

The patient will:
- express understanding of illness and treatment regimen
- remain hemodynamically stable
- remain free of complications.

Nursing interventions

- Provide emotional support.
- Give prescribed drugs.

Monitoring

- Vital signs
- Cardiac status
- Respiratory status
- Response to treatment

Patient teaching

Be sure to cover:
- the disorder, diagnosis, and treatment
- the importance of follow-up care and compliance with long-term therapy
- dosage, administration, and possible adverse effects of prescribed medications.

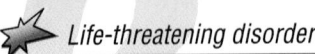

Rabies

Overview

Description

- An acute central nervous system (CNS) infection usually transmitted by animal bite
- Incubation period usually 20 to 90 days, possibly up to 19 years
- 70% of cases in the United States from raccoon, skunk, fox, or bat bite; vaccinations have reduced transmission from dogs
- Almost always fatal if symptoms occur, although prompt treatment may prevent fatal CNS invasion

Pathophysiology

- The rabies virus is transmitted through the bite of an infected animal that introduces the virus through the skin or mucous membrane.
- The virus begins to replicate in the striated muscle cells at the bite site.
- It then travels up the nerve to the CNS and replicates in the brain.
- Finally, it moves through the nerves into other tissues, including the salivary glands.

Causes

- Bite from a rabid animal
- Occasionally transmitted by airborne droplets and infected tissue transplants

Incidence

- Can affect anyone at any age
- Annually, an estimated 35,000 to 50,000 deaths worldwide

First aid for animal bites

- Immediately wash the bite vigorously with soap and water for at least 10 minutes to remove the animal's saliva.
- Flush the wound with an antiviral, followed by a clear-water rinse.
- Apply a sterile dressing.
- If possible, don't suture the wound, and don't immediately stop the bleeding (unless it's massive) because blood flow helps to clean the wound.
- Question the patient about the bite. Ask whether he provoked the animal (if so, chances are it isn't rabid) and whether he can identify it or its owner. (The animal may be confined for observation.)
- Consult local health authorities for treatment information.

Common characteristics

- Progressive signs and symptoms
- After incubation period, local or radiating pain or burning and coldness, pruritus, and tingling at the bite site
- Slight fever (100° to 102° F [37.8° to 38.9° C])
- Malaise
- Nervousness that progresses into agitation and cranial nerve dysfunction, causing ocular palsies
- Hyperesthesia
- Photophobia
- Sensitivity to loud noise
- Pupillary dilation
- Tachycardia
- Shallow respirations
- Excessive salivation, lacrimation, and perspiration
- Hydrophobia, during which forceful, painful pharyngeal muscle spasms expel liquids from the mouth and cause dehydration
- After about 3 days, gradual, generalized, flaccid paralysis that ultimately leads to peripheral vascular collapse, coma, and death

Assessment

History

- Animal bite
- Fever
- Malaise

Physical findings

- Burning at wound site
- Tachycardia
- Excessive salivation
- Shallow respirations
- Dilated pupils and photophobia

Test results

Laboratory

- Virus is isolated from the patient's saliva or throat; examination of blood shows fluorescent rabies antibody (FRA).
- White blood cell count is elevated with increased polymorphonuclear and large mononuclear cells.
- Urinary glucose, acetone, and protein levels are elevated.

Other

- Animal should be confined and observed for 10 days by a veterinarian. (If the animal appears rabid, it should be killed and its brain tissues tested for FRA and Negri bodies.)

Complications

- Paralysis
- Coma
- Death

Treatment

General

○ Immediate wound treatment (see *First aid for animal bites*)

Medication

○ Tetanus-diphtheria prophylaxis, if needed
○ Passive immunization with rabies immune globulin and active immunization with human diploid cell vaccine as soon as possible (if not previously immunized)
○ Vaccine booster (if already immunized)

Nursing considerations

Key outcomes

The patient will:
○ remain hemodynamically stable
○ express understanding of the treatment regimen
○ express concerns regarding infection.

Nursing interventions

○ When injecting the rabies vaccine, rotate injection sites on the upper arm or thigh.
○ Cooperate with public health authorities to determine the animal's vaccination status. If the animal is proven rabid, help identify others at risk.
○ Provide aggressive supportive care (even after onset of coma).
○ Follow standard precautions.
○ Provide emotional support.

Monitoring

○ Injection site reactions
○ Cardiac and pulmonary function

Patient teaching

Be sure to cover:
○ the need for vaccination of household pets that may be exposed to rabid wild animals
○ importance of not touching wild animals, especially if they appear ill or overly docile (a possible sign of rabies)
○ prophylactic rabies vaccine for high-risk people, such as farm workers, forest rangers, spelunkers (cave explorers), and veterinarians.

Radiation exposure

Overview

Description

- Exposure to excessive radiation that causes tissue damage
- Damage varies with amount of body area exposed, length of exposure, dosage absorbed, distance from the source, and presence of protective shielding
- Can result from cancer radiotherapy, working in a radiation facility, or other exposure to radioactive materials
- Can be acute or chronic

Pathophysiology

- Ionization occurs in the molecules of living cells.
- Electrons are removed from atoms. Charged atoms or ions form and react with other atoms to cause cell damage.
- Rapidly dividing cells are the most susceptible to radiation damage. Highly differentiated cells are more resistant to radiation.

Causes

- Exposure to radiation through inhalation, ingestion, or direct contact

Risk factors

- Cancer
- Employment in a radiation facility

Incidence

- Unknown

Common characteristics

- Nausea
- Diarrhea
- General weakness
- Immunosuppression
- Infections

Complications

- Leukemia
- Thyroid cancer
- Fetal growth retardation or genetic defects in offspring (from exposure during childbearing years)
- Decreased fertility
- Shortened life span
- Anemia
- Malignant neoplasms
- Bone necrosis and fractures

Assessment

History

Acute hematopoietic radiation toxicity
- Bleeding from the skin, genitourinary tract, and GI tract
- Nosebleeds
- Hemorrhage
- Increased susceptibility to infection

GI radiation toxicity
- Intractable nausea, vomiting, and diarrhea

Cerebral radiation toxicity
- Nausea, vomiting, and diarrhea
- Lethargy

Cardiovascular radiation toxicity
- Hypotension, shock, and cardiac arrhythmias

Physical findings

Acute hematopoietic radiation toxicity
- Petechiae
- Pallor
- Weakness
- Oropharyngeal abscesses

GI radiation toxicity
- Mouth and throat ulcers and infection
- Circulatory collapse and death

Cerebral radiation toxicity
- Tremors
- Seizures
- Confusion
- Coma and death

Generalized radiation exposure
- Signs of hypothyroidism
- Cataracts
- Skin dryness, erythema, atrophy, and malignant lesions
- Alopecia
- Brittle nails

Test results

Laboratory
- White blood cell, platelet, and lymphocyte counts are decreased.
- Serum potassium and chloride levels are decreased.

Imaging
- X-rays may reveal bone necrosis.

Diagnostic procedures
- Bone marrow studies may show blood dyscrasia.

Other
- Geiger counter helps determine if radioactive material was ingested or inhaled and evaluates the amount of radiation in open wounds.

Treatment

General

○ Management of life-threatening injuries
○ Symptomatic and supportive treatment
○ Based on the type and extent of radiation injury
○ High-protein, high-calorie diet
○ Activity as tolerated by clinical status

Medication

○ Chelating agents
○ Potassium iodide
○ Aluminum phosphate gel
○ Barium sulfate

Nursing considerations

Key outcomes

The patient will:
○ maintain an acceptable weight
○ maintain normal fluid volume
○ remain free from signs and symptoms of infection.

Nursing interventions

○ Implement appropriate respiratory and cardiac support measures.
○ Give prescribed I.V. fluids and electrolytes.
○ For skin contamination, wash the patient's body thoroughly with mild soap and water.
○ Debride and irrigate open wounds, as ordered.
○ For ingested radioactive material, perform gastric lavage and whole-bowel irrigation, and administer activated charcoal, as ordered.
○ Dispose of contaminated clothing properly.
○ Dispose of contaminated excrement and body fluids according to facility policy.
○ Use strict sterile technique.

Monitoring

○ Intake and output
○ Fluid and electrolyte balance
○ Vital signs
○ Signs and symptoms of hemorrhage
○ Nutritional status

Patient teaching

Be sure to cover:
○ the injury process, diagnosis, and treatment
○ effects of radiation exposure
○ how to prevent a recurrence
○ skin care
○ wound care
○ need for follow-up care.

Discharge planning

○ Refer the patient to resource and support services.
○ If the patient was exposed to significant amounts of radiation, provide a referral to genetic counseling resources.

Rape-trauma syndrome

Overview

Description

- Syndrome that occurs after rape (sexual intercourse without consent) or attempted rape and causes varying degrees of physical and psychological trauma
- Refers to the victim's short- and long-term reactions and the methods used to cope with trauma
- Carries a good prognosis if the victim receives physical and emotional support and counseling to help deal with feelings

Pathophysiology

- Rape causes psychological and physiologic reactions.
- Early stage (short-term) and late stage (long-term) reactions can occur.

Causes

- Rape or attempted rape

Incidence

- Affects all ages (reported victims from ages 2 months to 97 years)
- Most common in women ages 16 to 19 (about 8% of American women experience rape or attempted rape)
- Usually perpetrated by family member if victim is a child

Common characteristics

- Signs of physical trauma, depending on length of the attack and whether additional physical violence occurred
- Tearfulness, crying
- Withdrawal
- Anxiousness

Complications

- Lasting psychiatric problems, such as depression, guilt, anxiety, and suicidal ideation
- Sexually transmitted disease (STD)
- Unwanted pregnancy

Assessment

History

- Early stage:
  - Disbelief
  - Panic
  - Severe anxiety
  - Anger
  - Self-blame
  - Humiliation
  - Depression
- Late stage
  - Anxiety
  - Nightmares
  - Flashbacks
  - Depression
  - Anger
  - Disinterest in sex
  - Anorgasmia
  - Suicidal ideation
- Rape or attempted rape
- Time the victim arrived at the facility
- Date and time of alleged rape
- Time the victim was examined
- Whether the victim was pregnant at the time of the attack
- Date of last menstrual period
- Details of obstetric and gynecologic history
- Victim's statements (recorded in the first person, using quotation marks)
- Objective information provided by others

 Alert

Be aware that your assessment notes may be used as evidence if the rapist goes to trial.

Physical findings

- Sore throat
- Difficulty swallowing
- Vaginal pain
- Rectal pain
- Pain from other injuries incurred during the assault
- Early stage:
  - Reddened (sore) throat
  - Mouth irritation
  - Ecchymoses
  - Rectal pain and bleeding
  - Lacerations, contusions, and abrasions to vulva, cervix, and vaginal walls
  - Lacerations and contusions in a male victim
  - Outward calm
  - Compliance
  - Glibness
  - Talkativeness

Test results

Laboratory
- STD screening tests may reveal positive results.
- Rapid plasma reagin card test may show positive for syphilis.
- Urine pregnancy test may be positive 0 to 3 weeks after missed period.
- Serum human chorionic gonadotropin test becomes positive 24 to 48 hours after implantation.
- Drug screen (if symptoms warrant) may be positive.
- Serum ethanol level (if symptoms warrant) may be elevated.

Alert

If the rape occurred within 7 days, the following specimens may be obtained for legal purposes: blood; samples for deoxyribonucleic acid testing (should be collected within 48 hours); hairs of a different color than the victim's or that are obviously out of place; fibers; soiled or torn material; body fluids, such as blood or semen, that don't belong to the victim; and specimens from the cervical canal, throat, or rectum.

Treatment

General

○ Treatment of physical injuries
○ Crisis intervention and counseling
○ Follow-up gynecologic examination after 7 to 14 days; for male patient, follow-up urologic examination
○ Emergency contraception such as the Copper-T intrauterine device
○ Activity based on injuries

Medication

○ Tetanus prophylaxis
○ STD prophylaxis
○ Emergency contraceptive pills

Nursing considerations

Key outcomes

The patient will:
○ remain free from signs and symptoms of infection
○ express relief of pain
○ report absence of or reduction in anxiety
○ discuss feelings related to the rape and its effect on self-esteem.

Nursing interventions

○ Don't leave the patient alone unless requested.
○ Place the patient's clothing in paper, not plastic, bags. Label each bag and its contents.
○ Collect and label fingernail scrapings and foreign material obtained by combing the patient's pubic hair.
○ Label all specimens with the patient's name, physician's name, and site from which the specimen was obtained.
○ Note the name of the person to whom specimens were given.
○ Report the rape if required by state law.
○ Encourage the patient to express feelings.
○ Provide emotional support.

Monitoring

○ Mental status
○ Vital signs
○ Signs and symptoms of shock

Patient teaching

Be sure to cover:
○ the disorder, diagnosis, and treatment
○ verbal and written instructions regarding treatment
○ administration, dosage, and possible adverse reactions to medications.

Discharge planning

○ Encourage the patient to get follow-up care.
○ Refer the patient to resource and support services.

Raynaud's phenomenon

Overview

Description

- Primary arteriospastic disorder
- Causes episodic vasospasms in the small peripheral arteries and arterioles in response to cold exposure or stress
- Typically occurs in three phases
- Diagnosis requires exclusion of secondary causes
- More than half of patients have Raynaud's disease
- Also called *vasospastic arterial disease*

Pathophysiology

- Blood flow to digits decreases in response to stress or cold.
- Proposed explanations for decreased digital blood flow include an antigen-antibody immune response (most probable theory), intrinsic vascular wall hyperactivity to cold, ineffective basal heat production, and increased vasomotor tone from sympathetic stimulation or stress.

Causes

Primary causes
- Unknown

Secondary causes
- Collagen vascular disease
- Arterial occlusive disease
- Neurologic disorders
- Blood dyscrasias
- Trauma
- Drugs
- Pulmonary hypertension (see *Causes of Raynaud's phenomenon*)

Incidence

- More common in females, particularly between late adolescence and age 40

Common characteristics

- Occurs bilaterally
- Usually affects the hands or, less commonly, the feet; rarely, the earlobes and tip of nose

Complications

- Ischemia
- Gangrene
- Amputation

Assessment

History

- Altered skin color in response to cold or stress
- Numbness and tingling (second stage)
- Throbbing, burning, painful sensation (third stage)

Physical findings

- First stage — marked pallor of affected skin areas
- Second stage — cyanosis of affected skin areas
- Third stage — red, warm skin
- Between attacks — normal appearance of affected areas (occasionally, coolness and excessive perspiration of these areas)
- In long-standing disease — trophic changes, such as sclerodactylia and ulcerations

Test results

Diagnostic procedures
- Arteriography and digital photoplethysmography may aid diagnosis.

Treatment

General

- Smoking cessation
- Biofeedback therapy
- Avoidance of activities involving exposure to cold and mechanical or chemical injury

Medication

- Phenoxybenzamine
- Nifedipine
- Reserpine
- Guanethidine combined with prazosin

Surgery

- Sympathectomy, if conservative treatment fails to prevent ischemic ulcers

Nursing considerations

Key outcomes

The patient will:
- describe feeling increased comfort and decreased pain
- maintain adequate skin temperature in affected areas
- maintain adequate collateral circulation
- maintain skin integrity
- perform normal activities to the extent possible
- demonstrate effective coping skills.

Nursing interventions

- Evaluate the patient's occupation and its effect on symptom occurrence.
- Help the patient identify stress triggers and use effective coping strategies.
- Provide psychological support and reassurance.

Monitoring

- Response to treatment
- Signs and symptoms of skin breakdown
- Signs and symptoms of infection

In primary or idiopathic Raynaud's phenomenon, more than half of patients have Raynaud's disease. Raynaud's phenomenon may also occur secondary to the following diseases and conditions as well as with the use of certain drugs.

Collagen vascular disease
○ Dermatomyositis
○ Polymyositis
○ Rheumatoid arthritis
○ Scleroderma
○ Systemic lupus erythematosus
Arterial occlusive disease
○ Acute arterial occlusion
○ Atherosclerosis of the extremities
○ Thoracic outlet syndrome
○ Thromboangiitis obliterans
Neurologic disorders
○ Carpal tunnel syndrome
○ Stroke
○ Intervertebral disk disease
○ Poliomyelitis
○ Spinal cord tumors
○ Syringomyelia
Blood dyscrasias
○ Cold agglutinins
○ Cryofibrinogenemia

○ Myeloproliferative disorders
○ Waldenström's disease
Trauma
○ Cold injury
○ Electric shock
○ Hammering
○ Keyboarding
○ Piano playing
○ Vibration injury
Drugs
○ Beta-adrenergic blockers
○ Bleomycin
○ Cisplatin
○ Ergot derivatives such as ergotamine
○ Methysergide
○ Vinblastine
Other
○ Pulmonary hypertension

Patient teaching

Be sure to cover:
○ avoidance of exposure to cold
○ importance of wearing mittens or gloves in cold weather and when handling cold items or defrosting the freezer
○ avoidance of stress and cigarette smoking
○ need to inspect skin frequently and to seek immediate care for evidence of skin breakdown or infection
○ prescribed medications and possible adverse reactions, including which ones to report to the physician
○ importance of follow-up care.

Discharge planning

○ Refer the patient to a smoking-cessation program or a support group, as indicated.

Reiter's syndrome

Overview

Description

○ Self-limiting syndrome associated with polyarthritis, urethritis, mucocutaneous lesions, and conjunctivitis (or, less commonly, uveitis)

Pathophysiology

○ Infection is thought to trigger an aberrant and hyperactive immune response that causes inflammation in involved target organs.

Causes

○ Unknown
○ Typically follows venereal or enteric infection, especially with *Mycoplasma, Shigella, Campylobacter, Salmonella, Yersinia,* or *Chlamydia*
○ May involve genetic susceptibility

Incidence

○ Most common in men ages 20 to 40, especially those positive for human immunodeficiency virus
○ Rare in women and children

Common characteristics

○ Polyarthritis (dominant feature)

Complications

○ Ankylosing spondylitis
○ Persistent joint pain and swelling
○ Anterior uveitis, glaucoma, blindness
○ Prostatitis and hemorrhagic cystitis
○ Cardiomyopathy, pericarditis
○ Pulmonary edema
○ Vertebral inflammation
○ Foot deformity and chronic heel pain

Assessment

History

○ Initially, dysuria, hematuria, urinary urgency and frequency, and mucopurulent penile discharge with swelling and reddening of the urethral meatus
○ Possible suprapubic pain, fever, and anorexia with weight loss

Physical findings

○ Small, painless ulcers on glans penis
○ Asymmetrical and extremely variable polyarticular arthritis, usually in weight-bearing joints of the legs and sometimes in the lower back or sacroiliac joints
○ Warm, erythematous, painful joints
○ Muscle wasting near affected joints
○ Swollen, sausagelike appearance of fingers and toes
○ Skin lesions (keratoderma blennorrhagicum)

○ Thick, opaque, brittle nails with keratic debris accumulation under nails
○ Painless, transient ulcerations on the buccal mucosa, palate, and tongue
○ Patches of scaly skin on the palms, soles, scalp, or trunk

Test results

Laboratory
○ Human leukocyte antigen (HLA) test is positive for HLA B27.
○ White blood cell (WBC) count and erythrocyte sedimentation rate are elevated.
○ Complete blood count and anemia panel show mild anemia.
○ Many WBCs (mostly polymorphonuclear leukocytes) appear in urethral discharge and synovial fluid.
○ Synovial fluid is grossly purulent with high complement and protein levels.
○ Cultures of urethral discharge and synovial fluid are used to rule out other possible causes of symptoms.

Imaging
○ During the first few weeks of the syndrome, X-rays are normal. Later they may show osteoporosis in inflamed areas. If inflammation persists, X-rays may show small joint erosion, periosteal proliferation (new bone formation) of involved joints, and calcaneal spurs.

Treatment

General

○ Physical therapy
○ Padded or supportive shoes
○ High-calorie, high-protein diet
○ During acute stages, weight-bearing restrictions or complete bed rest

Medication

○ Nonsteroidal anti-inflammatory drugs (NSAIDs)
○ Cytotoxic agents
○ Corticosteroids

Surgery

○ Surgical reconstruction of joints if medical management doesn't prevent severe joint damage

Nursing considerations

Key outcomes

The patient will:
○ express feelings of increased energy
○ express feelings of increased comfort and decreased pain
○ attain the highest degree of mobility possible within confines of the disease.

Nursing interventions

○ Follow standard precautions.
○ Give prescribed analgesics as needed.
○ Provide a high-calorie, high-protein diet.
○ Provide frequent rest periods.
○ Develop an exercise regimen with the physical therapist.
○ Maintain a nonjudgmental attitude.

Monitoring

○ Response to medications
○ Complications

Patient teaching

Be sure to cover:
○ the disorder, diagnosis, and treatment
○ importance of using condoms and avoiding multiple sex partners
○ how to avoid exposure to enteric pathogens (such as via anal intercourse)
○ drug dosages and possible adverse reactions
○ importance of taking NSAIDs with meals or milk
○ maintaining normal daily activities and moderate exercise
○ good posture and body mechanics
○ use of a firm mattress.

Discharge planning

○ If the patient has severe or chronic joint impairment, arrange for occupational counseling.

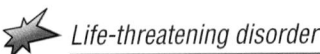

Relapsing fever

Overview

Description

○ An acute infectious disease caused by *Borrelia* spirochetes
○ Transmitted to humans by lice or ticks and characterized by relapses and remissions
○ Primary *Borrelia* reservoirs in rodents and other wild animals
○ Secondary reservoir possible in people, requiring no transmission by ordinary contagion and allowing possible congenital infection and transmission by contaminated blood
○ Mortality rate for untreated louseborne relapsing fever usually above 10%, possibly up to 50% in an epidemic
○ With treatment, excellent prognosis for both louseborne and tickborne relapsing fevers
○ Also called *tick, fowl-nest, cabin,* or *vagabond fever* or *bilious typhoid*

Pathophysiology

○ Inoculation takes place when the victim crushes the louse, causing its infected blood or body fluid to enter victim's bitten or abraded skin or mucous membranes.
○ Because tick bites are virtually painless and most *Ornithodoros* ticks feed at night but do not imbed themselves in the victim's skin, many people are bitten unknowingly.

Causes

○ Bite from body louse (*Pediculus humanus corporis*) that carries *Borrelia* spirochete, which typically occurs in epidemics during wars, famines, and mass migrations
○ Cold weather and crowded living conditions, which favor the spread of body lice
○ Bite from tick that carries one of three species of *Borrelia* most closely identified with tick carriers: *B. hermsii* (associated with *Ornithodoros hermsi*), *B. turicatae* (associated with *O. turicata*), or *B. parkeri* (associated with *O. parkeri*)

Incidence

○ Most common in indigent victims already suffering from other infections and malnutrition
○ Louseborne disease most common in North and Central Africa, Europe, Asia, and South America; no cases in the United States since 1900
○ Tickborne disease in the United States most prevalent in Texas and other western states, usually during the summer, when ticks and their hosts (chipmunks, goats, and prairie dogs) are most active; occasional cold-weather outbreaks in people such as campers who sleep in tick-infested cabins

Common characteristics

○ Incubation period 5 to 15 days (average 7 days)
○ Fever 105° F (40.5° C)
○ Prostration
○ Headache
○ Severe myalgia
○ Arthralgia
○ Diarrhea
○ Vomiting
○ Coughing
○ Eye or chest pain

Complications

○ Nephritis
○ Bronchitis
○ Pneumonia
○ Endocarditis
○ Seizures
○ Cranial nerve lesions
○ Paralysis
○ Coma
○ Death

Assessment

History

○ Recent travel to an epidemic or louse-infested area
○ Recent exposure to tick-infested area
○ Fever
○ Headache
○ Malaise
○ Arthralgia
○ Attacks that subside and recur

Physical findings

○ Splenomegaly
○ Hepatomegaly
○ Lymphadenopathy
○ Transient petechial rash over torso during febrile periods

Test results

Laboratory
○ During febrile periods, spirochetes may appear in blood smears using Wright's or Giemsa stain.
○ In severe infection, spirochetes appear in urine and cerebrospinal fluid.
○ White blood cell (WBC) count may reach 25,000/µl; lymphocytes and erythrocyte sedimentation rate may increase.
○ Syphilis test may show a false-positive result.

Treatment

General
- Supportive therapy
- Activity, as tolerated
- Diet, as tolerated

Medication
- Antipyretics
- Doxycycline or erythromycin

 Alert

Antibiotics shouldn't be given at the height of a severe febrile attack because they may cause Jarisch-Herxheimer reaction, resulting in malaise, rigors, leukopenia, flushing, fever, tachycardia, rising respiratory rate, and hypotension. This reaction, which is caused by toxic by-products from massive spirochete destruction, can mimic septic shock and may prove fatal. Antibiotics should be postponed until the fever subsides.

Nursing considerations

Key outcomes
The patient will:
- maintain a normal body temperature
- verbalize accurate information about the disease
- express increased comfort and decreased pain
- attain the highest degree of mobility possible.

Nursing interventions
- Give tepid sponge baths and antipyretics.
- Encourage fluid intake.
- Administer antibiotics carefully. Document and report any hypersensitive reactions (rash, fever, anaphylaxis), especially a Jarisch-Herxheimer reaction.
- Report all cases of louseborne or tickborne relapsing fever to the local public health department as required by law.

Monitoring
- Vital signs
- Level of consciousness

Patient teaching

Be sure to cover:
- symptoms of relapsing fever in family members and in others who may have been exposed to ticks or lice along with the victim
- proper hand-washing technique
- prevention for travelers going to tick-infested areas, such as wearing clothing that covers as much skin as possible and tucking pant legs into boots or socks.

Renal calculi

Overview

Description

- Formation of calculi ("stones") anywhere in the urinary tract
- Most common in the renal pelvis or calyces
- Vary in size; may be single or multiple (see *Variations in renal calculi*)
- Necessitate hospitalization in roughly 1 of every 1,000 Americans

Pathophysiology

- Calculi form when substances normally dissolved in the urine, such as calcium oxalate and calcium phosphate, precipitate.
- Large, rough calculi may occlude the opening to the ureteropelvic junction.
- The frequency and force of peristaltic contractions increase, causing pain.

Causes

- Unknown

Risk factors

- Dehydration
- Infection
- Urine pH changes
- Urinary tract obstruction
- Immobilization
- Metabolic factors

Incidence

- Affect more men than women
- Rare in blacks and children

Common characteristics

- Flank pain
- Nausea, vomiting

Complications

- Renal parenchymal damage
- Renal cell necrosis
- Hydronephrosis
- Complete ureteral obstruction

Assessment

History

- Classic renal colic pain — severe pain that travels from the costovertebral angle to the flank and then to the suprapubic region and external genitalia
- With calculi in the renal pelvis and calyces — relatively constant, dull pain
- Pain of fluctuating intensity; may be excruciating at its peak
- Nausea, vomiting
- Fever, chills
- Anuria (rare)

Physical findings

- Hematuria
- Abdominal distention

Test results

Laboratory
- 24-hour urine collection shows calcium oxalate, phosphorus, and uric acid excretion levels.
- Urinalysis shows increased urine specific gravity, hematuria, crystals, casts, and pyuria.

Imaging
- Kidneys-ureters-bladder (KUB) radiography reveals most renal calculi.
- Excretory urography helps confirm the diagnosis and determines calculi size and location.
- Kidney ultrasonography can detect obstructive changes and radiolucent calculi not seen on KUB.

Treatment

General

- Percutaneous ultrasonic lithotripsy
- Extracorporeal shock wave lithotripsy
- Vigorous hydration (more than 3 qt [3 L]/day)
- Dietary restrictions based on stone composition

Medication

- Antibiotics
- Analgesics
- Diuretics
- Methenamine mandelate
- Allopurinol (for uric acid calculi)
- Ascorbic acid

Surgery

- Parathyroidectomy for hyperparathyroidism
- Cystoscopy

Nursing considerations

Key outcomes

The patient will:
- maintain fluid balance
- report increased comfort
- identify risk factors that increase calculus formation and modify lifestyle accordingly
- demonstrate the ability to manage urinary elimination problems.

Renal calculi vary in size and type. Small calculi may remain in the renal pelvis or pass down the ureter. A staghorn calculus (a cast of the calyceal and pelvic collecting system) may develop from a calculus that stays in the kidney.

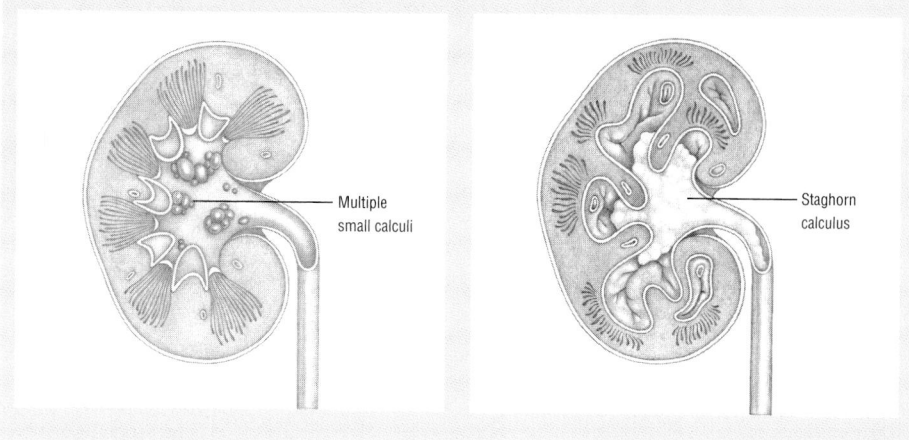

Multiple small calculi

Staghorn calculus

Nursing interventions

○ Provide I.V. fluids, as ordered; force fluids as needed.
○ Strain all urine and save solid material for analysis.
○ Encourage ambulation to aid spontaneous calculus passage.

Monitoring

○ Intake and output
○ Daily weight
○ Pain control
○ Catheter function and drainage
○ Signs and symptoms of infection

Patient teaching

Be sure to cover:
○ the disorder, diagnosis, and treatment
○ prescribed diet and importance of compliance
○ drug therapy
○ ways to prevent recurrences
○ how to strain urine for stones
○ immediate return visit to hospital for fever, uncontrolled pain, or vomiting.

Discharge planning

○ Patients who don't meet admission criteria should arrange for a follow-up with a urologist in 2 to 3 days.

Renal failure, acute

Overview

Description
- Sudden interruption of renal function resulting from obstruction, reduced circulation, or renal parenchymal disease
- Classified as prerenal failure, intrarenal failure (also called *intrinsic* or *parenchymal failure*), or postrenal failure
- Usually reversible with medical treatment
- If not treated, may progress to end-stage renal disease, uremia, and death
- Normally occurs in three distinct phases: oliguric, diuretic, and recovery

Oliguric phase
- This phase may last a few days or several weeks.
- Urine output drops below 400 ml/day.
- Fluid volume excess, azotemia, and electrolyte imbalance occur.
- Local mediators are released, causing intrarenal vasoconstriction.
- Medullary hypoxia causes cellular swelling and adherence of neutrophils to capillaries and venules.
- Hypoperfusion occurs.
- Cellular injury and necrosis occur.
- Reperfusion causes reactive oxygen species to form, leading to further cellular injury.

Diuretic phase
- Renal function is recovered.
- Urine output gradually increases.
- Glomerular filtration rate improves, although tubular transport systems remain abnormal.

Recovery phase
- This phase may last 3 to 12 months, or longer.
- The patient gradually returns to normal or near-normal renal function.

Pathophysiology
Prerenal failure
- Prerenal failure is caused by impaired blood flow.
- Decrease in filtration pressure causes decline in glomerular filtration rate.
- Failure to restore blood volume or blood pressure may cause acute tubular necrosis (ATN) or acute cortical necrosis.

Intrarenal failure
- A severe episode of hypotension, commonly associated with hypovolemia, is often a significant contributing event.
- Cell swelling, injury, and necrosis — a form of reperfusion injury that may also be caused by nephrotoxins — results from ischemia-generated toxic oxygen-free radicals and anti-inflammatory mediators.

Postrenal failure
- Postrenal failure usually occurs with urinary tract obstruction that affects the kidneys bilaterally such as prostatic hyperplasia.

Causes
Prerenal failure
- Hypovolemia
- Hemorrhagic blood loss
- Loss of plasma volume
- Water and electrolyte losses
- Hypotension or hypoperfusion

Intrarenal failure
- ATN
- Glomerulopathies
- Malignant hypertension
- Coagulation defects

Postrenal failure
- Obstructive uropathies, usually bilateral
- Ureteral destruction
- Bladder neck obstruction

Incidence
- Seen in 5% of hospitalized patients

Common characteristics
- Vary with renal failure phase

Complications
- Renal shutdown
- Electrolyte imbalance
- Metabolic acidosis
- Acute pulmonary edema
- Hypertensive crisis
- Infection

Assessment

History
- Predisposing disorder
- Recent fever, chills, or central nervous system problem
- Recent GI problem

Physical findings
- Oliguria or anuria, depending on renal failure phase
- Tachycardia
- Bibasilar crackles
- Irritability, drowsiness, or confusion
- Altered level of consciousness
- Bleeding abnormalities
- Dry, pruritic skin
- Dry mucous membranes
- Uremic breath odor

Test results
Laboratory
- Blood urea nitrogen, serum creatinine, and potassium levels are elevated.
- Hematocrit, blood pH, bicarbonate, and hemoglobin levels are decreased.
- Urine casts and cellular debris are present, and specific gravity is decreased.
- In glomerular disease, proteinuria and urine osmolality are close to serum osmolality level.

- Urine sodium level is below 20 mEq/L, caused by decreased perfusion in oliguria.
- Urine sodium level is above 40 mEq/L from an intrarenal problem in oliguria.
- Urine creatinine clearance is used to measure glomerular filtration rate and estimate the number of remaining functioning nephrons.

Imaging

The following imaging tests may show the cause of renal failure:
- kidney ultrasonography
- kidney-ureter-bladder radiography
- excretory urography renal scan
- retrograde pyelography
- computed tomography scan
- nephrotomography.

Diagnostic procedures
- Electrocardiography shows tall, peaked T waves; a widening QRS complex; and disappearing P waves if hyperkalemia is present.

Treatment

General
- Hemodialysis or peritoneal dialysis (if appropriate)
- High-calorie, low-protein, low-sodium, and low-potassium diet
- Fluid restriction
- Rest periods when fatigued

Medication
- Supplemental vitamins
- Diuretics
- In hyperkalemia, hypertonic glucose-and-insulin infusions, sodium bicarbonate, sodium polystyrene sulfonate

Surgery
- Creation of vascular access for hemodialysis

Nursing considerations

Key outcomes
The patient will:
- avoid complications
- maintain fluid balance
- maintain hemodynamic stability
- verbalize risk factors for decreased tissue perfusion and modify lifestyle appropriately
- demonstrate the ability to manage urinary elimination problems.

Nursing interventions
- Give prescribed drugs.
- Encourage the patient to express feelings.
- Provide emotional support.
- Identify patients at risk for and take steps to prevent ATN. (See *Preventing acute tubular necrosis.*)

Preventing acute tubular necrosis

Acute tubular necrosis occurs mainly in elderly hospitalized patients. Contributing causes include aminoglycoside therapy and exposure to industrial chemicals, heavy metals, and contrast media. Patients who have been exposed must receive adequate hydration; monitor their urinary output closely.

To prevent acute tubular necrosis, make sure every patient is well hydrated before surgery or after X-rays that use a contrast medium. Administer mannitol, as ordered, to a high-risk patient before and during these procedures. Carefully monitor a patient receiving a blood transfusion, and stop the transfusion immediately if signs of transfusion reaction (fever, rash, and chills) occur.

Monitoring
- Intake and output
- Daily weight
- Renal function studies
- Vital signs
- Effects of excess fluid volume
- Dialysis access site

Patient teaching

Be sure to cover:
- the disorder, diagnosis, and treatment
- administration, dosages, and possible adverse reactions to medications
- recommended fluid allowance
- compliance with diet and drug regimen
- daily weight and importance of immediately reporting changes of 3 lb or more
- signs and symptoms of edema and importance of reporting them to the physician.

Discharge planning
- Encourage follow-up care with nephrologist.

Renal failure, chronic

Overview

Description
- The end result of gradually progressive loss of renal function
- Symptoms sparse until more than 75% of glomerular filtration lost, worsening as renal function declines
- Fatal unless treated; to sustain life, may require maintenance dialysis or kidney transplantation

Pathophysiology
- Nephron destruction eventually causes irreversible renal damage.
- Disease may progress through the following stages: reduced renal reserve, renal insufficiency, renal failure, and end-stage renal disease.

Causes
- Chronic glomerular disease
- Chronic infections such as chronic pyelonephritis
- Congenital anomalies such as polycystic kidney disease
- Vascular diseases
- Obstructive processes such as calculi
- Collagen diseases such as systemic lupus erythematosus
- Nephrotoxic agents
- Endocrine disease

Incidence
- Affects about 2 of every 100,000 people
- Can occur at all ages but more common in adults
- Affects more men than women
- Affects more Blacks than Whites

Common characteristics
- Fatigue
- Decreasing urine output
- Increasing edema
- Electrolyte imbalance
- Fluid overload

Complications
- Anemia
- Peripheral neuropathy
- Lipid disorders
- Platelet dysfunction
- Pulmonary edema
- Electrolyte imbalances
- Sexual dysfunction

Assessment

History
- Predisposing factor
- Dry mouth
- Fatigue
- Nausea
- Hiccups
- Muscle cramps
- Fasciculations, twitching
- Infertility, decreased libido
- Amenorrhea
- Impotence
- Pathologic fractures

Physical findings
- Decreased urine output
- Hypotension or hypertension
- Altered level of consciousness
- Peripheral edema
- Cardiac arrhythmias
- Bibasilar crackles
- Pleural friction rub
- Gum ulceration and bleeding
- Uremic fetor
- Abdominal pain on palpation
- Poor skin turgor
- Pale, yellowish bronze skin color
- Thin, brittle fingernails and dry, brittle hair
- Growth retardation (in children)

Test results
Laboratory
- Blood urea nitrogen, serum creatinine, sodium, and potassium levels are elevated.
- Arterial blood gas (ABG) values show decreased arterial pH and bicarbonate levels.
- Hematocrit and hemoglobin level are low; red blood cell (RBC) survival time decreases.
- Mild thrombocytopenia and platelet defects appear.
- Aldosterone secretion is increased.
- Hyperglycemia and hypertriglyceridemia occur.
- High-density lipoprotein levels are decreased.
- ABG values show metabolic acidosis.
- Urine specific gravity is fixed at 1.010.
- Patient has proteinuria, glycosuria, and urinary RBCs, leukocytes, casts, and crystals.

Imaging
- Kidneys-ureters-bladder radiography, excretory urography, nephrotomography, renal scan, and renal arteriography show reduced kidney size.

Diagnostic procedures
- Renal biopsy allows histologic identification of the underlying pathology.
- Electroencephalography shows changes suggesting metabolic encephalopathy.

Treatment

General
- Hemodialysis or peritoneal dialysis
- Low-protein (with peritoneal dialysis, high-protein), high-calorie, low-sodium, low-phosphorus, and low-potassium diet
- Fluid restriction

○ Rest periods when fatigued

Medication

○ Loop diuretics
○ Cardiac glycosides
○ Antihypertensives
○ Antiemetics
○ Iron and folate supplements
○ Erythropoietin
○ Antipruritics
○ Supplementary vitamins and essential amino acids

Surgery

○ Creation of vascular access for dialysis
○ Possible kidney transplant

Nursing considerations

Key outcomes

The patient will:
○ avoid complications
○ maintain fluid balance
○ report feelings of increased comfort
○ maintain hemodynamic stability
○ demonstrate the ability to manage urinary elimination problems
○ perform activities of daily living within confines of the disease.

Nursing interventions

○ Give prescribed drugs.
○ Perform meticulous skin care.
○ Encourage the patient to express feelings.
○ Provide emotional support.

Monitoring

○ Renal function studies
○ Vital signs
○ Intake and output
○ Daily weight
○ Signs and symptoms of fluid overload
○ Signs and symptoms of bleeding

Patient teaching

Be sure to cover:
○ the disorder, diagnosis, and treatment
○ dietary changes
○ fluid restrictions
○ dialysis site care, as appropriate
○ importance of wearing or carrying medical identification.

Discharge planning

○ Refer the patient to resource and support services.

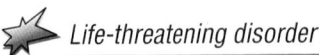 *Life-threatening disorder*

Respiratory acidosis

Overview

Description

- Acid-base disturbance characterized by reduced alveolar ventilation, as shown by hypercapnia (partial pressure of arterial carbon dioxide [$PaCO_2$] above 45 mm Hg)
- Carries varying prognosis, depending on severity of underlying disturbance and the patient's general clinical condition
- Can be acute or chronic

Pathophysiology

- Depressed ventilation causes respiratory acidosis.
- Carbon dioxide is then retained, and hydrogen ion concentration increases.
- Respiratory acidosis results.

Causes

- Central nervous system (CNS) trauma
- CNS-depressant drugs
- Chronic metabolic alkalosis
- Neuromuscular disease
- Airway obstruction
- Parenchymal lung disease
- Chronic obstructive pulmonary disease
- Asthma
- Severe acute respiratory distress syndrome
- Chronic bronchitis
- Large pneumothorax
- Extensive pneumonia
- Pulmonary edema

Incidence

- Affects males and females equally

Common characteristics

- Headache
- Shortness of breath
- Nausea and vomiting

Complications

- Shock
- Respiratory arrest
- Cardiac arrest

Assessment

History

- Predisposing factor
- Headache
- Shortness of breath
- Nausea and vomiting

Physical findings

- Diaphoresis
- Bounding pulses
- Rapid, shallow respirations
- Tachycardia
- Hypotension
- Papilledema
- Mental status changes
- Asterixis (tremor)
- Depressed deep tendon reflexes

Test results

Laboratory

- Arterial blood pH is below 7.35, and $PaCO_2$ is above 45 mm Hg (hypercapnia)

Treatment

General

- Correction of the condition causing alveolar hypoventilation
- Possible mechanical ventilation
- Possible dialysis
- I.V. fluid administration
- Possible need for parenteral nutrition
- Activity as tolerated

Medication

- Oxygen
- Bronchodilators
- Antibiotics
- Sodium bicarbonate
- Drug therapy for the underlying condition

Surgery

- Bronchoscopy

Nursing considerations

Key outcomes

The patient will:
- maintain a patent airway
- maintain adequate ventilation
- maintain fluid balance
- maintain adequate cardiac output
- demonstrate effective coping strategies.

Nursing interventions

- Give prescribed drugs and oxygen.
- Provide adequate fluids.
- Maintain a patent airway.
- Perform tracheal suctioning, as needed.

Monitoring

- Vital signs
- Intake and output
- Neurologic status
- Respiratory status
- Arterial blood gas values

○ Serum electrolyte values
○ Mechanical ventilator settings

 Alert

Be aware that pulse oximetry, used to monitor oxygen saturation, won't reveal increasing carbon dioxide levels.

Patient teaching

Be sure to cover:
○ the disorder, diagnosis, and treatment
○ supplemental oxygen
○ prescribed drugs and possible adverse effects
○ how to perform coughing and deep-breathing exercises
○ signs and symptoms of acid-base imbalance and when to notify the physician.

Discharge planning
○ Refer the patient for home oxygen therapy if indicated.

Respiratory distress syndrome

Overview

Description

○ Respiratory disorder that involves widespread alveolar collapse
○ Most common cause of neonatal death
○ If mild, subsides slowly after about 3 days
○ Also called *RDS* or *hyaline membrane disease*

Pathophysiology

○ In neonates born before the 27th week of gestation, immaturity of alveoli and capillary blood supply lead to alveolar collapse from lack of surfactant (a lipoprotein normally present in alveoli and respiratory bronchioles).
○ Surfactant deficiency causes widespread atelectasis, resulting in inadequate alveolar ventilation and shunting of blood through collapsed lung areas.
○ Hypoxia and acidosis result.
○ Compensatory grunting occurs, producing positive end-expiratory pressure (PEEP) that helps prevent further alveolar collapse.

Causes

○ Surfactant deficiency stemming from preterm birth

Incidence

○ Almost exclusively affects neonates born before the 27th gestational week; occurs in about 60% of those born before the 28th week
○ Most common in neonates of mothers with diabetes, neonates delivered by cesarean birth, and neonates delivered suddenly after antepartum hemorrhage

Common characteristics

○ Preterm birth
○ Labored breathing within minutes to hours after birth

Complications

○ Respiratory insufficiency
○ Shock
○ Bronchopulmonary dysplasia
○ Death

Assessment

History

○ Preterm birth
○ Cesarean birth
○ Maternal history of diabetes or antepartum hemorrhage

Physical findings

○ Rapid, shallow respirations
○ Intercostal, subcostal, or sternal retractions
○ Nasal flaring
○ Audible expiratory grunting
○ Pallor
○ Frothy sputum
○ Low body temperature
○ Diminished air entry and crackles
○ Possible hypotension, peripheral edema, and oliguria
○ Possible apnea, bradycardia, and cyanosis

Test results

Laboratory
○ Partial pressure of arterial oxygen (Pao_2) is decreased; partial pressure of arterial carbon dioxide may be normal, decreased, or increased; and arterial pH is decreased.
○ Lecithin-sphingomyelin ratio showing prenatal lung development and RDS risk

Imaging
○ Chest X-rays may show a fine reticulonodular pattern and dark streaks, indicating air-filled, dilated bronchioles.

Treatment

General

○ Aggressive management, assisted by mechanical ventilation with PEEP or continuous positive airway pressure (CPAP) administered by a tight-fitting face mask or, when necessary, an endotracheal tube
○ For a neonate who can't maintain adequate gas exchange, high-frequency oscillation ventilation
○ Radiant warmer or Isolette
○ Warm, humidified, oxygen-enriched gases given by oxygen hood or mechanical ventilation
○ Tube feedings or total parenteral nutrition

Medication

○ I.V. fluids and sodium bicarbonate
○ Pancuronium bromide
○ Prophylactic antibiotics
○ Diuretics
○ Surfactant replacement therapy
○ Vitamin E
○ Antenatal corticosteroids

Surgery

○ Possible tracheostomy

Nursing considerations

Key outcomes

The patient will:
- maintain adequate ventilation
- maintain a patent airway
- remain free from infection
- maintain intact skin integrity.

The patient's family will:
- identify factors that increase the risk of neonatal injury.

Nursing interventions

- Give prescribed drugs.
- Check the umbilical catheter for arterial or venous hypotension, as appropriate.
- Suction, as necessary.
- Change the transcutaneous PaO_2 monitor lead placement site every 2 to 4 hours.
- Adjust PEEP or CPAP settings as indicated by arterial blood gas (ABG) values.
- Implement measures to prevent infection.
- Provide mouth care every 2 hours.
- Encourage parents to participate in the infant's care.
- Encourage parents to ask questions and to express their fears and concerns.
- Advise parents that full recovery may take up to 12 months.
- Offer emotional support.

 Alert

In a neonate on a mechanical ventilator, watch carefully for signs of barotrauma and accidental disconnection from the ventilator. Check ventilator settings frequently. Be alert for signs of complications of PEEP or CPAP therapy, such as decreased cardiac output, pneumothorax, and pneumomediastinum.

Monitoring

- Vital signs
- ABG values
- Intake and output
- Central venous pressure
- Signs and symptoms of infection
- Thrombosis
- Decreased peripheral circulation
- Pulse oximetry
- Daily weight
- Skin color
- Respiratory status
- Skin integrity

 Alert

Watch for evidence of complications from oxygen therapy: lung capillary damage, decreased mucus flow, impaired ciliary functioning, and widespread atelectasis. Also be alert for signs of patent ductus arteriosus, heart failure, retinopathy, pulmonary hypertension, necrotizing enterocolitis, and neurologic abnormalities.

Patient teaching

Be sure to cover (with the parents):
- the disorder, diagnosis, and treatment
- drugs and possible adverse effects
- explanations of respiratory equipment, alarm sounds, and mechanical noise
- potential complications
- when to notify the physician.

Discharge planning

- Refer the parents to pastoral counselors and social worker, as indicated.
- Refer the patient for follow-up care with a neonatal ophthalmologist, as indicated.

Respiratory syncytial virus infection

Overview

Description

- Virus that's the leading cause of lower respiratory tract infection in infants and young children and upper respiratory infections in adults
- Suspected cause of fatal respiratory diseases in infants
- Can cause serious illness in immunocompromised adults, institutionalized elderly people, and patients with underlying cardiopulmonary disease
- Also known as *RSV*

Pathophysiology

- The virus attaches to cells, eventually resulting in necrosis of the bronchiolar epithelium; in severe infection, peribronchiolar infiltrate of lymphocytes and mononuclear cells occurs.
- Intra-alveolar thickening and filling of the alveolar spaces with fluid results.
- Narrowing of the airway passages on expiration prevents air from leaving the lungs, causing progressive overinflation.

Causes

- Respiratory syncytial virus, a subgroup of myxoviruses resembling paramyxovirus
- Transmitted from person to person by respiratory secretions
- Probably spread to infants and young children by school-age children, adolescents, and young adults with mild reinfections

Incidence

- Almost exclusively affects infants and young children, especially those in day care settings
- Highest among infants ages 1 to 6 months, peaking between ages 2 and 3 months
- Annual epidemics during winter and spring

Common characteristics

- Rhinorrhea, low-grade fever, and mild systemic symptoms accompanied by cough and wheezing
- Tachypnea, shortness of breath
- Cyanosis
- Apneic episodes
- Reinfection common; produces milder symptoms than primary infection

Complications

- Pneumonia and progressive pneumonia
- Bronchiolitis
- Croup
- Otitis media
- Respiratory failure
- Sudden infant death syndrome
- Residual lung damage

Assessment

History

- Nasal congestion
- Coughing
- Wheezing
- Malaise
- Sore throat
- Earache
- Dyspnea
- Fever

Physical findings

- Nasal and pharyngeal inflammation
- Otitis media
- Severe respiratory distress (nasal flaring, retraction, cyanosis, and tachypnea)
- Wheezes, rhonchi, and crackles

Test results

Laboratory

- Cultures of nasal and pharyngeal secretions show respiratory syncytial virus.
- Serum respiratory syncytial virus antibody titers are elevated.
- Arterial blood gas values show hypoxemia and respiratory acidosis.
- In dehydration, blood urea nitrogen levels are elevated.

Treatment

General

- Respiratory support
- Adequate nutrition
- Avoidance of overhydration
- Rest periods when fatigued

Medication

- Ribavirin

Surgery

- Possible tracheostomy

Nursing considerations

Key outcomes

The patient will:
- maintain a respiratory rate within 5 breaths/minute of baseline
- express or indicate feelings of increased comfort while maintaining adequate air exchange
- cough effectively
- maintain adequate fluid volume.

Nursing interventions

○ Institute contact isolation.
○ Perform percussion, drainage, and suction when necessary.
○ Give prescribed oxygen.
○ Use a croup tent, as needed.
○ Place the patient in semi-Fowler's position.
○ Observe for signs and symptoms of dehydration, and administer I.V. fluids accordingly.
○ Promote bed rest.
○ Offer diversional activities tailored to the patient's condition and age.

Monitoring

○ Respiratory status
○ Fluid and electrolyte status

Patient teaching

Be sure to cover (with the parents):
○ the disorder, diagnosis, and treatment
○ how the infection spreads
○ preventive measures (RSV immune globulin)
○ drugs and possible adverse effects
○ importance of a nonsmoking environment in the home
○ follow-up care.

Retinal detachment

Overview

Description

- Partial or complete separation of the sensory retina from the underlying pigment epithelium
- May be primary or secondary
- Commonly occurs spontaneously
- Usually involves only one eye; may occur in the other eye later
- Rarely heals spontaneously; usually can be reattached successfully with surgery
- Carries varying prognosis depending on the retinal area affected

Pathophysiology

- A hole or tear in the retina allows the liquid vitreous to seep between the retinal layers.
- Liquid separates the sensory retinal layer from its choroidal blood supply. (See *Understanding retinal detachment*.)

Causes

- Intraocular inflammation
- Trauma
- Age-related degenerative changes
- Tumors
- Systemic disease
- Traction placed on the retina by vitreous bands or membranes
- Hereditary factors, usually related to myopia

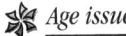 **Age issue**

In a child, retinal detachment can result from retinopathy of prematurity, tumors (retinoblastomas), or trauma.

Risk factors

- Myopia
- Cataract surgery
- Trauma

Understanding retinal detachment

Traumatic injury or degenerative changes cause retinal detachment by allowing the retina's sensory tissue layers to separate from the retinal pigment epithelium. This permits fluid—from the vitreous, for example—to seep into the space between the retinal pigment epithelium and the rods and cones of the tissue layers.

The pressure, which results from the fluid entering the space, balloons the retina into the vitreous cavity away from choroidal circulation. Separated from its blood supply, the retina can't function. Without prompt repair, the detached retina can cause permanent vision loss.

Incidence

- Affects twice as many men as women
- More common with increased age

Common characteristics

- Painless vision loss
- Sensation of floaters or of looking through a veil, curtain, or cobweb

Complications

- Severe vision impairment
- Blindness

Assessment

History

- Sensation of seeing floaters and flashes
- Painless vision loss, described as sensation of looking through a veil, curtain, or cobweb (which may obscure objects in a particular area of the visual field)

Physical findings

- Visual field loss

Test results

Imaging
- Ocular ultrasonography may be used to examine the retina if the lens is opaque and shows intraocular and intraorbital pathology. It also commonly detects retinal detachments, characteristically producing a dense, sheetlike echo on a B-mode scan.

Diagnostic procedures
- Direct ophthalmoscopy shows folds or discoloration in the usually transparent retina.
- Indirect ophthalmoscopy shows retinal tears.

Treatment

General

- Varies with location and severity of detachment
- Nothing by mouth before surgery
- Bed rest before surgery
- Restriction of eye movements before surgery by patching affected eye
- Positioning of the patient's head to allow gravity to pull the detached retina closer to the choroid

Medication

- Antiemetics
- Analgesics
- Mydriatics
- Cycloplegics
- Steroidal eyedrops
- Antibiotic eyedrops

Surgery

- Cryothermy
- Laser therapy

○ Scleral buckling (may be followed by vitreous replacement with silicone, oil, air, or gas)
○ Diathermy

Nursing considerations

Key outcomes

The patient will:
○ avoid harm or injury
○ express feelings and concerns
○ regain the previous level of visual functioning.

Nursing interventions

○ Prepare the patient for surgery.
○ Give prescribed antibiotics and cycloplegic or mydriatic eyedrops.
○ In macular involvement, maintain bed rest to prevent further retinal detachment.
○ Postoperatively, position the patient as directed.
○ Give prescribed antiemetics as indicated.
○ Give prescribed analgesics.
○ Discourage activities that increase intraocular pressure.
○ With retrobulbar injection, apply a protective eye patch.
○ Apply cold compresses.
○ Avoid putting pressure on the eye.
○ Provide encouragement and emotional support.

Monitoring

○ Localized corneal edema and perilimbal congestion after laser therapy
○ Persistent pain
○ Vital signs
○ Visual acuity
○ Response to treatment

Patient teaching

Be sure to cover:
○ the disorder, diagnosis, and treatment
○ leg and deep-breathing exercises
○ possible persistence of blurred vision for several days after laser therapy
○ importance of avoiding driving, bending, heavy lifting, and other activities that affect intraocular pressure for several days after surgery
○ avoidance of activities that could cause eye trauma
○ how to instill eyedrops
○ importance of wearing sunglasses
○ applying cold compresses
○ drugs and possible adverse effects
○ signs and symptoms of increasing ocular pressure and infection
○ early symptoms of retinal detachment.

Reye's syndrome

Overview

Description

- An acute childhood illness that causes fatty infiltration of the liver with concurrent hyperammonemia, encephalopathy, and increased intracranial pressure (ICP)
- Possible fatty infiltration of the kidneys, brain, and myocardium
- Variable prognosis depending on the severity of central nervous system depression

Pathophysiology

- Damaged hepatic mitochondria disrupt the urea cycle, which normally changes ammonia to urea for excretion from the body.
- This results in hyperammonemia, hypoglycemia, and an increase in serum short-chain fatty acids, leading to encephalopathy.
- Simultaneously, fatty infiltration is found in renal tubular cells, neuronal tissue, and muscle tissue, including the heart.

Causes

- Viral infection
- Associated with aspirin use

Incidence

- Linked to aspirin use
- Usually increased during influenza outbreaks

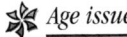 **Age issue**

Reye's syndrome is most common in children ages 4 to 12, with peak incidence at age 6.

Common characteristics

- Five-stage development, signs and symptoms varying in severity with the degree of encephalopathy and cerebral edema
- Possible atypical presentation for infants
- Brief recovery period after initial viral infection, during which child doesn't seem seriously ill
- A few days later, intractable vomiting, lethargy, rapidly changing mental status (mild to severe agitation, confusion, irritability, delirium), hyperactive reflexes, and rising blood pressure, respiratory rate, and pulse rate

Complications

- Increased ICP
- Coma
- Seizures
- Respiratory failure

Assessment

History

- Viral infection
- Aspirin use
- Vomiting
- Change in mental status

Physical findings

- Hyperactive reflexes
- Increased blood pressure
- Tachycardia
- Lethargy

Test results

Laboratory

- Low or absent serum salicylate level rules out aspirin overdose.
- Liver-function studies show aspartate aminotransferase and alanine aminotransferase levels elevated to twice normal; bilirubin level is usually normal.
- Cerebrospinal fluid (CSF) analysis reveals a white blood cell count of less than 10; with coma, CSF pressure increases.
- Coagulation studies result in prolonged prothrombin and partial thromboplastin times.
- Blood values show elevated serum ammonia levels; normal or, in 15% of cases, low serum glucose levels; and increased serum fatty acid and lactate levels.

Diagnostic procedures

- Liver biopsy reveals fatty droplets uniformly distributed throughout cells.

Other

- History of a recent viral disorder with typical signs and symptoms strongly suggests Reye's syndrome.

Treatment

- Dictated by stage of the syndrome (see *Stages of treatment for Reye's syndrome*)

Nursing considerations

Key outcomes

The patient will:

- maintain adequate ventilation
- maintain joint mobility and range of motion
- maintain skin integrity
- remain hemodynamically stable.

Nursing interventions

- Maintain seizure precautions.
- Provide skin and mouth care.
- Perform or assist with range-of-motion exercises.

Signs and symptoms	Baseline treatment
Stage I Vomiting, lethargy, hepatic dysfunction	• To decrease intracranial pressure (ICP) and brain edema, give I.V. fluids at two-thirds of the maintenance dose. Also give an osmotic diuretic or furosemide. • To treat hypoprothrombinemia, give vitamin K; if vitamin K proves unsuccessful, give fresh frozen plasma. • Monitor serum ammonia and blood glucose levels and plasma osmolality every 4 to 8 hours to check progress.
Stage II Hyperventilation, delirium, hepatic dysfunction, hyperactive reflexes	• Continue baseline treatment.
Stage III Coma, hyperventilation, decorticate rigidity, hepatic dysfunction	• Continue baseline and seizure treatment. • Monitor ICP with a subarachnoid screw or other invasive device. • Provide endotracheal intubation and mechanical ventilation to control partial pressure of carbon dioxide ($Paco_2$). A paralyzing agent, such as pancuronium I.V. may help maintain ventilation. • Give mannitol I.V. or glycerol by nasogastric tube.
Stage IV Deepening coma; decerebrate rigidity; large, fixed pupils; minimal hepatic dysfunction	• Continue baseline and supportive care. • If all previous measures fail, some pediatric centers use barbiturate coma, decompressive craniotomy, hypothermia, or an exchange transfusion.
Stage V Seizures, loss of deep tendon reflexes, flaccidity, respiratory arrest, ammonia level > 300 mg/dl	• Continue baseline and supportive care.

Monitoring

○ Vital signs
○ Intake and output
○ ICP
○ Respiratory status
○ Cardiovascular status
○ Level of consciousness

Patient teaching

Be sure to cover:
○ using a nonsalicylate analgesic and an antipyretic such as acetaminophen for children.

Discharge planning

○ Refer parents to the National Reye's Syndrome Foundation for more information.

Rhabdomyolysis

Overview

Description

○ Breakdown of muscle tissue, causing myoglobinuria
○ Usually follows major muscle trauma, especially a muscle crush injury
○ Good prognosis if contributing causes are stopped or disease is checked before damage is irreversible

Pathophysiology

○ Muscle trauma that compresses tissue causes ischemia and necrosis.
○ The ensuing local edema further increases compartment pressure and tamponade; pressure from severe swelling causes blood vessels to collapse, leading to tissue hypoxia, muscle infarction, neural damage in the area of the fracture, and release of myoglobin from the necrotic muscle fibers into the circulation.

Causes

○ Traumatic injury
○ Prescription and nonprescription drugs (see *Drugs that may cause rhabdomyolysis*)
○ Familial tendency
○ Strenuous exertion, such as long-distance running
○ Infection, especially severe infection
○ Anesthetics that cause intraoperative rigidity
○ Heat stroke
○ Electrolyte disturbances
○ Cardiac arrhythmias
○ Excessive muscular activity associated with status epilepticus, electroconvulsive therapy, or high-voltage electrical shock

Risk factors

○ Alcohol use
○ Recent soft tissue compression

Drugs that may cause rhabdomyolysis

The use of these drugs may cause rhabdomyolysis:
aminocaproic acid
amphotericin B
anesthetic and paralytic agents
antihistamines
caffeine
corticosteroids
cyclic antidepressants
fibric acid derivatives
lovastatin
neuroleptics
propofol
quinine
salicylates
selective serotonin reuptake inhibitors
simvastatin
theophylline

○ Seizure activity

Incidence

○ Greater occurrence in males than females
○ May occur at any age

Common characteristics

○ Tenderness, swelling, and muscle weakness from muscle trauma and pressure
○ Dark, reddish-brown urine from myoglobin

Complications

○ Renal failure
○ Amputation

Assessment

History

○ Muscle trauma or breakdown
○ Muscle pain
○ Presence of any risk factors

Physical findings

○ Dark, reddish-brown urine
○ Tense, tender muscle compartment (compartment syndrome)

Test results

Laboratory
○ Urine myoglobin level exceeds 0.5 mg/dl (evident with only 200 g of muscle damage).
○ Creatinine kinase level is elevated (0.5 to 0.95 mg/dl) from muscle damage.
○ Serum potassium, phosphate, creatinine, and creatine levels are elevated.
○ Hypocalcemia occurs in early stages, hypercalcemia in later stages.
○ Intracompartmental venous pressure measurements (using a wick catheter, needle, or slit catheter inserted into the muscle) are elevated.
Imaging
○ Computed tomography, magnetic resonance imaging, and bone scintigraphy are used to detect muscle necrosis.

Treatment

General

○ For underlying disorder
○ Prevention of renal failure
○ Bed rest

Medication

○ Anti-inflammatory agents
○ Corticosteroids (in extreme cases)
○ Analgesics

Surgery

○ Immediate fasciotomy and debridement if compart-ment venous pressure exceeds 25 mm Hg

Nursing considerations

Key outcomes

The patient will:
○ maintain normal renal function
○ express increased comfort and decreased pain
○ verbalize understanding of the disorder and treat-ment.

Nursing interventions

○ Give prescribed I.V. fluids and diuretics.
○ Measure intake and output accurately.
○ Promote comfort measures.

Monitoring

○ Intake and output
○ Urine myoglobins
○ Renal studies
○ Pain control

Patient teaching

Be sure to cover:
○ the disorder, diagnosis, and treatment
○ the need for prolonged, low-intensity training as op-posed to short bursts of intense exercise.

Rheumatic fever and rheumatic heart disease

Overview

Description

○ Systemic inflammatory disease of childhood that occurs 2 to 6 weeks following an inadequately treated upper respiratory tract infection with group A beta-hemolytic streptococci
○ Principally involves the heart, joints, central nervous system, skin, and subcutaneous tissues
○ In rheumatic heart disease, early acute phase that may affect endocardium, myocardium, or pericardium, possibly followed later by chronic valvular disease
○ Commonly recurs

Pathophysiology

○ Rheumatic fever appears to be a hypersensitivity reaction in which antibodies produced to combat streptococci react and produce lesions at specific tissue sites.
○ Antigens of group A streptococci bind to receptors in the heart, muscle, brain, and synovial joints, causing an autoimmune response.
○ Because the antigens are similar to the body's own cells, antibodies may attack healthy body cells by mistake.

Causes

○ Group A beta-hemolytic streptococcal pharyngitis

Incidence

○ In the United States, most common in northern states
○ Worldwide, 15 to 20 million new cases each year

Common characteristics

○ Familial tendency
○ Most common during cool, damp weather in winter and early spring

Complications

○ Destruction of mitral and aortic valves
○ Severe pancarditis
○ Pericardial effusion
○ Heart failure
○ Systemic emboli

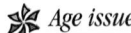 **Age issue**

In children, mitral insufficiency is the major consequence of rheumatic heart disease.

Assessment

History

○ Recent streptococcal infection
○ Recent history of low-grade fever spiking to at least 100.4° F (38° C) in late afternoon, along with unexplained epistaxis and abdominal pain
○ Migratory joint pain (polyarthritis)

Physical findings

○ Swelling, redness, and signs of effusion, most commonly in the knees, ankles, elbows, and hips
○ With pericarditis: sharp, sudden pain that usually starts over the sternum and radiates to the neck, shoulders, back, and arms; increases with deep inspiration and decreases when the patient sits up and leans forward
○ With heart failure caused by severe rheumatic carditis: dyspnea, right upper quadrant pain, and a hacking, nonproductive cough
○ Skin lesions, such as erythema marginatum, typically on the trunk and extremities
○ Subcutaneous nodules, 3 mm to 2 cm in diameter, that are firm, movable, and nontender occurring near tendons or bony prominences of joints, persisting for several days to weeks
○ With left-sided heart failure: edema and tachypnea, bibasilar crackles, and ventricular or atrial gallop
○ Transient chorea up to 6 months after original streptococcal infection
○ Pericardial friction rub
○ Heart murmurs and gallops

Test results

Laboratory
○ During acute phase, white blood cell count and erythrocyte sedimentation rate are elevated.
○ During inflammation, complete blood count shows slight anemia.
○ C-reactive protein test is positive, especially during acute phase.
○ In severe carditis, cardiac enzyme levels are increased.
○ Antistreptolysin-O titer is elevated in 95% of patients within 2 months of onset.
○ Throat cultures show group A beta-hemolytic streptococci.
Imaging
○ Chest X-rays show normal heart size (except with myocarditis, heart failure, and pericardial effusion).
○ Echocardiography helps evaluate valvular damage, chamber size, and ventricular function and detects pericardial effusion.
Diagnostic procedures
○ Electrocardiography reveals no diagnostic changes, but 20% of patients show a prolonged PR interval.
○ Cardiac catheterization evaluates valvular damage and left ventricular function in severe cardiac dysfunction.

Treatment

General

○ Dietary sodium restriction, if indicated
○ Bed rest during acute phase
○ Gradual activity increase, as tolerated

Medication

○ Antibiotics
○ Salicylates
○ Corticosteroids

Surgery

○ Commissurotomy, valvuloplasty, or heart valve replacement

Nursing considerations

Key outcomes

The patient will:
○ maintain adequate ventilation
○ maintain hemodynamic stability
○ avoid arrhythmias
○ carry out activities of daily living without weakness or fatigue
○ express feelings about diminished capacity to perform usual roles.

Nursing interventions

○ Find out if the patient has ever had a hypersensitivity reaction to penicillin. Warn the parents (if appropriate) that such a reaction is possible.
○ Give prescribed antibiotics on time.
○ Stress the importance of bed rest. Provide a bedside commode.
○ Position the patient upright.
○ Provide analgesics and oxygen, as needed.
○ Allow the patient to express feelings and concerns.
○ Help the parents overcome any guilt feelings they may have about their child's illness.
○ Encourage the parents and child to vent their frustrations during the long recovery. If the child has severe carditis, help them prepare for permanent changes in the child's lifestyle.

Monitoring

○ Vital signs
○ Heart rhythm
○ Heart and breath sounds

Patient teaching

Be sure to cover:
○ the disorder, diagnosis, and treatment
○ the importance of resuming activities of daily living slowly and scheduling frequent rest periods as instructed by the physician

○ what to do if signs of an allergic reaction to penicillin occur
○ the importance of reporting early signs and symptoms of left-sided heart failure, such as dyspnea and a hacking, nonproductive cough, and immediately reporting signs of recurrent streptococcal infection
○ keeping the child away from people with respiratory tract infections
○ transient nature of chorea
○ compliance with prolonged antibiotic therapy and follow-up care
○ the need for prophylactic antibiotics before any dental work or invasive procedures.

Rheumatoid arthritis

Overview

Description

- Chronic, systemic, symmetrical inflammatory disease
- Primarily attacks peripheral joints and surrounding muscles, tendons, ligaments, and blood vessels
- Marked by spontaneous remissions and unpredictable exacerbations
- Potentially crippling

Pathophysiology

- Cartilage damage resulting from inflammation triggers further immune responses, including complement activation.
- Complement, in turn, attracts polymorphonuclear leukocytes and stimulates release of inflammatory mediators, which exacerbates joint destruction.

Causes

- Unknown
- Possible influence of infection (viral or bacterial), hormonal factors, and lifestyle

Incidence

- Strikes three times as many women as men
- Can occur at any age; peak onset between ages 35 and 50

Common characteristics

- Stiff, swollen joints

Complications

- Fibrous or bony ankylosis
- Soft-tissue contractures
- Joint deformities
- Sjögren's syndrome
- Spinal cord compression
- Carpal tunnel syndrome
- Osteoporosis
- Recurrent infections
- Hip joint necrosis

Assessment

History

- Insidious onset of nonspecific symptoms, including fatigue, malaise, anorexia, persistent low-grade fever, weight loss, and vague articular symptoms
- Later, more specific localized articular symptoms, commonly in the fingers
- Bilateral and symmetrical symptoms, which may extend to the wrists, elbows, knees, and ankles
- Stiff joints
- Stiff, weak, or painful muscles
- Numbness or tingling in the feet or weakness or loss of sensation in the fingers
- Pain on inspiration
- Shortness of breath

Physical findings

- Joint deformities and contractures
- Painful, red, swollen arms
- Foreshortened hands
- Boggy wrists
- Rheumatoid nodules
- Leg ulcers
- Eye redness
- Joints that are warm to the touch
- Pericardial friction rub
- Positive Babinski's sign

Test results

Laboratory

- Rheumatoid factor test is positive in 75% to 80% of patients, as indicated by a titer of 1:160 or higher.
- Synovial fluid analysis shows increased volume and turbidity but decreased viscosity and complement (C3 and C4) levels, with white blood cell count possibly exceeding 10,000/µl.
- Serum globulin levels are elevated.
- Erythrocyte sedimentation rate is elevated.
- Complete blood count shows moderate anemia and slight leukocytosis. (See *Classifying rheumatoid arthritis*.)

Imaging

- In early stages, X-rays show bone demineralization and soft-tissue swelling. Later, they help determine the extent of cartilage and bone destruction, erosion, subluxations, and deformities and show the characteristic pattern of these abnormalities.
- Magnetic resonance imaging and computed tomography scan may provide information about the extent of damage.

Other

- Synovial tissue biopsy shows inflammation.

Treatment

General

- Adequate sleep (8 to 10 hours every night)
- Splinting
- Range-of-motion (ROM) exercises and carefully individualized therapeutic exercises
- Moist heat application
- Frequent rest periods between activities

Medication

- Salicylates
- Nonsteroidal anti-inflammatory drugs
- Antimalarials (hydroxychloroquine)
- Gold salts
- Penicillamine
- Corticosteroids
- Antineoplastic agents

Surgery

- Metatarsal head and distal ulnar resectional arthroplasty and insertion of silastic prosthesis between the metacarpophalangeal and proximal interphalangeal joints
- Arthrodesis (joint fusion)
- Synovectomy
- Osteotomy
- Repair of ruptured tendon
- In advanced disease, joint reconstruction or total joint arthroplasty

Nursing considerations

Key outcomes

The patient will:
- express feelings of increased comfort and decreased pain
- attain the highest degree of mobility possible within the confines of the disease
- maintain skin integrity
- verbalize feelings about limitations
- express an increased sense of well-being.

Nursing interventions

- Give prescribed analgesics, and watch for adverse reactions.
- Perform meticulous skin care.
- Supply adaptive devices, such as a zipper-pull, easy-to-open beverage cartons, lightweight cups, and unpackaged silverware.

After total knee or hip arthroplasty
- Give prescribed blood replacement products, antibiotics, and pain medication.
- Have the patient perform active dorsiflexion; immediately report inability to do so.
- Supervise isometric exercises every 2 hours.
- After total hip arthroplasty, check traction for pressure areas and keep the head of the bed raised 30 to 45 degrees.
- Change or reinforce dressings, as needed, using aseptic technique.
- Have the patient turn, cough, and breathe deeply every 2 hours.
- After total knee arthroplasty, keep the leg extended and slightly elevated.
- After total hip arthroplasty, keep the hip in abduction. Watch for and immediately report inability to rotate the hip or bear weight on it, increased pain, or a leg that appears shorter.
- Assist patient in activities, keeping the weight on the unaffected side.

Monitoring

- Joint mobility and pain level
- Skin integrity
- Vital signs and daily weight
- Sensory disturbances
- Serum electrolyte, hemoglobin, and hematocrit levels

Classifying rheumatoid arthritis

A patient who meets four of seven American College of Rheumatology criteria is classified as having rheumatoid arthritis. She must experience the first four criteria for at least 6 weeks, and a physician must observe the second through fifth criteria.
- Morning stiffness in and around the joints that lasts for 1 hour before full improvement
- Arthritis in three or more joint areas, with at least three joint areas (as observed by a physician) exhibiting soft-tissue swelling or joint effusions, not just bony overgrowth (the 14 possible areas involved include the right and left proximal interphalangeal, metacarpophalangeal, wrist, elbow, knee, ankle, and metatarsophalangeal joints)
- Arthritis of hand joints, including the wrist, the metacarpophalangeal joint, or the proximal interphalangeal joint
- Arthritis that involves the same joint areas on both sides of the body
- Subcutaneous rheumatoid nodules over bony prominences
- Demonstration of abnormal amounts of serum rheumatoid factor by any method that produces a positive result in less than 5% of patients without rheumatoid arthritis
- Radiographic changes, usually on posteroanterior hand and wrist radiographs, must show erosions or unequivocal bony decalcification localized in or most noticeable adjacent to the involved joints

- Activity tolerance
- Complications of corticosteroid therapy

Patient teaching

Be sure to cover:
- the disorder, diagnosis, and treatment
- chronic nature of rheumatoid arthritis and possible need for major lifestyle changes
- importance of a balanced diet and weight control
- importance of adequate sleep
- sexual concerns.

If the patient requires total knee or hip arthroplasty, be sure to cover:
- preoperative and surgical procedures
- postoperative exercises, with supervision
- deep-breathing and coughing exercises to perform after surgery
- performing frequent ROM leg exercises after surgery
- use of a constant-passive-motion device after total knee arthroplasty, or placement of an abduction pillow between the legs after total hip arthroplasty
- how to use a trapeze to move about in bed
- drug dosages and possible adverse effects.

Discharge planning

- Refer patient for physical and occupational therapy.
- Refer patient to the Arthritis Foundation.

Rocky Mountain spotted fever

Overview

Description

- Acute infectious, febrile, rash-producing illness associated with outdoor activities
- Fatal in about 5% of patients

Pathophysiology

- Infecting organism multiplies in endothelial cells and spreads via the bloodstream.
- Focal areas of infiltration lead to thrombosis and leakage of red blood cells into surrounding tissue.

Causes

- Rickettsia rickettsii, transmitted by the wood tick (Dermacentor andersoni) in the western United States and by the dog tick (D. variabilis) in the eastern United States; enters humans or small animals with the prolonged bite (4 to 6 hours) of an adult tick
- Occasionally, inhalation or contact of abraded skin with tick excreta or tissue juices

Incidence

- Endemic throughout the continental United States, but most common in southeastern and south-central regions
- Particularly prevalent in children ages 5 to 9
- Increased occurrence in spring and summer

Common characteristics

- Fever, headache, mental confusion, and myalgia
- Macular papular rash on palms and soles in about 90% of patients
- Rash, evident in about 15% of patients on day 1 and in nearly half of patients by day 3, starting at the wrists, ankles, or forehead and spreading to the remainder of the extremities and trunk
- Within 2 days, rash seen over the entire body (including scalp, palms, and soles)

Complications

- Lobar pneumonia
- Otitis media
- Parotitis
- Disseminated intravascular coagulation
- Renal failure
- Meningoencephalitis
- Hepatic injury
- Death
- Enterocolitis

Assessment

History

- Recent exposure to ticks or tick-infested areas, or a known tick bite
- Abrupt symptom onset, including persistent fever (temperature of 102° to 104° F [38.9° to 40° C]); generalized, excruciating headache; and aching in bones, muscles, joints, and back

Physical findings

- Erythematous macules, 1 to 5 mm in diameter, becoming maculopapules that blanch with pressure
- Frank hemorrhage at the center of maculopapules, creating petechia that don't blanch with pressure
- Bronchial cough
- Tachypnea
- Altered level of consciousness
- Decreased urine output; dark urine
- Tachycardia
- Hypotension
- Hepatomegaly, splenomegaly
- Generalized pitting edema
- Abdominal tenderness

Test results

Laboratory
- Serologic tests may be negative in initial stages.
- Indirect immunofluorescence assay has diagnostic titer of 64 or greater, detectable between days 7 and 14 of the illness.
- Latex agglutination diagnostic titer is 128 or greater 1 week after onset.
- Platelet count, white blood cell count, and fibrinogen levels are decreased.
- Prothrombin time and partial thromboplastin time are prolonged.
- Serum protein levels (especially albumin) are decreased.
- Hyponatremia and hypochloremia occur, related to increased aldosterone excretion.
- Serum creatinine, blood urea nitrogen, and potassium levels are elevated.
- Hepatic function is abnormal.
- Cerebrospinal fluid analysis shows mild mononuclear pleocytosis with slightly elevated protein content.
- Immunohistologic examination of cutaneous biopsy of a rash lesion shows *R. rickettsii.*

Treatment

General

- Careful tick removal
- Careful fluid administration
- Intubation and mechanical ventilation, if needed
- Hemodialysis, if needed
- Treatment of hemorrhage and thrombocytopenia, if needed

- Small, frequent meals
- Parenteral nutrition, if the patient can't receive oral intake
- Bed rest until condition improves

Medication

- Doxycycline (drug of choice), tetracycline, or chloramphenicol (in pregnant women)
- Anticonvulsants

Nursing considerations

Key outcomes

The patient will:
- maintain hemodynamic stability
- remain afebrile
- exhibit improved or healed lesions or wounds
- maintain adequate fluid volume
- maintain normal white blood cell count and differential
- report increased comfort and decreased pain.

Nursing interventions

- Give prescribed drugs.
- Provide oxygen therapy and assisted ventilation for pulmonary complications as ordered.
- Offer mentholated lotions if the rash itches.
- Turn the patient frequently.
- Encourage incentive spirometry and deep breathing.
- Plan care to promote adequate rest periods.

Monitoring

- Vital signs
- Fluid and electrolyte status
- Respiratory status
- Neurologic status

Patient teaching

Be sure to cover:
- the disorder, diagnosis, and treatment
- importance of reporting recurrent symptoms immediately
- preventive strategies, including avoiding tick-infested areas, whole-body inspection (including scalp) every 3 to 4 hours for attached ticks, protective clothing, and insect repellent
- correct tick removal technique using tweezers or forceps and steady traction.

Discharge planning

- Refer the patient to an infectious disease specialist if needed.

Rosacea

Overview

Description

- Chronic adult skin disorder that affects the skin and eyes
- Produces flushing and dilation of small blood vessels in the face, especially the nose and cheeks
- May cause papules and pustules, but without the characteristic comedones of acne vulgaris
- Usually spreads slowly; rarely subsides spontaneously
- Commonly more severe in men and usually associated with rhinophyma (dilated follicles and thickened, bulbous skin on the nose)

Pathophysiology

- Vascular reactivity leads to varying degrees of papules, pustules, and hyperplasia of the sebaceous glands.

Causes

- Unknown
- Factors that cause flushing:
  - Drinking hot beverages
  - Using tobacco or alcohol
  - Eating spicy foods
  - Engaging in physical activity
  - Being exposed to extreme heat or cold or to sunlight

Incidence

- Most common in white women ages 30 to 50

Common characteristics

- Flushed areas on cheeks, nose, forehead, and chin
- Ocular involvement (50% of cases)

Complications

- Decreased self-esteem
- Rosacea fulminans

Lupoid or granulomatous rosacea

Firm yellow, brownish, or reddish cutaneous papules or nodules characterize the variant form called lupoid or granulomatous rosacea. The lesions are less inflammatory that those of rosacea. Often the surrounding skin is relatively normal looking, but sometimes it's red and thickened diffusely. Usually, the lesions are monomorphic in each patient, affecting the cheeks and periorificial areas. Other signs or symptoms of rosacea aren't needed to make the diagnosis of this form of rosacea. Diascopy with a glass spatula reveals the lupoid character of the infiltrations. Lupoid or granulomatous rosacea may scar the skin.

With ocular involvement
- Blepharitis
- Conjunctivitis
- Uveitis
- Keratitis

Assessment

History

- Facial flushing
- Gritty feeling in eyes
- Facial edema
- Predisposing or aggravating factors
- Complaints of burning or stinging of face

Physical findings

- Flushed areas on the cheeks, nose, forehead, and chin, usually starting across the central oval of the face (see *Lupoid or granulomatous rosacea*)
- Telangiectasia with pustules and papules
- Rhinophyma (thickened and disfigured noses) (in severe rosacea)
- Dry skin appearance
- Facial edema
- Ocular rosacea:
  - Conjunctival infection
  - Chalazion
  - Cpiscleritis

Test results

- Rosacea is confirmed by observation of typical vascular and acneiform lesions without comedones.

Diagnostic procedures

- Skin biopsy may be done to rule out other diseases such as lupus erythematosus.

Treatment

General

- Identification and avoidance of aggravating factors, such as hot beverages, alcohol, and spicy foods
- Avoidance of physical activities involving sunlight or exposure to extreme heat or cold
- Facial massage

Medication

- Topical azelaic acid
- Topical sodium sulfacetamide
- Topical metronidazole
- Oral doxycycline (for ocular involvement)
- Corticosteroids

Surgery

- Electrosurgery
- Laser therapy

Nursing considerations

Key outcomes

The patient will:
○ exhibit improved or healed wounds or lesions
○ report feelings of increased comfort
○ demonstrate an appropriate skin care regimen
○ report feelings of improved self-image.

Nursing interventions

○ Give prescribed drugs.
○ Encourage patient to express feelings.
○ Offer emotional support and reassurance.
○ Assist with identification of triggers.

Monitoring

○ Adverse reactions to prescribed drugs
○ Complications
○ Response to treatment

Patient teaching

Be sure to cover:
○ the disorder, diagnosis, and treatment
○ drugs and possible adverse effects
○ aggravating factors
○ stress reduction techniques
○ meticulous hand-washing and personal hygiene
○ ways to prevent infection
○ signs and symptoms of infection
○ when to notify the physician
○ use of noncomedogenic, high-factor sunscreen when exposed to sunlight and wind.

Roseola infantum

Overview

Description
○ Common acute, benign, presumably viral illness characterized by fever with subsequent rash (see *Incubation and duration of common rash-producing infections*)
○ Also known as *exanthema subitum*

Pathophysiology
○ Human herpesvirus (HHV) type 6B, which causes the disorder, is similar to cytomegalovirus.
○ HHV-6 shows persistent and intermittent or chronic shedding in the normal population, resulting in the unusually early infection of children.
○ HHV-6 is thought to be latent in salivary glands and blood.

Causes
○ HHV-6B
○ May be transmitted by saliva and possibly by genital secretions

Incidence
○ Affects infants and young children, typically from age 6 months to 3 years
○ Affects both sexes equally
○ Occurs year-round, but most common in spring and fall

Common characteristics
○ Incubation period of 10 to 15 days
○ High fever with rash appearing after the fever breaks

Complications
○ Encephalopathy
○ Thrombocytopenic purpura
○ Febrile seizures
○ Meningitis
○ Hepatitis

Incubation and duration of common rash-producing infections

Infection	Incubation (days)	Duration (days)
Roseola	5-15	3-6
Varicella	10-14	7-14
Rubeola	13-17	5
Rubella	6-18	3
Herpes simplex	2-12	7-21

Assessment

History
○ Abruptly increasing, unexplainable fever that peaks between 103° and 105° F (39.4° and 40.5° C) for 3 to 5 days and then drops suddenly
○ Anorexia
○ Irritability
○ Listlessness
○ Cough

Physical findings
○ When temperature drops abruptly, maculopapular, nonpruritic rash appears that blanches with pressure
○ Profuse rash on the trunk, arms, and neck; mild rash on the face and legs; fades within 24 hours
○ Nagayama spots (red papules on soft palate and uvula)
○ Periorbital edema

Test results
○ Usually, roseola infantum is diagnosed from clinical observation.
Laboratory
○ Causative organism is present in saliva.
○ HHV-6 is isolated in peripheral blood.
○ Complete blood count shows leukopenia and relative lymphocytosis as temperature increases.
○ Immunofluorescence or enzyme immunoassays may show seroconversion during the convalescent phase.

Treatment

General
○ Supportive and symptomatic
○ Increased fluid intake
○ Rest until fever subsides

Medication
○ Antipyretics
○ Anticonvulsants

Nursing considerations

Key outcomes
The patient will:
○ regain a normal body temperature
○ maintain adequate fluid volume
○ maintain adequate nutritional intake
○ exhibit improved or healed lesions or wounds.

Nursing interventions
○ Give tepid sponge baths and prescribed antipyretics.
○ Replace fluids and electrolytes, as needed.
○ Institute seizure precautions.
○ Provide emotional support to parents.

Monitoring

○ Neurologic status
○ Fluid and electrolyte status
○ Vital signs, especially temperature

Patient teaching

Be sure to cover:
○ the disorder, diagnosis, and treatment
○ methods to reduce fever:
  – tepid sponge baths
  – dressing the child in lightweight clothing
  – keeping a comfortable room temperature
  – use of antipyretics
○ importance of adequate fluid intake
○ no need for isolation
○ reassurance that brief febrile seizures won't cause brain damage and will stop as the fever subsides.

Rotavirus

Overview

Description

- Self-limiting intestinal illness that causes mild to severe diarrhea in children
- Causes hospitalization of about 55,000 children each year in the United States and kills more than 600,000 children worldwide

Pathophysiology

- Rotavirus invades and damages the cells of the intestinal mucosa.
- Damage decreases viable absorptive surface, causing an imbalance of secretion and absorption that results in diarrhea.

Causes

- Infection with rotavirus, a member of the Reoviridae family
- Transmitted primarily by the fecal-oral route through ingestion of contaminated water or food or through contact with contaminated surfaces (see *Spreading rotavirus infection*)

Incidence

- Highest among infants and young children; affects most children in the United States by age 2
- Winter seasonal pattern seen in the United States and other temperate climate countries, with annual epidemics from November to April

Common characteristics

- Vomiting and watery diarrhea for 3 to 8 days
- Fever
- Abdominal pain

Complications

- Severe dehydration and shock
- Skin breakdown
- Worsening of other conditions such as cystic fibrosis

Spreading rotavirus infection

Rotavirus infection is contagious. Rotavirus particles pass in the stool of infected persons before and after they have symptoms of the illness. A child can catch a rotavirus infection if he puts his fingers in his mouth after touching something that has been contaminated by the stool of an infected person. Usually this happens when the child forgets to wash his hands often enough, especially before eating and after using the toilet. Because of the widespread nature of rotavirus and the fact that almost 100% of children get rotavirus illness, total prevention of the spread of rotavirus is nearly impossible.

Assessment

History

- Fever, nausea, and vomiting followed by diarrhea

Physical findings

- Diarrhea
- Signs of dehydration, such as:
  - Tachycardia
  - Hypotension
  - Dry mucous membranes
  - Concentrated urine
  - Poor tear production
  - Poor skin turgor
  - Oliguria
  - Sunken eyeballs
  - Sunken anterior fontanel
- Rectal excoriation

Test results

Laboratory
- Rapid antigen detection shows rotavirus in stool.

Treatment

General

- Small, frequent meals
- Increased fluid intake
- Rest periods when fatigued
- Skin care

Medication

- None (antibiotics and antimotility drugs contraindicated)

Nursing considerations

Key outcomes

The patient will:
- maintain adequate nutritional status
- maintain normal electrolyte levels
- maintain adequate fluid volume
- exhibit improved or healed lesions or wounds
- verbalize or demonstrate increased energy.

Nursing interventions

- Institute enteric precautions.
- Enforce strict hand-washing and careful cleaning of all equipment, including toys.
- Implement measures to ensure adequate hydration.
- Clean the patient's perineum thoroughly to prevent skin breakdown.
- Be aware that breast-fed infants can continue to breast-feed without restrictions. Bottle-fed infants can use lactose-free soybean formulas.

Monitoring

○ Intake and output (including stools)
○ Skin integrity

Patient teaching

Be sure to cover (with the parents):
○ the disorder, diagnosis, and treatment
○ proper hand-washing technique
○ instructions on diaper changing and thorough cleaning of the perineum and all affected surfaces
○ the importance of notifying the physician of increased diarrhea or signs of dehydration.

Rubella

Overview

Description

○ Acute, mildly contagious viral disease that causes a distinctive maculopapular rash (resembling measles or scarlet fever) and lymphadenopathy
○ Self-limiting with an excellent prognosis, except for congenital rubella, which can have disastrous consequences
○ Transmitted through contact with blood, urine, stools, or nasopharyngeal secretions of an infected person; also can be transmitted transplacentally
○ Communicable from about 10 days before until 5 days after rash appears
○ Also called *German measles*

Pathophysiology

○ A ribonucleic acid virus enters the bloodstream, usually through the respiratory route.
○ The incubation period lasts 18 days, with a duration of 12 to 23 days.
○ The rash is thought to result from virus dissemination to the skin.

Causes

○ Rubella virus (a togavirus) spread by direct contact or contaminated airborne respiratory droplets

Incidence

○ Occurs worldwide
○ Most common among children ages 5 to 9, adolescents, and young adults
○ Epidemics seen in institutions, colleges, and military populations
○ Flourishes during spring, with limited outbreaks in schools and workplaces

---

Giving the rubella vaccine

Know how to manage rubella immunization before giving the vaccine. First, ask about allergies, especially to neomycin. If the person has this allergy or has had a reaction to any immunization in the past, check with the physician before giving the vaccine.

If the person is a woman of childbearing age, ask if she's pregnant. If she is or thinks she may be, don't give the vaccine.

Give the vaccine at least 3 months after any administration of immune globulin or blood. These substances may have antibodies that could neutralize the vaccine.

Don't vaccinate an immunocompromised person, a person with immunodeficiency disease, or a person receiving immunosuppressant, radiation, or corticosteroid therapy. Instead, administer immune serum globulin, as ordered, to prevent or reduce infection.

Common characteristics

○ Rash covering the trunk and body; begins to fade in the opposite order in which it appeared by the end of day 2
○ Rash subsiding on the face; on the trunk may be confluent and hard to distinguish from scarlet fever rash
○ Rash disappearing on day 3

Complications

○ Arthritis
○ Postinfectious encephalitis
○ Thrombocytopenic purpura
○ Congenital rubella
In fetal infection (rare after 20th week of gestation)
○ Intrauterine death
○ Spontaneous abortion
○ Congenital malformations of major organ systems

Assessment

History

○ Inadequate immunization, exposure to a person with rubella infection within the previous 2 to 3 weeks, or recent travel to an endemic area without reimmunization
○ In a child, absence of prodromal symptoms
○ In an adolescent or adult, headache, malaise, anorexia, coryza, sore throat, and cough preceding rash onset
○ Polyarthralgias and polyarthritis (in some adults)

Physical findings

○ Rash accompanied by low-grade fever (99° to 101° F [37.2° to 38.3° C]) that may reach 104° F (40° C)
○ Exanthematous, maculopapular, mildly pruritic rash; typically begins on the face, and spreads rapidly, covering the trunk and limbs within hours
○ Small, red, petechial macules on the soft palate (Forschheimer spots) preceding or accompanying the rash
○ Coryza
○ Conjunctivitis
○ Suboccipital, postauricular, and postcervical lymph node enlargement

Test results

○ Usually, the diagnosis is made from clinical observation.
Laboratory
○ Cultures of throat, blood, urine, and cerebrospinal fluid isolate the rubella virus; convalescent serum shows a fourfold increase in antibody titers.
○ ELISA for immunoglobulin (Ig) M antibodies reveals rubella-specific IgM antibody.
○ In congenital rubella, rubella-specific IgM antibody is present in umbilical cord blood.

Treatment

General

○ Isolation precautions
○ Small, frequent meals
○ Increased fluid intake
○ Rest until fever subsides
○ Skin care

Medication

○ Antipyretics
○ Analgesics

Nursing considerations

Key outcomes

The patient will:
○ remain free from signs and symptoms of infection
○ exhibit improvement or healing of lesions or wounds
○ express or demonstrate feelings of increased comfort and decreased pain.

Nursing interventions

○ Give prescribed drugs.
○ Institute isolation precautions until 5 days after the rash disappears. Keep an infant with congenital rubella in isolation for 3 months, until three throat cultures are negative.
○ Keep the patient's skin clean and dry.
○ Ensure that the patient receives care only from nonpregnant hospital workers who are not at risk for rubella. As ordered, administer immune globulin to nonimmunized people who visit the patient. (See *Giving the rubella vaccine.*)
○ Report confirmed rubella cases to local public health officials.
○ Refer the patient to an infectious disease specialist if congenital rubella is confirmed.
○ Provide parents of an infant with congenital rubella with support, counseling, and referrals, as needed.

Monitoring

○ Vital signs
○ Skin for signs of exanthem
○ Auditory impairment in congenital rubella

Patient teaching

Be sure to cover (with the parents):
○ the disorder, diagnosis, and treatment
○ ways to reduce fever
○ devastating effects of rubella on an unborn neonate
○ importance of people with rubella avoiding pregnant women
○ avoidance of aspirin in a child receiving rubella vaccine.

Rubeola

Overview

Description

- Acute, highly contagious infection causing a characteristic rash
- In the United States, a usually excellent prognosis
- Can be severe or fatal in patients with impaired cell-mediated immunity
- Mortality highest in children under age 2 and in adults
- Also called *measles* or *morbilli*

Pathophysiology

- Virus invades the respiratory epithelium and spreads via the blood stream to the reticuloendothelial system, infecting all types of white blood cells.
- Viremia and viruria develop, leading to infection of the entire respiratory tract, which spreads to the integumentary system.
- In measles encephalitis, focal hemorrhage, congestion, and perivascular demyelination occur.

Causes

- Rubeola virus
- Spread by direct contact or by contaminated airborne respiratory droplets, with portal of entry in the upper respiratory tract

Incidence

- Affects mostly preschool children
- In temperate zones, most commonly seen in late winter and early spring

Common characteristics

- Fever, Koplik's spots, and characteristic red, blotchy, rash that begins on the face and becomes generalized
- Peak communicability from 1 to 2 days before symptom onset until 4 days after the rash appears

Complications

- Secondary bacterial infection
- Autoimmune reaction
- Bronchitis
- Otitis media
- Pneumonia
- Encephalitis

Assessment

History

- Inadequate immunization and exposure to someone with measles in the past 14 days
- Photophobia
- Malaise
- Anorexia
- Coryza
- Hoarseness
- Hacking cough

Physical findings

- Temperature peaking at 103° to 105° F (39.4° C to 40.5° C)
- Periorbital edema
- Conjunctivitis
- Koplik's spots (tiny, bluish gray specks, surrounded by red halo) on oral mucosa opposite the molars, which may bleed
- Pruritic rash starting as faint macules behind the ears and on the neck and cheeks, becoming papular and erythematous, and rapidly spreading over the face, neck, eyelids, arms, chest, back, abdomen, and thighs
- Fading of rash when it reaches the feet 2 to 3 days later, occurring in the same sequence it appeared, leaving brown discoloration that disappears in 7 to 10 days
- Severe cough
- Rhinorrhea
- Lymphadenopathy

Test results

Laboratory

- The measles virus appears in blood, nasopharyngeal secretions, and urine during the febrile period.
- Serum antibodies appear within 3 days after rash onset and reach peak titers 2 to 4 weeks later.

Treatment

General

- Respiratory isolation precautions
- Use of vaporizer
- Warm environment
- Small, frequent meals
- Increased fluid intake
- Rest until symptoms improve
- Skin care

Medication

- Antipyretics

Nursing considerations

Key outcomes

The patient will:
- remain free from signs and symptoms of infection
- exhibit improved or healed lesions or wounds
- remain free from complications related to oral mucous membrane trauma.

The patient's family will:
- communicate an understanding of the patient's special dietary needs.

Nursing interventions
○ Institute respiratory isolation measures for 4 days after rash onset.
○ Follow standard precautions.
○ Give prescribed drugs.
○ Encourage bed rest during the acute period.
○ If photophobia occurs, darken the room or provide sunglasses.
○ To prevent disease spread, administer measles vaccine, as ordered and needed.
○ Report measles cases to local health authorities.

Monitoring
○ Vital signs
○ Skin for signs of exanthem
○ Eyes for conjunctivitis
○ Mental status
○ Signs and symptoms of pneumonia
○ Ears for otitis media

Patient teaching

Be sure to cover (with the parents):
○ the disorder, diagnosis, and treatment
○ supportive measures, isolation, bed rest, and increased fluids
○ instructions on cleaning a vaporizer (if used) and the importance of changing the water every 8 hours
○ early signs and symptoms of complications that should be reported.

Saint Louis encephalitis

Overview

Description

○ Acute inflammatory disease of short duration that involves the brain, spinal cord, and meninges following the bite of an infected mosquito (mosquitoes infective for life)
○ Usually asymptomatic, but severe infection may have acute onset
○ Incubation period of 4 to 21 days
○ No person-to-person transmission
○ No chronic infection or reports of relapsing infection
○ Also known as *SEV, SLEV, mosquito-borne encephalitis, arbovirus,* and *viral encephalitis*

Pathophysiology

○ The virus is found in common birds, such as sparrows, finches, blue jays, robins, and doves.
○ Culex mosquitoes feed on these birds, contract the virus, and then pass it on to human hosts through a bite.
○ A primary viremia follows reproduction of the virus at the site of inoculation.
○ In subclinical disease, the pathogen is cleared by the liver, spleen, and lymph nodes before invasion of the central nervous system.
○ Secondary viremia occurs with continued viral replication, which overwhelms the liver, spleen, and lymph nodes.
○ The virus then invades the central nervous system, including the brain and spinal cord.

Causes

○ Transmitted by the bite of an infected mosquito
○ Laboratory-acquired infections possible through infected blood, cerebrospinal fluid (CSF), urine, and exudates

Risk factors

○ Human immunodeficiency virus infection
○ Age older than 70 (tenfold increased risk of clinical illness)
○ Travel to endemic areas
○ Participation in outdoor activities
○ Low socioeconomic status

Incidence

○ Occurs in North, South, and Central America and the Caribbean; major health problem in the United Sates
○ Highest incidence in late summer or early fall
○ Higher incidence in males, probably because of more outdoor exposure
○ Highly susceptible individuals: elderly people, those living in crowded conditions, those living in low-income areas, those working outside or participating in outdoor activities in endemic areas

Common characteristics

○ Symptoms usually mild
○ In severe infections
  – Acute onset of headache
  – High fever
  – Nausea
  – Myalgia
  – Malaise
  – Meningeal signs of stupor
  – Coma
  – Seizures (especially in infants)
  – Spastic paralysis
  – Death
○ In children, possible urinary tract symptoms

Complications

○ Acute encephalitis
○ Death
○ Movement disorders and motor deficits
○ Seizures and coma
○ Cranial nerve palsies

 Alert

Patients with atherosclerosis, heart disease, and hypertension have an increased risk of death from this infection.

Assessment

History

○ Exposure to infected insect
○ Onset of encephalitis characterized by:
  – Malaise
  – Fever
  – Cough and sore throat, followed by common symptoms of headache, nausea, vomiting, confusion, disorientation, irritability, tremors, and possible seizures

Physical findings

○ Temperature elevation
○ Normal neurological exam
○ 5% of patients present in a deep coma
○ Cranial nerve palsies in about 25% of patients
○ Possibly ataxia
○ Possibly seizures (infrequent, but more common in children)

Test results

Laboratory
○ One of the following will be present: A fourfold increase in the antivirus antibody titer between the acute and the convalescent periods; virus isolation from tissue, blood, or CSF; or specific immunoglobulin M antibody.

○ Pyuria or proteinuria occurs.
○ Sodium level is decreased.
○ CSF pressure is normal to mildly elevated, blood glucose level is normal, and protein level is normal to mildly elevated; CSF white blood cell count usually is less than 200/μl.

Treatment

General

○ Supportive
○ Management of seizures or neurological symptoms
○ Diet as tolerated
○ Bed rest

Medication

○ Antipyretics
○ Analgesics

Nursing considerations

Key outcomes

The patient will:
○ remain safe from falls caused by ataxia or seizures
○ accept comfort measures
○ maintain adequate nutrition and fluid intake.

Nursing interventions

○ Give prescribed drugs.
○ Encourage nutritional intake.
○ Encourage fluids and lying flat after lumbar puncture.
○ Assist with ambulation, as needed.
○ Frequently reposition the unconscious patient.
○ Encourage range-of-motion (ROM) exercises (passive ROM exercises if the patient is unconscious).

Monitoring

○ Vital signs
○ Level of consciousness
○ Skin breakdown
○ Seizure activity
○ Complications of lumbar puncture, if performed

Patient teaching

Be sure to cover:
○ the disorder, diagnosis, and treatment.
○ mosquito bite prevention, such as:
  – staying inside between dusk and dark
  – wearing long pants and long-sleeved shirts when outside
  – spraying exposed skin with insect repellent
  – avoiding areas of standing water where mosquitoes congregate.

Discharge planning

○ Encourage follow-up appointments, as needed.

Salmonella infection

Overview

Description

○ One of the most common intestinal infections in the United States
○ Occurs as enterocolitis, bacteremia, localized infection, typhoid fever, or paratyphoid fever
○ Nontyphoid forms, usually mild to moderate illness with low mortality
○ Typhoid fever most severe form; usually lasts from 1 to 4 weeks and confers lifelong immunity, although patient may become a carrier

Pathophysiology

○ Invasion occurs across the small intestinal mucosa, altering the plasma membrane and entering the lamina propria.
○ Invasion activates cell-signaling pathways, which alter electrolyte transport, and may cause diarrhea.
○ Some salmonella produce a molecule that increases electrolyte and fluid secretion.

Causes

○ Gram-negative bacilli of the genus *Salmonella* (member of the Enterobacteriaceae family)
  – Typhoid fever: *S. typhi*
  – Enterocolitis: *S. enteritidis*
  – Bacteremia: *S. choleresis*
○ Nontyphoidal infection — usually, ingestion of contaminated water or food or inadequately processed food, especially eggs, chicken, turkey, and duck
○ Contact with infected person or animal
○ Ingestion of contaminated dry milk, chocolate bars, or pharmaceuticals of animal origin

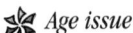 *Age issue*

Salmonella infection may occur in children younger than age 5 and from fecal-oral spread.

○ Typhoid fever — usually, drinking water contaminated by excretions of a carrier

Incidence

○ Increasing in the United States due to travel to endemic areas, especially the borders of Mexico
○ Lifelong immunity after initial attack of typhoid fever, but patient may become a carrier
○ Paratyphoid fever rare in the United States

Common characteristics

○ Nontyphoidal forms — usually, mild to moderate illness, with low mortality
○ Enterocolitis and bacteremia — especially common (and more virulent) among infants, elderly people, and those already weakened by other infections, especially human immunodeficiency virus infection

Complications

○ Dehydration
○ Hypovolemic shock
○ Abscess formation
○ Sepsis
○ Toxic megacolon

Assessment

History

○ With enterocolitis, possible report of contaminated food eaten 6 to 48 hours before onset of symptoms
○ With bacteremia, patient usually reveals immunocompromised condition, especially acquired immunodeficiency syndrome
○ With typhoid fever, possible ingestion of contaminated food or water, typically 1 to 2 weeks before symptoms develop

Physical findings

○ Fever
○ Abdominal pain
○ With enterocolitis, severe diarrhea
○ With typhoidal infection, headache, increasing fever, and constipation

Test results

Laboratory

○ Blood culture in typhoid or paratyphoid fever and bacteremia shows causative organism in most cases.
○ Stool culture in typhoid or paratyphoid fever and enterocolitis shows causative organism.
○ Other culture specimens (urine, bone marrow, pus, and vomitus) show causative organism.
○ Presence of *S. typhi* in stools 1 or more years after treatment indicates that the patient is a carrier (about 3% of patients).
○ Widal's test, an agglutination reaction against somatic and flagellar antigens, suggests typhoid fever with a fourfold increase in titer.
○ Complete blood count (CBC) shows transient leukocytosis during the first week of typhoidal salmonella infection.
○ CBC shows leukopenia during the third week of typhoidal salmonella infection.
○ CBC shows leukocytosis with local infection.

Treatment

General

○ Usually no treatment
○ Possible hospitalization for severe diarrhea
○ Fluid and electrolyte replacement
○ High-calorie fluids
○ Activity as tolerated

Medication

○ Antimicrobials
○ Antidiarrheals

 Alert

Don't give antipyretics. They may mask fever and lead to hypothermia. Instead, promote heat loss by applying tepid, wet towels to the patient's groin and axillae.

Surgery

○ Surgical drainage of localized abscesses

Nursing considerations

Key outcomes

The patient will:
○ regain and maintain fluid and electrolyte balance
○ return to a normal elimination pattern
○ conserve energy while carrying out daily activities
○ report adequate pain relief
○ experience no further weight loss.

Nursing interventions

○ Follow enteric precautions until three consecutive stool cultures are negative — the first one 48 hours after antibiotic treatment ends, followed by two more at 24-hour intervals.
○ Watch closely for signs of bowel perforation.
○ Maintain adequate I.V. fluid and electrolyte therapy, as ordered.
○ Provide good skin and mouth care.
○ Apply mild heat to relieve abdominal cramps.
○ Report salmonella cases to public health officials.

Monitoring

○ Fluid and electrolyte status
○ Vital signs
○ Daily weight

Patient teaching

Be sure to cover:
○ the disorder, diagnosis, and treatment
○ the need for close contacts to obtain a medical examination and treatment if cultures are positive
○ how to prevent salmonella infections
○ the need to be vaccinated (for those at high risk for contracting typhoid fever, such as laboratory workers and travelers)
○ the importance of proper hand-washing
○ the need to avoid preparing food or pouring water for others until salmonella infection is eliminated.

Preventing recurrence of salmonella infection

To prevent salmonella infection from recurring, follow these teaching guidelines:
○ Explain the causes of salmonella infection.
○ Show the patient how to wash his hands by wetting them under running water, lathering with soap and scrubbing, rinsing under running water with his fingers pointing down, and drying with a clean towel or paper towel.
○ Tell the patient to wash his hands after using the bathroom and before eating.
○ Tell him to cook foods thoroughly — especially eggs and chicken — and to refrigerate them at once.
○ Teach him how to avoid cross-contaminating foods by cleaning preparation surfaces with hot, soapy water and drying them thoroughly after use; cleaning surfaces between foods when preparing more than one food; and washing his hands before and after handling each food.
○ Tell the patient with a positive stool culture to avoid handling food and to use a separate bathroom or clean the bathroom after each use.
○ Tell the patient to report dehydration, bleeding, or recurrence of signs of salmonella infection.

Discharge planning

○ Arrange for follow-up with an infectious disease specialist or a gastroenterologist as needed. (See *Preventing recurrence of salmonella infection*.)

Sarcoidosis

Overview

Description

- A multisystemic, granulomatous disorder that characteristically produces lymphadenopathy, pulmonary infiltration, and skeletal, liver, eye, or skin lesions
- May be acute (usually resolves within 2 years) or chronic
- Chronic, progressive sarcoidosis (uncommon) associated with pulmonary fibrosis and progressive pulmonary disability

Pathophysiology

- An excessive inflammatory process begins in the alveoli, bronchioles, and blood vessels of the lungs.
- Monocyte-macrophages accumulate in the target tissue where they induce the inflammatory process.
- CD4+ T-lymphocytes and sensitized immune cells form a ring around the inflamed area.
- Fibroblasts, mast cells, collagen fibers, and proteoglycans encase the inflammatory and immune cells, causing granuloma formation.

Causes

- Exact cause unknown
- Possible causes:
  - Hypersensitivity response to atypical mycobacteria, fungi, and pine pollen
  - Chemicals
  - T-cell abnormalities
  - Lymphokine production abnormalities

Incidence

- Most common in people ages 20 to 40
- In the United States, predominant occurrence among Blacks
- Affects twice as many women as men
- Incidence slightly higher in families, suggesting genetic predisposition

Common characteristics

- Pain in the wrists, ankles, and elbows
- Malaise
- Unexplained weight loss
- Shortness of breath on exertion
- Substernal pain

Complications

- Pulmonary fibrosis
- Pulmonary hypertension
- Cor pulmonale

Assessment

History

- Pain in the wrists, ankles, and elbows
- General fatigue and malaise
- Unexplained weight loss
- Breathlessness and dyspnea
- Nonproductive cough
- Substernal pain

Physical findings

- Erythema nodosum
- Punched out lesions on the fingers and toes
- Cranial or peripheral nerve palsies
- Extensive nasal mucosal lesions
- Anterior uveitis
- Glaucoma and blindness occasionally in advanced disease
- Bilateral hilar and paratracheal lymphadenopathy
- Splenomegaly
- Arrhythmias

Test results

Laboratory
- Arterial blood gas (ABG) analysis shows a decreased partial pressure of arterial oxygen and increased carbon dioxide levels.

Imaging
- Chest X-rays show bilateral hilar and right paratracheal adenopathy, with or without diffuse interstitial infiltrates.

Diagnostic procedures
- Kveim-Siltzbach skin test shows granuloma development at the injection site in 2 to 4 weeks when positive.
- Lymph node, skin, or lung biopsy shows noncaseating granulomas with negative cultures for mycobacteria and fungi.
- Pulmonary function tests show decreased total lung capacity and compliance and reduced diffusing capacity.

Treatment

General

- None needed for asymptomatic sarcoidosis
- Protection from sunlight
- Low-calcium diet for hypercalcemia
- Reduced-sodium, high-calorie diet
- Adequate fluids
- Activity as tolerated

Medication

- Corticosteroids

Nursing considerations

Key outcomes

The patient will:

○ maintain adequate ventilation
○ demonstrate effective coping mechanisms
○ express an understanding of the illness
○ perform activities of daily living within confines of the illness
○ remain free from signs and symptoms of infection.

Nursing interventions

○ Give prescribed drugs.
○ Administer supplemental oxygen.
○ Provide a nutritious, high-calorie diet.
○ Encourage oral fluid intake.
○ Provide a low-calcium diet for hypercalcemia.
○ Provide emotional support.
○ Provide comfort measures.
○ Include the patient in care decisions whenever possible.

Monitoring

○ Vital signs
○ Intake and output
○ Daily weight
○ Respiratory status
○ Chest X-ray results
○ Sputum production
○ ABG results
○ Cardiac rhythm

 Alert

Because corticosteroids may induce or worsen diabetes mellitus, test the patient's blood by fingersticks for glucose and acetone at least every 12 hours at the beginning of corticosteroid therapy. Also, watch for other adverse effects, such as fluid retention, electrolyte imbalance (especially hypokalemia), moon face, hypertension, and personality changes.

Patient teaching

Be sure to cover:

○ the disorder, diagnosis, and treatment
○ drugs and possible adverse effects
○ when to notify the physician
○ steroid therapy
○ the need for regular follow-up examinations
○ the importance of wearing a medical identification bracelet
○ infection prevention.

Discharge planning

○ Refer a patient with failing vision to community support and resource groups such as the American Foundation for the Blind, if necessary.

Scabies

Overview

Description

- Transmissible skin infestation with *Sarcoptes scabiei* var. *hominis* (itch mite)
- Characterized by burrows, severe pruritus, and excoriations

Pathophysiology

- Mites burrow into the skin on contact, progressing 2 to 3 mm per day.
- Females live about 4 to 6 weeks and lay about 40 to 50 eggs, which hatch in 3 to 4 days.
- Pruritus occurs only after sensitization to the mite develops. With initial infestation, sensitization requires several weeks. With reinfestation, sensitization develops within 24 hours.
- Dead mites, eggs, larvae, and their excrement trigger an inflammatory eruption of the skin in infested areas.

Causes

- Direct (skin to skin) contact or contact with contaminated articles for up to 48 hours (see *Scabies: Cause and effect*)

Risk factors

- Overcrowded living conditions
- Poor hygiene
- Sexual promiscuity
- Day-care or institutional settings

Incidence

- Common in children and young adults
- Common in elderly and debilitated patients

Scabies: Cause and effect

Infestation with *Sarcoptes scabiei*—the itch mite— causes scabies. This mite (shown enlarged below) has a hard shell and measures a microscopic 0.1 mm.

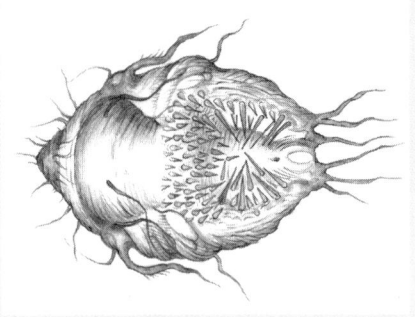

- Occurs worldwide
- Can be endemic

Common characteristics

- Burrows
- Severe pruritus
- Excoriations

Complications

- Excoriations
- Secondary bacterial infection
- Abscess formation
- Septicemia

Assessment

History

- Predisposing factors
- May be asymptomatic initially
- Intense pruritus that's more severe at night

Physical findings

- Characteristic gray-brown, threadlike burrows (0.5 to 1 cm long) with tiny papule or vesicle at one end
- Common sites: flexor surfaces of wrists, elbows, axillary folds, waistline, nipples in females, and genitalia

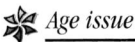 *Age issue*

In infants, the burrows may appear on the head and neck.

- Papules, vesicles, crusting, abscess formation, and cellulites with secondary infection

Test results

Laboratory
- Wound culture demonstrates secondary bacterial infection.

Diagnostic procedures
- Mineral oil burrow-scraping reveals mites, nits, or eggs, and feces or scybala.
- Punch biopsy may help to confirm the diagnosis.

Other
- Resolution of infestation with therapeutic trial of a pediculicide confirms the diagnosis.

Treatment

General

- Bathing with soap and water

Medication

- Scabicides
- 6% to 10% sulfur solution
- Systemic antibiotics
- Antipruritics

Alert

Avoid the use of topical steroids, which may potentiate the infection.

 Age issue

When treating infants, include the head in treatment.

Nursing considerations

Key outcomes

The patient will:
○ exhibit resolution of infestation
○ report relief of pruritus
○ avoid complications
○ demonstrate understanding of proper skin care regimen.

Nursing interventions

○ Trim patient's fingernails short.
○ Give prescribed drugs.
○ Isolate the patient until treatment is completed.
○ Practice meticulous hand-washing.
○ Sterilize blood pressure cuffs in a gas autoclave before using on other patients.
○ Decontaminate linens, towels, clothing, and personal articles.
○ Disinfect the patient's room after discharge.
○ If the patient is a child, notify his school of the infestation.
○ Encourage verbalization of feelings.
○ Observe wound and skin precautions for 24 hours after treatment with a scabicide.

Monitoring

○ Response to treatment
○ Complications
○ Neurologic status

 Alert

Prolonged use of scabicides may lead to excessive central nervous system stimulation and seizures.

Patient teaching

Be sure to cover:
○ the disorder, diagnosis, and treatment
○ identification of characteristic lesions
○ modes of transmission
○ mite resistance to scabicides
○ assessment of close personal contacts for infestation
○ successful treatment for infestation with good hygiene and scabicides

○ prevention of transmission and recurrence
○ proper application of the prescribed scabicide.

Scarlet fever

Overview

Description

- A hypersensitivity reaction that usually follows strep-tococcal pharyngitis
- May follow other streptococcal infections, such as wound infections, urosepsis, and puerperal sepsis
- Also known as *scarlatina*

Pathophysiology

- After infection, an erythrogenic toxin is produced, re-sulting in a hypersensitivity reaction.
- Replication site is the tonsils and pharynx.
- Inflammatory reaction occurs.

Causes

- Group A beta-hemolytic streptococci transmitted by direct contact with infected person or droplet spread; indirectly by contact with contaminated arti-cles or ingestion of contaminated food

Incidence

- Most common in children ages 3 to 15; peak inci-dence ages 4 to 8
- Infection rate is increased in overcrowded situations
- Males and females are affected equally

Common characteristics

- Incubation period commonly lasting 2 to 4 days, may last 1 to 7 days
- High fever
- Pharyngitis
- Rash

Complications

- Severe disseminated toxic illness
- Septicemia
- Rheumatic heart disease
- Liver damage
- Otitis media
- Peritonsillar and retropharyngeal abscess
- Sinusitus
- Glomerulonephritis
- Meningitis
- Brain abscess

Assessment

History

- Possible contact with person with a sore throat
- Sore throat
- Headache
- Chills
- Anorexia
- Abdominal pain

- Malaise
- Likely high temperature (100° to 103° F [37.8° to 39.4° C])
- Characteristic rash 12 to 48 hours after onset of fever

Physical findings

- Inflamed and heavily coated tongue, progressing to strawberry-like tongue
- Tongue that peels and becomes beefy red, returning to normal by the end of the second week
- Red and edematous uvula, tonsils, and posterior oropharynx, with mucopurulent exudate
- Fine, erythematous rash, appears first on the upper chest and back, spreading to the neck, abdomen, legs, and arms
- Rash resembling sunburn with goose bumps; blanch-es with pressure
- Flushed face; circumoral pallor
- Tachycardia

Test results

Laboratory
- Pharyngeal culture is positive for group A beta-hemolytic streptococci.
- Complete blood count reveals increased white blood cell count and eosinophilia during the second week.

Treatment

General

- Increased fluid intake
- Rest periods when fatigued
- Appropriate skin care

Medication

- Antibiotics
- Antipyretics

Nursing considerations

Key outcomes

The patient will:
- have moist and pink mucous membranes without le-sions
- chew and swallow without discomfort
- have no signs or symptoms of infection
- express feelings of increased comfort or absence of pain at rest.

Nursing interventions

- Implement respiratory secretion precautions for 24 hours after starting antibiotic therapy.
- Offer frequent oral fluids and oral hygiene.
- Give prescribed drugs.
- Provide skin care to relieve discomfort from the rash.
- Provide warm liquids or cold foods to ease sore throat pain.

○ Use a cool mist humidifier to keep the air moist and prevent the throat from getting too dry and more sore.

Monitoring

○ Adverse drug reactions
○ Response to treatment
○ Complications
○ Body temperature
○ Rash
○ Nutritional status
○ Signs and symptoms of dehydration

Patient teaching

Be sure to cover:
○ the disorder, diagnosis, and treatment
○ the need to take oral antibiotics for the prescribed length of time to prevent serious complications
○ proper disposal of purulent discharge
○ follow-up care
○ when to notify the physician
○ drugs and possible adverse effects
○ prevention of scarlet fever and strep throat.

Schizophrenia

Overview

Description

- Disturbances in thought content and form, perception, affect, language, social activity, sense of self, volition, interpersonal relationships, and psychomotor behavior
- Five types recognized by the *DSM-IV-TR:* catatonic, paranoid, disorganized, residual, and undifferentiated
- Insidious onset and poor outcome
- Can progress to social withdrawal, perceptual distortions, chronic delusions, and hallucinations
- Up to one-third of patients having only one psychotic episode
- Some patients having no disability between periods of exacerbation; others needing continuous institutional care
- Worsening prognosis with each acute episode

Pathophysiology

- A biochemical hypothesis holds that schizophrenia results from excessive activity at dopaminergic synapses.
- Other neurotransmitter alterations may also contribute to schizophrenic symptoms.
- Structural abnormalities of the intraventricular system, temporal lobe abnormalities, decreased volume of the amygdala and hippocampus of the limbic system, structural changes in prefrontal white matter, and increased volume of the basal ganglia have been found.

Causes

- Exact cause unknown
- May result from a combination of genetic, biological, cultural, and psychological factors

Risk factors

- Familial history
- Gestational and birth complications
- Prenatal nutritional deficiencies

Incidence

- Affects about 0.85% of people worldwide, with a lifetime prevalence of 1% to 1.5%
- Close relatives of patients up to 50 times more likely to develop schizophrenia; the closer the degree of biological relatedness, the higher the risk
- Higher incidence among lower socioeconomic groups

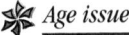 *Age issue*

The onset of schizophrenia usually occurs during late adolescence.

Common characteristics

- Change in emotional expression
- Inappropriate behavior
- Inaccurate interpretation of events
- Ineffective communication

Complications

- Suicide
- Impairment of health
- Impairment of social functioning

Assessment

History

- Possible long-standing psychiatric illness with repeated episodes
- Decreased social functioning

Physical findings

- Decreased emotional expression
- Impaired concentration

DSM-IV-TR criteria

Diagnosis depends on identifying two or more of the following signs and symptoms for a significant portion of time during a 1-month period (or only one symptom if delusions are bizarre, hallucinations consist of a voice issuing a running commentary, or hallucinations consist of two or more voices conversing with each other):

- delusions
- prominent hallucinations
- disorganized speech
- grossly disorganized or catatonic behavior
- negative symptoms (flat affect or inability to make decisions or speak).

In addition, one or more major areas of functioning (work, relationships, and self-care) are markedly below previous level, and the disturbance isn't due to a substance, medical condition, or schizoaffective or mood disorder.

Treatment

General

- Psychotherapy
- Social skills training
- Family therapy
- Vocational counseling

Medication

- Antipsychotic drugs (neuroleptic drugs)
- Antidepressants
- Anxiolytics

Nursing considerations

Key outcomes

The patient will:
- identify internal and external factors that trigger delusional episodes
- identify and perform activities that decrease delusions
- remain free from injury
- participate with his family in care and prescribed therapies
- demonstrate effective social interaction skills.

Nursing interventions

- Evaluate the patient's ability to carry out activities of daily living.
- Maintain a safe environment, minimizing stimuli.
- Give prescribed drugs.
- Adopt an accepting and consistent approach.
- Avoid promoting dependence.
- Reward positive behavior.
- Provide reality-based explanations for distorted body images or hypochondriacal complaints.
- Set limits on inappropriate behavior.
- Offer simple and matter-of-fact explanations about environmental safeguards, drugs, and policies.
- Build trust; be honest and dependable. Don't threaten, and don't promise what you can't fulfill.

Monitoring

- Suicidal ideation
- Homicidal ideation
- Effects of drug regimen
- Weight

Patient teaching

Be sure to cover:
- the disorder, diagnosis, and treatment
- drug administration, dosage, and possible adverse effects
- how family members can recognize an impending relapse, and ways to manage symptoms.

Discharge planning

- Refer the patient to appropriate community resources and support services.

Schistosomiasis

Overview

Description
○ A slowly progressive disease caused by blood flukes of the class *Trematoda*
○ Three major types: *Schistosoma mansoni* and *S. japonicum* that infect intestinal tract; *S. haematobium* that infects urinary tract (see *Types of schistosomes*)
○ Degree of infection determines intensity of illness
○ Also known as *bilharziasis*

Pathophysiology
○ Larvae penetrate the skin or mucous membranes and eventually work their way to the liver's venous portal circulation. They mature in 1 to 3 months and migrate to other parts of the body.
○ The female cercariae (the final larval stage) lay spiny eggs in blood vessels surrounding the large intestine or bladder.
○ After penetrating the mucosa of these organs, the eggs are excreted in feces or urine.
○ If the eggs hatch in fresh water, the first-stage larvae (miracidia) penetrate freshwater snails, which act as passive intermediate hosts. Cercariae produced in snails escape into water and begin a new life cycle.

Causes
○ Contamination with *Schistosoma* larvae transmitted by bathing, swimming, wading, or working in water

Types of schistosomes

Species and incidence	Signs and symptoms
Schistosoma mansoni Western hemisphere, particularly Puerto Rico, Lesser Antilles, Brazil, and Venezuela; also Nile delta, Sudan, and central Africa	Irregular fever, malaise, weakness, abdominal distress, weight loss, diarrhea, ascites, hepatosplenomegaly, portal hypertension, fistulas, and intestinal stricture
Schistosoma japonicum Affects men more than women; particularly prevalent among farmers in Japan, China, and the Philippines.	Irregular fever, malaise, weakness, abdominal distress, weight loss, diarrhea, ascites, hepatosplenomegaly, portal hypertension, fistulas, and intestinal stricture
Schistosoma haematobium Africa, Cyprus, Greece, India	Terminal hematuria, dysuria, uretal colic; with secondary infection — colicky pain, intermittent flank pain, vague GI complaints, and total renal failure

Incidence
○ Not common in the United States
○ Most prevalent in children and adolescents

Common characteristics
○ Initially, a transient, pruritic rash at the site of cercariae penetration, along with fever, myalgia, and cough
○ Later, hepatomegaly, splenomegaly, and lymphadenopathy

Complications
○ Portal hypertension
○ Pulmonary hypertension
○ Heart failure
○ Ascites
○ Hematemesis from ruptured esophageal varices
○ Renal failure
○ Flaccid paralysis
○ Seizures
○ Skin abscesses

Assessment

History
○ Recent travel to endemic areas
○ Fever
○ Myalgia
○ Cough

Physical findings
○ Rash at site of contamination
○ Hepatomegaly
○ Splenomegaly
○ Lymphadenopathy

Test results
Laboratory
○ Ova appear in the urine or stool.
○ White blood cell count shows eosinophilia.
Diagnostic procedures
○ Mucosal lesion biopsy confirms infection.

Treatment

General
○ Supportive
○ Fluid replacement
○ Diet as tolerated
○ Activity as tolerated

Medication
○ Praziquantel

Nursing considerations

Key outcomes

The patient will:
- remain hemodynamically stable
- avoid complications
- express an understanding of the disorder and treatment.

Nursing interventions

- Encourage fluid intake.
- Provide support.
- Encourage activity.

Monitoring

- Vital signs
- Comfort level
- Response to treatment

Patient teaching

Be sure to cover:
- the disorder, diagnosis, and treatment
- avoiding possibly contaminated water or, if the patient must enter the water, the need to wear protective clothing and dry off thoroughly once leaving the water. (See *Schistosomal dermatitis*.)

Discharge planning

- Before discharge, tell the patient to schedule a follow-up visit between 3 and 6 months after treatment. (If this checkup reveals any living eggs, treatment may be resumed.)

Schistosomal dermatitis

Schistosomal dermatitis, also known as *swimmer's itch* or *clam digger's itch,* affects those who bathe in and camp along freshwater lakes in the eastern and western United States. It's caused by schistosomal cercariae that are harbored by migratory birds and penetrate the skin, causing a pruritis papular rash. Initially mild, the reaction grows more severe with repeated exposure. Treatment consists of 5% copper sulfate solution as an antipruritic and 2% methylene blue as an antibacterial agent.

Scleroderma

Overview

Description

- Connective tissue disease characterized by inflammatory, degenerative, and fibrotic changes in skin, blood vessels, synovial membranes, skeletal muscles, and internal organs; thickening of tissues
- May affect the visceral organs or remain localized to the skin when the connective tissues of many organs, including the heart, kidney, GI tract, and lungs, are involved
- Cutaneous lesions usually on the face, hands, neck, and upper chest
- Also known as *systemic sclerosis*

Pathophysiology

- The skin atrophies, and infiltrates containing CD4+ T cells surround the blood vessels; inflamed collagen fibers become edematous, losing strength and elasticity.
- The dermis becomes tightly bound to the underlying structures, resulting in atrophy of the affected dermal appendages and destruction of the distal phalanges by osteoporosis.
- As the disease progresses, atrophy can affect other areas.

Causes

- Unknown
- Possible causes:
  - Systemic exposure to silica dust, polyvinyl chloride, or organic solvents
  - Anticancer agents such as bleomycin or nonopioid analgesics such as pentazocine
  - Fibrosis due to an abnormal immune system response
  - Underlying vascular cause with tissue changes initiated by inconsistent perfusion
  - Asymptomatic or common viral infections

Incidence

- Rarely occurs in children or men younger than age 35
- Affects women three to four times more often than men, especially between ages 30 and 50
- Peak incidence from ages 50 to 60

Common characteristics

- Skin thickening in face and fingers

Complications

- Related to thickening of tissues:
  - Slowly healing ulcerations on fingertips or toes leading to gangrene
  - Decreased food intake and weight loss due to GI symptoms
  - Arrhythmias and dyspnea
  - Malignant hypertension
  - Respiratory failure
  - Renal failure
  - Esophageal or intestinal obstruction or perforation
- Raynaud's phenomenon
- Pulmonary fibrosis

Assessment

History

- Pain, stiffness, and swelling of fingers and joints (later symptoms)
- Frequent reflux, heartburn, dysphagia, and bloating after meals due to GI dysfunction
- Diarrhea, constipation, and malodorous floating stool

Physical findings

- Skin thickening, commonly limited to the distal extremities and face, but possibly involving internal organs
- CREST syndrome (a benign subtype of limited systemic sclerosis): calcinosis, Raynaud's phenomenon, esophageal dysfunction, sclerodactyly, and telangiectasia
- Patchy skin changes with a teardrop-like appearance known as *morphea* (localized scleroderma)
- Band of thickened skin on the face or extremities that severely damages underlying tissues, causing atrophy and deformity (linear scleroderma)
- Raynaud's phenomenon (blanching, cyanosis, and erythema of the fingers and toes); progressive phalangeal resorption that may shorten the fingers (early symptoms)
- Taut, shiny skin over the entire hand and forearm due to skin thickening
- Tight and inelastic facial skin, causing a masklike appearance and "pinching" of the mouth
- Thickened skin over proximal limbs and trunk (diffuse systemic sclerosis)
- Abdominal distention

Test results

Laboratory
- Erythrocyte sedimentation rate is slightly elevated, rheumatoid factor is positive in 25% to 35% of patients, and antinuclear antibody is positive.
- Urinalysis shows proteinuria, microscopic hematuria, and casts.

Imaging
- Hand X-rays show terminal phalangeal tuft resorption, subcutaneous calcification, and joint space narrowing and erosion.
- Chest X-rays show bilateral basilar pulmonary fibrosis.
- GI X-rays show distal esophageal hypomotility and stricture, duodenal loop dilation, small-bowel malabsorption pattern, and large diverticula.

Diagnostic procedures

○ Pulmonary function studies show decreased diffusion and vital capacity.
○ Electrocardiogram shows nonspecific abnormalities related to myocardial fibrosis and possible arrhythmias.
○ Skin biopsy shows changes consistent with disease progression, such as marked thickening of the dermis and occlusive vessel changes.

Treatment

General

○ Physical therapy
○ Heat therapy
○ Hemodialysis
○ Lanolin emollients
○ Soft, bland foods
○ Possible enteral feedings
○ Regular exercise, as tolerated
○ Frequent rest periods

Medication

○ Immunosuppressants
○ Vasodilators
○ Antihypertensives
○ Antacids
○ Histamine-2 receptor antagonist or proton pump inhibitor
○ Broad-spectrum antibiotics
○ Angiotensin-converting enzyme inhibitor

Surgery

○ Digital sympathectomy or, rarely, cervical sympathetic blockade
○ Digital plaster cast
○ Possible surgical debridement
○ Renal transplant

Nursing considerations

Key outcomes

The patient will:
○ express feelings of increased comfort and decreased pain
○ attain the highest degree of mobility possible within the confines of disease
○ state feelings about limitations
○ express an increased sense of well-being
○ regain and maintain skin integrity.

Nursing interventions

○ Avoid using fingersticks for blood tests.
○ Provide heat therapy to relieve joint stiffness.
○ Elevate the head of the bed to help relieve GI symptoms.
○ Provide meticulous skin care.
○ Encourage oral fluid intake.
○ Provide a soft, bland diet with frequent small meals.

○ Administer oxygen, as ordered, for pulmonary complications.

Monitoring

○ Intake and output
○ Possible adverse reactions to prescribed drugs
○ Daily weight
○ End organ damage such as renal failure
○ Skin integrity
○ Nutritional status
○ Vital signs, especially blood pressure
○ Renal function
○ Electrocardiograms
○ Pulmonary function
○ Abdominal distention

Patient teaching

Be sure to cover:
○ the disorder, diagnosis, and treatment
○ how to assess skin for changes
○ avoiding cold weather and cigarette smoking
○ reporting abnormal bleeding or bruising and any nonhealing abrasions
○ the importance of staying as active as possible, with frequent rest periods
○ follow-up care.

Discharge planning

○ Refer the patient to physical therapy and occupational therapy as needed.
○ Refer the patient to a smoking-cessation program, if needed.
○ Refer the patient to the Scleroderma Foundation.

Scoliosis

Overview

Description

- Lateral curvature of the spine that's apparent on frontal projection, measures greater than 10 degrees, and is associated with vertebral rotation
- Right thoracic curve most common
- Classified as nonstructural (flexible spinal curve, with temporary straightening when patient leans sideways) or structural (fixed deformity)

Pathophysiology

- The vertebrae rotate, forming the convex part of the curve.
- The rotation causes rib prominence along the thoracic spine and waistline asymmetry in the lumbar spine.
- Severity of spinal deformity dictates physiological impairment.

Causes

- Nonstructural scoliosis:
  - Leg-length discrepancies
  - Poor posture
  - Paraspinal inflammation
  - Acute disk disease
- Structural scoliosis: no known cause
- Neuromuscular scoliosis: may be caused by muscular dystrophy, polio, cerebral palsy, or spinal muscular atrophy
- Neurofibromatosis (Recklinghausen's disease)
- Traumatic scoliosis: may result from vertebral fractures or disk disease
- Local inflammation and infection

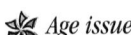 *Age issue*

Degenerative scoliosis may develop in older patients with osteoporosis and degenerative joint disease of the spine.

Risk factors

- Congenital or neuromuscular problem

Incidence

- Idiopathic
- Less than 1% of school-age children affected
- Seen at growth spurts between ages 10 and 13
- Affects females 7 times more than males
- Infantile scoliosis: most common in boys ages 1 to 3
- Juvenile scoliosis: affects boys and girls ages 3 to 10 about equally
- Adolescent scoliosis: occurs after age 10 and during adolescence

Common characteristics

- Fatigue
- Backache
- Dyspnea
- Change in appearance
- Kyphosis

Complications

- Debilitating back pain
- Severe deformity
- With thoracic curve exceeding 60 degrees, possible reduced pulmonary function
- With thoracic curve exceeding 80 degrees, increased risk of cor pulmonale in middle age

Assessment

History

- Familial history
- Detected during community or school scoliosis screening
- Hemlines look uneven
- Pant legs appear unequal in length
- One hip higher than the other
- Backache, fatigue, and dyspnea

Physical findings

- Signs of scoliosis (see *Testing for scoliosis*)

Test results

Imaging
- Spinal X-ray studies confirm scoliosis and determine the degree of curvature and flexibility of the spine; they also determine skeletal maturity, predict remaining bone growth, and differentiate nonstructural from structural scoliosis.

Other
- Bone growth studies may help determine skeletal maturity.

Treatment

General

- Close observation
- Brace
- Spinal orthoses
- Functional strengthening program
- Gradually increased activity
- No vigorous sports
- Prescribed exercise regimen
- Swimming, but no diving

Surgery

- Posterior spinal fusion and internal stabilization (rods and spinal hardware)

Testing for scoliosis

When assessing the patient for an abnormal spinal curve, use this screening test for scoliosis. Have the patient remove her shirt and stand as straight as she can with her back to you. Instruct her to distribute her weight evenly on each foot. While the patient does this, observe both sides of her back from neck to buttocks. Look for these signs:

- uneven shoulder height and shoulder blade prominence
- unequal distance between the arms and the body
- asymmetrical waistline
- uneven hip height
- a sideways lean.

With the patient's back still facing you, ask the patient to do the "forward-bend" test. In this test, the patient places her palms together and slowly bends forward, remembering to keep her head down. As she complies, check for these signs:

- asymmetrical thoracic spine or prominent rib cage (rib hump) on either side
- asymmetrical waistline.

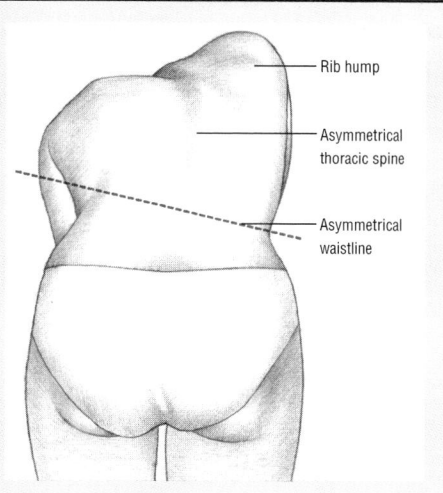

Rib hump

Asymmetrical thoracic spine

Asymmetrical waistline

Nursing considerations

Key outcomes

The patient will:
- experience feelings of increased comfort and decreased pain
- maintain joint mobility and range of motion (ROM)
- achieve the highest level of mobility possible
- express positive feelings about self
- demonstrate measures to prevent injury to self.

Nursing interventions

- Promote self-care while allowing adequate time.
- Give prescribed drugs.
- Encourage deep-breathing exercises.
- Promote active ROM arm exercises.

Monitoring

- Response to analgesia
- Skin around the cast edge daily
- Sensation, movement, color, and pulses
- Intake and output
- Urine specific gravity
- Abdominal distention and bowel sounds
- Skin breakdown

 Alert

Watch for signs of cast syndrome (nausea, abdominal pressure, and vague abdominal pain), which may result from hyperextension of the spine.

Patient teaching

Be sure to cover:
- the disorder, diagnosis, and treatment
- brace care
- skin care
- safe body mechanics
- cast care, if needed
- the signs of cast syndrome
- the prescribed drug regimen
- adverse drug reactions
- relaxation techniques.

Septic arthritis

Overview

Description

- Inflammation of a synovial membrane
- Usually caused by bacteria
- Usually affects a single joint
- May have sudden onset
- Also known as *infectious arthritis*

Pathophysiology

- Bacteria invade a joint, and inflammation of the synovial lining results.
- Organisms invade the joint cavity, and effusion and pyogenesis follow.
- Eventual bone and cartilage destruction result.

Causes

- Bacteria spread from a primary site of infection
- Gram-positive cocci
- *Staphylococcus aureus*
- *Streptococcus pyogenes*
- *Streptococcus pneumoniae*
- *Streptococcus viridans*
- Gram-negative cocci
- *Neisseria gonorrhoeae*
- *Haemophilus influenzae*
- Gram-negative bacilli
- *Escherichia coli*
- Salmonella
- Pseudomonas
- Fungi or mycobacteria (rare cause)

Risk factors

- Concurrent bacterial infection
- Serious chronic illness
- Alcoholism
- Advanced age
- Immune system depression
- History of immunosuppressive therapy
- I.V. drug abuse
- Recent articular trauma
- Arthroscopy and joint surgery
- Intra-articular injections
- Local joint abnormalities

Incidence

- Gram-positive cocci more common in children age 2 and older and adults
- *H. influenzae* most common in children younger than age 2

Common characteristics

- Joint inflammation
- Severe pain
- Pseudoparalysis of affected area
- Warmth and erythema of affected area

Complications

- Osteomyelitis
- Loss of joint cartilage
- Ankylosis
- Fatal septicemia

Assessment

History

- Abrupt onset of intense pain in the affected joint
- Fever and chills

Physical findings

- Affected joint kept in a flexed position
- Redness and edema over the affected joint
- Severely reduced range of motion (ROM)
- Warmth and extreme tenderness over the involved joint
- Chills

Test results

Laboratory

- Synovial fluid analysis shows pus or watery, cloudy fluid of decreased viscosity, typically with 50,000/µl or more white blood cells (WBCs) containing primarily neutrophils; also a low glucose level.
- Gram stain or culture of the fluid identifies the causative organism.
- Countercurrent immunoelectrophoresis measures bacterial antigens in body fluids and guides treatment.
- Positive blood cultures confirm the diagnosis even with negative synovial culture.
- WBC count is elevated with many polymorphonuclear cells.
- Erythrocyte sedimentation rate is increased.
- C-reactive protein level is elevated.
- Lactic assay distinguishes septic from nonseptic arthritis.

Imaging

- X-rays may show distention of the joint capsule, narrowing of the joint space, and erosion of bone.
- Radioisotope joint scan may show infection or inflammation, especially in less accessible joints.

Diagnostic procedures

- Arthrocentesis allows collection of a synovial fluid specimen for analysis.
- Biopsy of the synovial membrane confirms the diagnosis and identifies the causative organism.

Treatment

General

- Based on antimicrobial susceptibilities and the patient's age
- Drainage by repeated closed-needle aspiration, arthroscopy, or arthrotomy
- Exercise, as tolerated
- Joint immobilization

Medication

○ Analgesics
○ Parenteral antibiotic

Surgery

○ Reconstructive surgery for severe joint damage
○ Possible open surgical drainage

Nursing considerations

Key outcomes

The patient will:
○ express feelings of increased comfort and decreased pain
○ maintain joint mobility and ROM
○ perform activities of daily living within confines of the disorder.

Nursing interventions

○ Practice strict sterile technique.
○ Check splints or traction regularly.
○ Maintain proper alignment.
○ Assist with ROM exercises.
○ Give prescribed drugs for pain.
○ Allow adequate time for and promote self-care.

Monitoring

○ Signs and symptoms of joint inflammation
○ Vital signs and fever pattern
○ Pain levels
○ Response to pain medications
○ Condition after joint aspiration

Patient teaching

Be sure to cover:
○ the disorder, diagnosis, and treatment
○ the etiology of the disease
○ the role of I.V. drug use
○ the prevention of recurrence
○ prescribed drugs
○ adverse drug reactions
○ the exercise regimen
○ rest periods
○ home I.V. therapy, if required
○ avoiding aggravating factors.

Discharge planning

○ Refer the patient to drug counseling, if appropriate.
○ Refer the patient to Alcoholics Anonymous, if appropriate.

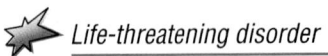

Severe acute respiratory syndrome

Overview

Description

- Severe viral infection that may progress to pneumonia
- Believed to be less infectious than influenza
- Incubation period estimated to range from 2 to 7 days (average, 3 to 5 days)
- Not highly contagious when protective measures are used
- Also known as *SARS*

Pathophysiology

- Coronaviruses cause diseases in pigs, birds, and other animals.
- A theory suggests that a coronavirus may have mutated, allowing transmission to and infection of humans.

Causes

- A new type of coronavirus known as *SARS-associated coronavirus* (SARS-CoV)

Risk factors

- Close contact with an infected person
- Contact with aerosolized (exhaled) droplets and bodily secretions from an infected person
- Travel to endemic areas

Incidence

- More common in adults than children
- Outbreaks in China, Hong Kong, Toronto, Singapore, Taiwan, and Vietnam, with many other countries reporting smaller numbers of cases
- Affects all races
- Affects both sexes equally

Common characteristics

- Fever greater than 100.4° F (38° C)
- Dry cough
- Shortness of breath or other respiratory difficulties
- Headache
- Muscular stiffness
- Loss of appetite
- Malaise
- Confusion
- Rash
- Diarrhea
- Sore throat

Complications

- Respiratory difficulties
- Severe thrombocytopenia (low platelet count)
- Death

Assessment

History

- Contact with a person known to have SARS
- Travel to an endemic area

Physical findings

- Non-productive cough
- Rash
- High fever
- Diarrhea
- Respiratory distress in later stages

Test results

Laboratory
- Antibodies to coronavirus are detected.
- Sputum Gram's stain and culture isolates coronavirus.
- Platelet count may be low.

Imaging
- Changes in chest X-rays indicate pneumonia (infiltrates).

Diagnostic procedures
- SARS-specific polymerase chain reaction test detects SARS-CoV RNA.
- Antibody testing via enzyme-linked immunosorbent assay and the immunofluorescent antibody test is in development.

Treatment

General

- Symptomatic treatment
- Isolation for hospitalized patients
- Strict respiratory and mucosal barrier precautions
- Quarantine of exposed people to prevent spread
- Diet as tolerated
- Activity as tolerated
- Global surveillance and reporting of suspected cases to national health authorities

Medication

- Antivirals
- Combination of steroids and antimicrobials

Nursing considerations

Key outcomes

The patient will:
- remain in isolation as recommended
- practice good hygiene to prevent further transmission
- maintain good nutritional status
- maintain a patent airway.

Nursing interventions

○ Give prescribed drugs.
○ Encourage adequate nutritional intake.
○ Observe, record, and report nature of rash.
○ Maintain proper isolation technique.
○ Collect laboratory specimens, as needed.

Monitoring

○ Vital signs
○ Nutritional status
○ Respiratory status
○ Complications

Patient teaching

Be sure to cover:
○ the importance of frequent hand-washing
○ covering mouth and nose when coughing or sneezing
○ avoiding close personal contact with friends and family.
○ the importance of not going to work, school, or other public places until 10 days after fever and respiratory symptoms resolve
○ wearing a surgical mask when around other people or, if the patient can't wear one, mask wearing by those in contact with the patient
○ not sharing silverware, towels, or bedding until they have been washed in soap and hot water
○ using disposable gloves and household disinfectant to clean any surface that might have been exposed to the patient's body fluids.

Discharge planning

○ Refer the patient for follow-up, as needed.

Severe combined immunodeficiency disease

Overview

Description

○ Disorder that involves deficient or absent cell-mediated (T-cell) and humoral (B-cell) immunity
○ Predisposes patient to infection from all classes of microorganisms during infancy
○ Also known as *SCID* and *graft-versus-host disease*

Pathophysiology

○ Three types of SCID have been identified:
  – Reticular dysgenesis, the most severe type, in which the hematopoietic stem cell fails to differentiate into lymphocytes and granulocytes
  – Swiss-type agammaglobulinemia, in which the hematopoietic stem cell fails to differentiate into lymphocytes alone
  – Enzyme deficiency, such as adenosine deaminase deficiency, in which the buildup of toxic products in the lymphoid tissue causes damage and subsequent dysfunction.

Causes

○ Transmitted as autosomal recessive trait but may be X-linked
○ Possible enzyme deficiency
○ Failure of thymus or bursa equivalent to develop normally or possible defect in thymus and bone marrow (responsible for T- and B-cell development)

Incidence

○ Affects more males than females
○ Occurs in 1 of every 100,000 to 500,000 births

Common characteristics

○ Frequent infections in the first few months after birth

Complications

○ Without treatment, infection within 1 year of birth causes death
○ Pneumonia
○ Oral ulcers
○ Failure to thrive
○ Dermatitis

Assessment

History

○ Extreme susceptibility to infection within the first few months after birth, but probably no sign of gram-negative infection until about age 6 months because of protection by maternal immunoglobulin G

Physical findings

○ Emaciated appearance and failure to thrive
○ Assessment findings dependant on the type and site of infection
○ Signs of chronic otitis media and sepsis
○ Signs of the usual childhood diseases such as chickenpox

Test results

○ Defective humoral immunity is difficult to detect before an infant reaches age 5 months.
Laboratory
○ Tests show a severely diminished or absent T-cell number and function.
Imaging
○ A chest X-ray characteristically shows bilateral pulmonary infiltrates.
Diagnostic procedures
○ Lymph node biopsy that shows an absence of lymphocytes can be used to confirm diagnosis.

Treatment

General

○ Strict protective isolation (germ-free environment)
○ Gene therapy (experimental)

Medication

○ Immunoglobulin
○ Antibiotic therapy

Surgery

○ Histocompatible bone marrow transplantation
○ Fetal thymus and liver transplantation

Nursing considerations

Key outcomes

The patient will:
○ demonstrate age-appropriate skills and behaviors
○ not experience chills, fever, and other signs of illness.
The parents will:
○ establish eye, physical, and verbal contact with the infant or child
○ develop adequate coping mechanisms and support systems.

Nursing interventions

○ If infection develops, provide prompt and aggressive drug therapy and supportive care, as ordered.
○ Watch for adverse effects of any drugs given.
○ Avoid vaccinations, and give only irradiated blood products if a transfusion is ordered.

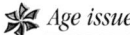 *Age issue*

Although SCID infants must remain in strict protective isolation, try to provide a stimulating atmosphere to promote growth and development.

○ Encourage parents to visit their child often, to hold him, and to bring him toys that can be easily sterilized.
○ Maintain a normal day and night routine, and talk to the child as much as possible.
○ If parents can't visit, call them often to report on the infant's condition.
○ Provide emotional support for the family.

Monitoring

○ Signs and symptoms of infection
○ Growth and development
○ Skin integrity
○ Respiratory status
○ Response to treatment
○ Complications
○ Signs and symptoms of transplant rejection
○ Social interaction

Patient teaching

Be sure to cover:
○ the disorder, diagnosis, and treatment
○ the proper technique for strict protective isolation
○ the signs and symptoms of infection and the need to notify a physician promptly
○ drug administration, dosage, purpose, and adverse effects.

Discharge planning

○ Encourage the parents to seek genetic counseling.

Shigellosis

Overview

Description

- An acute intestinal infection caused by the bacteria *Shigella*, a short, nonmotile, gram-negative rod
- Can be classified into four groups:
  - Group A, which is caused by *S. dysenteriae,* is most common in Central America, and causes particularly severe infection and septicemia
  - Group B, which is caused by *S. flexneri* and, together with Group D, is responsible for 90% of shigellosis cases
  - Group C, which is caused by *S. boydii* and occurs internationally
  - Group D, which is caused by *S. sonnei*
- Also known as *bacillary dysentery*

Pathophysiology

- Highly contagious aerobic, nonmotile, glucose-fermenting, gram-negative rods cause diarrhea after ingestion of as few as 180 organisms.
- Rods invade the colonic epithelium and produce enterotoxin, which enhances virulence.

Causes

- Transmission of *Shigella* bacteria through the fecal-oral route, by direct contact with contaminated objects, or through ingestion of contaminated food or water
- Occasional transmission by housefly vector

Incidence

- Most common in children ages 1 to 4; many adults acquire illness from children
- Endemic in North America, Europe, and the tropics; in the United States, about 23,000 cases annually, usually in children or elderly, debilitated, or malnourished people
- Commonly occurs among confined populations such as those in mental institutions; also common in hospitals

Common characteristics

- High fever (especially in children)
- Acute self-limiting diarrhea with tenesmus (ineffectual straining at stool)
- Electrolyte imbalance and dehydration

Complications

- Electrolyte imbalance (especially hypokalemia)
- Metabolic acidosis
- Shock

Assessment

History

- Crowded living conditions
- Close contact with someone who has acute diarrhea
- Fever
- Diarrhea
- Tenesmus

Physical findings

- Pus in stools
- Signs of dehydration
- Decreased blood pressure
- Hyperactive bowel sounds
- Abdominal tenderness
- Abdominal distention
- Rapid, thready pulse

Test results

Laboratory

- Microscopic examination of stools reveals mucus, red blood cells, and polymorphonuclear leukocytes.
- Direct immunofluorescence with specific antisera may reveal *Shigella.*

Diagnostic procedures

- Sigmoidoscopy or proctoscopy may reveal typical superficial ulcerations.

Treatment

General

- Enteric precautions
- Low-residue diet
- Replacement of fluids and electrolytes with I.V. infusions of normal saline solution (with electrolytes)

Medication

- Antibiotics (questionable value, but may be used)

 Alert

Antidiarrheals that slow intestinal motility are contraindicated in shigellosis because they delay fecal excretion of Shigella and prolong fever and diarrhea.

 Alert

A vaccine to help prevent shigellosis is currently under development.

Nursing considerations

Key outcomes

The patient will:
○ maintain hemodynamic stability
○ regain and maintain normal fluid and electrolyte balance
○ experience no further weight loss.

Nursing interventions

○ Give prescribed I.V. fluids.
○ Maintain enteric precautions until microscopic bacteriologic studies confirm that the stool specimen is negative.

Monitoring

○ Vital signs
○ Comfort level
○ Intake and output

Patient teaching

Be sure to cover:
○ the disorder, diagnosis, and treatment
○ prevention of infecting others.

⭐ *Life-threatening disorder*

Shock, cardiogenic

Overview

Description

○ A condition of diminished cardiac output that severely impairs tissue perfusion
○ The most lethal form of shock
○ Sometimes called *pump failure*

Pathophysiology

○ Left ventricular dysfunction initiates a series of compensatory mechanisms that attempt to increase cardiac output.
○ As cardiac output decreases, aortic and carotid baroreceptors activate sympathetic nervous responses.
○ Responses increase heart rate, left ventricular filling pressure, and peripheral resistance to flow to enhance venous return to the heart.
○ This action initially stabilizes the patient but later causes deterioration with increasing oxygen demands on the already compromised myocardium.
○ These events consist of a cycle of low cardiac output, sympathetic compensation, myocardial ischemia, and even lower cardiac output.

Causes

○ Myocardial infarction (MI) (most common)
○ Myocardial ischemia
○ Papillary muscle dysfunction
○ End-stage cardiomyopathy
○ Myocarditis
○ Acute mitral or aortic insufficiency
○ Ventricular septal defect
○ Ventricular aneurysm

Incidence

○ Typically affects patients in whom area of MI involves 40% or more of left ventricular muscle mass (a group in which mortality may exceed 85%.)

Common characteristics

○ Previous disorder that decreases left ventricular function

Complications

○ Multiple organ dysfunction
○ Death

Assessment

History

○ Disorder, such as MI or cardiomyopathy, that severely decreases left ventricular function
○ Anginal pain

Physical findings

○ Urine output less than 20 ml/hour
○ Pale, cold, clammy skin
○ Decreased sensorium
○ Rapid, shallow respirations
○ Rapid, thready pulse
○ Mean arterial pressure of less than 60 mm Hg in adults
○ Gallop rhythm, faint heart sounds and, possibly, a holosystolic murmur
○ Jugular vein distention
○ Severe anxiety
○ Decreased level of consciousness (LOC)
○ Pulmonary crackles

Test results

Laboratory
○ Serum enzyme measurements show elevated levels of creatine kinase, lactate dehydrogenase, aspartate aminotransferase, and alanine aminotransferase.
○ Troponin levels are elevated.
Imaging
○ Cardiac catheterization and echocardiography may reveal other conditions that can lead to pump dysfunction and failure, such as cardiac tamponade, papillary muscle infarct or rupture, ventricular septal rupture, pulmonary emboli, venous pooling, and hypovolemia.
Diagnostic procedures
○ Pulmonary artery pressure monitoring reveals increased pulmonary artery pressure and pulmonary artery wedge pressure, reflecting an increase in left ventricular end-diastolic pressure (preload) and heightened resistance to left ventricular emptying (afterload) caused by ineffective pumping and increased peripheral vascular resistance.
○ Invasive arterial pressure monitoring shows systolic arterial pressure less than 80 mm Hg caused by impaired ventricular ejection.
○ Arterial blood gas (ABG) analysis may show metabolic and respiratory acidosis and hypoxia.
○ Electrocardiography demonstrates possible evidence of acute MI, ischemia, or ventricular aneurysm.

Treatment

General

○ Intra-aortic balloon pump (IABP)
○ Possible parenteral nutrition or tube feedings
○ Bed rest

Medication

○ Vasopressors
○ Inotropics
○ Vasoconstrictors
○ Analgesics; sedatives
○ Osmotic diuretics
○ Vasodilators
○ Oxygen

Surgery

○ Possible ventricular assist device
○ Possible heart transplant

Nursing considerations

Key outcomes

The patient will:
○ maintain adequate cardiac output and hemodynamic stability
○ develop no complications of fluid volume excess
○ maintain adequate ventilation
○ express feelings and develop adequate coping mechanisms.

Nursing interventions

○ Administer oxygen therapy.
○ Follow IABP protocols and policies.

 Alert

When a patient is on an IABP, move him as little as possible. Never place the patient in a sitting position higher than 45 degrees (including for chest X-rays) because the balloon may tear through the aorta and cause immediate death. Assess pedal pulses and skin temperature and color. Check the dressing on the insertion site frequently for bleeding, and change it according to facility protocol. Also check the site for hematoma or signs of infection, and culture any drainage.

○ Monitor the patient for cardiac arrhythmias.
○ Plan your care to allow frequent rest periods, and provide as much privacy as possible. Allow the patient's family to visit and comfort him as much as possible.
○ Provide explanations and reassurance for the patient and his family as appropriate.
○ Prepare the patient and his family for a possibly fatal outcome, and help them find effective coping strategies.

Monitoring

○ ABG levels (acid-base balance) and pulse oximetry
○ Complete blood count and electrolyte levels
○ Vital signs and peripheral pulses
○ Cardiac status
○ Hemodynamics
○ Intake and output

○ Respiratory status
○ LOC

Patient teaching

Be sure to cover:
○ the disorder, diagnosis, and treatment
○ explanations and reassurance for patient and his family
○ the possibly fatal outcome.

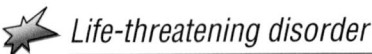 *Life-threatening disorder*

Shock, hypovolemic

Overview

Description

○ Reduced intravascular blood volume causing circulatory dysfunction and inadequate tissue perfusion resulting from loss of blood, plasma, or fluids
○ Potentially life-threatening

Pathophysiology

○ When fluid is lost from the intravascular space, venous return to the heart is reduced.
○ This decreases ventricular filling, which leads to a drop in stroke volume.
○ Cardiac output falls, causing reduced perfusion to tissues and organs.
○ Tissue anoxia prompts a shift in cellular metabolism from aerobic to anaerobic pathways.
○ This produces an accumulation of lactic acid, resulting in metabolic acidosis.

Causes

○ Acute blood loss (about one-fifth of total volume)
○ Intestinal obstruction
○ Burns
○ Peritonitis
○ Acute pancreatitis
○ Ascites
○ Dehydration, as from excessive perspiration, severe diarrhea, protracted vomiting, diabetes insipidus, diuresis, or inadequate fluid intake
○ Diuretic abuse

Checking for early hypovolemic shock

Orthostatic vital signs and tilt test results can help in assessing for the possibility of impending hypovolemic shock.
Orthostatic vital signs
Measure the patient's blood pressure and pulse rate while he's lying in a supine position, sitting, and standing. Wait at least 1 minute between each position change. A systolic blood pressure decrease of 10 mm Hg or more between positions or a pulse rate increase of 10 beats/minute or more is a sign of volume depletion and impending hypovolemic shock.
Tilt test
With the patient lying in a supine position, raise his legs above heart level. If his blood pressure increases significantly, the test is positive, indicating volume depletion and impending hypovolemic shock.

Incidence

○ Depends on cause
○ Affects all ages
○ More frequent and less tolerated in elderly patients
○ Affects males and females equally

Common characteristics

○ Pallor, tachycardia, hypotension
○ Cool skin
○ Altered level of consciousness

Complications

○ Acute respiratory distress syndrome
○ Acute tubular necrosis and renal failure
○ Disseminated intravascular coagulation
○ Multiple organ dysfunction

Assessment

History

○ Disorders or conditions that reduce blood volume, such as GI hemorrhage, trauma, and severe diarrhea and vomiting
○ Patient with cardiac disease: possible anginal pain because of decreased myocardial perfusion and oxygenation

Physical findings

○ Pale, cool, clammy skin
○ Decreased sensorium
○ Rapid, shallow respirations
○ Urine output usually less than 20 ml/hour
○ Rapid, thready pulse
○ Mean arterial pressure less than 60 mm Hg in adults (in chronic hypotension, mean pressure may fall below 50 mm Hg before signs of shock)
○ Orthostatic vital signs and tilt test results consistent with hypovolemic shock (see *Checking for early hypovolemic shock*)

Test results

Laboratory
○ Hematocrit is low, and hemoglobin levels and red blood cell and platelet counts are decreased.
○ Serum potassium, sodium, lactate dehydrogenase, creatinine, and blood urea nitrogen levels are elevated.
○ Urine specific gravity (greater than 1.020) and urine osmolality are increased.
○ The pH and partial pressure of arterial oxygen are decreased, and partial pressure of arterial carbon dioxide is increased.
○ Aspiration of gastric contents through a nasogastric tube identifies internal bleeding.
○ Occult blood tests are positive.
○ Coagulation studies show coagulopathy from disseminated intravascular coagulation.

Imaging
○ X-rays (chest or abdominal) help to identify internal bleeding sites.

Diagnostic procedures
○ Gastroscopy helps to identify internal bleeding sites.
○ Invasive hemodynamic monitoring shows reduced central venous pressure, right atrial pressure, pulmonary artery pressure, pulmonary artery wedge pressure, and cardiac output.

Treatment

General

○ In severe cases, an intra-aortic balloon pump, ventricular assist device, or pneumatic antishock garment
○ Oxygen administration
○ Bleeding control by direct application of pressure and related measures
○ Possible parenteral nutrition or tube feedings
○ Bed rest

Medication

○ Prompt and vigorous blood and fluid replacement
○ Positive inotropes
○ Possibly diuretics

Surgery

○ Possibly, to correct underlying problem

Nursing considerations

Key outcomes

The patient will:
○ maintain adequate cardiac output
○ maintain hemodynamic stability
○ maintain adequate ventilation
○ express feelings and develop adequate coping mechanisms
○ regain adequate fluid volume.

Nursing interventions

○ Check for a patent airway and adequate circulation. If blood pressure and heart rate are absent, start cardiopulmonary resuscitation.
○ Obtain type and crossmatch, as ordered.
○ Give prescribed I.V. solutions or blood products.
○ Insert an indwelling urinary catheter.
○ Give prescribed oxygen.
○ Provide emotional support to the patient and family.

Monitoring

○ Vital signs and peripheral pulses
○ Cardiac rhythm
○ Coagulation studies for signs of impending coagulopathy
○ Complete blood count and electrolyte measurements
○ Arterial blood gas levels

○ Intake and output
○ Hemodynamics

Patient teaching

Be sure to cover:
○ the disorder, diagnosis, and treatment
○ all procedures and their purpose
○ the risks associated with blood transfusions
○ the purpose of all equipment such as mechanical ventilation
○ dietary restrictions
○ drugs and possible adverse effects.

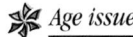
Shock, septic

Overview

Description

○ Low systemic vascular resistance and an elevated cardiac output
○ Probably a response to infections that release microbes or an immune mediator

Pathophysiology

○ Initially, the body's defenses activate chemical mediators in response to the invading organisms.
○ The release of these mediators results in low systemic vascular resistance and increased cardiac output.
○ Blood flow is unevenly distributed in the microcirculation, and plasma leaking from capillaries causes functional hypovolemia.
○ Diffuse increase in capillary permeability occurs.
○ Eventually, cardiac output decreases, and poor tissue perfusion and hypotension cause multisystem dysfunction syndrome and death.

Causes

○ Any pathogenic organism
○ Gram-negative bacteria, such as *Escherichia coli, Klebsiella pneumoniae, Serratia, Enterobacter,* and *Pseudomonas,* most common causes (up to 70% of cases)

Incidence

○ Possible in any person with impaired immunity

✳ *Age issue*

Neonates and elderly people are at greatest risk for septic shock.

○ About two-thirds of cases in hospitalized patients (most have underlying diseases)

Common characteristics

○ Hyperdynamic or warm phase
○ Hypodynamic or cold phase

Complications

○ Disseminated intravascular coagulation
○ Renal failure
○ Heart failure
○ GI ulcers
○ Abnormal liver function
○ Death

Assessment

History

○ Possible disorder or treatment that can cause immunosuppression
○ Possibly, previous invasive tests or treatments, surgery, or trauma
○ Possible fever and chills (although 20% of patients possibly hypothermic)

Physical findings

Hyperdynamic or warm phase
○ Peripheral vasodilation
○ Skin possibly pink and flushed or warm and dry
○ Altered level of consciousness (LOC) reflected in agitation, anxiety, irritability, and shortened attention span
○ Respirations rapid and shallow
○ Urine output below normal
○ Rapid, full, bounding pulse
○ Blood pressure normal or slightly elevated

Hypodynamic or cold phase
○ Peripheral vasoconstriction and inadequate tissue perfusion
○ Pale skin and possible cyanosis
○ Decreased LOC; possible obtundation and coma
○ Respirations possibly rapid and shallow
○ Urine output possibly less than 25 ml/hour or absent
○ Rapid, weak, thready pulse
○ Irregular pulse if arrhythmias are present
○ Cold, clammy skin
○ Hypotension
○ Crackles or rhonchi if pulmonary congestion is present

Test results

Laboratory
○ Blood cultures are positive for the causative organism.
○ Complete blood count shows the presence or absence of anemia and leukopenia, severe or absent neutropenia, and usually the presence of thrombocytopenia.
○ Blood urea nitrogen and creatinine levels are increased, and creatinine clearance is decreased.
○ Prothrombin time and partial thromboplastin time are abnormal.
○ Serum lactate dehydrogenase levels are elevated, with metabolic acidosis.
○ Urine studies show increased specific gravity (more than 1.02), increased osmolality, and decreased sodium levels.
○ Arterial blood gas (ABG) analysis demonstrates increased blood pH and partial pressure of arterial oxygen and decreased partial pressure of arterial carbon dioxide with respiratory alkalosis in early stages.

Diagnostic procedures
○ Invasive hemodynamic monitoring shows:
  – increased cardiac output and decreased systemic vascular resistance in warm phase
  – decreased cardiac output and increased systemic vascular resistance in cold phase.

Treatment

General
○ Removal of I.V., intra-arterial, or urinary drainage catheters whenever possible
○ In patients immunosuppressed from drug therapy, drugs discontinued or reduced, if possible
○ Mechanical ventilation if respiratory failure occurs
○ Fluid volume replacement
○ Possible parenteral nutrition or tube feedings
○ Bed rest

Medication
○ Antimicrobial
○ Granulocyte transfusions
○ Colloid or crystalloid infusions
○ Oxygen
○ Diuretics
○ Vasopressors
○ Antipyretics

Nursing considerations

Key outcomes
The patient will:
○ maintain adequate cardiac output
○ maintain hemodynamic stability
○ maintain adequate ventilation
○ show no signs of infection
○ express feelings and develop adequate coping mechanisms
○ maintain adequate fluid volume.

Nursing interventions
○ Remove any I.V., intra-arterial, or urinary drainage catheters, and send them to the laboratory to culture for the presence of the causative organism.
○ Give prescribed I.V. fluids and blood products.

 Alert

A progressive drop in blood pressure accompanied by a thready pulse generally signals inadequate cardiac output from reduced intravascular volume. Notify a physician immediately and increase the infusion rate.

○ Administer appropriate antimicrobial I.V. drugs.
○ Notify a physician if urine output is less than 30 ml/hour.
○ Administer prescribed oxygen.

○ Provide emotional support to the patient and his family.
○ Document the occurrence of a nosocomial infection, and report it to the infection-control practitioner.

Monitoring
○ ABG levels and pulse oximetry
○ Intake and output
○ Vital signs and peripheral pulses
○ Hemodynamics
○ Cardiac rhythm
○ Heart and breath sounds

Patient teaching

Be sure to cover:
○ the disorder, diagnosis, and treatment
○ all procedures and their purpose (to ease the patient's anxiety)
○ risks associated with blood transfusions
○ all equipment and its purpose
○ drugs and possible adverse effects
○ possible complications.

Silicosis

Overview

Description

- Progressive pneumonoconiosis disease characterized by nodular lesions, commonly leading to fibrosis
- Classified according to severity of pulmonary disease and rapidity of onset and progression
- Usually a simple, asymptomatic illness
- Considered an industrial disease
- Prognosis good unless complications occur

Pathophysiology

- Small particles of mineral dust are inhaled and deposited in the respiratory bronchioles, alveolar ducts, and alveoli.
- The surface of these particles generates silicon-based radicals that lead to the production of hydroxy, hydrogen peroxide, and other oxygen radicals that damage cell membranes and inactivate essential cell proteins.
- Alveolar macrophages ingest the particles, become activated, and release cytokines, such as tumor necrosis factor and others that attract other inflammatory cells.
- The inflammation damages resident cells and the extracellular matrix.
- Fibroblasts are stimulated to produce collagen, resulting in fibrosis.

Causes

- Silica dust due to:
    - manufacture of ceramics (flint) and building materials (sandstone)
    - mixed form in construction materials (cement)
    - powder form (silica flour), in paints, porcelain, scouring soaps, and wood fillers
    - mining of gold, lead, zinc, and iron.

Incidence

- Highest incidence in those who work around silica dust, such as foundry workers, boiler scalers, and stone cutters
- Acute silicosis possible after 1 to 3 years in sand blasters, tunnel workers, and others exposed to high concentrations of respirable silica
- Accelerated silicosis possible in those exposed to lower concentrations of free silica, usually after about 10 years of exposure
- More common in those ages 40 to 75
- More common in males than in females

Common characteristics

- Dyspnea on exertion
- Dry cough, especially in the morning

Complications

- Pulmonary fibrosis
- Cor pulmonale
- Cardiac or respiratory failure
- Pulmonary tuberculosis
- Lung infection
- Pneumothorax

Assessment

History

- Long-term exposure to silica dust
- Dyspnea on exertion
- Dry cough, especially in the morning

Physical findings

- Decreased chest expansion
- Tachypnea
- Lethargy
- Decreased mentation
- Areas of increased and decreased resonance
- Medium crackles, wheezing
- Diminished breath sounds

 Alert

Assess patient for the presence of an intensified ventricular gallop on inspiration, which is a hallmark of cor pulmonale.

- Hemoptysis

Test results

Laboratory
- Arterial blood gas analysis shows:
    - normal partial pressure of oxygen in simple silicosis (may be significantly decreased in late stages or complicated disease)
    - normal partial pressure of carbon dioxide in early stages of the disease. (Hyperventilation may cause it to decrease; partial pressure of arterial carbon dioxide may increase if restrictive lung disease develops.)

Imaging
- Chest X-rays in simple silicosis show small, discrete, nodular lesions distributed throughout both lung fields, although they typically concentrate in the upper lung.
- Lung nodes may appear enlarged and show eggshell calcification.
- Chest X-rays in complicated silicosis show one or more conglomerate masses of dense tissue.

Diagnostic procedures
- Pulmonary function tests show:
    - reduced forced vital capacity (FVC) in complicated silicosis
    - reduced forced expiratory volume in 1 second (FEV_1) with obstructive disease

– reduced FEV_1 with a normal or high ratio of FEV_1 to FVC in complicated silicosis
– reduced diffusing capacity for carbon monoxide when fibrosis destroys alveolar walls and obliterates pulmonary capillaries or when it thickens the alveocapillary membrane.

Treatment

General

○ Relief of respiratory symptoms
○ Management of hypoxia and cor pulmonale
○ Prevention of respiratory tract infections
○ Steam inhalation and chest physiotherapy
○ Increased fluid intake
○ High-calorie, high-protein diet
○ Regular exercise program, as tolerated

Medication

○ Bronchodilators
○ Oxygen
○ Antibiotics
○ Anti-inflammatory agents

Surgery

○ Possible tracheostomy
○ Possible lung transplantation
○ Whole lung lavage

Nursing considerations

Key outcomes

The patient will:
○ maintain adequate ventilation
○ use energy conservation techniques
○ express an understanding of the illness
○ demonstrate effective coping mechanisms
○ maintain adequate caloric intake.

Nursing interventions

○ Give prescribed drugs.
○ Perform chest physiotherapy.
○ Provide a high-calorie, high-protein diet.
○ Provide small, frequent meals.
○ Provide frequent mouth care.
○ Ensure adequate hydration.
○ Encourage daily exercise as tolerated.
○ Provide diversional activities as appropriate.
○ Provide frequent rest periods.
○ Help with adjustment to the lifestyle changes associated with a chronic illness.
○ Include the patient and family in care decisions whenever possible.

Monitoring

○ Vital signs
○ Intake and output
○ Daily weight
○ Respiratory status

○ Activity tolerance
○ Complications
○ Changes in mentation
○ Sputum production
○ Breath sounds

Patient teaching

Be sure to cover:
○ the disorder, diagnosis, and treatment
○ drugs and possible adverse effects
○ when to notify a physician
○ the need to avoid crowds and people with known infections
○ home oxygen therapy, if needed
○ transtracheal catheter care, if needed
○ postural drainage and chest percussion
○ coughing and deep-breathing exercises
○ the need to consume a high-calorie, high-protein diet
○ adequate hydration
○ the risk of tuberculosis
○ energy conservation techniques.

Discharge planning

○ Refer the patient for influenza and pneumococcus immunizations, as needed.
○ Refer the patient to a smoking-cessation program, if indicated.
○ Refer the patient for tuberculosis testing, if indicated.

Sinusitis

Overview

Description

- Inflammation of the paranasal sinuses
- Usually follows upper respiratory infections
- May be acute, subacute, chronic, allergic, or hyperplastic
- In hyperplastic sinusitis, a combination of purulent acute sinusitis and allergic sinusitis or rhinitis
- For all types, prognosis good

Pathophysiology

- Impairment in drainage of sinuses and retention of secretions result in inflammation.

Causes

- Bacterial infections (common)
- Viral infections
- Fungal infections (uncommon)
- Any condition that interferes with sinus drainage and ventilation
- Swimming in contaminated conditions
- Immunocompromised states
- Diabetes
- Blood dyscrasias
- Allergic rhinitis
- Orofacial trauma
- Endotracheal intubation

Risk factors

- Anatomic abnormalities
- Viral upper respiratory infection
- Allergies
- Overuse of topical decongestants
- Asthma

Incidence

- Affects 16% of population annually
- Affects all ages
- Affects both sexes equally

Common characteristics

- Nasal congestion
- Purulent nasal discharge
- Facial pain specific to affected sinus
- Fever

Complications

- Meningitis
- Cavernous and sinus thrombosis
- Bacteremia or septicemia
- Brain abscess
- Osteomyelitis
- Mucocele
- Orbital cellulitis or abscess

Assessment

History

- Nasal congestion
- Nasal discharge, clear turning purulent
- Sore throat
- Localized headache
- Generalized malaise; fatigue
- Pain specific to the affected sinus (see *Locating the paranasal sinuses*)
- Vague facial discomfort
- Nonproductive cough

Physical findings

- Edematous nasal mucosa
- Low-grade fever
- Edema over sinuses
- Enlarged turbinates
- Mucosal lining thickening
- Mucosal polyps (hyperplastic sinusitis)
- Pain and pressure over affected sinus areas with palpation

Test results

Laboratory
- Culture and sensitivity testing of purulent nasal drainage shows the causative bacterial organism.

Imaging
- Sinus X-rays show cloudiness in affected sinus, air-fluid levels, or thickened mucosal lining.
- Ultrasonography and computed tomography scanning show recurrent or chronic sinusitis, unresolved sinusitis.

Diagnostic procedures
- Transillumination of sinuses may be diminished.
- Sinus endoscopy shows purulent nasal drainage, nasal edema, and obstruction of ostia.

Treatment

General

- Depends on type of sinusitis
- Indirect drainage of ethmoid and sphenoid sinuses
- Steam inhalation
- Local heat applications
- Adequate rest periods

Medication

- Antibiotics
- Analgesics
- Vasoconstrictors
- Corticosteroids
- Antihistamines

Surgery

- Antral puncture to remove purulent material
- Sinus irrigation

Nursing considerations

Key outcomes

The patient will:
○ express feelings of increased comfort
○ exhibit an adequate breathing pattern
○ show no signs of infection
○ express an understanding of the condition and treatment
○ develop no complications.

Nursing interventions

○ Encourage oral fluid intake.
○ Elevate head of the bed no more than 30 degrees.
○ Encourage expression of concerns.
○ Apply warm compresses.
○ Give prescribed drugs.
○ Encourage use of humidifiers.

 Alert

Watch for and report vomiting, chills, fever, edema of the forehead or eyelids, blurred or double vision, and personality changes.

After surgery
○ Place the patient in semi-Fowler's position.
○ Apply ice compresses over the nose and iced saline gauze over the eyes for 24 hours.
○ Frequently change the mustache dressing or drip pad.
○ Provide meticulous and frequent mouth care.

Monitoring

○ Complications
○ Response to treatment
○ Pain control
○ Nasal discharge
After surgery
○ Excessive drainage or bleeding
○ Consistency, amount, and color of drainage
○ Vital signs

Patient teaching

Be sure to cover:
○ the disorder, diagnosis, and treatment
○ prescribed drugs
○ potential adverse reactions
○ cautions against driving a motor vehicle or consuming alcohol while taking antihistamines or analgesics
○ the need to complete the full course of prescribed antibiotics
○ the need to leave nasal packing in place for 12 to 24 hours after surgery
○ the need to breathe through the mouth and refrain from blowing the nose and sneezing
○ the need to refrain from smoking for at least 2 or 3 days after surgery

Locating the paranasal sinuses

The location of a patient's sinusitis pain indicates the affected sinus. For example, an infected maxillary sinus can cause tooth pain. (*Note:* The sphenoid sinus, which lies under the eye and above the soft palate, isn't depicted here.)

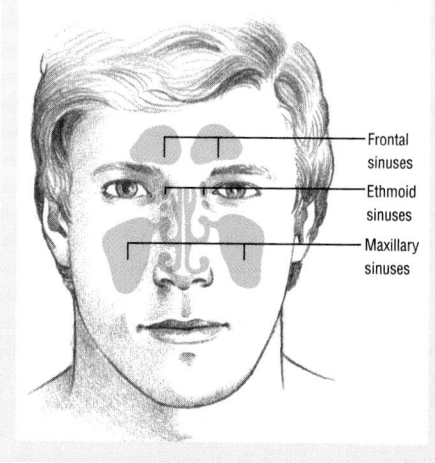

Frontal sinuses
Ethmoid sinuses
Maxillary sinuses

○ signs and symptoms of complications
○ importance of medical follow-up
○ proper hand-washing technique
○ avoidance of bending and stooping during the acute phase
○ avoidance of contact with an infected person.

Sjögren's syndrome

Overview

Description

○ Connective tissue disease that's the most common autoimmune disorder after rheumatoid arthritis
○ May be primary disorder or associated with other inflammatory connective tissue disorders

Pathophysiology

○ Lymphocytic infiltration of exocrine glands causing tissue damage resulting in xerostomia and dry eyes
○ Immunologic activation

Causes

○ Unknown
○ Possible genetic and environmental factors
○ Immunologic activation

Incidence

○ Affects more women (about 90%) than men
○ Mean age of occurrence is 50

Common characteristics

○ Dry eyes and mouth

Complications

○ Corneal ulceration or perforation
○ Epistaxis
○ Deafness
○ Otitis media
○ Splenomegaly
○ Renal tubular necrosis

Assessment

History

○ Xerophthalmia or xerostomia
○ Gritty, sandy eye along with redness, burning, photosensitivity, eye fatigue, itching, and mucoid discharge
○ Difficulty swallowing and talking; an abnormal taste or smell sensation (or both); thirst; ulcers of the tongue, mouth, and lips (especially at the corners of the mouth); and severe dental caries

---

Diagnosing Sjögren's syndrome

For a diagnosis of Sjögren's syndrome, the patient must have the following:
○ keratoconjunctivitis sicca
○ diminished salivary gland flow
○ a positive salivary gland biopsy, showing mononuclear cell infiltration
○ the presence of autoantibodies in a serum sample, indicating a systemic autoimmune process.

○ Possible epistaxis, hoarseness, chronic nonproductive cough, recurrent otitis media, and frequent respiratory tract infections
○ Possible dyspareunia
○ Generalized itching, fatigue, recurrent low-grade fever, and arthralgia or myalgia

Physical findings

○ Mouth ulcers, dental caries and, possibly, enlarged salivary glands
○ Palpable purpura
○ Palpable lymph node enlargement
○ Dry, sticky, erythematous oral mucosa

Test results

Laboratory
○ Erythrocyte sedimentation rate is elevated in more than 90% of patients.
○ Complete blood count shows mild anemia and leukopenia in about 30% of patients.
○ Serum protein electrophoresis shows hypergammaglobulinemia in about 50% of patients.
○ Typically, 75% to 90% of patients test positive for rheumatoid factor, and between 50% and 80% of patients test positive for antinuclear antibodies.

Diagnostic procedures
○ For a diagnosis of Sjögren's syndrome, symptoms must meet specific criteria. (See *Diagnosing Sjögren's syndrome*.)
○ Tests supporting the diagnosis include measuring eye involvement with the Schirmer's test and a slit-lamp examination with rose bengal dye.
○ Labial biopsy (to detect lymphoid foci), a simple procedure with minimal risk, is the only specific diagnostic technique.
○ Salivary gland involvement may be evaluated by measuring the volume of parotid saliva, by secretory sialography, and by salivary scintigraphy.
○ Salivary gland biopsy results typically show lymphocytic infiltration in Sjögren's syndrome; lower lip biopsy findings show salivary gland infiltration by lymphocytes.

Treatment

General

○ Meticulous oral hygiene
○ Humidifier
○ Unscented skin lotions
○ Frequent dental care
○ Avoidance of sugar, tobacco, alcohol, and spicy, salty, or highly acidic foods
○ Increased oral fluid intake for mouth dryness

Medication

○ Pilocarpine and cevimeline
○ Preservative-free artificial tears and sustained-release cellulose capsules
○ Artificial salivas

○ Glucocorticoids or other immunosuppressive agents for extraglandular manifestations such as systemic vasculitis
○ Saline nasal sprays
○ Vaginal lubricants
○ Nonsteroidal anti-inflammatory drugs
○ Antifungal agents
○ Ophthalmic lubricants

Nursing considerations

Key outcomes

The patient will:
○ express feelings of increased comfort
○ have pink and moist oral mucosa
○ demonstrate oral hygiene practices
○ acknowledge problems in sexual function.

Nursing interventions

○ Instill artificial tears as often as every 30 minutes to prevent eye damage, and instill an eye ointment at bedtime.
○ Provide plenty of fluids, especially water, for the patient to drink, and sugarless chewing gum or candy.

Monitoring

○ Response to treatment
○ Extraglandular manifestations
○ Complications

Patient teaching

Be sure to cover:
○ the disorder, diagnosis, and treatment
○ the instillation of eye drops and ointments
○ the need for sunglasses to protect the eyes
○ the need to keep the face clean and to avoid rubbing the eyes
○ avoidance of saliva-decreasing drugs, such as atropine derivatives, antihistamines, anticholinergics, and antidepressants
○ meticulous oral hygiene and regular dental visits
○ high-calorie, protein-rich liquid supplements to prevent malnutrition if mouth lesions make eating painful
○ the need to consume a nutritious diet
○ avoidance of sugar, tobacco, alcohol, and spicy, salty, or highly acidic foods
○ the need to humidify the home and work environments
○ use of normal saline solution, in drop or spray form, to relieve nasal dryness
○ avoidance of prolonged hot showers and baths and the use of moisturizing lotions on dry skin. (Suggest use of a water-soluble gel as a vaginal lubricant.)

Skull fracture

Overview

Description

- Break in the integrity of the skull bone
- May be simple (closed) or compound (open)
- May displace bone fragments
- May be linear (common hairline break, without displacement of structures), comminuted (splintering or crushing the bone into several fragments), or depressed (a fracture that pushes the bone toward the brain)

 Alert

Because possible damage to the brain is the first concern, rather than the fracture itself, a skull fracture is considered a neurosurgical condition.

- Classified according to location, such as cranial vault fracture and basilar fractures

 Alert

Because of the danger of grave cranial complications and meningitis, basilar fractures are usually far more serious than vault fractures.

Pathophysiology

- Trauma to the head causes a fracture at certain anatomic sites:
  - Parietal bone
  - Squama of temporal bone
  - Foramen magnum
  - Petrous temporal ridge
  - Inner parts of the sphenoid wings at the skull base
  - Middle cranial fossa
  - Cribriform plate
  - Roof of orbits in the anterior cranial fossa
  - Bony areas between the mastoid and dural sinuses in the posterior cranial fossa

Causes

- Head trauma

Incidence

- Simple linear fracture most common, especially in children younger than age 5
- May occur at any age

Common characteristics

- Persistent, localized headache
- Scalp wounds — abrasions, contusions, lacerations, or avulsions
- Signs of brain injury — agitation and irritability, loss of consciousness, labored respirations, abnormal deep tendon reflexes, and altered pupillary and motor response

In sphenoidal fracture
- Blindness

In temporal fracture
- Unilateral deafness or facial paralysis

In basilar fracture
- Hemorrhage from the nose, pharynx, or ears
- Blood under the periorbital skin (raccoon eyes) and conjunctiva
- Battle's sign (supramastoid ecchymosis)
- Cerebrospinal fluid (CSF) or brain tissue leakage from the nose or ears

Complications

- Epilepsy
- Hydrocephalus
- Organic brain syndrome
- Headaches, giddiness, fatigability, neuroses, and behavior disorders

Assessment

History

- Head trauma
- Headache
- Loss of consciousness

Physical findings

- Decreased pulse and respirations
- Altered level of consciousness (LOC)
- Scalp wound
- Bleeding in the periorbital area, nose, pharynx, ears, or under the conjunctivae
- CSF leakage from the nose or ears; halo sign on pillowcase (a blood-tinged spot surrounded by a lighter ring)

Test results

Laboratory
- Reagent strips turn blue if CSF is present.

Imaging
- Computed tomography scan and magnetic resonance imaging show fracture, intracranial hemorrhage from ruptured blood vessels, and swelling.

Treatment

General

- Depends on type and severity of fracture
- Supportive
- Cleaning and debridement of wounds
- Diet as tolerated; nothing by mouth if surgery is necessary
- Limited activity

Medication

○ Mild analgesics
○ Prophylactic antibiotics
○ Dexamethasone (basilar and vault fractures)

 Alert

Don't give the patient opioids or sedatives because they may depress respirations, increase carbon dioxide levels, lead to increased intracranial pressure, and mask changes in neurologic status.

Surgery

○ Craniotomy to elevate or remove fragments that have been driven into the brain and to extract foreign bodies and necrotic tissue, thereby reducing the risk of infection and further brain damage (severe injury)

Nursing considerations

Key outcomes

The patient will:
○ remain neurologically and hemodynamically stable
○ express increased comfort and decreased pain
○ relate fears and feelings related to traumatic event.

Nursing interventions

○ Establish and maintain a patent airway.

 Alert

Nasal airways are contraindicated in patients with possible basilar skull fractures. Intubation may be necessary.

○ Suction through the mouth, not the nose, to prevent the introduction of bacteria.
○ Position the patient with a head injury for proper secretion drainage. Elevate the head of the bed 30 degrees if intracerebral injury is suspected.
○ Apply appropriate dressings; control bleeding as necessary.
○ Institute seizure precautions.

Monitoring

○ Vital signs
○ Neurological status
○ Comfort level

Patient teaching

Be sure to cover:
○ preoperative and postoperative care, if appropriate
○ need to watch closely for changes in mental status, LOC, or respirations
○ use of mild analgesics as opposed to opioids
○ wound care.

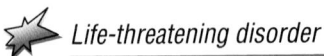

Life-threatening disorder

Smallpox

Overview

Description

○ Acute, highly contagious infectious disease caused by the poxvirus variola
○ Associated with tremendous morbidity and mortality
○ Two related viruses:
  – *Variola major* (classic smallpox), with a case mortality rate of 20% to 50%
  – *Variola minor* (alastrim), a clinically milder form with mortality less than 1%
○ Eliminated worldwide in 1980 (World Health Organization declaration) as a result of a global vaccination and eradication program; routine smallpox vaccination stopped; variola virus, preserved in two research laboratories, remains unlikely but potential source of infection; humans were sole reservoir of infection; no carrier state
○ Potential for use in bioterrorism and biological warfare; classified as category-A biological disease, transmitted human to human with no known treatment
○ Also known as *variola*

Pathophysiology

○ Poxviruses are characterized by a large double-stranded deoxyribonucleic acid (DNA) genome and a brick-shaped morphology.
○ Poxviruses are the only DNA viruses that replicate in cytoplasm.
○ The virus is spread through direct contact or inhalation of respiratory droplets.
○ The incubation period is 7 to 19 days. Illness onset is in 10 to 14 days, with onset of the characteristic rash in 2 to 4 days. Fever and macular rash appear after an average incubation period of 12 days, with a progression to typical vesicular and pustular lesions over 1 or 2 weeks.
○ It's most contagious during the first week of illness (before the eruptive period) and during the time between lesion development and scab disappearance.

Causes

○ Poxvirus variolae

Incidence

○ Last known case in the United States reported in 1949
○ Last case of endemic smallpox reported in Africa in 1977
○ Affected people of all ages
○ In temperate zones, incidence highest during winter
○ In tropics, incidence highest during hot, dry months

Common characteristics

○ Fever
○ Maculopapular rash

Complications

○ Secondary bacterial infections
○ Encephalitis
○ Bleeding abnormalities
○ Death

Assessment

History

○ Influenza-type symptoms
○ High fever, chills
○ Rash
○ Malaise
○ Headache, backache
○ Abdominal pain
○ Nausea, vomiting

Physical findings

○ After average incubation period of 12 days:
  – Fever
  – Macular rash
  – Progression to typical vesicular and pustular lesions, and then crusted scabs
  – Centrifugal distribution to rash; starts on the face and extremities; moves to the trunk

Test results

Laboratory
○ Culture of aspirate from vesicles and pustules shows presence of variola.
○ Electron microscopy of vesicular scrapings shows presence of variola.

Treatment

General

○ Home treatment if possible to reduce spread
○ No current treatment other than supportive
○ Strict isolation
○ Diet as tolerated
○ I.V. fluids
○ Activity as tolerated

Medication

○ Antibiotics
○ Antipruritics
○ Antihistamines
○ Analgesics

Nursing considerations

Key outcomes

The patient will:
○ maintain adequate nutrition
○ verbalize feelings of fear and anxiety
○ demonstrate effective coping mechanisms
○ maintain tissue perfusion and cellular oxygenation
○ maintain balanced fluid status
○ maintain skin integrity.

Nursing interventions

○ Give prescribed drugs.
○ Report any case of smallpox to the appropriate pub-
lic health office.
○ Institute strict exposure precautions, including isola-
tion and airborne, contact, and standard precau-
tions.
○ Autoclave all laundry and hospital waste before laun-
dering or incinerating.
○ Provide meticulous skin care.
○ Encourage verbalization of fears and concerns.
○ Provide adequate hydration.
○ Provide a well-balanced diet.
○ Assist in the development of effective coping mecha-
nisms.
○ Provide adequate rest periods.

Monitoring

○ Vital signs
○ Intake and output
○ Complications
○ Fluid and electrolyte status
○ Signs and symptoms of secondary bacterial infection

Patient teaching

Be sure to cover:
○ the disorder, diagnosis, and treatment
○ drugs and possible adverse effects
○ when to notify the physician
○ isolation precautions
○ hydration
○ skin lesion care.

Discharge planning

○ Refer those in direct contact with an infected person
for pre-exposure and postexposure vaccination if
more than 3 years have passed since last vaccination.

Spinal injury

Overview

Description
○ Fractures, contusions, or compressions of the spine
○ Most common sites: C5, C6, C7, T12, and L1 vertebrae

Pathophysiology
○ Injury causes microscopic hemorrhages.
○ All of the gray matter is filled with blood.
○ Necrosis results.
○ Edema causes spinal cord compression.
○ Blood supply is further decreased.
○ Long-term scarring and meningeal thickening occur.
○ Nerves are blocked or tangled.
○ Sensory and motor deficits occur.

Causes
Serious injury
○ Motor vehicle accident
○ Fall
○ Diving into shallow water
○ Gunshot and related wound
Less serious injury
○ Improper lifting of heavy object
○ Minor fall
○ Neoplastic lesion
○ Osteoporosis

Incidence
○ Most common between ages 15 and 35

Common characteristics
○ Based on severity and location of injury:
  – Muscle spasm or back pain (worsens with movement)
  – Mild paresthesia to quadriplegia
  – Shock
  – Loss of motor function, muscle flaccidity
  – Bladder and bowel atony
  – Loss of perspiration below the level of the injury
  – Respiratory impairment

Complications
○ Paralysis
○ Death
○ Autonomic dysreflexia
○ Spinal shock
○ Neurogenic shock

Assessment

History
○ Muscle spasm
○ Back or neck pain
○ In cervical fractures, point tenderness

Physical findings
○ Level of injury and any spinal cord damage located by neurologic assessment
○ Limited movement and activities that cause pain
○ Surface wounds
○ Pain location
○ Loss of sensation below the level of injury
○ Deformity

Test results
Imaging
○ Spinal X-rays, myelography, computed tomography, and magnetic resonance imaging scans can indicate the location of the fracture and the site of the compression.

Treatment

General
○ Stabilization of spine and prevention of cord damage
○ Hemodynamic support
○ Application of a hard cervical collar
○ Wound care (if appropriate)
○ Chemotherapy and radiation for neoplastic lesion
○ Aspiration precautions
○ Skeletal traction with skull tongs
○ Bed rest on a firm surface
○ Rotation bed with cervical traction (if appropriate)
○ Splinting: thoracic lumbar sacral orthotics

Medication
○ Corticosteroids
○ Analgesics
○ Muscle relaxants
○ Chemotherapy for neoplastic lesion

Surgery
○ Decompression of spinal cord
○ Stabilization of spinal column

Nursing considerations

Key outcomes
The patient will:
○ express feelings of increased comfort and decreased pain
○ develop effective coping mechanisms
○ attain the highest degree of mobility
○ maintain a patent airway and adequate ventilation
○ show no sign of aspiration.

Nursing interventions
○ Apply a hard cervical collar.
○ Immobilize the patient.
○ Comfort and reassure the patient.
○ Give prescribed drugs.
○ Provide wound care, if appropriate.
○ Provide diversionary activities.
○ Provide proper skin care.

Monitoring

○ Neurologic changes
○ Respiratory status
○ Changes in skin sensation and loss of muscle strength
○ Skin integrity
○ Hydration and nutritional status
○ Pain control

Patient teaching

Be sure to cover:
○ the disorder, diagnosis, and treatment
○ traction methods used
○ exercises to maintain physical mobility
○ drug administration, dosage, and possible adverse effects
○ the prescribed home care regimen
○ the importance of follow-up examinations.

Discharge planning

○ Refer the patient to the appropriate rehabilitation center.
○ Refer the patient to resource and support services.

Sprains and strains

Overview

Description

- Sprain — complete or incomplete tear in supporting ligaments surrounding a joint
- Strain — acute or chronic injury to a muscle or tendinous attachment
- Classified as mild, moderate, or severe (see *Classifying sprains and strains*)

Pathophysiology

Sprain
- A ligament tear causes bleeding.
- A hematoma forms.
- Inflammatory exudates follow.
- Granulation tissue develops.
- Collagen forms.
- Swelling or stretching of nerves or vessels occurs.
- Persistent laxity and chronic joint instability result.

Strain
- Strains result from the same process as sprains.
- New tendon or muscle eventually becomes strong enough to withstand normal muscle strain.

Causes

- Fall
- Motor vehicle accident
- Trauma
- Excessive or new exercise
- Sport injury

Common characteristics

Sprain
- Localized pain
- Swelling and warmth

Classifying sprains and strains

The guide below will help you classify the severity of sprains and strains.

Sprains
- Grade 1 (mild): minor or partial ligament tear with normal joint stability and function
- Grade 2 (moderate): partial tear with mild joint laxity and some function loss
- Grade 3 (severe): complete tear or incomplete separation of ligament from bone, causing total joint laxity and function loss

Strains
- Grade 1 (mild): microscopic muscle or tendon tear (or both) with no loss of strength
- Grade 2 (moderate): incomplete tear with bleeding into muscle tissue and some loss of strength
- Grade 3 (severe): complete rupture, usually resulting from separation of muscle from muscle, muscle from tendon, or tendon from bone (usually stems from sudden, violent movement or direct injury)

- Progressive loss of motion
- Ecchymosis

Strain
- Pain
- Inflammation
- Erythema
- Ecchymosis
- Elevated skin temperature

Risk factors

- Participation in sports

Incidence

- More common in athletes (occurs in 80% of athletes)
- More common in men than in women

Complications

Sprain
- Avulsion fracture

Strain
- Complete rupture of muscle tendon unit
- Deep vein thrombosis

Assessment

History

- Physical activity
- Similar past injury
- Systemic disease with high risk factors
- Local pain that worsens during joint movement
- Loss of mobility
- Sharp, transient pain and rapid swelling
- Stiffness, soreness, and generalized tenderness

Physical findings

- Ecchymosis
- Swelling
- Point tenderness

Test results

Imaging
- X-ray results are used to rule out fractures and confirm damage to ligaments.

Treatment

General

- RICE — rest, ice, compression (wrapping in an elastic bandage), and elevation to affected area
- Rehabilitation or exercise program
- Nothing by mouth if surgery scheduled
- Limited activity and weight bearing to injured area, based on extent of injury
- Elevation of affected joint above the level of the heart for 48 to 72 hours
- Range-of-motion (ROM) exercises

Medication

○ Vitamin C supplements
○ Nonsteroidal anti-inflammatory drugs
○ Analgesics
○ Cox-2 inhibitors

Surgery

○ Based on extent of injury

Nursing considerations

Key outcomes

The patient will:
○ attain the highest possible level of mobility
○ express feelings of increased comfort and decreased pain
○ identify factors that increase the potential for injury.

Nursing interventions

○ Apply ice intermittently.
○ Apply an elastic bandage or air cast.
○ Give prescribed drug.
○ Elevate the extremity.

Monitoring

○ Edema
○ Response to treatment
○ Pain control
○ Complications
○ Adverse effects of drugs
○ ROM

Patient teaching

Be sure to cover:
○ the disorder, diagnosis, and treatment
○ how to apply ice intermittently for the first 12 to 48 hours
○ how to reapply elastic bandage or air cast
○ crutch-gait training
○ avoidance of further injury to the joint
○ drug administration, dosage, and possible adverse effects.

Spurious polythemia

Overview

Description

- Blood disorder characterized by an increased hematocrit and a normal or low red blood cell (RBC) total mass
- Results from diminished plasma volume and subsequent hemoconcentration
- Also known as *relative polycythemia, stress erythrocytosis, stress polycythemia, benign polycythemia, Gaisböck's disease,* or *pseudopolycythemia*

Pathophysiology

- Conditions that promote severe fluid loss decrease plasma volume and lead to hemoconcentration.
- Nervous stress causes hemoconcentration by an unknown mechanism. This form of erythrocytosis (chronically elevated hematocrit) is particularly common in the middle-aged man who is a chronic smoker and has a type A personality (tense, hard driving, and anxious).
- In many patients, an increased hematocrit merely reflects a normally high RBC mass and low plasma volume. This is particularly common in patients who don't smoke, aren't obese, and have no history of hypertension.

Causes

- Dehydration
- Hemoconcentration from stress
- High-normal RBC mass and low-normal plasma volume
- Hypertension
- Thromboembolic disease
- Elevated serum cholesterol and uric acid
- Familial tendency
- Pregnancy

Incidence

- Usually affects middle-aged people
- More common in men than in women

Common characteristics

- Headaches or dizziness
- Ruddy appearance
- Slight hypertension
- Tendency to hyperventilate when recumbent
- Cardiac or pulmonary disease

Complications

- Thromboemboli

Assessment

History

- Headaches
- Dizziness
- Cardiac or pulmonary disease
- Fatigue
- Diaphoresis
- Dyspnea
- Claudication

Physical findings

- Ruddy appearance
- Short neck
- Hepatosplenomegaly
- Slight hypertension
- Hypoventilation when recumbent

Test results

Laboratory
- Hemoglobin and hematocrit are increased.
- RBC count is increased.
- RBC mass is normal or decreased
- Arterial oxygen saturation is normal.
- Bone marrow is normal.
- Plasma volume is decreased or normal.
- Hyperlipidemia may be present.
- Uricosuria may be present.

Treatment

General

- Appropriate fluids and electrolytes to correct dehydration
- Cessation of dietary diuretics such as caffeine
- Low-cholesterol, low-fat diet
- Adequate hydration
- Adequate exercise

Medication

- Antidiarrheals, if needed

Nursing considerations

Key outcomes

The patient will:
- express feelings of increased energy
- exhibit adequate ventilation
- express feelings of increased comfort
- maintain normal fluid volume.

Nursing interventions

- Give prescribed I.V. fluids.
- Encourage adequate fluid intake.
- Encourage activity.
- Provide emotional support.

○ Provide dietary counseling if appropriate.

Monitoring
○ Intake and output
○ Blood studies
○ Response to treatment

Patient teaching

Be sure to cover:
○ the disorder, diagnosis, and treatment
○ changing the patient's work habits, if appropriate
○ the need for proper relaxation
○ dietary restrictions
○ importance of proper hydration
○ recognizing and reporting of signs and symptoms of increasing polycythemia and thromboembolism.

Discharge planning
○ Refer the patient to a smoking-cessation program, if necessary.
○ Emphasize the need for follow-up examinations every 3 to 4 months after leaving the hospital.

Squamous cell carcinoma

Overview

Description

○ Invasive tumor arising from keratinizing epidermal cells

Pathophysiology

○ Transformation from a premalignant lesion to squamous cell carcinoma may begin with induration and inflammation of an existing lesion.
○ When squamous cell carcinoma arises from normal skin, the nodule grows slowly on a firm, indurated base. If untreated, this nodule eventually ulcerates and invades underlying tissues. (See *Squamous cell carcinoma nodule.*)

Causes

○ Unknown
○ Actinic damage from solar ultraviolet radiation
○ Ionizing radiation
○ Chemical carcinogens
○ Burns, scars
○ Ulcerations

Risk factors

○ Overexposure to the sun's ultraviolet rays
○ Radiation therapy
○ Ingestion of herbicides containing arsenic
○ Chronic skin irritation and inflammation
○ Exposure to local carcinogens (such as tar and oil)
○ Hereditary diseases (such as xeroderma pigmentosum and albinism)

Squamous cell carcinoma nodule

An ulcerated nodule with an indurated base and a raised, irregular border is a typical lesion in squamous cell carcinoma.

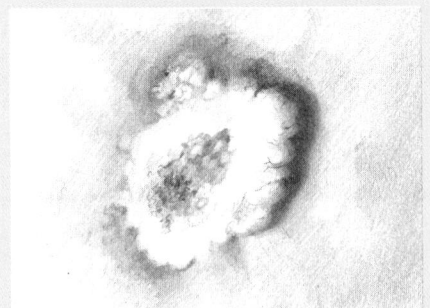

○ Presence of premalignant lesions (such as actinic keratosis or Bowen's disease)
○ Rarely, develops on site of smallpox vaccination, psoriasis, or chronic discoid hippus erythematosus

Common characteristics

○ Chronic skin ulceration

Incidence

○ Most common in fair-skinned, light-eyed, and light-haired people
○ Risk greatly increased by outdoor employment and residence in sunny, warm climate

Complications

○ Lymph node involvement
○ Visceral metastasis

Assessment

History

○ Areas of chronic ulceration, especially on sun-damaged skin
○ Pain, malaise, anorexia, fatigue, and weakness

Physical findings

○ Lesions on the face, ears, or dorsa of the hands and forearms, and on other sun-damaged skin areas (lesions possibly scaly and keratotic with raised, irregular borders; in late disease, lesions growing outward or exophytic and friable and tending toward chronic crusting)

Test results

Diagnostic procedures
○ Excisional biopsy allows a definitive diagnosis.

Treatment

General

○ Determined by size, shape, location, and invasiveness of tumor and condition of underlying tissue
○ Radiation therapy for older or debilitated patients
○ High-protein, high-calorie diet

Medication

○ Chemotherapy
○ Topical corticosteroids

Surgery

○ Wide surgical excision, curettage, and electrodesiccation
○ Cryosurgery

Nursing considerations

Key outcomes

The patient will:
○ express positive feelings about self
○ experience feelings of increased energy
○ exhibit improved or healed lesions or wounds
○ express feelings of increased comfort.

Nursing interventions

○ Encourage verbalization and provide emotional support.
○ Deliver appropriate wound care.
○ Provide periods of rest between procedures if the patient fatigues easily.
○ Provide small, frequent meals and a high-protein, high-calorie diet.

Monitoring

○ Wound site
○ Adverse effects of radiation therapy, such as nausea, vomiting, hair loss, malaise, and diarrhea
○ Pain control

Patient teaching

Be sure to cover:
○ the disorder, diagnosis, and treatment
○ drug administration, dosage, and possible adverse effects
○ information about skin examination
○ the importance of follow-up skin surveillance
○ avoidance of excessive sun exposure to prevent recurrence; the need to use strong sunscreen.

Discharge planning

○ Refer the patient to resource and support services.

Stomatitis

Overview

Description
- Inflammation of oral mucosa; may extend to the buccal mucosa, lips, palate, and tongue
- Common infection occurring alone or as part of systemic disease
- Two main types: acute herpetic stomatitis and aphthous stomatitis
- Usually heals spontaneously, without scarring, in 10 to 14 days

Pathophysiology
- Stomatitis is an inflammatory reaction that may cause loss of the oral epithelium as a protective barrier.

Causes
Acute herpetic stomatitis
- Herpes simplex virus

Aphthous stomatitis
- Unknown (autoimmune and psychosomatic causes under investigation)

Risk factors
- Smoking
- Poor oral hygiene
- Stress
- Poor nutrition
- Chemotherapy
- Immunosuppression

Looking at aphthous stomatitis

In aphthous stomatitis, numerous small, round vesicles appear. They soon break and leave shallow ulcers with red areolae.

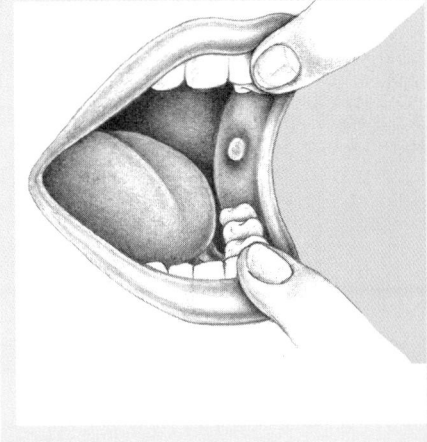

Incidence
Acute herpetic stomatitis
- Common in children ages 1 to 3

Aphthous stomatitis
- Common in young girls and female adolescents

Common characteristics
- Painful gums
- Ulcers on gum papillae

Complications
- Dysphagia
- Sepsis (in immunocompromised patient)
- Ocular or central nervous system involvement (herpetic stomatitis)

Assessment

History
- Burning mouth pain
- Malaise
- Lethargy
- Anorexia
- Irritability
- Fever
- Extreme tenderness of the oral mucosa

Physical findings
Herpetic stomatitis
- Bleeding and swollen gums
- Papulovesicular ulcers in the mouth and throat
- Submaxillary lymphadenitis

Aphthous stomatitis
- Slight swelling of the mucous membrane
- Single or multiple shallow ulcers with whitish centers and red borders, about 2 to 5 mm in diameter (see *Looking at aphthous stomatitis*)

Test results
Laboratory
- Smear of ulcer exudate identifies the causative organism in Vincent's angina (painful pseudomembranous ulceration of gums, oral mucous membranes, pharynx, and tonsils).
- Viral cultures performed on fluid and herpetic vesicles in acute herpetic stomatitis identify the virus.

Treatment

General
- Symptom relief
- Nonantiseptic warm-water mouth rinses
- Ice
- Soft-bristled toothbrush
- Smoking cessation
- Soft, pureed, or liquid diet, as tolerated; avoidance of salty, spicy foods
- Activity as tolerated

Medication

○ I.V. fluids (severe cases)

Acute herpetic stomatitis

○ Topical anesthetic solutions
○ Topical corticosteroids
○ Acyclovir

Aphthous stomatitis

○ Topical anesthetic coating agent

Nursing considerations

Key outcomes

The patient will:

○ show improvement or complete healing of lesions or wounds
○ avoid complications
○ express feelings of increased comfort and decreased pain
○ demonstrate good oral hygiene practices.

Nursing interventions

○ Advise using a sponge instead of a toothbrush for brushing teeth.
○ Suggest rinsing with hydrogen peroxide or normal saline mouthwash.
○ Give prescribed analgesics.
○ Develop a meal plan based on soft, liquid, or pureed foods.
○ Offer iced drinks.

Monitoring

○ Lesion state
○ Response to treatment
○ Complications

Patient teaching

Be sure to cover:

○ the infection and expected course
○ the importance of good oral hygiene
○ the proper application of topical drugs
○ recommended dietary changes
○ adverse effects of prescribed drugs
○ (with aphthous stomatitis) the need to avoid such precipitating factors as stress and fatigue.

Discharge planning

○ Refer the patient to a smoking-cessation program, if appropriate.

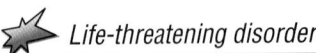 *Life-threatening disorder*

Streptococcus pneumoniae infection, drug-resistant

Overview

Description

○ Infections caused by *Streptococcus pneumoniae* among leading causes of illness and death among people who are young, old, and debilitated
○ Also known as *DRSP*
○ Seven serotypes (6A, 6B, 9V, 14, 19A, 19F, and 23F) accounting for most DRSP
○ Vaccine available for the 23 most common serotypes
○ Commonly resistant to penicillin; also resistant to erythromycin, co-trimoxazole, vancomycin, tetracycline, chloramphenicol, and ofloxacin
○ In pneumonias caused by resistant strains, death rate twice as high as in those sensitive to antibiotics

Pathophysiology

○ DRSP can affect people by colonization or infection.
○ People who carry *S. pneumoniae* as part of their normal flora but remain asymptomatic may unknowingly spread the infection.
○ Disease results when bacteria multiply locally (otitis media), multiply after aspiration (pneumonia), or invade a sterile site (central nervous system or blood).

Causes

○ Abuse of antimicrobial agents
○ Increasing prevalence of strains resistant to multiple drug classes

Risk factors

○ Contact with infected respiratory droplets or direct or indirect contact with objects freshly soiled with respiratory discharge
○ Populations at risk:
  – Elderly people
  – Children age 2 and older
  – Blacks
  – Native Americans
  – People with autoimmune disorders
  – Nursing home residents
  – Child-care workers

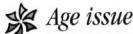 *Age issue*

The Advisory Committee on Immunization Practices recommends the S. pneumoniae *vaccine be given to people age 2 and older with certain medical conditions and to all people age 65 and older.*

Incidence

○ 3% to 35% of pneumococcal illness due to drug-resistant strains

Common characteristics

○ DRSP can cause:
  – bacteremia
  – meningitis
  – otitis media
  – peritonitis
  – pneumonia
  – sinusitis.

Complications

○ Colonized people not commonly detected or treated
○ Treatment failures, prolonged hospitalization, recurrent disease, and increased cost
○ Death in 14% of adults with invasive disease
○ Neurologic sequelae after meningitis
○ Hearing impairment from recurrent otitis media
○ Developmental delay in children with recurrent otitis media

Assessment

History

○ Member of high-risk population
○ Recent exposure to respiratory secretions of infected person
○ Recent antimicrobial use

Physical findings

In meningitis
○ Fever
○ Stiff neck
○ Drowsiness
○ Rash
○ Seizures
○ Increased white blood cells in cerebrospinal fluid (CSF)

In otitis media
○ High fever (101.3° F [38.5° C])
○ Irritability
○ Possibly effusion
○ Bulging tympanic membrane that's red, opaque, white, yellow, or purple and immobile on pneumatic otoscope

In pneumonia
○ Fluid-filled tissue and lobes
○ Shaking chills
○ Cough
○ Rust- or green-colored mucus
○ High fever
○ Diaphoresis
○ Elevated pulse and respirations
○ Bluish lips and nailbeds
○ Confusion or delirium

Test results

Laboratory
- Bacteria are isolated from a fluid sample (blood, CSF, sputum, respiratory drops, ear).

Imaging
- Chest X-rays display pneumonia.

Diagnostic procedures
- Lumbar puncture is performed for suspected meningitis.

Treatment

General
- Supportive, symptomatic care
- Activity as tolerated
- Diet as tolerated

Medication
- Analgesics
- Antibiotics
- Vancomycin (meningitis)

Nursing considerations

Key outcomes
The patient will:
- report resolution of symptoms
- have normal vital signs
- have adequate oxygen levels
- have normal laboratory values.

Nursing interventions
- Give prescribed drugs.
- Provide rest periods as needed.
- Provide emotional support.

Monitoring
- Seizures
- Vital signs
- Intake and output
- Complications after lumbar puncture

Patient teaching

Be sure to cover:
- the importance of covering the mouth and nose while sneezing or coughing
- regular hand-washing
- taking the entire prescription of antibiotic for any infection
- never giving a prescribed antibiotic to anyone else
- importance of reporting to a physician a change in symptoms.

Discharge planning
- Refer the patient for follow-up, as needed.
- Recommend to the patient that close contacts receive the *S. pneumoniae* vaccine.

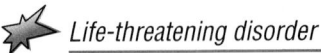

Stroke

Overview

Description

○ Sudden impairment of blood circulation to the brain
○ Third most common cause of death in the United States
○ Affects 500,000 people each year, causing death in half
○ Most common cause of neurologic disability
○ About 50% of stroke survivors permanently disabled
○ Recurrences possible within weeks, months, or years
○ Also known as *cerebrovascular accident* or *brain attack*

Pathophysiology

○ The oxygen supply to the brain is interrupted or diminished.
○ In thrombotic or embolic stroke, neurons die from lack of oxygen.
○ In hemorrhagic stroke, impaired cerebral perfusion causes infarction.

Causes

Cerebral thrombosis
○ Most common cause of stroke
○ Obstruction of a blood vessel in the extracerebral vessels
○ Site possibly intracerebral
Cerebral embolism
○ Second most common cause of stroke
○ History of rheumatic heart disease
○ Endocarditis
○ Posttraumatic valvular disease
○ Cardiac arrhythmias
○ Post open-heart surgery
Cerebral hemorrhage
○ Third most common cause of stroke
○ Chronic hypertension
○ Cerebral aneurysms
○ Arteriovenous malformation

Risk factors

○ History of transient ischemic attack
○ Heart disease
○ Smoking
○ Familial history of cerebrovascular disease
○ Obesity
○ Alcohol use
○ High red blood cell count
○ Cardiac arrhythmias
○ Diabetes mellitus
○ Gout
○ High serum triglyceride levels

○ Use of hormonal contraceptives in conjunction with smoking and hypertension
○ Elevated cholesterol and triglycerides

Incidence

○ Mostly affects older adults but can strike at any age
○ More common in men than in women
○ Affects Blacks and Hispanics more commonly than other groups

Common characteristics

○ Sudden unilateral weakness or numbness in limb
○ Sudden speech difficulties
○ Sudden vision disturbances
○ Sudden ataxia, gait disturbance
○ Sudden altered level of consciousness (LOC)
○ Sudden severe headache

Complications

○ Unstable blood pressure from loss of vasomotor control
○ Fluid and electrolyte imbalances
○ Malnutrition
○ Infections
○ Sensory impairment
○ Altered LOC
○ Aspiration
○ Contractures
○ Skin breakdown
○ Deep vein thrombosis
○ Pulmonary emboli
○ Depression

Assessment

History

○ Varying clinical features, depending on:
  – artery affected
  – severity of damage
  – extent of collateral circulation
○ One or more risk factors present
○ Sudden onset of hemiparesis or hemiplegia
○ Gradual onset of dizziness, mental disturbances, or seizures
○ Loss of consciousness or sudden aphasia

Physical findings

○ With stroke in left hemisphere, signs and symptoms on right side
○ With stroke in right hemisphere, signs and symptoms on left side
○ With stroke that causes cranial nerve damage, signs and symptoms on same side
○ Change in LOC
○ With conscious patient, anxiety along with communication and mobility difficulties
○ Urinary incontinence
○ Loss of voluntary muscle control
○ Hemiparesis or hemiplegia on one side of the body
○ Decreased deep tendon reflexes

- Hemianopsia on the affected side of the body
- With left-sided hemiplegia, problems with visuospatial relations
- Sensory losses

Test results

Laboratory
- Laboratory tests — including anticardiolipin antibodies, antiphospholipid, factor V (Leiden) mutation, antithrombin III, protein S, and protein C — may show increased thrombotic risk.

Imaging
- Magnetic resonance imaging and magnetic resonance angiography allow for evaluation of the location and size of the lesion.
- Cerebral angiography details the disruption of cerebral circulation and is the test of choice for examining the entire cerebral blood flow.
- Computed tomography scan detects structural abnormalities.
- Positron emission tomography provides data on cerebral metabolism and on cerebral blood flow changes.

Other
- Transcranial Doppler studies evaluate the velocity of blood flow.
- Carotid Doppler measures flow through the carotid arteries.
- Two-dimensional echocardiogram evaluates the heart for dysfunction.
- Cerebral blood flow studies measure blood flow to the brain.
- Electrocardiogram evaluates electrical activity in an area of cortical infarction.

Treatment

General
- Careful blood pressure management
- Pureed dysphagia diet or tube feedings, if indicated
- Physical, speech, and occupational rehabilitation
- Helping patient adapt to specific deficits

Medication
- Tissue plasminogen activator when the cause isn't hemorrhagic (emergency care within 3 hours of onset of the symptoms)
- Anticonvulsants
- Stool softeners
- Anticoagulants
- Analgesics
- Antidepressants
- Antiplatelets
- Lipid-lowering agents
- Antihypertensives

Surgery
- Craniotomy
- Endarterectomy
- Extracranial-intracranial bypass
- Ventricular shunts

Preventing stroke

To decrease the risk of another stroke, teach the patient and family members about the need to correct risk factors. For example, if the patient smokes, refer him to a smoking-cessation program. Teach the importance of maintaining an ideal weight and controlling diabetes and hypertension. Teach all patients to follow a low-cholesterol, low-salt diet; perform regular physical exercise; avoid prolonged bed rest; and minimize stress. Early recognition of signs and symptoms of complications or impending stroke is imperative, as is seeking prompt treatment.

Nursing considerations

Key outcomes
The patient will:
- maintain adequate ventilation
- remain free from injury
- achieve maximal independence
- maintain joint mobility and range of motion.

Nursing interventions
- Maintain a patent airway and oxygenation.
- Offer the urinal or bedpan every 2 hours.
- Insert an indwelling urinary catheter, if necessary.
- Ensure adequate nutrition.
- Provide careful mouth and eye care.
- Follow the physical therapy program, and assist the patient with exercise.
- Establish and maintain patient communication.
- Provide psychological support.
- Set realistic short-term goals.
- Protect the patient from injury and complications.
- Provide careful positioning to prevent aspiration and contractures.
- Give prescribed drugs.

Monitoring
- Neurologic, GI, and respiratory status
- Vital signs
- Fluid, electrolyte, and nutritional intake
- Development of deep vein thrombosis and pulmonary embolus

Patient teaching

Be sure to cover:
- the disorder, diagnosis, and treatment
- occupational and speech therapy programs
- the dietary and drug regimens
- adverse drug reactions
- stroke prevention. (See *Preventing stroke.*)

Discharge planning
- Refer patient to home care services, outpatient services, and speech and occupational rehabilitation programs as needed.

Strongyloidiasis

Overview

Description

○ A parasitic intestinal infection caused by the helminth *Strongyloides stercoralis*
○ Doesn't confer immunity; in people with autoimmune disorders, possibly overwhelming disseminated infection
○ Because threadworm's reproductive cycle may continue in untreated host for up to 45 years, autoinfection highly probable
○ Most patients recover, but death resulting from debilitating protein loss possible
○ Also called *threadworm infection*

Pathophysiology

○ Larvae develop from noninfective rhabdoid larvae in human feces.
○ The filariform larvae penetrate the human skin, usually at the feet, and then migrate by way of the lymphatic system to the bloodstream and the lungs.
○ Once they enter into pulmonary circulation, the filariform larvae break through the alveoli and migrate upward to the pharynx, where they are swallowed.
○ Larvae then lodge in the small intestine, where they deposit eggs that mature into noninfectious rhabdoid larvae.
○ These larvae migrate into the large intestine and are excreted in feces, starting the cycle again.
○ In autoinfection, rhabdoid larvae mature in the intestine to become infective filariform larvae.

Causes

○ Contact with soil that contains infective *S. stercoralis* filariform larvae

Incidence

○ Endemic to the tropics and subtropics
○ Universal susceptibility

Common characteristics

○ Erythematous maculopapular rash at the site of penetration that produces swelling and pruritus
○ Pulmonary signs including minor hemorrhage, pneumonitis, and pneumonia
○ Intestinal infection producing frequent, watery, and bloody diarrhea, accompanied by intermittent abdominal pain

Complications

○ Malnutrition
○ Anemia
○ Secondary bacterial infection
○ Perforated intestine
○ Septicemia

Assessment

History

○ Institutionalization
○ Autoimmune susceptibility
○ Cough
○ Abdominal pain and diarrhea
○ Recent travel to endemic area

Physical findings

○ Erythematous, pruritic rash at entrance site
○ Normal or hyperactive bowel sounds
○ Crackles

Test results

Laboratory
○ *S. stercoralis* larvae can be observed in a fresh stool specimen (2 hours after excretion, look like hookworm larvae).
○ Eosinophils and larvae may appear in sputum, with marked eosinophilia in disseminated strongyloidiasis (pulmonary phase).
○ Hemoglobin level is decreased.
○ In white blood cell count with differential, eosinophil count is 450 to 700/µl.

Imaging
○ Chest X-rays show alveolar or interstitial infiltrates or pulmonary effusions (pulmonary phase).

Treatment

General

○ High-protein diet
○ I.V. fluids
○ Blood transfusion

Medication

○ Thiabendazole

Nursing considerations

Key outcomes

The patient will:
○ experience no further weight loss
○ maintain normal fluid and electrolyte balance
○ express feelings of increased comfort and decreased pain.

Nursing interventions

○ Encourage high-protein diet.
○ Wear gloves when handling bedpans or giving perineal care, and dispose of feces promptly.
○ In pulmonary infection, reposition the patient frequently, encourage coughing and deep breathing, and administer oxygen, as ordered.

Monitoring
○ Intake and output
○ Response to treatment
○ Respiratory status
○ Amount and character of stools

Patient teaching

Be sure to cover:
○ the possibility that thiabendazole may cause mild nausea, vomiting, drowsiness, and giddiness
○ proper hand-washing technique, stressing the importance of washing hands before eating and after defecating
○ the need to wear shoes when in endemic areas.

Discharge planning
○ Check the patient's family and close contacts for signs of infection.
○ Emphasize the need for follow-up stool examination, continuing for several weeks after treatment.

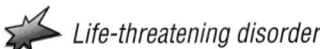

Subdural hematoma

Overview

Description

○ Meningeal hemorrhage resulting from accumulation of blood in subdural space
○ May be acute (less than 72 hours old), subacute (3 to 20 days old), or chronic (older than 20 days)
○ May be unilateral or bilateral

Pathophysiology

Acute
○ Blunt impact to the skull may cause a tear in connecting veins (rarely, arteries) in the cerebral cortex.
Chronic
○ Chronic subdural hematoma begins as a separation in the dura-arachnoid interface, which then is filled by cerebrospinal fluid (CSF).
○ Dural border cells proliferate around this CSF collection to produce a neomembrane.
○ Fragile new vessels grow into the membrane and hemorrhage.

Causes

○ Head trauma

Risk factors

Acute
○ Anticoagulation therapy
○ Age
Chronic
○ Alcoholism
○ Epilepsy
○ Coagulopathy
○ Arachnoid cysts
○ Anticoagulant therapy (including aspirin)
○ Cardiovascular disease (hypertension, arteriosclerosis)
○ Thrombocytopenia
○ Diabetes

Incidence

○ Acute type occurs in 5% to 25% of patients with severe head injuries.
○ Acute type is most common in people older than age 40; chronic type is most common in people older than age 50.
○ Both types occur more frequently in men than in women.

Common characteristics

○ Headache
○ Deteriorating mental status

○ Dilated, nonreactive pupil ipsilateral to the hematoma
○ Hemiparesis contralateral to the hematoma

Complications

○ Neurological impairment
○ Coma
○ Death

Assessment

History

○ Head trauma
○ Headache
○ Change in level of consciousness (LOC)

Physical findings

○ Dilated, nonreactive pupil ipsilateral to the hematoma
○ Hemiparesis contralateral to the hematoma
○ Balance problems
○ Altered LOC

Test results

Laboratory
○ CSF is yellow with relatively low protein (chronic subdural hematoma).
○ Coagulation studies may be abnormal.
Imaging
○ Computed tomography scan, X-rays, and arteriography reveal mass and altered blood flow in the area.

Treatment

General

○ Supportive treatment
○ Wound care
○ Fresh frozen plasma (to correct coagulation)
○ Adequate hydration
○ Diet based on extent of injury
○ Nothing by mouth if surgery is necessary
○ Bed rest initially, then activity as tolerated
○ Flat bed after evacuation of hematoma

Medication

○ If coagulation studies are abnormal, vitamin K, fresh frozen plasma, platelets, or clotting products
○ Analgesics (after extent of injury is determined)
○ Osmotic diuretics
○ Anticonvulsants
○ Prophylactic antibiotics (with surgery)

Surgery

○ Burr holes
○ Craniotomy

Nursing considerations

Key outcomes

The patient will:
- remain neurologically stable
- express feelings of increased comfort and decreased pain
- express an understanding of the disorder and treatment regimen.

Nursing interventions

- Provide appropriate wound care.
- Give prescribed drugs.
- Provide emotional support.
- Institute seizure precautions.

Monitoring

- Vital signs
- Neurologic status
- Wound healing
- Seizure activity
- Respiratory status

Patient teaching

Be sure to cover:
- importance of reporting changes in neurological status
- avoiding aspirin as a pain treatment
- observing for CSF drainage and signs of infection.

Discharge planning

- Refer the patient to physical therapy, occupational therapy, and speech therapy, as appropriate.
- Refer the patient to social services, as appropriate.

Substance abuse and dependence

Overview

Description

○ Use of a legal or an illegal substance that causes physical, mental, emotional, or social harm, such as opioids, stimulants, depressants, antianxiety agents, and hallucinogens
○ Number one health problem in the United States

Pathophysiology

○ Tolerance develops when a drug is administered long-term (such as an opioid for a cancer patient), with cross-tolerance developing.
○ Withdrawal occurs with abrupt discontinuation or administration of an antagonist due to rebound noradrenergic activity in the central nervous system (CNS).

Causes

○ Combination of low self-esteem, peer pressure, inadequate coping skills, and curiosity
○ May follow the use of prescribed drugs to relieve physical pain

Risk factors

○ Male gender
○ History of depression
○ History of other substance abuse disorders
○ Familial history
○ Peer pressure
○ Low socioeconomic status

Incidence

○ Can occur at any age
○ Experimentation common beginning in adolescence and preadolescence
○ Affects more than 18 million Americans who use alcohol and 5 million who use illicit drugs (fewer than one-fourth treated)

Common characteristics

○ Nutritional deficiency
○ Mood swings, anxiety, impaired memory, sleep disturbances, flashbacks, slurred speech, depression, and thought disorders
○ Physical signs of substance abuse (based on substance)
○ Withdrawal signs when substance not used

Complications

○ Cardiac and respiratory arrest
○ Intracranial hemorrhage
○ Acquired immunodeficiency syndrome
○ Subacute bacterial endocarditis
○ Hepatitis
○ Cirrhosis
○ Vasculitis
○ Septicemia
○ Thrombophlebitis
○ Pulmonary emboli
○ Gangrene
○ Malnutrition and GI disturbances
○ Respiratory infections
○ Musculoskeletal dysfunction
○ Trauma
○ Depression and increased risk of suicide
○ Psychosis
○ Toxic or allergic reactions
○ Impaired social and occupational functioning

Assessment

History

○ Abdominal pain, nausea, or vomiting
○ Painful injury or chronic illness
○ Feigned illnesses
○ Overdose
○ High tolerance to potentially addictive drugs
○ Amenorrhea
○ Suggestive behavior patterns or the presence of known risk factors
○ Mood swings, anxiety, impaired memory, sleep disturbances, flashbacks, slurred speech, depression, and thought disorders

Physical findings

○ Lacrimation (with opiate withdrawal)
○ Nystagmus (with CNS depressants and phencyclidine intoxication)
○ Drooping eyelids (with opiate or CNS depressant use)
○ Constricted pupils (with opiate use or withdrawal)
○ Dilated pupils (with hallucinogens or amphetamines)
○ Rhinorrhea (with opiate withdrawal or cocaine abuse)
○ Inflammation, atrophy, or perforation of the nasal mucosa (with drug sniffing)
○ Sweating (with opiates or CNS stimulants or drug withdrawal)
○ Sensation of bugs crawling on the skin (with alcohol withdrawal)
○ Excoriated skin
○ Needle marks or tracks
○ Cellulitis or abscesses
○ Thrombophlebitis
○ Fascial infection
○ Bilateral crackles and rhonchi (with smoking and inhaling drugs or by opiate overdose)
○ Cardiopulmonary signs of overdose (respiratory depression and hypotension)
○ Acute-onset hypertension
○ Cardiac arrhythmias

- ○ Hemorrhoids
- ○ Tremors, hyperreflexia, hyporeflexia, and seizures
- ○ Uncooperative, disruptive, or violent behavior

DSM-IV-TR criteria

- ○ Diagnosis is confirmed with at least three of the following criteria (some symptoms must have persisted for at least 1 month or have occurred repeatedly over a longer time):
  - – substance often taken in larger amounts or for a longer time than the patient intended
  - – persistent desire or one or more unsuccessful efforts to cut down or control substance use
  - – excessive time devoted to activities necessary to obtain the substance
  - – frequent intoxication or withdrawal symptoms when expected to fulfill major obligations at work, school, or home or when substance use is physically hazardous
  - – impaired social, occupational, or recreational activities
  - – continued substance use despite the recognition of a persistent or recurrent social, psychological, or physical problem that's caused or exacerbated by the use of the substance
  - – marked tolerance
  - – characteristic withdrawal symptoms
  - – substance commonly taken to relieve or avoid withdrawal symptoms.

Test results

Laboratory

- ○ Serum or urine drug screen reveals the substance.
- ○ Serum protein electrophoresis shows elevated serum globulin levels.
- ○ Serum glucose measurement shows hypoglycemia.
- ○ Complete blood count (CBC) shows leukocytosis.
- ○ Liver function is abnormal.
- ○ CBC shows elevated mean corpuscular hemoglobin levels.
- ○ Uric acid levels are elevated.
- ○ Blood urea nitrogen levels are decreased.

Treatment

General

- ○ Symptomatic treatment based on the drug ingested
- ○ Fluid replacement therapy
- ○ Symptomatic treatment for complications
- ○ Gastric lavage, induced emesis, activated charcoal instillation, forced diuresis and, possibly, hemoperfusion or hemodialysis
- ○ Detoxification (inpatient or outpatient)
- ○ Psychotherapy
- ○ Exercise
- ○ Relaxation techniques
- ○ Rehabilitation
- ○ Well-balanced diet
- ○ Monitored activity for safety

Medication

- ○ Detoxification with the same drug or a pharmacologically similar drug
- ○ Sedatives
- ○ Anticholinergics
- ○ Antidiarrheal agents
- ○ Antianxiety drugs
- ○ Anticonvulsants
- ○ Nutritional and vitamin supplements

Nursing considerations

Key outcomes

The patient will:
- ○ express his feelings related to self-esteem
- ○ join gradually in self-care and the decision-making process
- ○ engage in social interactions with others
- ○ participate with his family to identify and use support systems.

Nursing interventions

- ○ Maintain a quiet, safe environment.
- ○ Institute seizure precautions.
- ○ Set limits for dealing with demanding, manipulative behavior.

Monitoring

- ○ Vital signs
- ○ Suicide ideation
- ○ Visitors
- ○ Signs of complications
- ○ Nutrition
- ○ Effects of pharmacologic therapy

Patient teaching

Be sure to cover:
- ○ the disorder, diagnosis, and treatment
- ○ detoxification and rehabilitation, as appropriate
- ○ measures for preventing human immunodeficiency virus infection and hepatitis
- ○ measures for safer sex and birth control.

Discharge planning

- ○ Recommend participation in a drug-oriented self-help group.
- ○ Refer the patient to support services.

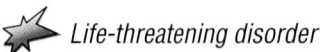

Sudden infant death syndrome

Overview

Description
○ Sudden death of an infant younger than age 1 year without identifiable cause
○ Also known as *SIDS* and *crib death*

Pathophysiology
Hypotheses
○ The infant may have damage to the respiratory control center in the brain from chronic hypoxemia.
○ The infant may not respond to increasing carbon dioxide levels. During an episode of apnea, carbon dioxide levels increase, but the child isn't stimulated to breathe. As apnea continues, high levels of carbon dioxide further suppress the ventilatory effort until the infant stops breathing.
○ The infant may have periods of sleep apnea and eventually die during one of these episodes.

Causes
○ Possibly viral
○ Hypoxia theory
○ Apnea theory
○ Possible *Clostridium botulinum* toxin
○ Possibly associated with diphtheria, tetanus, and pertussis vaccines

Incidence
○ About 7,000 SIDS deaths annually in United States
○ 2 in every 1,000 live births; about 60% male

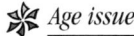 *Age issue*

SIDS occurs mostly between ages 1 and 4 months. Incidence declines rapidly between ages 4 and 12 months.

○ Increased incidence in non–breast-fed infants
○ Occurs most often in fall and winter
○ Slightly higher incidence in:
 – Preterm neonates
 – Inuit neonates
 – Disadvantaged Black neonates
 – Neonates of mothers younger than age 20
 – Neonates of multiple births

Common characteristics
○ Respiratory tract infections
○ Apnea

Complications
○ Always fatal

Assessment

History
○ Occasionally, respiratory tract infection
○ Possible abnormal hepatic or pancreatic function
○ Previous near-miss respiratory event in 60% of cases
○ With infant wedged in a crib corner or with blankets wrapped around head, suffocation ruled out by autopsy as the cause of death
○ With frothy, blood-tinged sputum found around infant's mouth or on crib sheets revealing a patent airway, aspiration of vomitus ruled out by autopsy as cause of death
○ No crying or signs of disturbed sleep by infant

Physical findings
○ Postmortem examination may show:
 – changes indicating chronic hypoxia, hypoxemia, and large airway obstruction
 – bruising; possible fractured ribs
 – blood in the infant's mouth, nose, or ears
 – mottled complexion; extremely cyanotic lips and fingertips
 – pooled blood in legs and feet
 – diaper possibly wet and full of stool.

Test results
Diagnostic procedures
○ Autopsy may show:
 – small or normal adrenal glands
 – enlarged thymus
 – petechiae over the visceral surfaces of the pleura, within the thymus, and in the epicardium
 – well-preserved lymphoid structures
 – signs of chronic hypoxemia
 – increased pulmonary artery smooth muscle
 – edematous, congestive, and fully expanded lungs
 – liquid blood in the heart
 – stomach curd inside the trachea.

Treatment

General
○ Emotional support for the family
○ Prevention for any surviving infant found apneic and any sibling with apnea; assessment with home apnea monitor until the at-risk infant passes age of vulnerability

Nursing considerations

Key outcomes
The family will:
○ use available support systems to assist in coping
○ share feelings about the event

- identify feelings of hopelessness regarding the current situation
- use effective coping strategies to ease spiritual discomfort.

Nursing interventions

- Ensure that both parents are present when the child's death is confirmed.
- Stay calm and allow the parents to express their feelings.
- Reassure the parents that they aren't to blame.
- Allow the parents to see the infant in a private room and to express their grief. Stay in the room with them, if appropriate.
- Offer to call clergy, friends, or relatives.
- Return the infant's belongings to the parents.
- Ensure that the parents receive the autopsy report promptly.

Monitoring

- Parents' reactions and coping mechanisms

Patient teaching

Be sure to cover:
- the need for an autopsy to confirm the diagnosis
- basic facts about SIDS
- information to help parents cope with pregnancy and the first year of a new infant's life, if they decide to have another child.

Discharge planning

- Refer the parents and family to community and health care facility support services.
- Refer the parents to a local SIDS parents' group.
- Advise the parents to contact the SIDS hot line (1-800-221-SIDS).
- Refer the parents to cardiopulmonary resuscitation classes, if appropriate.
- Refer the family to a home health nurse for continued support, if indicated.

Syndrome of inappropriate anitidiuretic hormone secretion

Overview

Description

○ Disease of the posterior pituitary marked by excessive release of antidiuretic hormone (ADH) (vasopressin)
○ Potentially life-threatening
○ Prognosis depends on underlying disorder and response to treatment
○ Also known as *SIADH*

Pathophysiology

○ Excessive ADH secretion occurs in the absence of normal physiologic stimuli for its release.
○ Excessive water reabsorption from the distal convoluted tubule and collecting ducts results in hyponatremia and normal to slightly increased extracellular fluid volume. (See *Understanding SIADH.*)

Causes

○ Oat cell carcinoma of the lung
○ Neoplastic diseases
○ Central nervous system disorders
○ Pulmonary disorders
○ Drugs
○ Miscellaneous conditions, such as myxedema and psychosis

Incidence

○ Common cause of hospital-acquired hyponatremia

Common characteristics

○ Increased water retention
○ Fluid and electrolyte imbalance
○ Hyponatremia

Complications

○ Water intoxication
○ Cerebral edema
○ Severe hyponatremia
○ Heart failure
○ Seizures
○ Coma
○ Death

Assessment

History

○ Possible clue to the cause
○ Cerebrovascular disease
○ Cancer
○ Pulmonary disease
○ Recent head injury
○ Anorexia, nausea, vomiting
○ Weight gain
○ Lethargy, headaches, emotional and behavioral changes

Physical findings

○ Tachycardia
○ Disorientation
○ Seizures and coma
○ Sluggish deep tendon reflexes
○ Muscle weakness

Test results

Laboratory
○ Serum osmolality levels are less than 280 mOsm/kg.
○ Serum sodium levels are less than 123 mEq/L.
○ Urine sodium levels are more than 20 mEq/L without diuretics.
○ Renal function tests are normal.

Treatment

General

○ Based primarily on symptoms
○ Correction of the underlying cause
○ Restricted water intake (500 to 1,000 ml/day)
○ High-salt, high-protein diet or urea supplements to enhance water excretion
○ Activity as tolerated

Medication

○ Demeclocycline or lithium for long-term treatment
○ Loop diuretics if fluid overload, history of heart failure, or resistance to treatment
○ 3% sodium chloride solution if serum sodium level is less than 120 or if the patient is seizing

Surgery

○ To treat underlying cause such as cancer

Nursing considerations

Key outcomes

The patient will:
○ develop no complications
○ remain alert and oriented to the environment
○ verbalize an understanding of the disorder and treatment regimen
○ maintain adequate fluid balance.

The events that produce the syndrome of inappropriate antidiuretic hormone (SIADH) secretion are depicted in this flowchart.

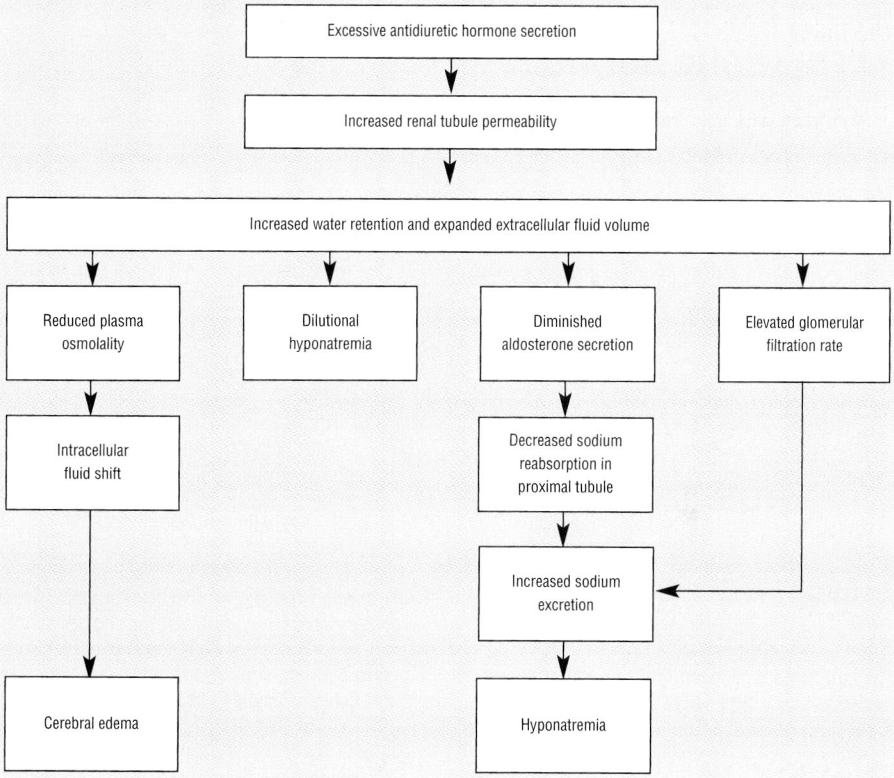

```
┌─────────────────────────────────────────┐
│ Excessive antidiuretic hormone secretion │
└─────────────────────────────────────────┘
                    ↓
┌─────────────────────────────────────────┐
│    Increased renal tubule permeability    │
└─────────────────────────────────────────┘
                    ↓
┌──────────────────────────────────────────────────────────────┐
│ Increased water retention and expanded extracellular fluid volume │
└──────────────────────────────────────────────────────────────┘
```

| Reduced plasma osmolality | Dilutional hyponatremia | Diminished aldosterone secretion | Elevated glomerular filtration rate |

| Intracellular fluid shift | | Decreased sodium reabsorption in proximal tubule | |

Increased sodium excretion

| Cerebral edema | | Hyponatremia |

Nursing interventions

○ Restrict fluids.
○ Provide comfort measures for thirst.
○ Reduce unnecessary environmental stimuli.
○ Orient as needed.
○ Provide a safe environment.
○ Institute seizure precautions as needed.
○ Give prescribed drugs.

Monitoring

○ Intake and output
○ Vital signs
○ Daily weight
○ Serum electrolytes, especially sodium
○ Response to treatment
○ Breath sounds
○ Heart sounds
○ Neurologic checks
○ Changes in level of consciousness

 Alert

Watch closely for signs and symptoms of heart failure, which may occur because of fluid overload.

Patient teaching

Be sure to cover:
○ the disorder, diagnosis, and treatment
○ fluid restriction
○ methods to decrease discomfort from thirst
○ prescribed drugs and possible adverse effects
○ self-monitoring techniques for fluid retention such as daily weight
○ signs and symptoms that require immediate medical intervention.

Syphilis

Overview

Description

○ Chronic, infectious, sexually transmitted disease
○ Untreated, progresses in four stages: primary, secondary, latent, and late (formerly called tertiary)

Pathophysiology

○ The infecting organism penetrates intact mucous membranes or abrasions in the skin, entering lymphatics and blood.
○ Systemic infection and systemic foci precede primary lesion development at the site of inoculation.
○ Organ involvement occurs from dissemination.

Causes

○ The spirochete *Treponema pallidum*
○ Transmission primarily through sexual contact during the primary, secondary, and early latent stages of infection
○ Prenatal transmission possible
○ Transmission by way of fresh blood transfusion (rare)

Incidence

○ In the United States, incidence highest in urban populations, especially in people between ages 15 and 39, drug users, and those infected with human immunodeficiency virus (HIV)
○ About 34,000 cases, in primary and secondary stages, reported in the United States annually

Complications

○ Cardiovascular disease
○ Irreversible neurologic disease
○ Irreversible organ damage
○ Membranous glomerulonephritis
○ With fetal infection:
  – Spontaneous abortion
  – Stillbirth
  – Low birth weight
  – Deafness

Assessment

History

○ Unprotected sexual contact with an infected person or with multiple or anonymous sexual partners

Physical findings

Primary syphilis
○ One or more chancres (small, fluid-filled lesions) on the genitalia; others on the anus, fingers, lips, tongue, nipples, tonsils, or eyelids

○ In female patient, possible chancres on cervix or vaginal wall
○ Unilateral or bilateral adenopathy

Secondary syphilis
○ Headache, malaise
○ Nausea, vomiting
○ Anorexia, weight loss
○ Sore throat, slight fever
○ Symmetrical mucocutaneous lesions
○ Rash possibly macular, papular, pustular, or nodular
○ Lesions uniform, well defined, and generalized
○ Macules typically erupting between rolls of fat on the trunk and proximally on the arms, palms, soles, face, and scalp
○ In warm, moist body areas, lesions enlarged and eroding, producing highly contagious, pink or grayish white lesions (condylomata lata)
○ Alopecia
○ Brittle and pitted nails
○ Generalized lymphadenopathy

Latent syphilis
○ Physical signs and symptoms absent except for possible recurrence of mucocutaneous lesions that resemble those of secondary syphilis

Late syphilis
○ Findings that vary with the involved organ
○ Three subtypes:
  – Neurosyphilis affecting meningovascular tissues: headache, vertigo, insomnia, hemiplegia, seizures, and psychological difficulties; if parenchymal tissue affected: paresis, alteration in intellect, paranoia, illusions, and hallucinations; in addition, Argyll Robertson pupil (a small, irregular pupil that's nonreactive to light but accommodates for vision), ataxia, slurred speech, trophic joint changes, positive Romberg's sign, and a facial tremor
  – Late benign: gummas (lesions that develop between 1 and 10 years after infection and may be a chronic, superficial nodule or a deep, granulomatous lesion that's solitary, asymmetrical, painless, indurated, and large or small) visible on the skin and mucocutaneous tissues; commonly affect bones and can develop in any organ
  – Cardiovascular: decreased cardiac output that may cause decreased urine output and decreased sensorium related to hypoxia, pulmonary congestion

Test results

Laboratory
○ Dark-field microscopy identifies *T. pallidum* from lesion exudate to provide an immediate syphilis diagnosis. (See *Identifying syphilis by dark-field microscopy.*)
○ Non-treponemal serologic tests include the Venereal Disease Research Laboratory (VDRL) slide test, the rapid plasma reagin (RPR) test, and the automated reagin test, detecting nonspecific antibodies.
○ Treponemal serologic studies include the fluorescent treponemal antibody absorption test, the *T. pallidum* hemagglutination assay, and the microhemagglutina-

tion assay, detecting the specific antitreponemal antibody and confirming positive screening results.
○ Cerebrospinal fluid examination identifies neurosyphilis when the total protein level is above 40 mg/dl, the VDRL slide test is reactive, and the white blood cell count exceeds 5 mononuclear cells/µl.

Treatment

General

○ Immediate examination of all sexual contacts
○ Avoidance of pregnancy until a good response to therapy is demonstrated
○ Hospitalization for symptomatic late syphilis
○ No sexual activity until cured

Medication

○ Antibiotics (penicillin being the treatment of choice)

Nursing considerations

Key outcomes

The patient will:
○ voice feelings about changes in sexual activity
○ express concern about self-concept, self-esteem, and body image
○ state infection risk factors
○ exhibit improved or healed lesions or wounds
○ report feelings of increased comfort.

Nursing interventions

○ Follow standard precautions.
○ Give prescribed drugs.
○ Promote rest and adequate nutrition.
○ In secondary syphilis, keep lesions clean and dry; dispose of contaminated materials properly.
○ Report all syphilis cases to the appropriate health authorities.

Monitoring

○ Neurologic status
○ Cardiovascular status
○ Complications
○ Response to treatment
○ Compliance with treatment

Patient teaching

Be sure to cover:
○ the disorder, diagnosis, and treatment
○ the importance of completing the prescribed course of therapy even after symptoms subside
○ the importance of informing, testing, and treating sexual partners
○ the need to refrain from sexual activity until treatment is completed and follow-up VDRL/RPR test results are normal

Identifying syphilis by dark-field microscopy

The presence of spiral-shaped bacteria (*Treponema pallidum*) on dark-field examination confirms the diagnosis of syphilis.

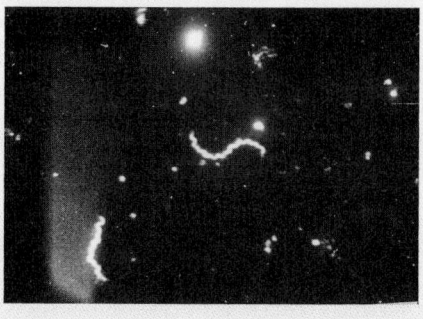

○ information for patient and sexual partners about HIV infection
○ risks to the fetus if the patient is contemplating pregnancy
○ following safer sex practices.

Discharge planning

○ As needed, obtain a physical or occupational therapy consultation.
○ Refer the patient for contact tracing.
○ Refer the patient to a specialist if congenital syphilis is suspected.
○ Consult a social worker to determine home care needs.

Systemic lupus erythematosus

Overview

Description
○ A chronic inflammatory autoimmune disorder that affects connective tissues
○ Two forms: discoid lupus erythematosus (DLE) and systemic lupus erythematosus (SLE)
○ Only the skin affected by DLE

Pathophysiology
○ The body produces antibodies, such as antinuclear antibodies (ANAs), against its own cells.
○ The formed antigen-antibody complexes suppress the body's normal immunity and damage tissues.
○ Patients with SLE produce antibodies against many different tissue components, such as red blood cells (RBCs), neutrophils, platelets, lymphocytes, and almost any organ or tissue in the body.

Causes
○ Unknown
○ Predisposing factors:
  – Stress
  – Streptococcal or viral infections
  – Exposure to sunlight or ultraviolet light
  – Injury
  – Surgery
  – Exhaustion
  – Emotional upsets
  – Immunization, pregnancy
  – Abnormal estrogen metabolism

Incidence
○ Affects women eight times more often than men (15 times more often during childbearing years)
○ Occurs worldwide; most prevalent among Asians and Blacks

Common characteristics
○ Recurrent seasonal remissions and exacerbations, especially during spring and summer

Complications
○ Pleurisy
○ Pleural effusions
○ Pericarditis, myocarditis, endocarditis
○ Coronary atherosclerosis
○ Renal failure
○ Seizures and mental dysfunction

Assessment

History
○ Onset acute or insidious; no characteristic clinical pattern
○ Possible fever, anorexia, weight loss, malaise, fatigue, abdominal pain, nausea, vomiting, diarrhea, constipation, rash, and polyarthralgia
○ Possible drug history with one of 25 drugs that can cause SLE-like reaction
○ Irregular menstruation or amenorrhea, particularly during flare-ups
○ Chest pain and dyspnea
○ Emotional instability, psychosis, organic brain syndrome, headaches, irritability, and depression
○ Oliguria, urinary frequency, dysuria, and bladder spasms

Physical findings
○ Joint involvement that resembles rheumatoid arthritis
○ Raynaud's phenomenon
○ Skin eruptions provoked or aggravated by sunlight or ultraviolet light
○ Tachycardia, central cyanosis, and hypotension
○ Altered level of consciousness, weakness of the extremities, and speech disturbances
○ Skin lesions
○ Butterfly rash over nose and cheeks
○ Patchy alopecia (common)
○ Vasculitis
○ Lymph node enlargement (diffuse or local and nontender)
○ Pericardial friction rub

Test results
Laboratory
○ Complete blood count with differential shows anemia and a reduced white blood cell (WBC) count, decreased platelet count, and elevated erythrocyte sedimentation rate; serum electrophoresis shows hypergammaglobulinemia.
○ ANA, anti-deoxyribonucleic acid, and lupus erythematosus cell test findings are positive in most patients with active SLE, but these are only slightly useful in diagnosing the disease. (ANA test is sensitive but not specific for SLE.)
○ Urine studies show RBCs, WBCs, urine casts, sediment, and significant protein loss (more than 3.5 g in 24 hours).
○ Blood studies demonstrate decreased serum complement (C3 and C4) levels, indicating active disease. (Leukopenia, mild thrombocytopenia, and anemia are also seen during active disease.)
○ C-reactive protein level is increased during flare-ups.
○ Rheumatoid factor is positive in 30% to 40% of patients.
Imaging
○ Chest X-rays may disclose pleurisy or lupus pneumonitis.

Diagnostic procedures

- Central nervous system (CNS) involvement may account for abnormal EEG results in about 70% of patients, but brain and magnetic resonance imaging scans may be normal in patients with SLE despite CNS disease.
- Electrocardiography may show a conduction defect with cardiac involvement or pericarditis.
- Renal biopsy shows progression of SLE and the extent of renal involvement.
- Skin biopsy shows immunoglobulin and complement deposition in the dermal-epidermal junction in 90% of patients.

Treatment

General

- Use of sunscreen with sun protection factor of at least 15
- No dietary restrictions unless renal failure occurs
- Regular exercise program

Medication

- Nonsteroidal anti-inflammatory drugs
- Topical corticosteroid creams
- Fluorinated steroids
- Antimalarials
- Corticosteroids
- Cytotoxic drugs
- Antihypertensives

Surgery

- Possible joint replacement

Nursing considerations

Key outcomes

The patient will:
- express feelings of increased comfort and decreased pain
- express feelings of increased energy
- maintain joint mobility and range of motion (ROM)
- maintain skin integrity
- maintain fluid balance.

Nursing interventions

- Provide a balanced diet.
- Provide bland, cool foods if the patient has a sore mouth.
- Provide a mouth rinse of normal saline solution after meals to assist healing of oral lesions.
- Apply heat packs to relieve joint pain and stiffness.
- Encourage regular exercise to maintain full ROM.
- Explain the expected benefit of prescribed drugs, and watch for adverse effects.
- Institute seizure precautions if you suspect CNS involvement.

- Warm and protect the patient's hands and feet if she has Raynaud's phenomenon.
- Support the patient's self-image.

Monitoring

- Signs and symptoms of organ involvement
- Urine, stools, and GI secretions for blood
- Scalp for hair loss and skin and mucous membranes for petechiae, bleeding, ulceration, pallor, and bruising
- Response to treatment
- Complications
- Nutritional status
- Joint mobility
- Seizure activity

Patient teaching

Be sure to cover:
- the disorder, diagnosis, and treatment
- ROM exercises and body alignment and postural techniques
- ways to avoid infection, such as avoiding crowds and people with known infections
- the need to notify a physician if fever, cough, or rash occurs or if chest, abdominal, muscle, or joint pain worsens
- the importance of eating a balanced diet and the restrictions associated with prescribed drugs
- prescribed drugs
- the importance of good skin care
- the benefits of exercise
- the importance of keeping regular follow-up appointments and contacting a physician if flare-ups occur
- the need to wear protective clothing and use a sunscreen
- how to perform meticulous mouth care.

Discharge planning

- Arrange for a physical therapy and occupational therapy consultation if musculoskeletal involvement compromises mobility.
- Refer the patient to a rheumatology specialist if she becomes pregnant.

Taeniasis

Overview

Description

○ A parasitic infestation by *Taenia saginata* (beef tapeworm), *T. solium* (pork tapeworm), *Diphyllobothrium latum* (fish tapeworm), or *Hymenolepis nana* (dwarf tapeworm)
○ Although usually a chronic, benign intestinal disease, dangerous systemic and central nervous system (CNS) symptoms possible if *T. solium* larvae invade the brain or striated muscle of vital organs
○ Also called *tapeworm disease* and *cestodiasis*

Pathophysiology

○ Gastric acid activates larvae, allowing them to mature, after ingestion of undercooked, bacteria-infested beef or pork.
○ Mature tapeworms fasten to the intestinal wall and produce ova that are passed in the feces.
○ A single tapeworm produces an average of 50,000 eggs per day and may live 25 years.

Causes

T. saginata
○ Uncooked or undercooked beef

T. solium
○ Uncooked or undercooked pork

D. latum
○ Uncooked or undercooked freshwater fish, such as pike, trout, salmon, and turbot

H. nana
○ No intermediate host
○ Person-to-person transmission via ova passed in stool
○ Inadequate hand-washing facilities

Incidence

T. saginata
○ Worldwide, but most prevalent in Europe and East Africa

T. solium
○ Incidence highest in Mexico and Latin America
○ Lowest incidence among Muslims and Jews

D. latum
○ Most prevalent in Finland, parts of the former Soviet Union, Japan, Alaska, Australia, the Great Lakes region of the United States, Switzerland, Chile, and Argentina

H. nana
○ Most common tapeworm in humans
○ Particularly prevalent among institutionalized mentally retarded children and in underdeveloped countries

Common characteristics

T. saginata
○ Crawling sensation in the perianal area caused by worm segments that have passed rectally

T. solium
○ Seizures
○ Headaches
○ Personality changes

D. latum
○ Anemia

H. nana
○ Dependent on patient's nutritional status and number of parasites
○ Commonly no symptoms with mild infestation
○ With severe infestation, anorexia, diarrhea, restlessness, dizziness, and apathy

Complications

○ Appendicitis
○ Obstruction of bile ducts and pancreatic duct

Assessment

History

○ Ingestion of raw or undercooked beef or pork
○ Occasionally, worm segments exiting through the anus and appearing on bed clothes
○ Increased hunger
○ Weight loss
○ Nausea
○ Abdominal pain (usually in the morning) relieved by eating
○ Pruritus ani

Physical findings

○ Weight loss
○ Intraocular larvae

Test results

Laboratory
○ Observation of tapeworm ova or body segments in feces (may require multiple specimens)

Treatment

General

○ Diet as tolerated
○ Activity as tolerated

Medication

○ Anthelmintics
○ High-dose glucocorticosteroids

During treatment for T. solium, *other health-related measures, such as laxative use and induced vomiting, are contraindicated because of the danger of autoinfection and systemic disease.*

Surgery
○ Possible if complications develop

Nursing considerations

Key outcomes
The patient will:
○ express understanding of illness
○ exhibit no signs of infection
○ regain or maintain optimal weight.

Nursing interventions
○ Dispose of the patient's excretions carefully. Wear gloves when giving personal care and handling fecal excretions, bedpans, and bed linens; wash your hands thoroughly and instruct the patient to do the same.
○ Tell the patient not to consume anything after midnight on the day niclosamide therapy begins because the drug must be taken on an empty stomach. After administering the drug, document passage of strobilae.

Monitoring
○ Stool specimens
○ Daily weight
○ Response to treatment

Patient teaching

Be sure to cover:
○ the diagnosis and treatment
○ expected response to treatment
○ preventing reinfection by washing hands thoroughly and cooking meat and fish thoroughly.

Discharge planning
○ After drug treatment, all types of tapeworm infestation require a follow-up laboratory examination of stool specimens during the next 3 to 5 weeks to check for any remaining ova or worm segments.
○ Persistent infestation typically requires a second course of medication.

Tay-Sachs disease

Overview

Description

○ Lipid storage disease that results from a congenital enzyme deficiency
○ Leads to progressive mental and motor deterioration
○ Always fatal, usually before age 5
○ Rare form occurs in patients between ages 20 and 30
○ No known cure

Pathophysiology

○ In this autosomal recessive disorder, the enzyme hexosaminidase A is absent or deficient.
○ Without hexosaminidase A, lipid pigments (ganglioside GM_2) accumulate and progressively destroy and demyelinate central nervous system cells.
○ The juvenile form typically appears between ages 2 and 5 as a progressive deterioration of psychomotor skills and gait.

Causes

○ Autosomal recessive disorder

Incidence

○ Affects fewer than 100 infants born yearly in the United States
○ About 100 times more common (about 1 in 3,600 live births) in those with Ashkenazic Jewish ancestry than in the general population
○ About 1 in 30 Ashkenazi Jews, French Canadians, and American Cajuns heterozygous carriers of gene for this disorder

Common characteristics

○ Progressive mental and motor deterioration
○ Blindness
○ Deafness
○ Inability to swallow
○ Cherry-red spot on the retina

Complications

○ Recurrent bronchopneumonia
○ Dementia
○ Blindness
○ Seizures
○ Paralysis
○ Death, usually before age 5

Assessment

History

○ Familial history of Tay-Sachs disease
○ Normal appearance at birth (but with possible exaggerated Moro's reflex)
○ Onset of clinical signs and symptoms between ages 5 and 6 months
○ Progressive deterioration
○ Psychomotor retardation
○ Blindness
○ Dementia

Physical findings

○ In 3- to 6-month-old infant:
 – Apathetic appearance
 – Augmented response to loud sounds
 – Progressive weakness of the neck, trunk, arm, and leg muscles that prevents child from sitting up or lifting head
 – Difficulty turning over
 – Inability to grasp objects
 – Progressive vision loss
○ By age 18 months:
 – Possible seizures
 – Generalized paralysis
 – Spasticity
 – Blindness
 – Holding eyes wide open and rolling eyeballs
 – Pupils always dilated
 – Decerebrate rigidity
 – Complete vegetative state
 – Head circumference possibly showing enlargement
 – Pupils nonreactive to light
 – Ophthalmoscopic examination possibly showing optic nerve atrophy and a distinctive cherry-red spot on the retina
○ In a child who survives bouts of recurrent bronchopneumonia: possible ataxia and progressive motor retardation between ages 2 and 8 years

Test results

Laboratory

○ Serum analysis shows deficient hexosaminidase A.
○ Amniocentesis or chorionic villus sampling allows prenatal diagnosis of hexosaminidase A deficiency.

Treatment

General

○ Supportive care
○ Suctioning
○ Postural drainage to remove secretions
○ Meticulous skin care
○ Long-term care in special facility
○ Tube feedings with nutritional supplements

○ Activity as tolerated
○ Active and passive range-of-motion exercises

Medication

○ Mild laxatives
○ Anticonvulsants

Nursing considerations

Key outcomes

The patient (or family, if appropriate) will:
○ avoid complications
○ maintain a patent airway
○ express understanding of the disease process and treatment regimen
○ seek outside sources to assist with coping and adjustment to the patient's situation.

Nursing interventions

○ Help the patient's family deal with progressive illness and death.
○ Prevent skin breakdown.
○ Provide adequate nutrition.
○ Maintain a patent airway.
○ Implement seizure precautions.
○ Give drug treatments.
○ Stress the importance of amniocentesis in future pregnancies.

Monitoring

○ Vital signs
○ Intake and output
○ Respiratory status
○ Nutritional status
○ Neurologic status
○ Response to treatment

Patient teaching

Be sure to cover:
○ the disorder, diagnosis, and treatment
○ how to perform suctioning when needed
○ how to perform postural drainage
○ how to give tube feedings
○ need for proper skin care to prevent breakdown.

Discharge planning

○ Refer the parents for genetic counseling.
○ Refer the parents to the National Tay-Sachs and Allied Diseases Association.
○ Refer the parents for psychological counseling if indicated.
○ Refer the siblings for screening to determine whether they're carriers.
○ If the siblings are adult carriers, refer them for genetic counseling; stress that the disease isn't transmitted to offspring unless both parents are carriers.

Tendinitis and bursitis

Overview

Description
Tendinitis
○ Inflammation affecting the tendons and tendon-muscle attachments
○ Most common sites:
  – Shoulder rotator cuff
  – Hip
  – Achilles tendon
  – Hamstring
  – Elbow
Bursitis
○ Painful inflammation of one or more bursae
○ Most common sites:
  – Subdeltoid
  – Subacromial
  – Olecranon
  – Trochanteric
  – Calcaneal
  – Prepatellar
○ May be septic, calcific, acute, or chronic

Pathophysiology
Tendinitis
○ Inflammation causes localized pain around the affected area.
○ Joint movement is restricted.
○ Swelling results from fluid accumulation.
○ Calcium deposits form in and around the tendon.
○ Further swelling and immobility result.
Bursitis
○ Bursae sacs hold lubricating synovial fluid.
○ Inflammation causes gradual pain and limits joint motion.

Causes
Tendinitis
○ Trauma (such as a strain during sports activity)
○ Musculoskeletal disorders (rheumatic diseases and congenital defects)
○ Postural malalignment
○ Abnormal body development
○ Hypermobility in calcific tendinitis
Bursitis
○ Recurring trauma from an inflammatory joint disease
○ Common stressors:
  – Repetitive kneeling
  – Jogging in worn-out shoes on hard asphalt surfaces
  – Prolonged sitting with crossed legs on hard surfaces
○ Septic bursitis: wound infection or bacterial invasion (see *Anatomy of tendons and bursae*)

Incidence
○ More common in elderly people

○ Common in those who perform activities that over-stress a tendon or repeatedly stress a joint

Common characteristics
○ Localized pain
○ Interrupted sleep
○ Limited movement
○ Crepitus over involved area
○ Swelling over involved area

Complications
○ Scar tissue with subsequent disability

Assessment

History
Tendinitis
○ Traumatic injury or strain from athletic activity
○ Concurrent musculoskeletal disorder
○ Palpable tenderness over the affected site
○ Referred tenderness in the related segment
○ Shoulder:
  – Localized pain that's most severe at night
  – Pain that usually interferes with sleep
  – Pain aggravated by heat
○ Elbow: pain when grasping objects or twisting the elbow
○ Hamstring: pain in the posterolateral aspect of the knee
○ Foot: pain over the Achilles tendon and on dorsiflexion
Bursitis
○ Unusual strain or injury 2 to 3 days before pain began
○ Pain that develops suddenly or gradually
○ Pain that may limit movement
○ Work or leisure activity that may involve repetitive action

Physical findings
Tendinitis
○ Shoulder: restricted shoulder movement (especially abduction)
○ Elbow: tenderness over the lateral epicondyle
○ Hamstring: palpable tenderness when knee flexed at a 90-degree angle
○ Foot: crepitus when the patient moves his foot
Bursitis
○ Tenderness over the affected site
○ Swelling with severe bursitis

Test results
Laboratory
○ Various serum and urine test results rule out other disorders.
Imaging
○ X-rays in tendinitis may show bony fragments, osteophyte sclerosis, or calcium deposits.
○ X-rays in calcific bursitis may show calcium deposits in the joint.

Tendons, like stiff rubber bands, hold the muscles in place and enable them to move the bones. Bursae are located at friction points around joints and between tendons, cartilage, or bone. Bursae keep these body parts lubricated so they move freely.

SHOULDER JOINT

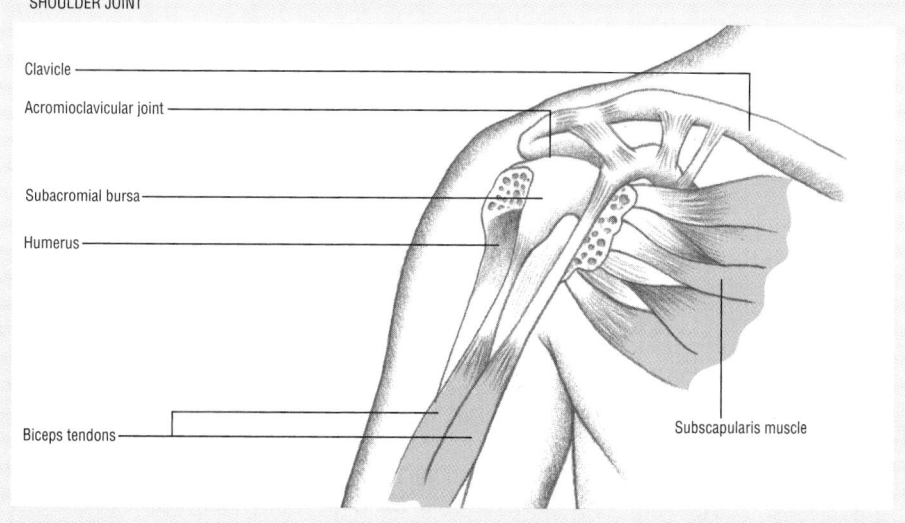

Clavicle

Acromioclavicular joint

Subacromial bursa

Humerus

Biceps tendons

Subscapularis muscle

○ Arthrography is usually normal in tendinitis with minor irregularities on the tendon under the surface.

Diagnostic procedures

○ Arthrocentesis may identify causative microorganisms and other causes of inflammation.

Treatment

General

○ Cold, heat, or ultrasound applications
○ No dietary restrictions
○ Resting the affected joint
○ Range-of-motion (ROM) exercises

Medication

○ Nonsteroidal anti-inflammatory drugs (NSAIDs)
○ Local anesthetics
○ Corticosteroids
○ Oral anti-inflammatory agents
○ Short-term analgesics

Nursing considerations

Key outcomes

The patient will:
○ have increased comfort and decreased pain
○ maintain joint mobility and ROM
○ perform activities of daily living
○ express understanding of the treatment regimen and disease process.

Nursing interventions

○ Apply cold or heat therapies, as ordered.
○ Promote self-care.
○ Give drug therapy.
○ Encourage use of active ROM exercises.

Monitoring

○ Severity and pattern of pain
○ Response to treatment
○ ROM

Patient teaching

Be sure to cover:
○ the disorder, diagnosis, and treatment
○ how to minimize GI distress from NSAIDs
○ adverse drug reactions
○ activities that promote rest and relaxation
○ strengthening exercises
○ the prescribed exercise regimen
○ need for proper sports equipment, shoes, and playing surfaces
○ use of cushioned shoes
○ application of cold packs
○ proper body mechanics.

Discharge planning

○ Refer the patient to a weight-management program, as appropriate.

Testicular cancer

Overview

Description

- Proliferation of cancerous cells in the testicles
- Most originating from germinal cells and about 40% becoming seminomas
- Prognosis dependent on cancer cell type and stage (with treatment, a more than 5-year survival rate)

Pathophysiology

- Testicular cancer spreads through the lymphatic system to the iliac, para-aortic, and mediastinal nodes.
- Metastases affect the lungs, liver, viscera, and bone.

Causes

- Exact cause unknown

Risk factors

- Cryptorchidism (see *Cryptorchidism and testicular cancer*)
- Mumps orchitis
- Inguinal hernia in childhood
- Maternal use of diethylstilbestrol (DES) or other estrogen-progestin combinations during pregnancy

Common characteristics

- Fullness of testes
- Lump in testes

Incidence

- Most common in men ages 20 to 40
- Rare in nonwhite men
- Accounts for less than 1% of all male cancer deaths
- Rare in children

Complications

- Back or abdominal pain from retroperitoneal adenopathy

Cryptorchidism and testicular cancer

In men with cryptorchidism (the failure of a testicle to descend into the scrotum), testicular tumors are about 50 times more common than in men with normal anatomic structure. A simple surgical procedure, called orchiopexy, can bring the testicle to its normal position in the scrotum and reduce the testicular cancer risk. Nevertheless, testicular tumors occur more commonly in a surgically descended testicle than in a naturally descended one.

What happens in orchiopexy
In orchiopexy, the surgeon incises the groin area and separates the testicle and its blood supply from surrounding abdominal structures. Then, he creates a "tunnel" into the scrotum to accommodate the descent of the testicle.

Reducing the risk further
After orchiopexy, urge the patient to examine his testicles monthly to detect a tumor at its earliest stage.

- Metastasis
- Ureteral obstruction

Assessment

History

- Previous injury to the scrotum
- Viral infection (such as mumps)
- Use of DES or other estrogen-progestin drugs by the patient's mother during pregnancy
- Feeling of heaviness or a dragging sensation in the scrotum
- Weight loss (late sign)
- Fatigue and weakness (late sign)

Physical findings

- Enlarged testes
- Gynecomastia
- Lethargic, thin, and pallid appearance (later stages)
- Palpable firm, smooth testicular mass
- Enlarged lymph nodes in surrounding areas

Test results

Laboratory
- Elevated levels of the proteins (tumor markers) human chorionic gonadotropin (HCG) and alpha-fetoprotein (AFP) suggest testicular cancer and can differentiate a seminoma from a nonseminoma.
- Elevated HCG and AFP levels indicate a nonseminoma.
- Elevated HCG and normal AFP levels indicate a seminoma.

Diagnostic procedures
- Biopsy confirms the diagnosis and can be used to stage the disease.

Treatment

General

- Varies with tumor cell type and stage
- Radiation therapy
- Autologous bone marrow transplantation for patients nonresponsive to standard therapy
- Well-balanced diet

Medication

- Chemotherapy
- Hormonal therapy

Surgery

- Orchiectomy and retroperitoneal node dissection

Nursing considerations

Key outcomes

The patient will:
- express positive feelings about himself
- report feeling less tension or pain

- avoid or minimize complications
- voice understanding of treatment
- express feelings and perceptions about change in sexual performance.

Nursing interventions
- Encourage verbalization and provide support.
- Administer drug therapy.
- Apply an ice pack to the scrotum.

Monitoring
- Wound site
- Vital signs
- Hydration and nutritional status
- Pain control
- Effects of medication
- Postoperative complications

Patient teaching

Be sure to cover:
- the disorder, diagnosis, and treatment
- reassurance that infertility and impotence usually don't follow unilateral orchiectomy
- sperm-banking procedures before the patient begins treatment, especially if infertility and impotence may result from surgery
- testicular self-examination.

Discharge planning
- Refer the patient to available resource and support services.

Testicular torsion

Overview

Description

- An abnormal twisting of the spermatic cord caused by rotation of a testis or the mesorchium (a fold in the area between the testis and epididymis)
- Causes strangulation and eventual infarction of the testis if untreated
- 90% of cases unilateral

Pathophysiology

- Normally, the tunica vaginalis envelops the testis and attaches to the epididymis and spermatic cord.
- In intravaginal torsion (the most common type of testicular torsion in adolescents), testicular twisting may result from an abnormality of the tunica, in which the testis is abnormally positioned, or from a narrowing of the mesentery support.
- In extravaginal torsion (most common in neonates), loose attachment of the tunica vaginalis to the scrotal lining causes spermatic cord rotation above the testis. A sudden forceful contraction of the cremaster muscle may precipitate this condition. (See *Extravaginal torsion.*)

Causes

- Congenital anomaly
- Trauma
- Sexual activity
- Undescended testicle
- Exercise

Extravaginal torsion

In extravaginal torsion, rotation of the spermatic cord above the testis causes strangulation and, eventually, infarction of the testis.

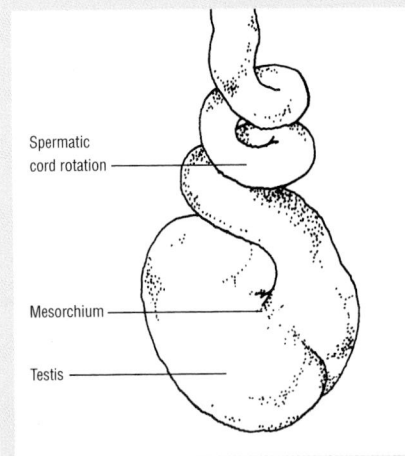

Spermatic cord rotation

Mesorchium

Testis

Incidence

- Most common between ages 12 and 18, but may occur at any age
- Occurs in 1 in 4,000 males younger than age 25

Common characteristics

- Excruciating pain in the affected testis or iliac fossa

Complications

- Loss of testicle
- Infarction of testicle
- Infection

Assessment

History

- Previous episodes of intermittent testicular pain that resolved spontaneously
- Sudden scrotal pain
- Nausea and vomiting
- Abdominal pain
- Fever

Physical findings

- Scrotal swelling
- Painful testicle
- Horizontal lie of the testicle
- Scrotal erythema
- Ipsilateral loss of the cremasteric reflex

Test results

Diagnostic procedures
- Doppler ultrasonography helps distinguish testicular torsion from strangulated hernia, undescended testes, or epididymitis.

Treatment

General

- Manual detorsion
- Nothing by mouth before surgery; diet as tolerated after surgery
- Activity as tolerated after surgery

Medication

- Analgesics

Surgery

- Immediate surgical repair by orchiopexy (fixation of a viable testis to the scrotum) or orchiectomy (excision of a nonviable testis); as with ovarian torsion in the female, preservation of the organ preferred

Nursing considerations

Key outcomes

The patient will:
- report increased comfort and decreased pain

○ express understanding of condition and treatment
○ develop no complications.

Nursing interventions

○ Promote the patient's comfort before and after surgery.
○ After surgery, administer drugs for pain.
○ Apply an ice bag with a cover to reduce edema.
○ Protect the wound from contamination.

Monitoring

○ Voiding
○ Scrotal swelling
○ Pain control

Patient teaching

Be sure to cover:
○ the disorder, diagnosis, and treatment
○ wound care.

Tetanus

Overview

Description

- An acute exotoxin-mediated infection
- Usually systemic, but possibly localized
- Up to 60% fatal in unimmunized patients
- Also known as *lockjaw*

Pathophysiology

- After the organism enters the body, local infection and tissue necrosis result.
- Toxins enter the bloodstream and lymphatics, eventually spreading to central nervous system tissue.
- The incubation period is 3 to 21 days.

Causes

- Anaerobic, spore-forming, gram-positive bacillus *Clostridium tetani*
- Transmission through puncture wounds, burns, or minor wounds contaminated by soil, dust, or animal excreta containing *C. tetani*

Incidence

- Occurs worldwide, but more prevalent in agricultural regions and developing countries that lack mass immunization programs
- One of the most common causes of neonatal deaths in developing countries
- In the United States, about 110 cases each year, all in patients who aren't immunized or whose immunization has expired
- About 75% of cases between April and September

Common characteristics

- Usually, a normal body temperature or a slight fever in the early stages; fever may increase as disease progresses
- Despite pronounced neuromuscular symptoms, normal cerebral and sensory function

Complications

- Pneumonia
- Airway obstruction
- Respiratory arrest
- Heart failure
- Fractures
- Cardiac arrhythmias
- Rhabdomyolysis
- Death

Assessment

History

- Inadequate immunization
- Recent wound or burn
- Pain or paresthesia at the site of injury
- Complaints of difficulty chewing or swallowing food

Physical findings

- Spasm and increased muscle tone near the wound (local infection)
- Irregular heartbeat and tachycardia
- Marked muscle hypertonicity
- Hyperactive deep tendon reflexes
- Profuse sweating, low-grade fever
- Painful, involuntary muscle contractions
- Rigid neck and facial muscles, resulting in lockjaw (trismus) and a grotesque, grinning expression (risus sardonicus)
- Rigid somatic muscles causing arched-back rigidity (opisthotonos)
- Intermittent tonic seizures

Test results

Laboratory
- Blood cultures and tetanus antibody tests are negative.
- Wound culture is positive in one-third of patients.
- Cerebrospinal fluid pressure is increased.

Diagnostic procedures
- Lumbar puncture (spinal tap) may show elevated cerebrospinal fluid pressure.

Treatment

General

- Airway maintenance
- Enteral or parenteral feeding
- Bed rest until recovery

Medication

- Tetanus immune globulin
- Tetanus antitoxin
- Tetanus toxoid immunization
- Muscle relaxants
- Neuromuscular blockers
- Antibiotics

Nursing considerations

Key outcomes

The patient will:
- maintain adequate fluid balance
- express feelings of increased comfort and decreased pain
- maintain tissue perfusion and cellular oxygenation
- have a patent airway and adequate ventilation
- show no signs of neurologic compromise.

Nursing interventions

○ Debride and clean the injury site.
○ Check the immunization history.
○ Maintain an adequate airway and ventilation.
○ Keep emergency airway equipment on standby.
○ Administer I.V. therapy as prescribed.
○ Minimize stimulation.
○ Perform range-of-motion exercises.

Monitoring

○ Response to treatment
○ Fluid and electrolyte status
○ Respiratory status
○ Cardiovascular status
○ Injury site
○ Complications
○ Deep tendon reflexes
○ Muscle tone

Patient teaching

Be sure to cover:
○ the disorder, diagnosis, and treatment
○ the importance of getting a booster dose of tetanus toxoid every 10 years
○ the need for tetanus prophylaxis in case of a skin injury or burn
○ the need to avoid external stimulation (evokes muscle spasms) and to keep the room dark and quiet
○ the potential outcomes.

Tetralogy of Fallot

Overview

Description
- A combination of four cardiac defects: ventricular septal defect (VSD); right ventricular outflow tract obstruction (pulmonary stenosis); right ventricular hypertrophy; and dextroposition of the aorta, with overriding of the VSD

Pathophysiology
- Blood shunts right to left through the VSD, permitting unoxygenated blood to mix with oxygenated blood, resulting in cyanosis.
- Condition sometimes coexists with other congenital heart defects, such as patent ductus arteriosus or atrial septal defect.

Causes
- Unknown
- Associated with fetal alcohol syndrome and thalidomide use during pregnancy

Incidence
- Accounts for about 10% of all congenital heart diseases
- Occurs equally in males and females

Common characteristics
- Cyanosis
- Blue spells, which are characterized by dyspnea; deep, sighing respirations; bradycardia; fainting; seizures; and loss of consciousness

Complications
- Cerebral abscesses
- Pulmonary thrombosis
- Venous thrombosis
- Cerebral embolism
- Infective endocarditis
- In females with tetralogy of Fallot who live to childbearing age, increased risk of spontaneous abortion, premature births, and low birth weight

Assessment

History
- Blue spells
- Diminished exercise tolerance
- Increasing dyspnea on exertion
- Growth retardation
- Eating difficulties

Physical findings
- Clubbing
- Cyanosis
- Dyspnea on exertion
- Loud systolic heart murmur (best heard along the left sternal border), which may diminish or obscure the pulmonic component of S_2
- Cardiac thrill at the left sternal border and an obvious right ventricular impulse
- Prominent inferior sternum

Test results
Laboratory
- Arterial oxygen saturation is diminished.
- Polycythemia is present. (Hematocrit may be more than 60%.)

Imaging
- Chest X-rays may demonstrate decreased pulmonary vascular marking, depending on the severity of the pulmonary obstruction, and a boot-shaped cardiac silhouette.
- Echocardiography identifies septal overriding of the aorta, the VSD, and pulmonary stenosis and detects the hypertrophied walls of the right ventricle.

Diagnostic procedures
- Electrocardiogram shows right ventricular hypertrophy, right axis deviation and, possibly, right atrial hypertrophy.
- Cardiac catheterization confirms the diagnosis by showing pulmonary stenosis, the VSD, and the overriding aorta and ruling out other cyanotic heart defects.

Treatment

General
- Prevention and treatment of complications
- During cyanotic spells, knee-chest position and administration of oxygen and morphine to improve oxygenation

Medication
- Beta blockers
- Prophylactic antibiotics

Surgery
- Palliative surgery is performed on infants with potentially fatal hypoxic spells. The goal of surgery is to enhance blood flow to the lungs to reduce hypoxia; this is commonly accomplished by joining the subclavian artery to the pulmonary artery (Blalock-Taussig procedure).
- Complete corrective surgery relieves pulmonary stenosis and closes the VSD, directing left ventricular outflow to the aorta.

Nursing considerations

Key outcomes
The patient and family will:
- maintain hemodynamic stability
- foster improved cardiac blood flow
- express understanding of condition and treatment.

Nursing interventions

○ Provide postoperative care.
○ Administer drug therapy.
○ Explain the disorder and its treatment to the patient's parents. Inform them that their child will set his own exercise limits and will know when to rest.

Monitoring

○ Vital signs
○ Blue spells
○ Oxygenation levels
○ Intake and output

Patient teaching

Be sure to cover:
○ how to recognize serious hypoxic spells, which can cause dramatically increased cyanosis; deep, sighing respirations; and loss of consciousness
○ preventing infective endocarditis and other infections, and keeping the child away from people with infections
○ following good dental hygiene, and watching for ear, nose, and throat infections and dental caries, all of which require immediate treatment.

Thalassemia

Overview

Description

- A group of genetic disorders characterized by defective synthesis in one or more of the polypeptide chains needed for hemoglobin production
- Most commonly occurring as a result of reduced or absent production of alpha or beta chains
- Affects hemoglobin production and impairs red blood cell (RBC) synthesis

Pathophysiology

In beta-thalassemia
- The fundamental defect is the uncoupling of alpha- and beta-chain synthesis.
- Beta-chain production is depressed — moderately in beta-thalassemia minor and severely in beta-thalassemia major (also called *Cooley's anemia*).
- Depression of beta-chain synthesis results in erythrocytes with reduced hemoglobin and accumulations of free-alpha chains.
- The free-alpha chains are unstable and easily precipitate in the cell; most erythroblasts that contain precipitates are destroyed by mononuclear phagocytes in the marrow, resulting in ineffective erythropoiesis and anemia.
- Some precipitate-carrying cells mature and enter the bloodstream but are destroyed prematurely in the spleen, resulting in mild hemolytic anemia.

Skull changes in thalassemia major

This illustration of an X-ray shows a characteristic skull abnormality in thalassemia major: diploetic fibers extending from internal lamina and resembling hair standing on end.

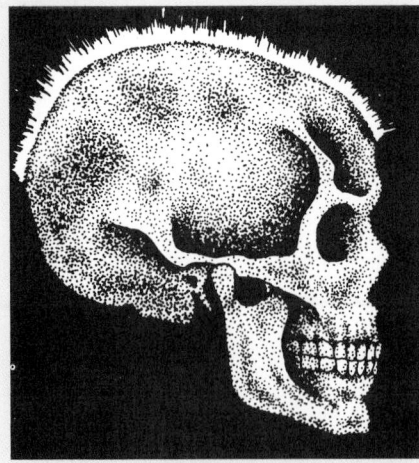

In alpha-thalassemia
- Four forms exist:
    - Alpha trait (the carrier trait), in which a single alpha-chain-forming gene is defective
    - Alpha-thalassemia minor, in which two genes are defective
    - Hemoglobin H disease, in which three genes are defective
    - Alpha-thalassemia major, in which all four alpha-chain–forming genes are defective; death is inevitable because alpha chains are absent and oxygen can't be released to the tissues

Causes

- Inherited autosomal recessive disorder

Incidence

- Second most common cause of microcytic anemia
- Alpha-thalassemia more common in Blacks and Asians
- Beta-thalassemia more common in Mediterranean populations

Common characteristics

- Anemia

Complications

- Iron overload from RBC transfusions
- Pathologic fractures
- Cardiac arrhythmias
- Liver failure
- Heart failure
- Death

Assessment

History

- Severity of anemia and symptoms range from mild to severe, including:
    - fatigue
    - shortness of breath
    - headache
    - angina.

Physical findings

- Pallor or bronze appearance
- Dyspnea on exertion
- Splenomegaly
- Hepatomegaly
- Tachycardia
- Systolic murmur (in moderate or severe anemia)

Test results

Laboratory
- Complete blood count shows decreased hemoglobin, hematocrit, and mean corpuscular volume.
- Serum iron level is normal or increased.
- Serum ferritin level is normal or increased.
- Total iron-binding capacity is normal.

○ Reticulocyte count is normal or increased.
○ Hemoglobin electrophoresis shows decreased alpha- or beta-hemoglobulin chains.

Imaging
○ In thalassemia major, X-rays of the skull and long bones show thinning and widening of the marrow space because of overactive bone marrow. Long bones may show areas of osteoporosis. The phalanges may also be deformed (rectangular or biconvex). The bones of the skull and vertebrae may appear granular. (See *Skull changes in thalassemia major.*)

Treatment

General

○ No treatment for mild or moderate forms
○ Iron supplements contraindicated in all forms
○ Avoidance of iron-rich foods
○ Avoidance of strenuous activities

Medication

○ Transfusions of packed RBCs
○ Desferal (chelation therapy)

Surgery

○ Splenectomy
○ Bone marrow transplantation

Nursing considerations

Key outcomes

The patient will:
○ develop no arrhythmias
○ remain hemodynamically stable
○ demonstrate age-appropriate skills and behaviors to the extent possible.

Nursing interventions

○ Administer blood transfusions, and watch for adverse reactions.
○ Provide an adequate diet, and encourage oral fluid intake.
○ Provide emotional support to help the patient and family cope with the chronic nature of the illness and the need for lifelong transfusions.

Monitoring

○ Transfusion reaction
○ Signs and symptoms of iron overload
○ Complications
○ Cardiac arrhythmias
○ Anemia symptom severity
○ Response to treatment

Patient teaching

Be sure to cover:
○ the disorder, diagnosis, and treatment
○ the importance of good nutrition
○ signs and symptoms of iron overload
○ follow-up care
○ with the parents of a young patient, various options for healthy physical and creative outlets. Such a child must avoid strenuous athletic activity. Reassure the parents that the child may be allowed to participate in less stressful activities.

Discharge planning

○ Refer the patient to a hematologist.
○ Refer the patient for genetic counseling.

Thrombocytopenia

Overview

Description
- A deficient number of circulating platelets
- The most common cause of hemorrhagic disorders

Pathophysiology
- Lack of platelets can cause inadequate hemostasis.
- Four mechanisms are responsible: decreased platelet production, decreased platelet survival, pooling of blood in the spleen, and intravascular dilation of circulating platelets.
- Megakaryocytes are giant cells in bone marrow that produce the marrow. Platelet production decreases when the number of megakaryocytes is reduced or when platelet production becomes dysfunctional.

Causes
- May be congenital or acquired
- Decreased or defective platelet production in the bone marrow
- Increased platelet destruction outside the marrow caused by an underlying disorder (such as cirrhosis of the liver, disseminated intravascular coagulation, or severe infection)
- Sequestration (hypersplenism, hypothermia) or platelet loss
- Transient occurrence after a viral infection (such as Epstein-Barr virus) or infectious mononucleosis

Incidence
- Acquired form more common

Common characteristics
- Sudden onset of petechiae or ecchymoses on skin
- Bleeding into any mucous membrane

Complications
In severe thrombocytopenia
- Hemorrhage
- Death

Assessment

History
- Sudden onset of petechiae and ecchymoses or bleeding into mucous membranes (GI, urinary, vaginal, or respiratory)
- Malaise, fatigue, and general weakness (with or without accompanying blood loss)
- In acquired thrombocytopenia, possible use of one or several offending drugs
- Menorrhagia

Physical findings
- Petechiae and ecchymoses, along with slow, continuous bleeding from any injuries or wounds
- In adults, blood-filled bullae in the mouth

Test results
Laboratory
- Platelet count is diminished to less than 100,000/µl in adults.
- Bleeding time is prolonged.
- Prothrombin and partial thromboplastin times are normal.

Diagnostic procedures
- In severe thrombocytopenia, a bone marrow study shows the number, size, and cytoplasmic maturity of the megakaryocytes (bone marrow cells that release mature platelets); study may show ineffective platelet production as the cause of thrombocytopenia and be used to rule out a malignant disease process.

Treatment

General
- Removal of the offending agents in drug-induced thrombocytopenia
- Well-balanced diet
- Rest periods between activities
- During active bleeding, strict bed rest

Medication
- Platelet transfusions
- Corticosteroids
- Immune globulin

Surgery
- Splenectomy

Nursing considerations

Key outcomes
The patient will:
- incur no injury
- experience no fever, chills, or other signs or symptoms of illness
- demonstrate use of protective measures, energy conservation, a balanced diet, and adequate rest
- demonstrate effective coping skills.

Nursing interventions
- Provide emotional support.
- Provide rest periods between activities.
- Provide a stool softener if necessary.
- Protect all areas of ecchymosis and petechiae from further injury.
- Take precautions against bleeding; protect the patient from trauma.
- Avoid invasive procedures.
- During active bleeding, maintain strict bed rest; keep the head of the bed elevated.

Monitoring

○ Daily platelet count
○ Bleeding
○ Ecchymoses and petechiae
○ Occult blood in stool, urine, and emesis
○ During corticosteroid therapy, fluid and electrolyte balance and signs and symptoms of infection, pathologic fractures, and mood changes

Patient teaching

Be sure to cover:
○ the disorder and its cause, if known and, if appropriate, reassurance that thrombocytopenia commonly resolves spontaneously
○ how to recognize and report signs of intracranial bleeding and other signs of bleeding
○ avoidance of straining with stools and coughing, both of which can lead to increased intracranial pressure
○ the function of platelets
○ in severe thrombocytopenia, an understanding that even minor bumps or scrapes may result in bleeding
○ how to control local bleeding
○ if thrombocytopenia is drug-induced, the importance of avoiding the offending drug
○ if the patient must receive long-term corticosteroid therapy, the need to watch for and report cushingoid symptoms and to discontinue corticosteroids gradually
○ avoidance of aspirin in any form as well as other drugs that impair coagulation
○ if the patient experiences frequent nosebleeds, using a humidifier at night
○ how to examine the skin for ecchymoses and petechiae
○ how to test stools for occult blood
○ the importance of wearing medical identification jewelry.

Thrombophlebitis

Overview

Description

○ Development of a thrombus that may cause vessel occlusion or embolization
○ An acute condition characterized by inflammation and thrombus formation
○ May occur in deep or superficial veins (see *Major venous pathways of the leg*)
○ Typically occurs at the valve cusps because venous stasis encourages accumulation and adherence of platelet and fibrin

Pathophysiology

○ Alteration in epithelial lining causes platelet aggregation and fibrin entrapment of red blood cells, white blood cells, and additional platelets.
○ The thrombus initiates a chemical inflammatory process in the vessel epithelium that leads to fibrosis, which may occlude the vessel lumen or embolize.

Major venous pathways of the leg

Thrombophlebitis can occur in any leg vein. It most commonly occurs at valve sites.

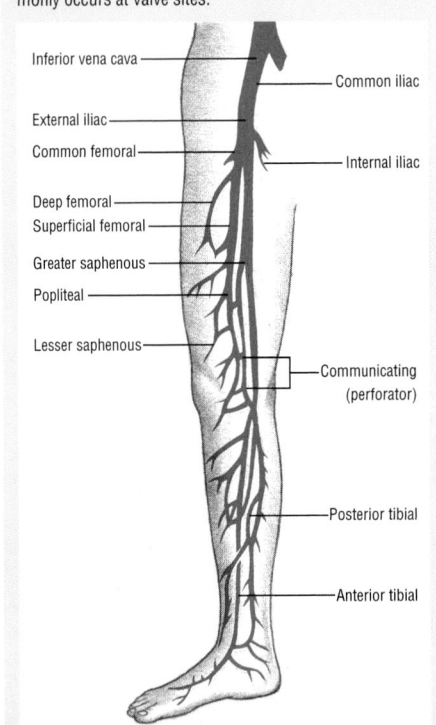

Inferior vena cava
Common iliac
External iliac
Common femoral
Internal iliac
Deep femoral
Superficial femoral
Greater saphenous
Popliteal
Lesser saphenous
Communicating (perforator)
Posterior tibial
Anterior tibial

Causes

○ May be idiopathic
○ Prolonged bed rest
○ Trauma
○ Surgery
○ Pregnancy and childbirth
○ Hormonal contraceptives such as estrogens
○ Neoplasms
○ Fracture of the spine, pelvis, femur, or tibia
○ Venous stasis
○ Venulitis

Incidence

○ Increasing with the use of subclavian vein catheters
○ Risk for developing deep vein thrombophlebitis dramatically increased after age 40

Common characteristics

○ Tenderness, erythema, and warmth over affected area
○ Swelling of affected leg

Complications

○ Pulmonary embolism
○ Chronic venous insufficiency

Assessment

History

○ Asymptomatic in up to 50% of patients with deep vein thrombophlebitis
○ Possible tenderness, aching, or severe pain in the affected leg or arm; fever, chills, and malaise

Physical findings

○ Redness, swelling, and tenderness of the affected leg or arm
○ Possible positive Homans' sign
○ Positive cuff sign
○ Possible warm feeling in affected leg or arm
○ Lymphadenitis in case of extensive vein involvement

Test results

Diagnostic procedures

○ Doppler ultrasonography shows reduced blood flow to a specific area and any obstruction to venous flow, particularly in iliofemoral deep vein thrombophlebitis.
○ Plethysmography shows decreased circulation distal to the affected area and is more sensitive than ultrasonography in detecting deep vein thrombophlebitis.
○ Phlebography confirms the diagnosis and shows filling defects and diverted blood flow.

Treatment

General

○ Application of warm, moist compresses to the affected area

- ○ Antiembolism stockings
- ○ Bed rest, with elevation of the affected extremity

Medication

- ○ Anticoagulants
- ○ Thrombolytics
- ○ Analgesics

Surgery

- ○ Simple ligation to vein plication, or clipping
- ○ Embolectomy
- ○ Caval interruption with transvenous placement of a vena cava filter

Nursing considerations

Key outcomes

The patient will:
- ○ maintain collateral circulation
- ○ express feelings of increased comfort and decreased pain
- ○ maintain tissue perfusion and cellular oxygenation
- ○ develop no signs or symptoms of infection.

Nursing interventions

- ○ Enforce bed rest and elevate the patient's affected arm or leg, but avoid compressing the popliteal space.
- ○ Apply warm compresses or a covered aquathermia pad.
- ○ Give prescribed analgesics.
- ○ Mark, measure, and record the circumference of the affected arm or leg daily, and compare this measurement with that of the other arm or leg.
- ○ Give prescribed anticoagulants.
- ○ Perform or encourage range-of-motion exercises.
- ○ Use pneumatic compression devices.
- ○ Apply antiembolism stockings.
- ○ Encourage early ambulation.

Monitoring

- ○ Signs and symptoms of bleeding
- ○ Vital signs
- ○ Partial thromboplastin time for patient on heparin therapy
- ○ Prothrombin time for patient on warfarin
- ○ Signs and symptoms of heparin-induced thrombocytopenia
- ○ Signs and symptoms of pulmonary embolism
- ○ Response to treatment

Patient teaching

Be sure to cover:
- ○ the disorder, diagnosis, and treatment
- ○ the importance of follow-up blood studies to monitor anticoagulant therapy

- ○ how to give injections (if the patient is being discharged on subcutaneous anticoagulation therapy)
- ○ the need to avoid prolonged sitting or standing to help prevent a recurrence
- ○ proper application and use of antiembolism stockings
- ○ the importance of adequate hydration
- ○ use of an electric razor and avoidance of products that contain aspirin.

Thyroid cancer

Overview

Description

- Proliferation of cancer cells in the thyroid gland
- The most common endocrine malignancy
- Papillary carcinomas: 50% of all cases
- Medullary cancer: may be associated with pheochromocytoma; curable when detected before it causes symptoms

Pathophysiology

- Papillary cancer is usually multifocal and bilateral. It metastasizes slowly into regional nodes of the neck, mediastinum, lungs, and other distant organs. It's the least virulent form of thyroid cancer.
- Follicular cancer is less common but is more likely to recur and metastasize to the regional lymph nodes and spread through blood vessels into the bones, liver, and lungs.
- Medullary (solid) carcinoma originates in the parafollicular cells derived from the last branchial pouch and contains amyloid and calcium deposits. It can produce calcitonin, histaminase, corticotropin (producing Cushing's syndrome), and prostaglandin E_2 and F_3 (producing diarrhea). Untreated medullary cancer grows rapidly, commonly metastasizing to bones, liver, and kidneys.
- Anaplastic carcinoma (giant and spindly cell cancer) resists radiation and is almost never curable by resection. This cancer metastasizes rapidly, causing death by invading the trachea and compressing adjacent structures.

Causes

- Previous exposure to radiation treatment in the neck area
- Prolonged secretion of thyroid-stimulating hormone (radiation or heredity)

Risk factors

- Familial predisposition (possibly inherited as an autosomal dominant trait)
- Chronic goiter

Incidence

- 1.2 to 2.6 per 100,000 cases in men
- 2.0 to 3.8 per 100,000 cases in women
- Nearly two times the number of cases in Iceland and Hawaii compared with Canada and the U.S. mainland
- Particularly common among Chinese males and Filipino females
- Rare in children

Common characteristics

- Painless nodule; hard nodule in an enlarged thyroid gland

- Palpable lymph nodes with an enlarged thyroid
- Hoarseness
- Dysphagia

Complications

- Dysphagia
- Stridor
- Hormone alterations
- Distant metastasis

Assessment

History

- Sensitivity to cold and mental apathy (hypothyroidism)
- Sensitivity to heat, restlessness, and overactivity (hyperthyroidism)
- Diarrhea
- Dysphagia
- Anorexia
- Irritability
- Ear pain

Physical findings

- Hard, painless nodule in an enlarged thyroid gland or palpable lymph nodes with thyroid enlargement
- Hoarseness and vocal stridor
- Disfiguring thyroid mass
- Bruits

Test results

Laboratory
- Calcitonin assay identifies silent medullary carcinoma. Measuring calcitonin level in a resting state and during calcium infusion (15 mg/kg over 4 hours) shows an elevated fasting calcitonin level and an abnormal response to calcium stimulation — a higher release of calcitonin from the node than from the rest of the gland — indicating medullary cancer.

Imaging
- Thyroid scan differentiates functional nodes, which are rarely malignant, from hypofunctional nodes, which are commonly malignant.
- Ultrasonography shows changes in the size of thyroid nodules after thyroxine suppression therapy and is used to guide fine-needle aspiration and to detect recurrent disease.
- Magnetic resonance imaging and computed tomography scans provide a basis for treatment planning because they show the extent of disease in the thyroid and surrounding structures.

Diagnostic procedures
- Fine-needle aspiration biopsy differentiates benign from malignant thyroid nodules.
- Histologic analysis stages the disease and thereby guides treatment plans.

Treatment

General

○ Radioisotope (^{131}I) therapy with external radiation (sometimes postoperatively in lieu of radical neck excision) or alone (for metastasis)
○ Soft diet with small frequent meals if dysphagia occurs

Medication

○ Suppressive thyroid hormone therapy
○ Chemotherapy

Surgery

○ Total or subtotal thyroidectomy with modified node dissection (bilateral or homolateral) on the side of the primary cancer (for papillary or follicular cancer)
○ Total thyroidectomy and radical neck excision (for medullary or anaplastic cancer)

Nursing considerations

Key outcomes

The patient will:
○ maintain current weight without further loss
○ express positive feelings about self
○ not aspirate
○ express feelings of increased comfort and decreased pain.

Nursing interventions

○ Encourage verbalization and provide support.
Before surgery
○ Prepare the patient for scheduled surgery.
○ Establish a way to communicate postoperatively.
After surgery
○ Keep the patient in semi-Fowler's position, with adequate neck support.
○ Keep a tracheotomy set and oxygen equipment nearby in case of respiratory obstruction.

Monitoring

○ Vital signs
○ Wound site
○ Pain control
○ Serum calcium levels (if the parathyroid glands were removed)
○ Postoperative complications
○ Hydration and nutritional status

Patient teaching

Be sure to cover:
○ the disorder, diagnosis, and treatment
○ (before surgery) the operation and postoperative procedures and positioning

○ treatments and home care
○ drug administration, dosage, and possible adverse effects.

Discharge planning

○ Refer the patient to available resource and support services.

Thyroiditis

Overview

Description

○ Several disorders that involve inflammation of the thyroid gland
○ Autoimmune (Hashimoto's) thyroiditis: the most common chronic inflammatory disease of the thyroid gland
○ Postpartum thyroiditis: a form of autoimmune thyroiditis that occurs within 1 year of delivery
○ Subacute thyroiditis: a transient inflammation of the thyroid gland that's probably viral in origin
○ Riedel's thyroiditis: a rare condition with unknown etiology that may be a variant of Hashimoto's thyroiditis
○ Supportive thyroiditis: an uncommon bacterial or fungal infection of the thyroid that's potentially very serious
○ Silent thyroiditis: a transient hyperthyroid condition that's characterized by a small painless goiter and may be autoimmune in origin

Pathophysiology

○ The inflammatory process has varying effects on thyroid hormone levels (may be low, normal, or high). Also, lymphocytes and leukocytes may infiltrate thyroid tissue.
○ Hashimoto's thyroiditis is thought to result from lymphocytic infiltration of the thyroid gland and formation of antibodies to thyroid antigens in the blood.
○ Riedel's thyroiditis causes intense fibrosis of the thyroid and surrounding structures.

Causes

○ Mumps
○ Influenza, coxsackievirus, or adenovirus infections
○ Tuberculosis
○ Syphilis
○ Actinomycosis
○ Bacterial infection
○ Sarcoidosis and amyloidosis

Incidence

○ More common in women than in men
○ Autoimmune thyroiditis most common in middle-age women; most common cause of sporadic goiter in children
○ Postpartum thyroiditis within 1 year of delivery

Common characteristics

○ Signs and symptoms of hyperthyroidism or hypothyroidism

Complications

○ Depending on type of inflammation:
  – Non-Hodgkin's lymphoma of the thyroid gland
  – Permanent hypothyroid or hyperthyroid condition
  – Abscess formation and rupture
  – Tracheal or esophageal compression, necrosis, and hemorrhage

Assessment

History

○ Recent viral or bacterial infection
○ Disorder, such as systemic lupus erythematosus, rheumatoid arthritis, pernicious anemia, or Graves' disease
○ Gradual onset of hypothyroid-like symptoms
○ Occasionally, symptoms of hyperthyroidism
○ Local pain or pain referred to the lower jaw, ear, or occiput
○ Dysphagia
○ Dyspnea
○ Asthenia, malaise

Physical findings

○ Enlargement of the thyroid gland (goiter)
○ Reddened skin over the thyroid gland
○ Indurated neck tissues
○ Small, firm, and finely nodular thyroid gland with a characteristic bandlike depression circling the gland
○ A small lymph node in the midline above the isthmus
○ Nodularity
○ Swelling and warmth of the overlying skin
○ Woody, hard enlargement that feels "anchored" to surrounding structures
○ Stridor

Test results

Laboratory

○ In autoimmune processes, serum thyroglobulin and microsomal antibody levels are increased.

HASHIMOTO'S THYROIDITIS

○ Thyroid-stimulating hormone (TSH) level is increased.
○ Triiodothyronine and thyroxine levels are normal or decreased.
○ Antimicrosomal and antithyroglobulin antibodies are increased.

SUBACUTE THYROIDITIS

○ Thyroid hormone levels may be elevated, suppressed, or normal depending on the phase of the disorder.
○ Protein-bound iodine levels are increased.
○ TSH levels are decreased in the thyrotoxic phase, failing to respond to thyrotropin-releasing hormone; in the hypothyroid phase, TSH levels are increased.
○ Radioactive iodine (^{131}I) uptake is decreased.
○ Erythrocyte sedimentation rate, white blood cell count, and hepatic enzyme levels are increased.
○ Thyroid antibody levels are transiently low.
○ Thyroglobin levels are increased.

RIEDEL'S THYROIDITIS

○ ^{131}I uptake is normal or decreased.
○ Antimicrosomal antibody levels are increased.

Imaging
○ Thyroid scan may show isolated areas of function or total failure to visualize the gland.
Diagnostic procedures
○ Fine-needle thyroid gland biopsy offers histologic confirmation.

Treatment

General
○ Varies with the type of thyroiditis
○ Activity, as tolerated

Medication
○ Thyroid hormone
○ Analgesics
○ Anti-inflammatory drugs
○ Beta-adrenergic blockers
○ Corticosteroids
○ Antibiotics

Surgery
○ Partial thyroidectomy

Nursing considerations

Key outcomes
The patient will:
○ maintain a patent airway
○ express feelings of increased comfort
○ consume adequate calories daily
○ express positive feelings about self
○ avoid complications.

Nursing interventions
○ Administer drug therapy.
○ Elevate the head of the bed 90 degrees during mealtimes and for 30 minutes afterward.
○ Keep suction equipment readily available.
○ Consult the dietitian.
○ Provide frequent mouth care.
○ Provide meticulous skin care.
○ Provide comfort measures.
○ Encourage oral fluid intake.
○ Encourage verbalization of feelings.
○ Offer emotional support.
○ Help develop effective coping strategies.

 Alert

After thyroidectomy, watch for signs of tetany secondary to accidental parathyroid injury during surgery. Keep 10% calcium gluconate available for I.V. use if needed. Check dressings frequently for excessive bleeding. Watch for signs of airway obstruction, such as difficulty talking or increased swallowing, and keep tracheotomy equipment handy.

Monitoring
○ Vital signs
○ Intake and output
○ Daily weight
○ Respiratory status
○ Signs and symptoms of hyperthyroidism or hypothyroidism
○ Neck circumference

Patient teaching

Be sure to cover:
○ the disorder, diagnosis, and treatment
○ drug administration, dosage, and possible adverse effects
○ when to notify the physician
○ signs and symptoms of respiratory distress
○ signs and symptoms of hyperthyroidism and hypothyroidism
○ long-term hormone replacement therapy after thyroidectomy
○ the importance of wearing or carrying medical identification.

Discharge planning
○ Refer the patient to a mental health professional for additional counseling if indicated.

Tonsillitis

Overview

Description
○ Inflammation of the tonsils
○ May be acute or chronic
○ Typical viral infection: mild and of limited duration

Pathophysiology
○ The inflammatory response to cell damage by viruses or bacteria results in hyperemia and fluid exudation.

Causes
○ Bacterial infection (group A beta-hemolytic streptococci)
○ Viral infection

Incidence

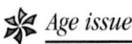 *Age issue*

Commonly affects children between ages 5 and 10.

○ Tonsils tending to hypertrophy during childhood and atrophy after puberty

Common characteristics
○ Sore throat
○ Enlarged tonsils

Complications
○ Chronic upper airway obstruction
○ Sleep disturbance, sleep apnea
○ Cor pulmonale
○ Failure to thrive
○ Eating or swallowing disorders
○ Speech abnormalities
○ Febrile seizures
○ Otitis media
○ Cardiac valvular disease
○ Peritonsillar abscesses
○ Glomerulonephritis
○ Bacterial endocarditis
○ Cervical lymph node abscesses

Assessment

History
○ Mild to severe sore throat
○ Young child possibly stops eating
○ Muscle and joint pain
○ Chills
○ Malaise
○ Headache
○ Pain, commonly referred to the ears
○ Constant urge to swallow
○ Constricted feeling in the back of the throat

Physical findings
○ Fever
○ Swollen, tender submandibular lymph nodes
○ Generalized inflammation of pharyngeal wall
○ Swollen tonsils projecting from between the pillars of the fauces and exuding white or yellow follicles
○ Purulent drainage with application of pressure to tonsillar pillars
○ Uvula possibly edematous and inflamed

Test results
Laboratory
○ Throat culture reveals the infecting organism.
○ Serum white blood cell count usually reveals leukocytosis.

Treatment

General
○ Symptom relief
○ Adequate fluid intake
○ Rest periods as needed

Medication
○ Aspirin or acetaminophen
○ Antibiotics

Surgery
○ Possible tonsillectomy

Nursing considerations

Key outcomes
The patient will:
○ express feelings of increased comfort
○ show no signs of aspiration
○ maintain effective breathing pattern
○ have balanced intake and output.

Nursing interventions
○ Encourage oral fluids.
○ Offer a child ice cream and flavored drinks and ices.
○ Provide humidification.
○ Encourage gargling to soothe the throat and remove debris from tonsillar crypts.
After surgery
○ Maintain a patent airway.
○ Prevent aspiration by side positioning.
○ Keep suction equipment readily available.
○ Provide water after gag reflex returns.
○ Later, encourage nonirritating oral fluids.
○ Avoid milk products and salty or irritating foods.
○ Provide analgesics for pain relief.
○ Encourage deep-breathing exercises.

Monitoring
○ Hydration status
○ Effect of pain medication

Before surgery
○ Bleeding abnormalities
After surgery
○ Vital signs
○ Signs and symptoms of bleeding
○ Respiratory status

 Alert

Immediately report excessive bleeding, increased pulse rate, or decreasing blood pressure.

 Alert

The greatest risk of bleeding is 7 to 10 days after surgery.

Patient teaching

Be sure to cover:
○ the disorder, diagnosis, and treatment
○ the importance of completing the entire course of antibiotics
○ avoidance of irritants
○ the need for soft foods for about 3 weeks after surgery to decrease risk of rebleeding
○ drug administration, dosage, and possible adverse effects
○ the possibility of throat discomfort and some bleeding after surgery
○ expectation of a white scab to form in the throat 5 to 10 days after surgery
○ the need to report bleeding, ear discomfort, or a fever that lasts 3 days or more.

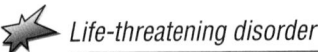
Life-threatening disorder

Toxic shock syndrome

Overview

Description

○ An inflammatory response syndrome linked to bacterial infections
○ An acute and life-threatening condition
○ Also called *TSS*

Pathophysiology

○ Toxic exoproteins are produced by infecting organisms.
○ TSST-1 is the most common toxin; staphylococcal enterotoxin B is the second most common.
○ For illness to develop, the patient must be infected with a toxigenic strain of *Staphylococcus aureus* and lack antibodies to that strain.

Causes

○ Penicillin-resistant *S. aureus*

Risk factors

○ Tampon use
○ Varicella infection
○ Streptococcal pharyngitis

Incidence

○ Affects 1 in 100,000
○ Primarily affects young people

Guidelines for diagnosing toxic shock syndrome

Toxic shock syndrome is typically diagnosed based on the following criteria.
○ Fever 102° F (38.9° C) or higher
○ Diffuse macular erythrodermal rash (sunburn rash)
○ Hypotension (systolic blood pressure 90 mm Hg or less in adults or below the 5th percentile for age)
○ Involvement of at least three organ systems:
  – GI (vomiting, diarrhea)
  – Muscular (myalgias or liver function test at least twice normal upper limit)
  – Mucous membrane hyperemia (conjunctiva, vagina, oropharyngeal)
  – Renal (blood urea nitrogen or creatinine level at least twice normal upper limit, or pyuria)
  – Hepatic (total serum bilirubin or aminotransferase level twice normal level)
  – Hematologic (thrombocytopenia)
  – Central nervous system (disorientation or change in level of consciousness)
○ Desquamation, especially of palms and soles, 1 or 2 weeks after onset of illness
○ Other conditions ruled out

○ Half of all cases in settings other than menstruation
○ Affects both sexes and all ages

Common characteristics

○ In the early convalescent period: fever, hypotension, rash, multiorgan dysfunction, and desquamation
○ Menstruation (the most common setting for TSS)
○ Bacteremia (in about 60% of patients)

Complications

○ Septic abortion
○ Musculoskeletal and respiratory infections
○ Staphylococcal bacteremia
○ Renal and myocardial dysfunction
○ Acute respiratory distress syndrome
○ Desquamation of the skin
○ Peripheral gangrene
○ Muscle weakness
○ Neuropsychiatric dysfunction

Assessment

History

○ Possible recent streptococcal infection
○ Possible tampon usage or menstruation
○ Intense myalgia, headache
○ Nausea, vomiting, and diarrhea
○ Sore throat
○ Dizziness

Physical findings

○ Fever (104° F [40° C] or higher)
○ Pharyngeal infection, strawberry tongue
○ Hypotension
○ Altered mental status
○ Macular erythroderma (generalized or local)
○ Peripheral edema
○ Vaginal hyperemia, purulent vaginal discharge

Test results

Laboratory
○ Isolation of *S. aureus* from vaginal discharge or infection site supports the diagnosis. (See *Guidelines for diagnosing toxic shock syndrome*.)
○ Blood urea nitrogen examination shows azotemia.
○ Urinalysis shows pyuria.
○ Serum albumin levels reveal hypoalbuminemia.
○ Serum calcium levels reveal hypocalcemia.
○ Serum phosphorus levels reveal hypophosphatemia.
○ Complete blood count shows leukocytosis or leukopenia.
○ Platelet count shows thrombocytopenia.
○ Serum creatinine level is increased.

Treatment

General

○ Aggressive fluid resuscitation
○ Correction of electrolyte imbalances

○ Supportive treatment such as possible ventilatory support
○ Identification and decontamination of toxin production site
○ Bed rest until acute phase resolved

Medication

○ Antibiotics
○ Inotropics
○ Vasopressors
○ I.V. immunoglobulin

Surgery

○ Examination and irrigation of recent surgical wounds

Nursing considerations

Key outcomes

The patient will:
○ maintain collateral circulation
○ attain and maintain hemodynamic stability
○ maintain adequate cardiac output
○ remain afebrile
○ have an adequate fluid volume.

Nursing interventions

○ Administer drug therapy.
○ Assess fluid balance and replace fluids I.V., as needed.
○ Reorient as needed.
○ Use appropriate safety measures to prevent injury.
○ Use standard precautions for any vaginal discharge and lesion drainage.

Monitoring

○ Cardiovascular status
○ Fluid and electrolyte status
○ Neurologic status
○ Vital signs
○ Pulmonary status
○ Response to treatment
○ Complications

Patient teaching

Be sure to cover:
○ the disorder, diagnosis, and treatment
○ the need to avoid using tampons, especially superabsorbent ones, because of the risk of recurrence
○ TSS prevention.

Toxoplasmosis

Overview

Description

- One of the most common parasitic infectious diseases
- Usually causes localized infection
- May produce significant generalized infection, especially in an immunodeficient patient
- Once infected, organism carried for life and acute infection can reactivate
- Congenital type characterized by lesions in the central nervous system (CNS); may result in stillbirth or serious birth defects

Pathophysiology

- After ingestion, parasites are released from latent cysts by the digestive process; they then invade the GI tract and multiply.
- Parasites disseminate to various organs, especially lymphatic tissue, skeletal muscle, myocardium, retina, placenta, and the CNS (most commonly).
- The parasite infects host cells, replicates, and then invades adjoining cells, resulting in cell death and focal necrosis surrounded by an acute inflammatory response.

Causes

- The protozoan *Toxoplasma gondii,* which exists in trophozoite forms in the acute stages of infection and in cystic forms (tissue cysts and oocysts) in latent stages
- Transmitted by ingestion of tissue cysts in raw or undercooked meat or by fecal-oral contamination from infected cats
- Congenital toxoplasmosis from transplacental transmission

Incidence

- Up to 70% of people in United States infected
- Occurs worldwide; less common in cold or hot, arid climates and at high elevations

Ocular toxoplasmosis

Ocular toxoplasmosis (active chorioretinitis) is characterized by focal necrotizing retinitis. It accounts for about 25% of all cases of granulomatous uveitis. Although usually the result of a congenital infection, it may not appear until adolescence or young adulthood, when infection is reactivated.

Symptoms include blurred vision, scotoma, pain, photophobia, and impairment or loss of central vision. Vision improves as inflammation subsides but usually without recovery of lost visual acuity. Ocular toxoplasmosis may subside after treatment with prednisone.

Common characteristics

- Fever
- Rash
- Constitutional symptoms

Complications

- Seizure disorder
- Vision loss (see *Ocular toxoplasmosis*)
- Mental retardation
- Deafness
- Generalized infection
- Stillbirth
- Congenital toxoplasmosis

Assessment

History

- Possible immunocompromised state, exposure to cat feces, or ingestion of poorly cooked meat
- Malaise
- Fatigue
- Myalgia
- Headache
- Sore throat
- Vomiting

Physical findings

- Fever (if generalized, possibly 106° F [41.1° C])
- Cough
- Dyspnea
- Cyanosis
- Coarse crackles
- Delirium, seizures
- Diffuse maculopapular rash (except on the palms, soles, and scalp)
- In an infant with congenital toxoplasmosis:
  - Hydrocephalus or microcephalus
  - Jaundice, purpura, rash
  - Strabismus, blindness
  - Epilepsy, mental retardation
  - Lymphadenopathy, splenomegaly, and hepatomegaly

Test results

Laboratory

- Specimens (such as bronchoalveolar lavage material from immunocompromised patients or lymph node biopsy) contain parasites.
- Intraperitoneal inoculation with blood or other body fluids into mice or tissue cultures shows isolation of parasites.
- Polymerase chain reaction detects parasite's genetic material (especially in detecting congenital infections in utero).

Treatment

General

○ No treatment in otherwise healthy patient who isn't pregnant
○ Rest periods when fatigued
○ Seizure precautions

Medication

○ Pyrimethamine plus sulfadiazine with leucovorin

Nursing considerations

Key outcomes

The patient will:
○ have normal vital signs
○ have an adequate fluid volume
○ report an increased energy level
○ develop no complications
○ maintain respiratory rate within 5 breaths/minute of baseline.

Nursing interventions

○ Give tepid sponge baths to decrease fever.
○ Administer drug therapy.
○ Provide chest physiotherapy, and administer oxygen, as needed. Assist ventilations if needed.
○ Institute seizure precautions.

 Alert

Don't palpate the patient's abdomen vigorously; this could lead to a ruptured spleen. For the same reason, discourage vigorous activity.

○ Report all cases of toxoplasmosis to the local public health department.

Monitoring

○ Neurologic status
○ Response to treatment
○ Complications

Patient teaching

Be sure to cover:
○ the disorder, diagnosis, and treatment
○ necessary drugs, including the need for frequent blood tests
○ the importance of regularly scheduled follow-up care
○ ways to prevent the spread of toxoplasmosis (washing hands after working with soil, cooking meat thoroughly and freezing promptly, covering children's sandboxes, and keeping flies away from food because flies transport oocysts)
○ the need for pregnant women to avoid cleaning and handling cat litter boxes, or to wear gloves.

Discharge planning

○ Refer the patient for follow-up with a neurologist or infectious disease specialist if needed.

Tracheoesophageal fistula and esophageal atresia

Overview

Description

○ Tracheoesophageal fistula: a developmental anomaly characterized by an abnormal connection between the trachea and the esophagus; usually accompanies esophageal atresia, in which the esophagus is closed off at some point

○ Malformations have numerous anatomic variations, most commonly, esophageal atresia with fistula to the distal segment

○ Two of the most serious surgical emergencies in neonates; requires immediate diagnosis and correction

Pathophysiology

○ Tracheoesophageal fistula and esophageal atresia result from failure of the embryonic esophagus and trachea to develop and separate correctly.

○ Respiratory system development begins at about day 26 of gestation.

○ Abnormal development of the septum during this time can lead to tracheoesophageal fistula.

○ The most common abnormality is type C tracheoesophageal fistula with esophageal atresia, in which the upper section of the esophagus terminates in a blind pouch, and the lower section ascends from the stomach and connects with the trachea by a short fistulous tract.

○ In type A atresia, both esophageal segments are blind pouches, and neither is connected to the airway.

○ In types B and D, the upper portion of the esophagus opens into the trachea; infants with this anomaly may experience life-threatening aspiration of saliva or food.

○ In type E (or H-type) tracheoesophageal fistula without atresia, the fistula may occur anywhere between the level of the cricoid cartilage and the midesophagus but usually is higher in the trachea than in the esophagus. Such a fistula may be as small as a pinpoint.

Causes

○ Congenital anomalies
○ Commonly found in infants with other anomalies, such as:
  – Congenital heart disease
  – Imperforate anus
  – Genitourinary abnormalities
  – Intestinal atresia

Incidence

○ Esophageal atresia in about 1 of 4,000 live births; about one-third of these neonates born prematurely

Common characteristics

Tracheoesophageal fistula
○ Type B (proximal fistula) and Type D (fistula to both segments): immediate aspiration of saliva into the airway and bacterial pneumonitis
○ Type E (or H-type): suspected with repeated episodes of pneumonitis, pulmonary infection, and abdominal infection; choking followed by cyanosis

Esophageal atresia
○ Type A: normal swallowing, excessive drooling, possible respiratory distress
○ Type C: seemingly normal swallowing followed shortly afterward by coughing, struggling, cyanosis, lack of breathing

Complications

○ Aspiration of secretions into the lungs leading to respiratory distress, pneumonia, or cessation of breathing
○ Death if untreated

After surgery
○ Abnormal esophageal motility
○ Recurrent fistulas
○ Pneumothorax
○ Esophageal stricture

Assessment

History

○ Coughing and choking after eating

Physical findings

○ Respiratory distress
○ Drooling

Test results

Imaging
○ Chest X-rays demonstrate the position of the catheter and can also show a dilated, air-filled upper esophageal pouch, pneumonia in the right upper lobe, or bilateral pneumonitis. Both pneumonia and pneumonitis suggest aspiration.
○ Abdominal X-rays show gas in the bowel in a distal fistula (type C) but none in a proximal fistula (type B) or in atresia without fistula (type A).
○ Cinefluorography allows visualization on a fluoroscopic screen. After a size 10 or 12 French catheter is passed through the patient's nostril into the esophagus, a small amount of contrast medium is instilled to define the tip of the upper pouch and to differentiate between overflow aspiration from a blind end

(atresia) and aspiration from passage of liquids through a tracheoesophageal fistula.

Other

○ A size 6 or 8 French catheter passed through the nose meets an obstruction (esophageal atresia) about 4″ to 5″ (10 to 12.5 cm) distal to the nostrils. Aspirate of gastric contents is less acidic than normal.

Treatment

General

○ I.V. fluids
○ Supine position with the head low to facilitate drainage or with the head elevated to prevent aspiration
○ After surgery: placement of a suction catheter in the upper esophageal pouch to control secretions and prevent aspiration

Medication

○ Antibiotics for superimposed infection

Surgery

○ Tracheoesophageal fistula and esophageal atresia require surgical correction and are usually surgical emergencies. The type and timing of the surgical procedure depend on the nature of the anomaly, the patient's general condition, and the presence of coexisting congenital defects.
○ In premature neonates (nearly 33% of infants with this anomaly) who are poor surgical risks, correction of combined tracheoesophageal fistula and esophageal atresia is done in two stages: first, gastrostomy (for gastric decompression, prevention of reflux, and feeding) and closure of the fistula; then, 1 to 2 months later, anastomosis of the esophagus.
○ Correction of esophageal atresia alone requires anastomosis of the proximal and distal esophageal segments in one or two stages. End-to-end anastomosis commonly produces postoperative stricture; end-to-side anastomosis is less likely to do so.
○ If the esophageal ends are widely separated, treatment may include a colonic interposition (grafting a piece of the colon) or elongation of the proximal segment of the esophagus by bougienage.

Nursing considerations

Key outcomes

The patient will:
○ develop no respiratory complications
○ remain hemodynamically stable.
   The parents or family will:
○ express understanding of disorder and treatment.

Nursing interventions

○ Administer oxygen as needed.

○ Perform pulmonary physiotherapy and suctioning, as needed.
○ Provide a humid environment.
○ Administer antibiotics and parenteral fluids.
○ Maintain gastrostomy tube feedings.
○ Offer the parents support and guidance in dealing with their infant's acute illness. Encourage them to participate in care and to hold and touch the infant as much as possible to facilitate bonding.

Monitoring

○ Respiratory status
○ Intake and output
After surgery
○ Chest tubes
○ Signs of complications

Patient teaching

Be sure to cover:
○ the disorder, diagnosis, and treatment
○ feeding procedures
○ recognizing and reporting complications
○ proper positioning.

Discharge planning

○ Instruct the parents that X-rays are required about 10 days after surgery, and again 1 and 3 months later, to evaluate the effectiveness of surgical repair.

Transposition of the great arteries

Overview

Description

- ○ Congenital heart defect in which the great arteries are reversed: aorta arising from right ventricle and pulmonary artery from left ventricle, producing two noncommunicating circulatory systems (pulmonary and systemic)
- ○ Commonly coexists with other congenital heart defects, such as ventricular septal defect (VSD), VSD with pulmonary stenosis (PS), atrial septal defect (ASD), and patent ductus arteriosus (PDA)

Pathophysiology

- ○ In transposition, oxygenated blood returning to the left side of the heart is carried back to the lungs by a transposed pulmonary artery; unoxygenated blood returning to the right side of the heart is carried to the systemic circulation by a transposed aorta.
- ○ Communication between the pulmonary and systemic circulations is necessary for survival. In infants with isolated transposition, blood mixes only at the patent foramen ovale and at the patent ductus arteriosus, resulting in slight mixing of unoxygenated systemic blood and oxygenated pulmonary blood.
- ○ In infants with concurrent cardiac defects, greater mixing of blood occurs.

Causes

- ○ Faulty embryonic development

Incidence

- ○ Accounts for about 5% of all congenital heart defects
- ○ Affects males two to three times more than females

Common characteristics

- ○ Within the first few hours after birth, neonates with transposition of the great arteries generally show cyanosis and tachypnea, which worsen with crying.
- ○ After several days or weeks, such neonates usually develop signs of heart failure (gallop rhythm, tachycardia, dyspnea, hepatomegaly, and cardiomegaly). S_2 is louder than normal because the anteriorly transposed aorta is directly behind the sternum; in many cases, however, no murmur can be heard during the first few days of life.

Complications

- ○ Heart failure
- ○ Cardiac arrhythmia
- ○ Eisenmenger's syndrome (irreversible and progressive pulmonary vascular obstructive disease)

Assessment

History

- ○ Diminished exercise tolerance
- ○ Fatigability
- ○ Coughing

Physical findings

- ○ Cyanosis
- ○ Clubbing of nailbeds
- ○ Pronounced murmurs if ASD, VSD, PDA, or PS is present

Test results

Laboratory

- ○ Arterial blood gas (ABG) measurements indicate hypoxia and secondary metabolic acidosis.

Imaging

- ○ Chest X-rays are normal in the first days of life. Within days to weeks, right atrial and right ventricular enlargement characteristically cause the heart to appear oblong. X-rays also show increased pulmonary vascular markings, except when pulmonary stenosis coexists.
- ○ Echocardiography demonstrates the reversed position of the aorta and pulmonary artery and records echoes from both semilunar valves simultaneously, due to aortic valve displacement. It also detects other cardiac defects.

Diagnostic procedures

- ○ Electrocardiogram typically reveals right axis deviation and right ventricular hypertrophy; it may be normal in a neonate.
- ○ Cardiac catheterization reveals decreased oxygen saturation in left ventricular blood and aortic blood; increased right atrial, right ventricular, and pulmonary artery oxygen saturation; and right ventricular systolic pressure equal to systemic pressure. Dye injection reveals the transposed vessels and the presence of any other cardiac defects.

Treatment

General

- ○ Atrial balloon septostomy (Rashkind procedure) during cardiac catheterization
- ○ Increased caloric density before correction; no dietary restrictions after correction
- ○ Activity, as tolerated

Medication

- ○ Inotropic agents
- ○ Loop diuretics
- ○ Prostaglandins
- ○ Prophylactic antibiotics

Surgery

One of three surgical procedures can correct transposition, depending on the defect's physiology:

- Mustard procedure replaces the atrial septum with a Dacron or pericardial partition that allows systemic venous blood to be channeled to the pulmonary artery, which carries the blood to the lungs for oxygenation and oxygenated blood returning to the heart to be channeled from the pulmonary veins into the aorta.
- Senning procedure accomplishes the same result using the atrial septum to create partitions to redirect blood flow.
- Arterial switch, or Jatene procedure, in which transposed arteries are surgically anastomosed to the correct ventricle. For this procedure to be successful, the left ventricle must be used to pump at systemic pressure, as it does in neonates or in children with a left ventricular outflow obstruction or large VSD. Surgery also corrects other heart defects.

Nursing considerations

Key outcomes

The patient will:
- maintain hemodynamic stability
- improve oxygenation
- have no signs of heart failure.

Nursing interventions

- Offer emotional support.
- Give digoxin and I.V. fluids, being careful to avoid fluid overload.
- After Mustard or Senning procedures, watch for signs of baffle obstruction such as marked facial edema.

Monitoring

- Vital signs
- ABG values
- Intake and output
- Central venous pressure
- Signs of heart failure

Patient teaching

Be sure to cover (with the parents):
- the disorder, diagnosis, and treatment
- how to recognize signs of heart failure and digoxin toxicity (poor feeding and vomiting)
- the importance of regular checkups to monitor cardiovascular status
- protecting the infant from infection and giving antibiotics.

Trichinosis

Overview

Description
- An infection caused by larvae of the intestinal roundworm *Trichinella spiralis*
- May produce multiple symptoms, such as respiratory, central nervous system (CNS), cardiovascular complications and, rarely, death
- Also known as *trichiniasis* or *trichinellosis*

Pathophysiology
- *T. spiralis* cysts are found primarily in swine, less commonly in dogs, cats, bears, foxes, wolves, and marine animals. These cysts result from the animals' ingestion of similarly contaminated flesh. In swine, such infection results from eating table scraps or raw garbage.
- After gastric juices free the worm from the cyst capsule, it reaches sexual maturity in a few days.
- The female roundworm burrows into the intestinal mucosa and reproduces.
- Larvae are then transported through the lymphatic system and the bloodstream. They become embedded as cysts in striated muscle, especially in the diaphragm, chest, arms, and legs.
- Human-to-human transmission doesn't take place.

Causes
- Ingestion of uncooked or undercooked meat that contains *T. spiralis* cysts

Incidence
- Occurs worldwide, especially in populations that eat pork or bear meat
- Affects both sexes equally

Common characteristics
- Usually mild and seldom produces symptoms; when symptoms occur, vary with the stage and degree of infection

Stage 1 (invasion)
- Occurs 1 week after ingestion
- Release of larvae and reproduction of adult *T. spiralis* causing:
  - Anorexia
  - Nausea
  - Vomiting
  - Diarrhea
  - Abdominal pain
  - Cramps

Stage 2 (dissemination)
- Occurs 7 to 10 days after ingestion
- Penetrates the intestinal mucosa and begins to migrate to striated muscle
- Signs and symptoms:
  - Edema, especially of the eyelids or face
  - Muscle pain, particularly in limbs
  - Occasionally, itching and burning skin, sweating, skin lesions, a temperature of 102° to 104° F (38.9° to 40° C), and delirium
  - In severe respiratory, cardiovascular, or CNS infections, palpitations and lethargy

Stage 3 (encystment)
- Occurs during convalescence, generally 1 week later
- Invades muscle fiber and becomes encysted

Complications
- Meningitis
- Subcortical infarcts
- Encephalitis
- Myocarditis with heart failure
- Nephritis
- Glomerulonephritis
- Sinusitis
- Pneumonia

Assessment

History
- Ingestion of raw or improperly cooked pork or pork products
- Myalgia
- Abdominal discomfort
- Diarrhea
- Constipation
- Anorexia
- Nausea

Physical findings
- Diffuse weakness
- Dyspnea on exertion
- Hoarseness
- Cough
- Abdominal distention
- Macular or petechial rash
- Periorbital edema

Test results
Laboratory
- Stools contain mature worms and larvae during the invasion stage.
- Diagnosis is confirmed by elevated acute and convalescent antibody titers (determined by flocculation tests 3 to 4 weeks after infection).
- Aspartate aminotransferase, alanine aminotransferase, creatine kinase, and lactate dehydrogenase levels are increased during the acute stages, and the eosinophil count is increased (up to 15,000/µl).
- Cerebrospinal fluid lymphocyte level (to 300/µl) is normal or increased, and protein levels are increased, indicating CNS involvement.

Diagnostic procedures
- Skeletal muscle biopsies can show encysted larvae 10 days after ingestion; if available, analyses of contaminated meat also show larvae.

○ Skin testing may show a positive histamine-like reactivity 15 minutes after intradermal injection of the antigen (within 17 to 20 days after ingestion); however, such a result may remain positive for up to 5 years after exposure.

Treatment

General

○ Supportive care as indicated
○ Diet as tolerated
○ Initially, bed rest with increased activity as tolerated

Medication

○ Antipyretics
○ Anthelmintics
○ Glucocorticoids
○ Analgesics

Nursing considerations

Key outcomes

The patient will:
○ report increased comfort and decreased pain
○ express an understanding of the disorder and its treatment
○ maintain adequate ventilation
○ maintain hemodynamic stability.

Nursing interventions

○ Reduce fever with alcohol rubs, tepid baths, hypothermia blankets, or antipyretics.
○ Relieve muscle pain with analgesics, enforced bed rest, and proper body alignment.
○ Frequently reposition the patient, and gently massage bony prominences to prevent pressure ulcers.
○ Report all cases of trichinosis to local public health authorities.

Monitoring

○ Response to treatment
○ Vital signs
○ Respiratory status

Patient teaching

Be sure to cover:
○ proper cooking and storing methods for all meat from carnivores
○ for travelers to foreign countries or poor areas of the United States, the importance of avoiding pork consumption; swine in these areas are commonly fed raw garbage.

Trichomoniasis

Overview

Description

○ A protozoal infection of the lower genitourinary tract
○ May be acute or chronic in females
○ Risk of recurrence minimized when sexual partners are treated concurrently

Pathophysiology

○ *Trichomonas vaginalis* — a tetraflagellated, motile protozoan — causes trichomoniasis in females by infecting the vagina, the urethra and, possibly, the endocervix, bladder, Bartholin's glands, or Skene's glands; in males, it infects the lower urethra and, possibly, the prostate gland, seminal vesicles, or epididymis.
○ *T. vaginalis* grows best when the vaginal mucosa is more alkaline than normal (pH about 5.5 to 5.8).

Causes

○ Usually transmitted by sexual intercourse; less commonly, by contaminated douche equipment or moist washcloths

Risk factors

○ Factors that raise the vaginal pH, such as
– use of hormonal contraceptives
– pregnancy
– bacterial overgrowth
– exudative cervical or vaginal lesions
– frequent douching, which disturbs lactobacilli that normally live in the vagina and maintain acidity.

Incidence

○ Affects about 15% of sexually active females and 10% of sexually active males

Common characteristics

○ About 70% of females and most males asymptomatic
○ In females: gray or greenish yellow and possibly profuse and frothy, malodorous vaginal discharge
○ In males: mild to severe transient urethritis, possibly with dysuria and urinary frequency

Complications

○ With pregnant women: preterm or low–birth-weight infant
○ Prostatitis
○ Epididymitis
○ Urethral stricture disease
○ Infertility

Assessment

History

○ Severe itching
○ Dyspareunia
○ Dysuria
○ Urinary frequency
○ Postcoital spotting, menorrhagia, or dysmenorrhea

Physical findings

○ Vaginal erythema, edema, and frank excoriation
○ Frothy, malodorous, greenish yellow vaginal discharge
○ Rarely, a thin, gray pseudomembrane over the vagina

Test results

Laboratory
○ Direct microscopic examination of vaginal or seminal discharge is decisive when it reveals *T. vaginalis*, a motile, pear-shaped organism. Examination of clear urine specimens may also reveal *T. vaginalis*.
Other
○ Cervical examination demonstrates punctate cervical hemorrhages, giving the cervix a strawberry appearance that's almost pathognomonic for this disorder.

Treatment

General

○ Abstinence from sexual intercourse until cured
○ Sitz baths to help relieve symptoms

Medication

○ Single 2-g dose of oral metronidazole given to both sexual partners

Nursing considerations

Key outcomes

The patient will:
○ express feelings of increased comfort and decreased pain
○ express understanding of the condition and treatment
○ discuss the impact of the disorder on self and significant others.

Nursing interventions

○ Instruct the patient to avoid using tampons.
○ Provide emotional support.
○ Practice standard precautions.

Monitoring

○ Response to treatment

Patient teaching

Be sure to cover:
- ○ the need to refer sexual partners for treatment
- ○ the need to avoid alcohol while taking metronidazole because alcohol may provoke a disulfiram-type reaction (confusion, headache, cramps, vomiting, and seizures)
- ○ the possibility that metronidazole may turn urine dark brown
- ○ the need to avoid over-the-counter douches and vaginal sprays because they can alter vaginal pH
- ○ the benefits of wearing loose-fitting, cotton underwear, which reduce the risk of genitourinary bacterial growth by allowing ventilation; bacteria flourish in a warm, dark, moist environment.

Tricuspid insufficiency

Overview

Description

- Heart condition in which the tricuspid valve doesn't function properly
- Also called *tricuspid regurgitation*

Pathophysiology

- The tricuspid valve is incompetent.
- Blood flows back into the right atrium.
- Fluid overload occurs in the atrium.
- Congestive failure occurs, and impedance to the pulmonary vasculature may result in hypoxemia, cyanosis, and polycythemia.

Causes

- Rheumatic heart disease
- Endocarditis
- Epstein's anomaly
- Prolapse
- Carcinoid heart disease
- Papillary muscle dysfunction
- Trauma
- Connective tissue disease

Incidence

- Affects both sexes equally
- Usually occurs in childhood

Common characteristics

- Dyspnea on exertion
- Peripheral edema
- Tachycardia
- Fatigue

Complications

- Heart failure
- Pulmonary edema
- Thromboembolism
- Endocarditis
- Arrhythmias

Identifying the murmur of tricuspid insufficiency

A high-pitched, blowing pansystolic murmur in the tricuspid area characterizes tricuspid insufficiency.

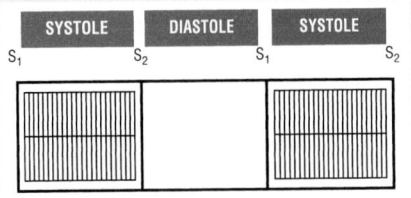

Assessment

History

- Occurrence of one of listed causes
- Orthopnea, dyspnea
- Fatigue
- Angina
- Palpitations

Physical findings

- Tachycardia
- Crackles in the lungs
- Hepatomegaly (right-sided failure)
- Jugular vein distention
- S_3
- Diminished peripheral pulses
- Ascites
- Atrial fibrillation
- Peripheral edema
- Pansystolic murmur (see *Identifying the murmur of tricuspid insufficiency*)

Test results

Imaging
- Chest X-rays show right atrial and ventricular enlargement.
- Echocardiography shows right ventricular dilation and prolapse or flailing of the tricuspid leaflets.

Diagnostic procedures
- Electrocardiogram shows right atrial hypertrophy, right or left ventricular hypertrophy, atrial fibrillation, and incomplete right bundle-branch block.
- Right-sided heart catheterization shows high atrial pressure, tricuspid insufficiency, and decreased or normal output.

Treatment

General

- Underlying cause
- Low-sodium diet
- Fluid restriction
- Activity as tolerated

Medication

- Diuretics
- Cardiac glycosides
- Anticoagulants
- Angiotensin-converting enzyme inhibitors
- Oxygen
- Prophylactic antibiotics before and after surgery or dental care to prevent endocarditis

Surgery

- Annuloplasty or valvuloplasty to reconstruct or repair the valve
- Valve replacement with a prosthetic valve

Nursing considerations

Key outcomes

The patient will:
- carry out activities of daily living without weakness or fatigue
- maintain hemodynamic stability
- maintain adequate ventilation.

Nursing interventions

- Administer oxygen.
- Watch for signs of heart failure or pulmonary edema.
- Alternate periods of activity and rest.
- Keep patient's legs eleveated to improve venous return to the heart.

Monitoring

- Vital signs and pulse oximetry
- Cardiac rhythm
- Pulmonary artery catheter readings
- Intake and output
- Adverse effects of drug therapy

Patient teaching

Be sure to cover:
- the disorder, diagnosis, and treatment
- dietary restrictions and drugs
- signs and symptoms that should be reported
- the importance of consistent follow-up care
- the need to elevate his legs when sitting.

Tricuspid stenosis

Overview

Description

○ Heart condition in which the tricuspid valve improperly functions, allowing backflow of blood into the right atrium and causing right atrial enlargement

Pathophysiology

○ Alterations in the structure of the tricuspid valve cause incompetence of the valve.
○ Restriction of blood flow into the right ventricle and, subsequently, to the pulmonary vasculature occurs.
○ Obstructed venous return results in hepatic enlargement, decreased pulmonary blood flow, peripheral edema, and right atrial enlargement.

Causes

○ Mitral and aortic valve disorders
○ Rheumatic heart disease
○ Carcinoid heart disease
○ Infective endocarditis
○ Endomyocardial fibrosis
○ Systemic lupus erythematosus
○ Tricuspid atresia

Incidence

○ Affects females slightly more often than males

Common characteristics

○ Dyspnea on exertion
○ Peripheral edema
○ Fatigue
○ Ascites

Complications

○ Heart failure
○ Pulmonary edema
○ Thromboembolism
○ Endocarditis
○ Arrhythmias

Assessment

History

○ Orthopnea
○ Dyspnea
○ Fatigue
○ Angina
○ Palpitations

Physical findings

○ Diastolic murmur (see *Identifying the murmur of tricuspid stenosis*)
○ Split S_1
○ Crackles in the lungs
○ Hepatomegaly (with right-sided failure)
○ Ascites

Test results

Imaging
○ Chest X-ray reveals cardiomegaly.
○ Echocardiography shows structure of the valves.
Diagnostic procedures
○ Electrocardiogram may show atrial fibrillation.

Treatment

General

○ Underlying cause
○ Low-sodium diet
○ Fluid restriction
○ Activity as tolerated

Medication

○ Diuretics
○ Inotropic agent
○ Angiotensin-converting enzyme inhibitors
○ Oxygen
○ Antibiotics before and after surgery or if infection is present

Surgery

○ Balloon valvoplasty
○ Pulmonary artery balloon angioplasty
○ Valvotomy

Nursing considerations

Key outcomes

The patient will:
○ carry out activities of daily living without weakness or fatigue
○ maintain hemodynamic stability
○ maintain adequate ventilation.

Nursing interventions

○ Administer oxygen.
○ Watch for signs of heart failure or pulmonary edema.
○ Alternate periods of activity and rest.

Identifying the murmur of tricuspid stenosis

A low, rumbling crescendo-decrescendo murmur in the tricuspid area characterizes tricuspid stenosis.

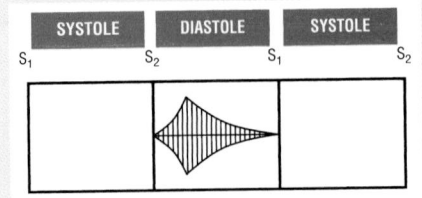

- When sitting in a chair, elevate legs to improve venous return to the heart.
- Elevate the head of the bed.
- Keep the patient on a low-sodium diet.
- If the patient has surgery, watch for hypotension, arrhythmias, and thrombus formation.

Monitoring

- Vital signs and pulse oximetry
- Cardiac rhythm
- Pulmonary artery catheter readings
- Intake and output
- Adverse effects of drug therapy

Patient teaching

Be sure to cover:
- the disorder, diagnosis, and treatment
- dietary restrictions
- prescribed drugs
- signs and symptoms that should be reported
- the importance of consistent follow-up care.

Trigeminal neuralgia

Overview

Description

- Painful disorder of the 5th cranial (trigeminal) nerve
- Right side of face affected more commonly than left
- Can subside spontaneously
- Remissions last from several months to years
- Also known as *tic douloureux*

Pathophysiology

- The trigeminal nerve has multiple branches. This nerve affects chewing movements and sensations of the face, scalp, and teeth. (See *Trigeminal nerve function and distribution.*)
- A trigger zone is stimulated, and interaction or short-circuiting of touch and pain fibers occurs.
- Paroxysmal attacks of excruciating facial pain result.

Causes

- Cause unknown
- Afferent reflex phenomenon
- Compression of the nerve root by:
  - Posterior fossa tumors
  - Middle fossa tumors
  - Vascular lesions
- Multiple sclerosis
- Herpes zoster

Trigeminal nerve function and distribution

Function
- Motor: chewing movements
- Sensory: sensations of face, scalp, and teeth (mouth and nasal chamber)

Distribution
- I   ophthalmic
- II maxillary
- III mandibular

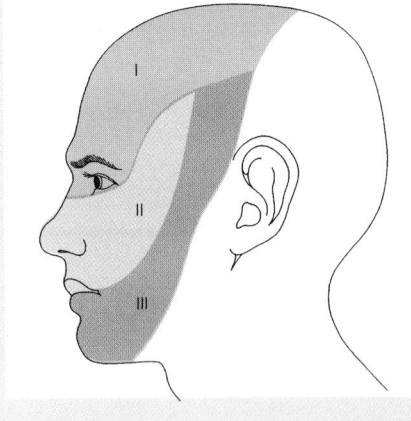

Incidence

- Affects those older than age 40
- Affects about 25% more women than men

Common characteristics

- Sudden onset of severe, throbbing pain
- Contortion of affected side of the face

Complications

- Excessive weight loss
- Depression
- Social isolation

Assessment

History

- Searing or burning facial pain that occurs in light-ninglike jabs
  - Lasts from 1 to 15 minutes (usually 1 or 2 minutes)
  - Localized in an area innervated by the trigeminal nerve
  - Initiated by a light touch to a hypersensitive area
- Attacks may follow:
  - draft of air
  - exposure to heat or cold
  - eating, smiling, and talking
  - drinking hot or cold beverages
  - a period that's free from pain.

Physical findings

- Favoring (splinting) of affected area
- Affected side of the face unwashed and unshaven
- Patient never touches affected area
- No impairment of sensory or motor function

Test results

Imaging
- Skull X-rays, computed tomography scan, and magnetic resonance imaging results rule out sinus or tooth infections and tumors.

Treatment

General

- Clinical trials investigating use of transmitter-receptor or ion channel-specific drugs
- No dietary restrictions
- No activity restrictions

Medication

- Anticonvulsants
- Analgesics

Surgery

- Microsurgery
- Radiosurgery with stereotactic technique

Nursing considerations

Key outcomes

The patient will:
- express feelings of increased comfort and decreased pain
- perform activities of daily living within confines of the disorder
- consume required caloric intake daily
- express feelings of increased energy and decreased fatigue
- perform routine roles.

Nursing interventions

- Provide emotional support.
- Provide nutritional management.
- Administer drug therapy.
- After microsurgery, provide postcraniotomy care.

Monitoring

- Characteristics of each attack
- Precipitating factors of each attack
- Response to medications
- Postoperatively, neurologic function and vital signs

Patient teaching

Be sure to cover:
- the disorder, diagnosis, and treatment
- preoperative teaching if indicated
- drugs and possible adverse effects
- nutritional management
- prevention of neuralgia attacks.

Trisomy 13 syndrome

Overview

Description

○ Third most common multiple malformation syndrome
○ In most affected infants, full trisomy 13 at birth; rarely, mosaic partial trisomy 13 syndrome (with varying phenotypes) or translocation types
○ Brain and facial abnormalities as well as major cardiac, GI, and limb malformations typical
○ Full trisomy 13 syndrome fatal
○ Also known as *Patau's syndrome*

Pathophysiology

○ About 75% of all cases result from chromosomal nondisjunction.
○ About 20% of cases result from chromosomal translocation, involving a rearrangement of chromosomes 13 and 14.
○ About 5% of cases are estimated to be mosaics; the clinical effects in these cases may be less severe.

Causes

○ Chromosomal abnormality

Risk factors

○ Advanced maternal age (mean maternal age about 31)

Incidence

○ Many trisomic zygotes spontaneously aborted (50% to 70% die within 1 month after birth and 85% by the first year)
○ Only isolated cases of survival beyond 5 years in full trisomy 13 patients; in all survivors, profound mental retardation
○ Estimated to affect 1 in 4,000 to 10,000 neonates

Common characteristics

○ Microcephaly
○ Varying degrees of holoprosencephaly
○ Sloping forehead with wide sutures and fontanel
○ Scalp defect at the vertex
○ Bilateral cleft lip with associated cleft palate
○ Flat, broad nose
○ Low-set ears and inner ear abnormalities
○ Polydactyl hands and feet
○ Club feet
○ Omphaloceles
○ Neural tube defects
○ Cystic hygroma
○ Genital abnormalities
○ Cystic kidneys
○ Hydronephrosis
○ Failure to thrive, seizures, apnea, and feeding difficulties

Complications

○ Congenital heart defects (common), especially hypoplastic left heart, ventricular septal defect, patent ductus arteriosus, or dextroposition, which may significantly contribute to the cause of death
○ Musculoskeletal abnormalities
○ Microphthalmia, cataracts, and other eye abnormalities

Assessment

History

○ Failure to thrive
○ Seizures
○ Apnea
○ Feeding difficulties

Physical findings

○ Sloping forehead with wide sutures and fontanel
○ Scalp defect at the vertex
○ Bilateral cleft lip with associated cleft palate
○ Flat, broad nose
○ Low-set ears and inner ear abnormalities
○ Polydactyl hands and feet
○ Club feet
○ Omphaloceles
○ Neural tube defects
○ Cystic hygroma
○ Genital abnormalities

Test results

Laboratory
○ Karyotype, done either prenatally or on peripheral blood lymphocytes or skin fibroblasts in a neonate or an aborted fetus, is diagnostic.
○ Results are abnormal (but not diagnostic) in multiple-marker maternal serum screening tests involving different combinations of alpha-fetoprotein, human chorionic gonadotropin (HCG) or free beta-HCG in some laboratories, and unconjugated estriol.

Imaging
○ Ultrasound usually reveals multiple abnormalities in the fetus.

Treatment

General

○ Supportive care

Nursing considerations

Key outcomes

The patient will:
○ function at the highest level possible
○ appear comfortable.

Nursing interventions

○ Maintain the infant's fluid balance.
○ Position the infant comfortably.
○ Allow adequate time for the parents to bond with and hold their child.
○ Provide emotional support to the family.

Monitoring

○ Intake and output
○ Safety
○ Growth

Patient teaching

Be sure to cover:
○ the disorder, diagnosis, and treatment
○ activities that can be carried out with the child
○ safety factors.

Discharge planning

○ Refer the parents of an affected infant for genetic counseling to explore the cause of the disorder and to discuss the risk of recurrence in future pregnancies.
○ Refer the parents to a social worker or grief counselor for additional support if needed.
○ Refer the parents to the Support Organization for Trisomy 18, 13, and Related Disorders (SOFT) national support program to allow them to interact with other parents of infants with trisomy 18 and trisomy 13.

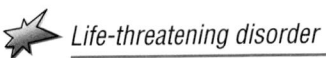 *Life-threatening disorder*

Trisomy 18 syndrome

Overview

Description

○ Second most common multiple malformation syndrome
○ In most affected infants, full trisomy 18, involving an extra (third) copy of chromosome 18 in each cell; partial trisomy 18 (with varying phenotypes) and translocation types also reported
○ Intrauterine growth retardation, congenital heart defects, microcephaly, and other malformations in most infants with this disorder
○ Full trisomy 18 syndrome generally fatal or extremely poor prognosis (30% to 50% of infants die within the first 2 months and 90% die within the first year; most surviving patients are profoundly mentally retarded.)
○ Also known as *Edwards' syndrome*

Pathophysiology

○ Most cases of trisomy 18 result from spontaneous meiotic nondisjunction, effecting an extra copy of chromosome 18 in each cell.

Causes

○ Chromosomal abnormality

Risk factors

○ Typically increases with maternal age (mean maternal age 32½)

Incidence

○ Incidence ranges from 1 in 3,000 to 8,000 neonates, with three to four females affected for every male.

Common characteristics

○ Growth retardation, which begins in utero and remains significant after birth
○ Initial hypotonia that may soon give way to hypertonia
○ Microcephaly and dolichocephaly
○ Micrognathia
○ Short, narrow nose with upturned nares
○ Unilateral or bilateral cleft lip and palate
○ Low-set, slightly pointed ears
○ Short neck
○ Conspicuous clenched hand with overlapping fingers (commonly seen on ultrasound)
○ Cystic hygroma
○ Choroid plexus cysts (also seen in some normal infants)

Complications

○ Congenital heart defects, such as ventricular septal defect, tetralogy of Fallot, transposition of the great vessels, and coarctation of the aorta (in 80% to 90% of patients), which may be the cause of death in many infants
○ Other congenital anomalies, such as diaphragmatic hernia, various renal defects, omphalocele, neural tube defects, genital and perineal abnormalities (including imperforate anus), and oligohydramnios

Assessment

History

○ Growth retardation, which begins in utero and remains significant after birth

Physical findings

○ Short, narrow nose with upturned nares
○ Unilateral or bilateral cleft lip and palate
○ Low-set, slightly pointed ears
○ Short neck
○ Conspicuous clenched hand with overlapping fingers (commonly seen on ultrasound)
○ Cystic hygroma
○ Choroid plexus cysts (also seen in some normal infants)

Test results

Laboratory
○ Karyotype, done either prenatally or on peripheral blood lymphocytes or skin fibroblasts in a neonate or an aborted fetus, is diagnostic.
○ Results are abnormal (but not diagnostic) in multiple-marker maternal serum screening tests involving different combinations of alpha-fetoprotein, human chorionic gonadotropin, and unconjugated estriol.
Imaging
○ Ultrasound commonly reveals variable abnormalities in the fetus.

Treatment

General

○ Emotional support for the family
○ Nutrition maintenance using gavage feedings

Nursing considerations

Key outcomes

The patient will:
○ function at the highest level possible
○ appear comfortable.

Nursing interventions
○ Allow adequate time for the parents to bond with and hold their child.
○ Provide emotional support to the family.

Monitoring
○ Intake and output
○ Growth

Patient teaching

Be sure to cover:
○ the disorder, diagnosis, and treatment
○ home care and feeding techniques.

Discharge planning
○ Refer the parents of a child affected with trisomy 18 syndrome for genetic counseling to explore the cause of the disorder and discuss the risk of recurrence in a future pregnancy.
○ Refer the parents to a social worker or grief counselor for additional support if needed.
○ Refer the parents to the Support Organization for Trisomy 18, 13, and Related Disorders (S.O.F.T.) national support program to allow them to interact with other parents of infants with trisomy 18 and trisomy 13.

Tuberculosis

Overview

Description

- ○ Acute or chronic lung infection characterized by pulmonary infiltrates and the formation of granulomas with caseation, fibrosis, and cavitation
- ○ Prognosis excellent with proper treatment and compliance
- ○ Also known as *TB*

Pathophysiology

- ○ Multiplication of the bacillus *Mycobacterium tuberculosis* causes an inflammatory process where deposited.
- ○ A cell-mediated immune response follows, usually containing the infection within 4 to 6 weeks.
- ○ The T-cell response results in the formation of granulomas around the bacilli, making them dormant. This confers immunity to subsequent infection.
- ○ Bacilli within granulomas may remain viable for many years, resulting in a positive purified protein derivative or other skin test for TB.
- ○ Active disease develops in 5% to 15% of those infected.
- ○ Transmission occurs when an infected person coughs or sneezes.

Causes

- ○ Exposure to *M. tuberculosis*
- ○ Sometimes, exposure to other strains of mycobacteria

Risk factors

- ○ Close contact with newly diagnosed TB patient
- ○ History of prior TB exposure
- ○ Multiple sexual partners
- ○ Recent immigration from Africa, Asia, Mexico, or South America
- ○ Gastrectomy
- ○ History of silicosis, diabetes, malnutrition, cancer, Hodgkin's disease, or leukemia
- ○ Drug and alcohol abuse
- ○ Residence in nursing home, mental health facility, or prison
- ○ Immunosuppression and use of corticosteroids
- ○ Homelessness

Incidence

- ○ Overall decrease in TB but greater among high-risk populations
- ○ Twice as common in men as in women
- ○ Four times as common in nonwhites as in whites
- ○ Higher incidence in Black and Hispanic men between ages 25 and 44
- ○ Highest incidence in people who live in crowded, poorly ventilated, unsanitary conditions

Common characteristics

- ○ Weakness and fatigue
- ○ Anorexia, weight loss
- ○ Low-grade fever
- ○ Night sweats

Complications

- ○ Massive pulmonary tissue damage
- ○ Respiratory failure
- ○ Bronchopleural fistulas
- ○ Pneumothorax
- ○ Pleural effusion
- ○ Pneumonia
- ○ Infection of other body organs by small mycobacterial foci
- ○ Liver involvement disease secondary to drug therapy

Assessment

History

In primary infection

- ○ May be asymptomatic after a 4- to 8-week incubation period
- ○ Weakness and fatigue
- ○ Anorexia, weight loss
- ○ Low-grade fever
- ○ Night sweats

In reactivated infection

- ○ Chest pain
- ○ Productive cough for blood, or mucopurulent or blood-tinged sputum
- ○ Low-grade fever

Physical findings

- ○ Dullness over the affected area
- ○ Crepitant crackles
- ○ Bronchial breath sounds
- ○ Wheezes
- ○ Whispered pectoriloquy

Test results

Laboratory

- ○ Tuberculin skin test is positive in both active and inactive tuberculosis.
- ○ Stains and cultures of sputum, cerebrospinal fluid, urine, abscess drainage, or pleural fluid show heat-sensitive, nonmotile, aerobic, acid-fast bacilli.

Imaging

- ○ Chest X-rays show nodular lesions, patchy infiltrates, cavity formation, scar tissue, and calcium deposits.
- ○ Computed tomography or magnetic resonance imaging shows presence and extent of lung damage.

Diagnostic procedures

- ○ Bronchoscopy specimens show heat-sensitive, nonmotile, aerobic, acid-fast bacilli in specimens.

Treatment

General

○ After 2 to 4 weeks, when disease is no longer infectious, resumption of normal activities while continuing to take medication
○ Well-balanced, high-calorie diet
○ Rest, initially; activity as tolerated

Medication

○ Antitubercular therapy for at least 6 months with daily oral doses of:
  – isoniazid
  – rifampin
  – pyrazinamide
  – ethambutol, added in some cases.
○ Second-line drugs include:
  – capreomycin
  – streptomycin
  – aminosalicylic acid (para-aminosalicylic acid)
  – pyrazinamide
  – cycloserine.

Surgery

○ For some complications

Nursing considerations

Key outcomes

The patient will:
○ maintain adequate ventilation
○ use support systems to assist with coping
○ identify measures to prevent or reduce fatigue
○ express an understanding of the illness
○ comply with treatment regimen.

Nursing interventions

○ Administer drug therapy.
○ Isolate the patient in a quiet, properly ventilated room, and maintain tuberculosis precautions.
○ Provide diversional activities.
○ Properly dispose of secretions.
○ Provide adequate rest periods.
○ Provide well-balanced, high-calorie foods.
○ Provide small, frequent meals.
○ Consult with dietitian if oral supplements are needed.
○ Perform chest physiotherapy.
○ Provide supportive care.
○ Include the patient in care decisions.

Monitoring

○ Vital signs
○ Intake and output
○ Daily weight
○ Complications
○ Adverse reactions
○ Visual acuity if taking ethambutol
○ Liver and kidney function tests

Preventing tuberculosis

Explain respiratory and standard precautions to a hospitalized patient with tuberculosis. Before discharge, tell him that he must take precautions to prevent spreading the disease, such as wearing a mask around others, until his physician tells him he's no longer contagious. He should tell all health care providers he sees, including his dentist and optometrist, that he has tuberculosis so that they can institute infection-control precautions.

Teach the patient other specific precautions to avoid spreading the infection. Tell him to cough and sneeze into tissues and to dispose of the tissues properly. Stress the importance of washing his hands thoroughly in hot, soapy water after handling his own secretions. Also instruct him to wash his eating utensils separately in hot, soapy water.

Patient teaching

Be sure to cover:
○ the disorder, diagnosis, and treatment
○ drugs and potential adverse effects
○ when to notify the physician
○ need for isolation
○ postural drainage and chest percussion
○ coughing and deep-breathing exercises
○ regular follow-up examinations
○ signs and symptoms of recurring TB
○ possible decreased hormonal contraceptive effectiveness while taking rifampin
○ need for a high-calorie, high-protein, balanced diet
○ TB prevention. (See *Preventing tuberculosis.*)

Discharge planning

○ Refer anyone exposed to an infected patient for testing and follow-up.
○ Refer patient to a support group, such as the American Lung Association.
○ Refer patient to a smoking-cessation program if indicated.

Tularemia

Overview

Description

- *Francisella tularensis* organism, a gram-negative pleomorphic bacterium, causing disease in humans and animals
- As few as 10 organisms able to cause disease
- Incubation period 3 to 4 days
- Six forms:
  - Ulceroglandular form
  - Glandular form
  - Oculoglandular form
  - Oropharyngeal form
  - Pneumonic form
  - Septicemic form

Pathophysiology

- The organism gains access to the host by skin or mucous membrane inoculation, inhalation, or ingestion.
- After inoculation a papule (that eventually evolves into an ulcer) and high fever develop.

Causes

- Bites of ticks and deerflies
- Eating or drinking contaminated food or water
- Contact with the blood of an infected animal, especially rabbits
- Breathing in the bacteria F. tularensis

Incidence

- About 200 cases in humans annually
- Occurs more commonly in the south-central and western United States

Common characteristics

- Ulcer and fever

Complications

- Pneumonia
- Lung abscess
- Respiratory failure
- Rhabdomyolysis
- Meningitis
- Pericarditis
- Osteomyelitis

Assessment

History

- Tick bite
- Exposure to contaminated food or water
- Exposure to contaminated blood
- Abrupt onset of fever, chills, headache, and malaise

Physical findings

Ulceroglandular
- Ulcers at the site of inoculation
- Swollen regional lymph nodes

Glandular
- Swollen regional lymph nodes

Oculoglandular
- Painful
- Red eye
- Purulent exudates
- Swollen submandibular, preauricular, or cervical lymph nodes

Oropharyngeal
- Sore throat
- Abdominal pain
- Nausea
- Vomiting
- Diarrhea
- Occasionally, GI bleeding

Pneumonic
- Dry cough
- Dyspnea
- Pleuritic chest pain

Septicemic
- Fever, chills, myalgia, malaise, and weight loss
- Absence of ulcer

Test results

- Serology for tularemia
- Chest X-ray
- May alter results of febrile or cold agglutins

Laboratory
- White blood cell count is normal or elevated.
- Blood or sputum cultures are positive for *F. tularensis*.

Treatment

General

- Proper skin care
- Increased fluid intake

Medication

- I.V., I.M., or oral antibiotics
- Antipyretics

Nursing considerations

Key outcomes

The patient will:
- regain normal temperature
- regain or maintain normal fluid balance.

Nursing interventions

- Give prescribed drugs.
- Replace lost fluids through diet or I.V. fluids.

Monitoring
○ Intake and output
○ Vital signs
○ Signs of dehydration

Patient teaching

Be sure to cover:
○ the disorder, diagnosis, and treatment
○ drugs and potential adverse effects
○ complications and when to notify the physician
○ preventive measures, such as using insect repellent containing DEET on skin, or treating clothing with repellent containing permethrin.

Ulcerative colitis

Overview

Description

- Episodic inflammatory chronic disease that causes ulcerations of the mucosa in the colon
- Condition begins in the rectum and sigmoid colon and may extend upward into the entire colon
- Rarely affects the small intestine, except for the terminal ileum
- Produces congestion, edema (leading to mucosal friability), and ulcerations
- Range of severity from mild, localized disorder to fulminant disease that causes many complications

Pathophysiology

- The disorder primarily involves the mucosa and the submucosa of the bowel.
- Crypt abscesses and mucosal ulceration may occur.
- The mucosa typically appears granular and friable.
- The colon becomes a rigid, foreshortened tube.
- In severe ulcerative colitis, areas of hyperplastic growth occur, with swollen mucosa surrounded by inflamed mucosa with shallow ulcers.
- Submucosa and the circular and longitudinal muscles may be involved.

Causes

- Cause unknown
- May be related to an abnormal immune response in the GI tract, possibly associated with genetic factors

Risk factors

- Stress (may increase severity of an attack)
- Family history
- Jewish ancestry

Incidence

- Primarily young adults, especially women
- More prevalent among Jews and higher socioeconomic groups
- About 1 in 1,000 persons affected
- Onset of symptoms commonly peaking between ages 15 and 30 and again between ages 50 and 70

Common characteristics

- Crampy lower abdominal pain
- Recurrent bloody diarrhea

Complications

- Nutritional deficiencies
- Perineal sepsis
- Anal fissure, anal fistula
- Perirectal abscess
- Perforation of the colon
- Hemorrhage, anemia
- Toxic megacolon
- Cancer
- Coagulation defects
- Erythema nodosum on the face and arms
- Pyoderma gangrenosum on the legs and ankles
- Uveitis
- Pericholangitis, sclerosing cholangitis
- Cirrhosis
- Cholangiocarcinoma
- Ankylosing spondylitis
- Strictures
- Pseudopolyps, stenosis, and perforated colon leading to peritonitis and toxemia
- Arthritis

Assessment

History

- Remission and exacerbation of symptoms
- Mild cramping and lower abdominal pain
- Recurrent bloody diarrhea as often as 10 to 25 times daily
- Nocturnal diarrhea
- Fatigue and weakness
- Anorexia and weight loss
- Nausea and vomiting

Physical findings

- Liquid stools with visible pus, mucus, and blood
- Possible abdominal distention
- Abdominal tenderness
- Perianal irritation, hemorrhoids, and fissures
- Jaundice
- Joint pain

Test results

Laboratory

- Stool specimen analysis reveals blood, pus, and mucus, but no pathogenic organisms.
- Other supportive laboratory tests show decreased serum levels of potassium, magnesium, hemoglobin, and albumin as well as leukocytosis and increased prothrombin time; an elevated erythrocyte sedimentation rate correlates with the severity of the attack.

Imaging

- Barium enema discloses the extent of disease and complications, such as strictures and carcinoma. This study isn't performed in a patient with active signs and symptoms.

Diagnostic procedures

- Sigmoidoscopy confirms rectal involvement in most cases by showing increased mucosal friability, decreased mucosal detail, and thick inflammatory exudates, edema, and erosions.
- Colonoscopy may be used to determine the extent of the disease and to evaluate the areas of stricture and pseudopolyps. This test isn't performed when the patient has active signs and symptoms.
- Biopsy, performed during colonoscopy, helps to confirm the diagnosis.

Treatment

General

- I.V. fluid replacement
- Blood transfusions (if needed)
- Nothing by mouth (if severe)
- Parenteral nutrition (with severe disease)
- Supplemental feedings
- Rest periods during exacerbations

Medication

- Corticotropin and adrenal corticosteroids
- Sulfasalazine
- Mesalamine
- Antispasmodics and antidiarrheals
- Fiber supplements

Surgery

- Treatment of last resort
- Proctocolectomy with ileostomy
- Pouch ileostomy
- Ileoanal reservoir with loop ileostomy
- Colectomy (after 10 years of active disease)

Nursing considerations

Key outcomes

The patient will:
- express feelings of increased comfort and decreased pain
- have normal fluid volume
- have intact skin
- exhibit no evidence of infection
- avoid or have only minimal complications
- maintain adequate caloric intake.

Nursing interventions

- Encourage verbalization and provide support.
- Provide diet therapy.
- Administer drug therapy.
- Give blood transfusions.
- Schedule care to allow for frequent rest periods.

Monitoring

- Response to treatment
- Fluid and electrolyte status
- Hemoglobin level and hematocrit
- Complications

After surgery
- Vital signs
- Wound site
- Pain level
- Bowel function
- Nasogastric tube function and drainage
- Skin integrity

Patient teaching

Be sure to cover:
- the disorder, diagnosis, and treatment
- all prescribed dietary changes
- need to avoid GI stimulants, such as caffeine, alcohol, and smoking
- drug administration, dosage, and possible adverse effects
- after a proctocolectomy and ileostomy, stoma care
- after a pouch ileostomy, procedures to insert the catheter and care for the stoma
- the need for regular physical examinations because of the increased risk of colorectal cancer.

Discharge planning

- Refer the patient to a smoking-cessation program if indicated.
- Refer the patient to an enterostomal therapist if appropriate.

Urinary tract infection, lower

Overview

Description

- Bacterial infection of the lower urinary tract system
- Two forms:
  - Cystitis (infection of the bladder)
  - Urethritis (infection of the urethra)
- Usually a ready response to treatment
- Possible recurring and resistant bacterial flare-ups during therapy
- Also known as *lower UTI*

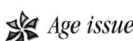 **Age issue**

In adult males and children, lower UTIs are typically associated with anatomic or physiologic abnormalities and require close evaluation.

Pathophysiology

- Local defense mechanisms in the bladder break down.
- Bacteria invade the bladder mucosa and multiply.
- Bacteria can't be readily eliminated by normal urination.
- The pathogen's resistance to prescribed antimicrobial therapy usually causes bacterial flare-up during treatment.
- Recurrent lower UTIs result from reinfection by the same organism or a new pathogen.

Causes

- Ascending infection by a single gram-negative, enteric bacterium, such as *Escherichia coli, Klebsiella, Proteus, Enterobacter, Pseudomonas,* and *Serratia*
- Simultaneous infection with multiple pathogens

Risk factors

- Natural anatomical variations
- Inadequate fluid consumption
- Trauma or invasive procedures
- Urinary catheter
- Urinary tract obstructions
- Vesicourethral reflux
- Urinary stasis
- Diabetes
- Bowel incontinence
- Immobility

Incidence

- Nearly 10 times more common in females than in males (except elderly males), probably because natural anatomic features facilitate infection
- Affects 10% to 20% of all females at least once

Common characteristics

- Urinary urgency and frequency
- Dysuria
- Cloudy, foul-smelling urine
- Mild fever

Complications

- Damage to the urinary tract lining
- Infection of adjacent organs and structures

Assessment

History

- Urinary urgency and frequency
- Bladder cramps or spasms
- Pruritus
- Feeling of warmth during urination
- Nocturia or dysuria
- Urethral discharge (in men)
- Lower back or flank pain
- Malaise and chills
- Nausea and vomiting

Physical findings

- Pain or tenderness over the bladder
- Hematuria
- Fever
- Cloudy, foul-smelling urine

Test results

Laboratory
- Microscopic urinalysis shows red blood cell and white blood cell counts greater than 10 per high-power field, suggesting lower UTI.
- Clean-catch urinalysis shows bacterial count of more than 100,000/ml, confirming UTI.
- Sensitivity testing determines appropriate antimicrobial drug.
- If the patient history and physical examination warrant, a blood test or a stained smear of urethral discharge rules out sexually transmitted disease.

Imaging
- Voiding cystourethrography or excretory urography may demonstrate congenital anomalies, predisposing the patient to recurrent UTIs.

Treatment

General

- Sitz baths or warm compresses
- Increased fruit juice intake, especially cranberry
- Increased fluid intake

Medication

- Antimicrobials

Surgery

○ In case of recurrent infections from infected renal calculi, chronic prostatitis, or structural abnormalities

Nursing considerations

Key outcomes

The patient will:
○ report increased comfort
○ identify risk factors that worsen the condition, and modify her lifestyle accordingly
○ demonstrate skill in managing the urinary elimination problem
○ complete the prescribed course of treatment.

Nursing interventions

○ Collect all urine specimens appropriately.
○ Administer drug therapy.
○ Encourage oral fluid intake unless contraindicated.
○ Use sitz baths or warm compresses, as needed.

Monitoring

○ Intake and output
○ Urine characteristics
○ Voiding patterns
○ Vital signs
○ Adverse effects of antimicrobial therapy

Patient teaching

Be sure to cover:
○ the disorder, diagnosis, and treatment
○ completing the prescribed course of antibiotic therapy
○ drug administration, dosage, and possible adverse effects
○ warm sitz baths to relieve perineal discomfort
○ proper cleaning after toileting.

Urticaria and angioedema

Overview

Description

○ Common allergic reactions
○ Occur separately or simultaneously
○ Urticaria: may be acute (present less than 6 weeks) or chronic (present at least 6 weeks)
○ Also known as *hives*

Pathophysiology

○ Urticaria is an episodic, rapidly occurring, usually self-limiting skin reaction. It involves only the superficial portion of the dermis, which erupts with local wheals surrounded by an erythematous flare.
○ Angioedema involves additional skin layers and produces deeper, larger wheals (usually on the hands, feet, lips, genitalia, and eyelids). It causes diffuse swelling of loose subcutaneous tissue and may affect the upper respiratory and GI tracts.
○ Several mechanisms and disorders may provoke urticaria and angioedema. They include immunoglobulin (Ig) E-induced release of mediators from cutaneous mast cells and binding of IgG or IgM to antigen, resulting in complement activation.

Causes

○ Unknown
○ Drug allergy
○ Food allergy
○ Insect bite
○ Occupational skin exposure
○ Inhalant allergens (animal dander, cosmetics)
○ Viral infection
○ Hormones
○ Thyroid abnormality
○ Rheumatological disease
○ Cholinergic trigger (heat, exercise, stress)

Incidence

○ Affect about 20% of general population at some time
○ More common after adolescence, with highest incidence in the 30s
○ Affect females more commonly than males

Common characteristics

○ Raised, red wheals
○ Diffuse edema
○ Pruritus

Complications

○ Skin abrasion and secondary infection
○ Laryngeal edema
○ Respiratory arrest
○ Severe abdominal colic

Assessment

History

○ Drug history including nonprescription preparations, such as vitamins, aspirin, and antacids
○ Reported commonly troublesome foods and environmental factors
○ Exposure to physical factors, such as cold, sunlight, exercise, and trauma (dermatographism)
○ Adverse reaction to iodinated contrast media used for diagnostic radiological studies

Physical findings

○ Distinct, raised, evanescent dermal wheals surrounded by a reddened flare
○ Nonpitting swelling of deep subcutaneous tissue on the eyelids, lips, genitalia, and mucous membranes that doesn't itch but may burn and tingle
○ Respiratory stridor and hoarseness
○ Anxiety, gasping for breath, and difficulty speaking
○ Abdominal colic with or without nausea and vomiting
○ Signs of anaphylaxis: hypotension, respiratory distress, stridor

Test results

Laboratory
○ Decreased serum levels of C1, C2, and C4 inhibitors confirm the diagnosis.
Diagnostic procedures
○ Diagnosis can be confirmed through careful skin testing with the suspected offending substance to see if a local wheal and flare result.

Treatment

General

○ Emergency measures if signs of anaphylaxis
○ Limited contact with triggering factors
○ Desensitization to the triggering antigen
○ Avoidance of food allergens

Medication

○ Antihistamines
○ Systemic glucocorticoids

Nursing considerations

Key outcomes

The patient will:
○ maintain a patent airway
○ express feelings of increased comfort and decreased pain
○ exhibit improved or healed lesions or wounds
○ avoid or have only minimal complications
○ correlate precipitating factors with appropriate skin care regimen.

Nursing interventions

○ Maintain a patent airway.
○ Reduce or minimize environmental exposure to offending allergens and irritants, such as wool and harsh detergents.
○ If food is a suspected cause, gradually eliminate foods from the diet, and watch for improvement.
○ Administer drug therapy.

Monitoring

○ Vital signs, with attention to respiratory status
○ Skin, for signs of secondary infection caused by scratching
○ Response to treatment

Patient teaching

Be sure to cover:
○ the disorder, diagnosis, and treatment
○ how to identify the cause by keeping a diary to record exposure to suspected offending substances and signs and symptoms that appear after exposure
○ how to monitor nutritional status and food replacements for nutrients lost by excluding allergy-provoking foods and beverages
○ the need to keep fingernails short to avoid abrading the skin when scratching
○ signs and symptoms that indicate a skin infection
○ use of an epinephrine emergency kit if anaphylaxis occurs.

Uterine bleeding, dysfunctional

Overview

Description

○ Abnormal endometrial bleeding without recognizable organic lesions
○ The indication for almost 25% of gynecologic surgical procedures
○ Prognosis varies with cause, but good prognosis with correction of hormonal imbalance or structural abnormality
○ Also known as *DUB*

Pathophysiology

○ Irregular bleeding is associated with hormonal imbalance and anovulation (failure of ovulation to occur).
○ When progesterone secretion is absent but estrogen secretion continues, the endometrium proliferates and becomes hypervascular.
○ When ovulation doesn't occur, the endometrium is randomly broken down, and exposed vascular channels cause prolonged and excessive bleeding.
○ In most cases of abnormal uterine bleeding, the endometrium shows no pathologic changes; however, in chronic unopposed estrogen stimulation (as from a hormone-producing ovarian tumor), the endometrium may show hyperplastic or malignant changes.

Causes

○ Usually an imbalance in the hormonal-endometrial relationship involving persistent and unopposed stimulation of the endometrium by estrogen
○ Disorders causing sustained high estrogen levels:
  – Polycystic ovary syndrome
  – Obesity (because enzymes present in peripheral adipose tissue convert the androgen androstenedione to estrogen precursors)
  – Immaturity of the hypothalamic-pituitary-ovarian mechanism (postpubertal teenagers)
  – Anovulation (women in their late 30s or early 40s)
○ Trauma (foreign object insertion or direct trauma)
○ Endometriosis
○ Coagulopathy, such as thrombocytopenia or leukemia (rare)
○ Drug-induced coagulopathy

Incidence

○ About 10% of women with normal ovulatory cycles
○ More episodes of abnormal bleeding among black women, possibly secondary to a higher incidence of leiomyomas and higher levels of estrogen
○ Most common in puberty and perimenopause

Common characteristics

○ Metrorrhagia (episodes of vaginal bleeding between menses)
○ Hypermenorrhea (heavy or prolonged menses, longer than 8 days, also incorrectly termed menorrhagia)
○ Chronic polymenorrhea (menstrual cycle less than 18 days) or oligomenorrhea (infrequent menses)
○ Fatigue from anemia
○ Oligomenorrhea and infertility from anovulation

Complications

○ Iron deficiency anemia (blood loss of more than 1.6 L over a short time)
○ Hemorrhagic shock
○ Right-sided heart failure (rare)
○ Endometrial adenocarcinoma from chronic estrogen stimulation

Assessment

History

○ Abnormal uterine bleeding
○ Fatigue
○ Infertility
○ Bleeding in response to a brief course of progesterone
○ Absence of body temperature changes during ovulatory cycle

Physical findings

○ Pallor
○ Signs of underlying disorder
○ Pelvic examination revealing uterine abnormality

Test results

Laboratory
○ Hemoglobin levels and hematocrit determine the need for blood transfusion or iron supplementation.
○ Serum progesterone levels are decreased.
Diagnostic procedures
○ Dilatation and curettage (D&C) or office endometrial biopsy rules out endometrial hyperplasia and cancer in women over age 35.

Treatment

General

○ Monitoring of bleeding episodes
○ Emotional support
○ Balanced diet
○ Rest periods when fatigued

Medication

○ High-dose estrogen-progestogen combination therapy (hormonal contraceptives); maintenance therapy with lower dose combination hormonal contraceptives

○ Progestogen therapy
○ I.V. estrogen followed by progesterone or combination hormonal contraceptives if the patient is young (more likely to be anovulatory) and severely anemic (if oral drug therapy is ineffective)
○ Iron supplementation or transfusions of packed cells or whole blood

Surgery

○ Endometrial biopsy to rule out endometrial adenocarcinoma (patients age 35 and older)
○ D&C (short-lived treatment and not clinically useful, but an important diagnostic tool) with hysteroscopy as an adjunct

Nursing considerations

Key outcomes

The patient will:
○ maintain hemodynamic stability
○ have normal menstrual cycles
○ express understanding of the disorder and its treatment.

Nursing interventions

○ Tell the patient to record the dates of the bleeding and the number of pads she saturates per day. Instruct the patient not to use tampons.
○ Offer reassurance and support.
○ Suggest to the patient that she minimize blood flow by avoiding strenuous activity and by lying down with her feet elevated.

Monitoring

○ Vital signs
○ Amount of bleeding
○ Hemoglobin levels
○ Response to treatment

Patient teaching

Be sure to cover:
○ the importance of following the prescribed hormonal therapy
○ the purpose and procedures of D&C or endometrial biopsy procedure if ordered
○ the need for regular checkups to assess the effectiveness of treatment
○ the importance of reporting abnormal bleeding immediately to help rule out major hemorrhagic disorders such as those that occur in abnormal pregnancy
○ having a Papanicolaou test and a pelvic examination annually.

Uterine cancer

Overview

Description

- Proliferation of cancer cells in the endometrium
- Most common gynecologic cancer
- Also known as *endometrial cancer*

Pathophysiology

- Uterine cancer is usually adenocarcinoma.
- Metastasis occurs late (usually from the endometrium to the cervix, ovaries, fallopian tubes, and other peritoneal structures). It may spread to distant organs, such as the lungs and the brain, by way of the blood or the lymphatic system; lymph node involvement can also occur.
- Less common uterine tumors include adenoacanthoma, endometrial stromal sarcoma, lymphosarcoma, mixed mesodermal tumors (including carcinosarcoma), and leiomyosarcoma.

Causes

- Exact cause unknown

Risk factors

- Low fertility index and anovulation
- History of infertility or failure of ovulation
- Abnormal uterine bleeding
- Obesity
- Hypertension
- Diabetes
- Nulliparity
- Familial tendency
- History of uterine polyps or endometrial hyperplasia
- Prolonged estrogen therapy with exposure unopposed by progesterone
- Tamoxifen therapy

Common characteristics

- Abnormal vaginal bleeding
- Lower abdominal bleeding

Incidence

- Most common in postmenopausal women between ages 60 and 70 (uncommon between ages 30 and 40 and rare before age 30)
- Most premenopausal patients having history of anovulatory menstrual cycles or other hormonal imbalances
- Annually about 33,000 new cases reported; about 5,500 eventually fatal

Complications

- Anemia
- Intestinal obstruction
- Ascites
- Increasing pain
- Hemorrhage

Assessment

History

- Presence of risk factors
- Spotting and protracted, heavy menses (in younger patient)
- In postmenopausal woman, possible bleeding beginning 12 or more months after menses stopped
- Vaginal discharge, initially watery, then increasingly blood streaked

Physical findings

- Palpable enlarged uterus (advanced disease)
- Abdominal tenderness

Test results

Diagnostic procedures
- Endometrial, cervical, or endocervical biopsy confirms the presence of cancer cells.
- Fractional dilatation and curettage are used to identify the problem when the disease is suspected but the endometrial biopsy result is negative.
- Multiple cervical biopsies and endocervical curettage pinpoint cervical involvement.
- Papanicolaou test result may be normal or show abnormal cells.

Other
- Schiller's test involves staining the cervix and vagina with an iodine solution that turns healthy tissues brown. (Cancerous tissues resist the stain.)

Treatment

General

- Radiation therapy
- Well-balanced diet

Medication

- Hormonal therapy
- Chemotherapy

Surgery

- Total abdominal hysterectomy, bilateral salpingo-oophorectomy or, possibly, omentectomy with or without pelvic or para-aortic lymphadenectomy
- Total pelvic exenteration

Nursing considerations

Key outcomes

The patient will:
- express positive feelings about self
- report feeling increased comfort and decreased pain
- (with partner) express feelings and perceptions about change in sexual performance
- experience no signs or symptoms of infection.

Nursing interventions
○ Encourage verbalization and provide support.
○ Administer drug therapy.
○ Encourage the patient to breathe deeply and cough.

Monitoring
After surgery
○ Wound site and drainage system
○ Vital signs
○ Postoperative complications
○ Pain control
Internal radiation therapy
○ Safety precautions (time, distance, and shielding)
○ Movement (limited while source is in place)
○ Vital signs
○ Complications from radiation therapy, such as skin
   reaction, vaginal bleeding, abdominal discomfort,
   and dehydration

Patient teaching

Be sure to cover:
○ the disorder, diagnosis, and treatment
○ preoperative and postoperative care
○ (if the patient is premenopausal) that removal of her
   ovaries will induce menopause
○ safety measures involved in internal radiation therapy
○ dietary modifications
○ drug administration, dosage, and possible adverse effects
○ importance of follow-up examinations with a gyne-
   cologist.

Discharge planning
○ Refer the patient to available resource and support
   services.

Uterine leiomyomas

Overview

Description

- Most common benign uterine tumors in women
- Tumors composed of smooth muscle that usually occur in the uterine corpus, although they may appear on the cervix or on the round or broad ligament
- Malignant (leiomyosarcoma) in less than 0.1% of patients
- Also known as *myomas, fibromyomas,* or *fibroids*

Pathophysiology

- Classified according to location, tumors may be located within the uterine wall (intramural) or protrude into the endometrial cavity (submucous) or from the serosal surface of the uterus (subserous).
- Size varies greatly.
- Tumors are usually firm and surrounded by a pseudocapsule composed of compressed but otherwise normal uterine myometrium.
- The uterine cavity may become larger, increasing the endometrial surface area. This can cause increased uterine bleeding.

Causes

- Unknown, but some factors implicated as regulators of leiomyoma growth include:
  - several growth factors including epidermal growth factor
  - steroid hormones, including estrogen and progesterone (typically arise after menarche and regress after menopause, implicating estrogen as a promoter of leiomyoma growth).

Incidence

- May affect three times as many Blacks as Whites; true incidence in either population unknown
- May occur at any age, but most common in women over age 30

Common characteristics

- Abnormal bleeding, typically menorrhagia with disrupted submucosal vessels (most common symptom)
- Pain only associated with torsion of a pedunculated (stemmed) subserous tumor or leiomyomas undergoing degeneration
- Pelvic pressure and impingement on adjacent viscera (indications for treatment, depending on severity) resulting in mild hydronephrosis

Complications

- Recurrent spontaneous abortion
- Preterm labor
- Malposition of the fetus
- Anemia secondary to excessive bleeding
- Bladder compression
- Infection (if tumor protrudes out of the vaginal opening)
- Secondary infertility (rare)
- Bowel obstruction

Assessment

History

- Abnormal menstrual bleeding
- Urinary frequency, urgency, or incontinence
- Abdominal cramping during menstruation

Physical findings

- Pelvic pressure
- Abdominal distention

Test results

Laboratory
- Blood studies show anemia from abnormal bleeding (may support diagnosis).

Imaging
- Ultrasound allows accurate assessment of the dimension, number, and location of tumors.
- Magnetic resonance imaging reveals calcified fibroids.

Diagnostic procedures
- Hysterosalpingography detects myomas.

Other
- Patient history reveals evidence.
- Bimanual examination shows enlarged, firm, nontender, and irregularly contoured uterus (also seen with adenomyosis and other pelvic abnormalities).
- Endometrial biopsy rules out endometrial cancer in patients over age 35 with abnormal uterine bleeding.
- Laparoscopy corroborates other testing.

Treatment

General

- Blood transfusions
- Activity as tolerated

Medication

- Gonadotropin-releasing hormone (Gn-RH) agonists to rapidly suppress pituitary gonadotropin release
- Nonsteroidal anti-inflammatories

Surgery

- Abdominal, laparoscopic, or hysteroscopic myomectomy
- Myolysis
- Uterine artery embolization (radiologic procedure) to block uterine arteries using small pieces of polyvinyl chloride
- Hysterectomy

Nursing considerations

Key outcomes

The patient will:
○ report increased comfort and decreased pain
○ relate understanding of the disorder and treatment and state feelings
○ return to normal menstrual periods.

Nursing interventions

○ Reassure the patient that she won't experience premature menopause if her ovaries are left intact.
○ In a patient with severe anemia from excessive bleeding, give iron supplements and blood transfusions.
○ Encourage the patient to verbalize her feelings and concerns related to the disease process and its effects on her lifestyle.

Monitoring

○ Comfort level
○ Amount of bleeding
○ Response to treatment

Patient teaching

Be sure to cover:
○ the disorder, diagnosis, and treatment
○ the importance of reporting abnormal bleeding or pelvic pain immediately
○ the importance of regular gynecologic examinations.

Vaginal cancer

Overview

Description
- Proliferation of cancer cells in the vagina
- Rarest gynecologic cancer
- Usually appears as squamous cell carcinoma, but occasionally as melanoma, sarcoma, or adenocarcinoma

Pathophysiology
- Because the vagina is a thin-walled structure with rich lymphatic drainage, vaginal cancer varies in severity, depending on its exact location and effect on lymphatic drainage.
- It may progress from an intraepithelial tumor to an invasive cancer.
- The upper third of the vagina is the most common site of vaginal cancer.

Causes
- Exact cause unknown

Risk factors
- Advanced age (most likely risk factor) combined with:
  - trauma
  - chronic pessary use
  - use of chemical carcinogens (such as those in some sprays and douches)
  - use of diethylstilbestrol (DES) by the patient's mother during pregnancy
  - previous cancer of the endometrium, vulva, or cervix.

Incidence
- Usually occurs in women in their early to middle 50s
- Rarely, rhabdomyosarcoma in children

Common characteristics
- Bloody vaginal drainage
- Urine retention

Complications
- Metastasis may affect the cervix, uterus, and rectum.

Assessment

History
- Presence of risk factors
- Bloody vaginal discharge
- Irregular or postmenopausal bleeding
- Urine retention or urinary frequency (if the lesion is close to the neck of the bladder)

Physical findings
- Ulcerated lesion in any area of the vagina

Test results

Laboratory
- Papanicolaou test shows abnormal cells.

Diagnostic procedures
- Biopsy identifies cancerous cells. Biopsy of the cervix and vulva may also be performed to rule out these areas as primary cancer sites.
- Colposcopy is used to locate lesions that may have been missed during the pelvic examination.

Other
- Lugol's solution painted on the suspected area helps to identify malignant areas by staining glycogen-containing normal tissue. (Abnormal tissue resists staining.)

Treatment

General
- Radiation therapy (preferred treatment for all stages of vaginal cancer)
- Well-balanced diet
- Limited activity with internal radiation therapy

Medication
- Topical chemotherapy with fluorouracil and laser surgery

Surgery
- May be recommended when tumor is so extensive that vagina's close proximity to the bladder and rectum allows only minimal tissue margins around resected vaginal tissue

Nursing considerations

Key outcomes
The patient will:
- express positive feelings about self
- experience feelings of increased comfort and decreased pain
- express feelings and perceptions about change in sexual performance (with partner)
- exhibit no signs or symptoms of infection.

Nursing interventions
- Encourage verbalization and provide support.
- Administer drug therapy.

Monitoring
- Response to treatment
- Vaginal discharge

Internal radiation therapy
- Safety measures (time, distance, and shielding)
- Limited movement
- Complications from radiation therapy

Patient teaching

Be sure to cover:
- the disorder, diagnosis, and treatment
- safety measures (for internal radiation therapy)
- importance of follow-up care
- importance of regular gynecologic check-ups
- potential adverse reactions to chemotherapy and ways to manage them
- signs and symptoms of infection and the need to report them to a physician immediately
- ways to avoid infection.

Discharge planning

- Refer the patient (and family) to American Cancer Society for resources and support services.

Vancomycin intermediate-resistant *Staphylococcus aureus*

Overview

Description

○ Staphylococci infection that has decreased susceptibility to vancomycin
○ Common in chronically ill patients; most likely developing in health care setting
○ Patient with methicillin-resistant *Staphylococcus aureus* (MRSA) normally most reliably and effectively treated with vancomycin; MRSA with decreased susceptibility to vancomycin possibly a sign that vancomycin-resistant strains are emerging
○ Also called *VISA* and *glycopeptide intermediate-resistant* Staphylococcus aureus

Pathophysiology

○ Genes encode resistance and are carried on plasmids that transfer themselves from cell to cell.
○ Resistance is mediated by enzymes that substitute a different molecule for the terminal amino acid so that vancomycin can't bind.

Causes

○ Colonized patient is more than 10 times as likely to become infected with the organism as uncolonized patient, such as through a breach in the immune system.
○ VISA enters a health care facility through an infected or colonized patient or a colonized health care worker.
○ It's spread during direct contact between the patient and caregiver or patient and patient; it may also be spread through patient contact with a contaminated surface such as an overbed table.

Incidence

○ First discovered in mid-1996
○ Four cases detected in the United States
○ Noted in patients receiving multiple courses of vancomycin for MSRA infections

Common characteristics

○ Causative organism can live for weeks on such surfaces as patient gowns, bed linens, and handrails
○ No specific symptoms; cultures found incidentally

Complications

○ Sepsis
○ Multisystem organ involvement
○ Death in the immunocompromised patient

Assessment

History

○ Possible breach in the immune system, surgery, or condition predisposing the patient to the infection
○ Multiple antibiotic use

Physical findings

○ The carrier patient is commonly asymptomatic but may exhibit signs and symptoms related to the primary diagnosis.
○ The patient may exhibit cardiac, respiratory, or other major symptoms.

Test results

Laboratory
○ Culture shows staphylococci with decreased susceptibility to vancomycin after 24-hour incubation.

Treatment

General

○ With an infection, possibly no treatment (Stop all antibiotics and simply wait for normal bacteria to repopulate and replace the strain.)
○ Colonized patient in contact isolation until culture-negative or discharged
○ Antimicrobial drugs (VISA isolates not susceptible to vancomycin generally are susceptible to other drugs.)
○ No dietary restrictions
○ Rest periods when fatigued

Medication

○ Antimicrobials

Nursing considerations

Key outcomes

The patient will:
○ maintain collateral circulation
○ attain hemodynamic stability
○ maintain adequate cardiac output
○ remain afebrile
○ have an adequate fluid volume.

Nursing interventions

○ Consider grouping infected patients together and having the same nursing staff care for them.
○ Institute contact isolation precautions.
○ Ensure judicious and careful use of antibiotics. Encourage physicians to limit the use of antibiotics.
○ Use infection-control practices, such as wearing gloves before and after contact with infectious body tissues and proper hand-washing, to reduce the spread of VISA.

Monitoring
○ Vital signs
○ Response to treatment
○ Complications

Patient teaching

Be sure to cover:
○ the disorder, diagnosis, and treatment
○ the need for family and friends to wear personal protective equipment when they visit the patient
○ how to dispose of protective equipment
○ drug administration, dosage, and possible adverse effects.

Vancomycin-resistant enterococcus

Overview

Description

- Mutation of a common bacterium
- Easily spread by direct person-to-person contact
- Also called *VRE*

Pathophysiology

- Genes encode resistance and are carried on plasmids that transfer themselves from cell to cell.
- Resistance is mediated by enzymes that substitute a different molecule for the terminal amino acid so that vancomycin can't bind.

Causes

- Enters health care facility through infected or colonized patient or colonized health care worker
- Spread through direct contact between patient and caregiver, between patients, or through contact with contaminated surfaces

Risk factors

- Immunocompromised condition
- Old age
- Indwelling catheter
- Major surgery
- Open wounds
- History of taking vancomycin or a third-generation cephalosporin
- History of enterococcal bacteremia, often linked to endocarditis
- Organ transplantation
- Prolonged or repeated hospital admissions
- Chronic renal failure
- Exposure to contaminated equipment or a VRE-positive patient.

Taking precautions at home

Tell the patient's caregivers to:
- wash their hands with soap and water after physical contact with the patient and before leaving the home
- use towels only once when drying hands after contact
- wear disposable gloves if they expect to come in contact with the patient's body fluids and to wash hands after removing the gloves
- change linens routinely and whenever they become soiled
- clean the patient's environment routinely and when it becomes soiled with body fluids
- tell physicians and other health care personnel caring for the patient that the patient is infected with an organism resistant to multiple drugs.

Incidence

- Reported in facilities in more than 40 states
- Rates as high as 14% in oncology units

Common characteristics

- No specific signs and symptoms
- May be found incidentally when culture results show the organism

Complications

- Sepsis

Assessment

History

- Possible breach in the immune system, surgery, or condition predisposing the patient to the infection
- Multiple antibiotic use

Physical findings

- Carrier commonly asymptomatic

Test results

Laboratory
- VRE is isolated from stool or a rectal swab.

Treatment

General

- With an infection, possibly no treatment
- Colonized patient placed in contact isolation until culture-negative or discharged
- Rest periods when fatigued

Medication

- Antimicrobials (VRE isolates not susceptible to vancomycin generally susceptible to other antimicrobial drugs)

Nursing considerations

Key outcomes

The patient will:
- remain afebrile
- have adequate fluid volume.

Nursing interventions

- Consider grouping infected patients together and having the same nursing staff care for them.
- Institute contact isolation precautions.
- Ensure judicious and careful use of antibiotics. Encourage physicians to limit the use of antibiotics.
- Use infection-control practices, such as wearing gloves and proper hand-washing techniques, to reduce the spread of VRE.

Monitoring
○ Vital signs
○ Response to treatment
○ Complications

Patient teaching

Be sure to cover:
○ the disorder, diagnosis, and treatment (see *Taking precautions at home*)
○ the need for family and friends to wear personal protective equipment when visiting the patient
○ how to dispose of protective equipment
○ drug administration, dosage, and possible adverse effects.

Varicella

Overview

Description

- An acute, highly contagious viral infection
- The same virus that causes chickenpox, thought to become latent until the sixth decade of life or later, causing herpes zoster (shingles)
- Transmission through direct contact (primarily with respiratory secretions, less commonly with skin lesions) and indirect contact (airborne)
- Commonly known as *chickenpox*

Pathophysiology

- Localized replication of the virus occurs (probably in the nasopharynx), leading to seeding of the reticuloendothelial system and development of viremia.
- Diffuse and scattered skin lesions result with vesicles involving the corium and dermis with degenerative changes (ballooning) and infection of localized blood vessels.
- Necrosis and epidermal hemorrhage result; vesicles eventually rupture and release fluid or are reabsorbed.
- Incubation period lasts 13 to 17 days.
- Infection is communicable from 48 hours before lesions erupt until after vesicles are crusted over.

Causes

- Varicella-zoster herpesvirus

Incidence

- Most common in children ages 5 to 9, but can occur at any age
- Congenital varicella possibly in infants whose mothers had acute infections in first or early second trimester
- Neonatal infection rare, probably because of transient maternal immunity
- Occurs worldwide; endemic in large cities with outbreaks occurring sporadically
- Equally affects all races and both sexes
- Seasonal distribution varies; in temperate areas, incidence higher during late winter and spring

Common characteristics

- Malaise
- Crops of macules progressing to vesicles
- Pruritus

Complications

- With scratching due to severe pruritus: infection, scarring, impetigo, furuncles, and cellulitis
- Reye's syndrome
- Pneumonia
- Myocarditis
- Bleeding disorders
- Arthritis
- Nephritis
- Hepatitis
- Acute myositis
- Congenital varicella-caused hypoplastic deformity, limb scarring, retarded growth, and central nervous system and eye problems

Assessment

History

- Recent exposure to someone with chickenpox
- Malaise
- Headache
- Anorexia

Physical findings

- Temperature 101° to 103° F (38.3° to 39.4° C)
- Crops of small, erythematous macules on the trunk or scalp
- Macules progressing to papules and then clear vesicles on an erythematous base (so-called dewdrops on rose petals)
- Vesicles becoming cloudy and breaking easily; then scabs forming
- Rash that spreads to face and, rarely, to extremities
- Rash containing a combination of red papules, vesicles, and scabs in various stages
- Ulcers on mucous membranes of the mouth, conjunctivae, and genitalia

Test results

Laboratory

- Virus can be isolated from vesicular fluid within the first 3 to 4 days of the rash.
- Giemsa stain distinguishes the varicella-zoster virus from the vaccinia-variola virus.
- Serum samples contain antibodies 7 days after onset of symptoms.
- Serologic testing differentiates rickettsial pox from varicella.

Treatment

General

- Strict isolation until all vesicles have crusted over; for congenital chickenpox, no isolation
- Increased fluid intake
- Rest periods when fatigued

Medication

- Antipruritics
- Antibiotics
- Analgesic and antipyretic
- Acyclovir
- Varicella-zoster immune globulin

Nursing considerations

Key outcomes

The patient will:
- report or demonstrate an increased energy level
- exhibit improved or healed lesions or wounds
- interact with family and peers to decrease feelings of isolation
- express or demonstrate increased comfort.

Nursing interventions

- Observe an immunocompromised patient for manifestations of complications, such as pneumonitis and meningitis, and report them immediately.
- Provide skin care comfort measures (calamine lotion, cornstarch, sponge baths, or showers).
- Administer varicella-zoster immune globulin if ordered to lessen the severity of the disease.
- Institute strict isolation measures until all skin lesions have crusted.
- Prevent exposure to pregnant women.

Monitoring

- Response to treatment
- Complications
- Skin integrity
- Signs and symptoms of dehydration
- Signs and symptoms of infection
- Adverse drug reactions

Patient teaching

Be sure to cover:
- the disorder, diagnosis, and treatment
- how to correctly apply topical antipruritic medications
- the importance of good hygiene and keeping the child's fingernails trimmed
- the need for the child to avoid scratching the lesions
- the parents' need to watch for and immediately report signs of complications (severe skin pain and burning that may indicate a serious secondary infection and require prompt medical attention)
- the need for parents to refrain from giving the child aspirin because of its association with Reye's syndrome
- signs and symptoms of Reye's syndrome and the need to immediately report them to a physician.

Varicocele

Overview

Description

○ A mass of dilated and tortuous varicose veins in the spermatic cord
○ Commonly described as a "bag of worms" (see *Taking a close look at a varicocele*)

Pathophysiology

○ Because of a valvular disorder in the spermatic vein, blood pools in the pampiniform venous plexus.
○ One function of the pampiniform plexus is to keep the testes slightly cooler than body temperature, which is the optimal temperature for sperm production.
○ Incomplete blood flow through the testes thus interferes with spermatogenesis.
○ Testicular atrophy may also occur because of the reduced blood flow.

Causes

○ Incompetent or congenitally absent valves in the spermatic veins
○ Tumor or thrombus obstructing the inferior vena cava (unilateral left-sided varicocele)

Taking a close look at a varicocele

Varicocele, an abnormal dilation of the veins of the spermatic cord, is asymptomatic, but it's important to identify and correct this condition in adolescent boys because it causes infertility.

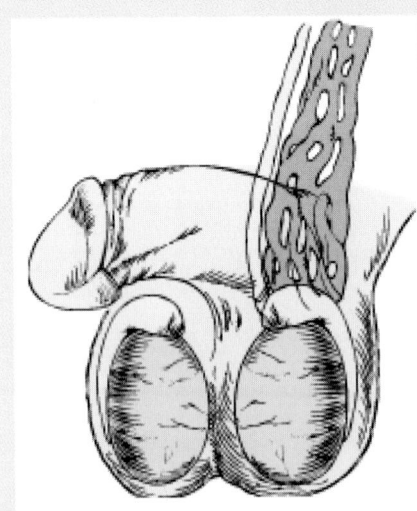

Incidence

○ Present in 30% of all men diagnosed with infertility
○ Occurs in the left spermatic cord 95% of the time
○ Occurs in 10% to 15% of all males, usually between ages 13 and 18

Common characteristics

○ Asymptomatic
○ Feeling of heaviness on the affected side
○ Testicular pain and tenderness on palpation

Complications

○ Infertility
○ Hydrocele

Assessment

History

○ Infertility
○ Feeling of heaviness on affected side

Physical findings

○ Palpation of "bag of worms" when the patient is upright
○ Drained, can't be felt when patient is recumbent
○ Testicular tenderness

Test results

Other
○ Physical examination confirms varicocele.

Treatment

General

○ Scrotal support to relieve discomfort

Surgery

○ Surgical repair or removal involving ligation of the spermatic cord at the internal inguinal ring (if infertility is an issue)

Nursing considerations

Key outcomes

The patient will:
○ express understanding of the disorder and its treatment
○ express feelings regarding effect on fertility
○ express feelings of increased comfort.

Nursing interventions

○ Promote the patient's comfort before and after surgery.
○ After surgery, administer drug therapy.
○ Apply an ice bag with a cover to reduce edema.

○ Protect the wound from contamination.
○ Allow the patient to perform as many normal daily activities as possible.

Monitoring

○ Intake and output
○ Comfort level
○ Wound healing

Patient teaching

Be sure to cover:
○ the disorder, diagnosis, and treatment
○ wound care.

Varicose veins

Overview

Description

- Dilated, tortuous veins, engorged with blood resulting from improper venous valve function
- Primary varicose veins originating in superficial veins (the saphenous veins and branches)
- Secondary varicose veins occurring in deep and perforating veins

Pathophysiology

- A weakened valve allows backflow of blood to the previous valve in a vein.
- If the valve can't hold the pooling blood, it becomes incompetent, allowing even more blood to flow backward.
- As the volume of venous blood builds, pressure in the vein increases and the vein becomes distended.
- As the vein stretches, it loses elasticity, enlarges, and becomes tortuous.
- Hydrostatic pressure increases, plasma is forced out into surrounding tissue, and edema results.

Causes

- Congenital weakness of the valves or venous wall
- Pregnancy
- Tight clothing
- Occupations that necessitate standing for an extended period
- Deep vein thrombosis
- Trauma

Incidence

- Common in middle adulthood
- Primary varicose veins: Family tendency, affect both legs, twice as common in women as men
- Secondary varicose veins: usually in only one leg

Common characteristics

- Dilated, purple, ropelike veins
- Edema of calves and ankles
- Venous stasis ulcers

Preventing varicose veins

Prevention of varicose veins involves identifying patients with increased risk factors, such as those in professions that require prolonged standing or time on the feet (such as nurses, surgeons, letter carriers, beauticians, teachers, and waiters). Other risk factors include obesity, heavy lifting, and pregnancy. People with these risk factors should be educated to rest their legs and elevate them periodically at work, wear supportive stockings, drink 2 to 3 qt (2 to 3 L) of fluid per day, and avoid crossing their legs.

Complications

- Venous insufficiency
- Venous stasis ulcers

Assessment

History

- May be asymptomatic
- Feeling of heaviness in the legs that worsens in the evening and in warm weather
- Leg cramps at night
- Diffuse, dull, aching leg pain after prolonged standing or walking
- Aching legs during menses
- Fatigue
- Exercise possibly relieving symptoms because venous return improves

Physical findings

- Dilated, purplish, ropelike veins, especially in the calf
- Orthostatic edema and stasis of the calves and ankles
- Nodules along affected veins and valve incompetence
- In chronic condition, venous stasis ulcers, which must be differentiated from arterial and diabetic ulcerations

Test results

Imaging

- Ascending and descending venography demonstrate venous occlusion and patterns of collateral flow.

Diagnostic procedures

- Photoplethysmography, a noninvasive test, characterizes venous blood flow by showing changes in the skin's circulation.
- Doppler ultrasonography quickly and accurately shows the presence or absence of venous backflow in deep or superficial veins.
- Venous outflow and reflux plethysmography can be used to detect deep venous occlusion.

Treatment

General

- Wearing elastic stockings
- Avoiding tight clothing
- For moderate varicose veins: wearing antiembolism stockings or elastic bandages
- For severe varicose veins: custom-fitted, surgical-weight stockings with graduated pressure
- Avoidance of prolonged standing
- Routine exercise
- Elevation of the legs

Medication

- Sclerotherapy

Surgery

- Stripping and ligation

Nursing considerations

Key outcomes

The patient will:
- ○ express understanding of disorder and treatment
- ○ maintain adequate distal and collateral circulation
- ○ express feelings of increased comfort and decreased pain
- ○ carry out activities of daily living without excess fatigue or discomfort.

Nursing interventions

- ○ After stripping and ligation or after injection of a sclerosing agent, administer analgesics as ordered to relieve pain.
- ○ Frequently check circulation in toes and observe elastic bandages for bleeding. When ordered, rewrap bandages at least once a shift, wrapping from toe to thigh, with the leg elevated. (See *Preventing varicose veins.*)

Monitoring

 Alert

Watch for signs and symptoms of complications, such as sensory loss in the leg, calf pain, and fever.

- ○ Response to treatment
- ○ Skin integrity
- ○ Pain control

Patient teaching

Be sure to cover:
- ○ the need to avoid wearing constrictive clothing
- ○ elevating the legs above heart level when possible and avoiding prolonged standing or sitting
- ○ how to put on the elastic, antiembolism, or compression stockings before getting out of bed in the morning (or lying with the legs raised for 1 minute before putting on the stockings)
- ○ how to avoid injury to the lower legs, ankles, and feet and the need to observe for altered skin integrity of those areas and to report any problems to the physician as soon as possible.

Vascular retinopathies

Overview

Description

○ Noninflammatory retinal disorders that result from interference with the blood supply to the eyes
○ Five distinct types: central retinal artery occlusion, central retinal vein occlusion, diabetic retinopathy, hypertensive retinopathy, and sickle cell retinopathy

Pathophysiology

○ When one of the arteries maintaining blood circulation in the retina becomes obstructed, the diminished blood flow causes visual deficits.

Causes

Central retinal artery occlusion
○ Idiopathic
○ Embolism
○ Atherosclerosis
○ Infection
○ Conditions that retard blood flow, such as carotid occlusion and heart valve vegetations
Central retinal vein occlusion
○ External compression of the retinal vein
○ Trauma
○ Diabetes
○ Thrombosis
○ Granulomatous diseases
○ Generalized and localized infections
○ Glaucoma
○ Atherosclerosis
Diabetic retinopathy
○ Juvenile or adult diabetes
Hypertensive retinopathy
○ Prolonged hypertensive disease
Sickle cell retinopathy
○ Impaired ability of the sickled cell to pass through the microvasculature, producing vasocclusion

Incidence

Central retinal vein occlusion
○ Most prevalent in elderly patients
Diabetic retinopathy
○ About 75% of patients with juvenile diabetes develop retinopathy within 20 years of onset of diabetes.
○ In adults with diabetes, incidence increases with the duration of diabetes; 80% of patients who have had diabetes for 20 to 25 years develop retinopathy. This condition is a leading cause of acquired adult blindness.
Sickle cell retinopathy
○ Occurs in 1% to 6% of sickle-cell patients

Common characteristics

Central retinal artery occlusion
○ Sudden, painless, unilateral loss of vision (partial or complete)

Central retinal vein occlusion
○ Reduced visual acuity, allowing perception of only hand movement and light within 3 to 4 months after occlusion
Diabetic retinopathy
NONPROLIFERATIVE DIABETIC RETINOPATHY
○ Changes in the lining of the retinal blood vessels that cause the vessels to leak plasma or fatty substances, which decrease or block blood flow (nonperfusion) within the retina
○ Microaneurysms and small hemorrhages
○ Significant loss of central visual acuity (necessary for reading and driving)
○ Diminished night vision
PROLIFERATIVE DIABETIC RETINOPATHY
○ Fragile new blood vessels on the disk and elsewhere in the fundus (neovascularization)
Hypertensive retinopathy
○ Based on the location of retinopathy, mild visual disturbances such as blurred vision resulting from retinopathy located near the macula
Sickle cell retinopathy
○ Optic disc changes
○ Macular changes

Complications

Central retinal artery occlusion
○ Permanent loss of vision
Central retinal vein occlusion
○ Secondary glaucoma
Diabetic retinopathy
PROLIFERATIVE DIABETIC RETINOPATHY
○ Vitreous hemorrhage with corresponding sudden vision loss
○ Macular distortion
○ Retinal detachment
Hypertensive retinopathy
○ Blindness
○ Mild, prolonged disease
○ Visual defects
Sickle cell retinopathy
○ Optic nerve neovascularization
○ Sickling crisis
○ Optic nerve and macular infarction

Assessment

History

○ Changes in visual acuity
○ Causative factors

Physical findings

○ Decreased visual acuity
○ Abnormal opthalmic examination

Test results

○ Appropriate diagnostic tests depend on the type of vascular retinopathy. (See *Diagnostic tests for vascular retinopathies.*)

Treatment

Central retinal artery occlusion

General
- ○ Immediate ocular massage
- ○ Anterior chamber paracentesis

Medication
- ○ Heparin (if the cause of the occlusion is the heart)

Central retinal vein occlusion

General
- ○ Laser photocoagulation

Medication
- ○ Aspirin

Diabetic retinopathy

General
- ○ Careful control of blood glucose levels
- ○ Eye examinations 3 to 4 times per year; annually for children with diabetes
- ○ Laser photocoagulation (proliferative diabetic retinopathy)
- ○ Diabetic diet
- ○ Regular exercise

Medication
- ○ Antidiabetic drugs or insulin as appropriate

Surgery
- ○ Vitrectomy for vitreous hemorrhage to restore vision

Hypertensive retinopathy

General
- ○ Control of blood pressure with appropriate drugs
- ○ Low-sodium, low-cholesterol diet
- ○ Regular exercise

Sickle cell retinopathy

General
- ○ Treatment of disease

Surgery
- ○ Laser retinal photocoagulation
- ○ Retinal cryotherapy
- ○ Vitrectomy or membranectomy

Nursing considerations

Key outcomes

The patient will:
- ○ maintain current health status
- ○ regain visual function
- ○ express understanding of the condition and its treatment.

Nursing interventions

- ○ Arrange for immediate ophthalmologic evaluation when a patient complains of sudden, unilateral loss of vision.
- ○ Encourage a patient with diabetes to comply with the prescribed regimen.

Diagnostic tests for vascular retinopathies

Central retinal artery occlusion
- ○ *Ophthalmoscopy (direct or indirect):* shows blockage of retinal arterioles during transient attack.
- ○ *Retinal examination:* within 2 hours of onset, shows clumps or segmentation in artery; later, milky white retina around disk caused by swelling and necrosis of ganglion cells caused by reduced blood supply; also shows cherry-red spot in macula that subsides after several weeks.
- ○ *Color Doppler tests:* evaluates carotid occlusion with no need for arteriography.

Central retinal vein occlusion
- ○ *Ophthalmoscopy (direct or indirect):* shows flame-shaped hemorrhages, retinal vein engorgement, white patches among hemorrhages, edema around the disk.
- ○ *Color Doppler tests:* confirm or rule out occlusion of blood vessels.

Diabetic retinopathy
- ○ *Indirect ophthalmoscopic examination:* shows retinal changes such as microaneurysms (earliest change), retinal hemorrhages and edema, venous dilation and beading, lipid exudates, fibrous bands in the vitreous, and growth of new blood vessels. Infarcts of the nerve fiber layer are observed.
- ○ *Fluorescein angiography:* shows leakage of flourescein from weak-walled vessels and "lights up" microaneurysms, differentiating them from true hemorrhages.

Hypertensive retinopathy
- ○ *Ophthalmoscopy (direct or indirect):* in early stages, shows hard, shiny deposits; flame-shaped hemorrhages; silver wire appearance of narrowed arterioles; and nicking of veins where arteries cross them (AV nicking). In late stages, shows cotton wool patches, lipid exudates, retinal edema, papilledema caused by ischemia and capillary insufficiency, hemorrhages, and microaneurysms in both eyes.

Sickle cell retinopathy
- ○ *Ocular examination and dilated retinal evaluation:* shows staged ocular symptoms.
  Stage 1: peripheral retinal arteriolar occlusion
  Stage 2: peripheral arteriovenous anastamoses
  Stage 3: neovascular fronds known as *seafans*
  Stage 4: vitreous hemorrhage and tearing of neovascular membranes
  Stage 5: severe vitreous traction and retinal detachment

Monitoring

- ○ Vital signs
- ○ Visual acuity

Patient teaching

Be sure to cover:
- ○ the disorder, diagnosis, and treatment
- ○ complying with therapy for underlying condition
- ○ obtaining recommended follow-up care.

Vasculitis

Overview

Description

○ Autoimmune condition that includes a broad spectrum of disorders characterized by blood vessel inflammation and necrosis
○ Clinical effects dependent on the vessels involved and reflective of tissue ischemia caused by blood flow obstruction

Pathophysiology

○ The process is initiated by excessive circulating antigen, which triggers the formation of soluble antigen-antibody complexes. The reticuloendothelial system can't effectively clear these complexes, which are deposited in blood vessel walls.
○ Increased vascular permeability (associated with the release of vasoactive amines by platelets and basophils) enhances this deposition. The deposited complexes activate the complement cascade and result in chemotaxis of neutrophils, which release lysosomal enzymes.
○ Vessel damage and necrosis result.

Causes

○ Several theories:
  – Follows serious infectious disease and may be related to high doses of antibiotics
  – Formation of autoantibodies directed at the body's own cellular and extracellular proteins, which can lead to the activation of inflammatory cells or cytotoxicity
  – Cell-mediated (T-cell) immune response
  – In atopic individuals, exposure to allergens

Incidence

○ Can affect a person at any age (except mucocutaneous lymph node syndrome, which affects only children)

Common characteristics

○ Based on affected blood vessel

Complications

○ Renal failure, renal hypertension, glomerulitis
○ Fibrous scarring of the lung tissue
○ Stroke
○ GI bleeding, intestinal obstruction
○ Myocardial infarction and pericarditis
○ Rupture of mesenteric aneurysms

Assessment

History

○ Varied findings, depending on blood vessels involved

Polyarteritis nodosa
○ Fever
○ Weight loss
○ Malaise
○ Headache
○ Abdominal pain
○ Myalgias

Physical findings

Polyarteritis nodosa (depends on body system)
○ Hypertension (renal)
○ Arthritic changes (musculoskeletal)
○ Rash, purpura, nodules, and cutaneous infarcts (skin)
○ Altered mental status and seizures (central nervous system)
○ Respiratory distress, peripheral edema, hepatomegaly, peripheral vasoconstriction (cardiovascular)

Test results

Diagnostic procedures
○ Not all vasculitis disorders can be diagnosed definitively through specific tests. The most useful general diagnostic procedure is biopsy of the affected vessel.

Treatment

General

○ Avoidance of antigenic drugs
○ Avoidance of antigenic foods
○ Avoidance of offending environmental substances

Medication

○ Corticosteroids
○ Antihypertensives
○ Analgesics
○ Immunosuppressive agents
○ Antineoplastics

Nursing considerations

Key outcomes

The patient will:
○ express feelings of increased comfort and decreased pain
○ express positive feelings about self
○ attain hemodynamic stability
○ demonstrate adequate ventilation
○ avoid complications.

Nursing interventions

○ Assess for dry nasal mucosa. Instill nose drops to lubricate the mucosa and minimize crusting; irrigate nasal passages with warm normal saline solution.
○ Keep the patient well hydrated (about 3 qt [3 L] of fluid daily).
○ Make sure that a patient with decreased visual acuity has a safe environment.

- Regulate environmental temperature to prevent additional vasoconstriction caused by cold.
- Provide emotional support to the patient and family.

Monitoring

- Vital signs and neurologic status
- Signs and symptoms of organ involvement
- Laboratory values
- GI disturbances and renal function tests
- Intake and output
- Daily weight

Patient teaching

Be sure to cover:
- the disorder, diagnosis, and treatment
- how to recognize adverse effects of drug therapy, watch for signs of bleeding, and report any of these findings to the physician
- the importance of wearing warm clothes and gloves when going outside in cold weather.

Discharge planning

- Refer the patient to a smoking-cessation program if appropriate.

Ventricular septal defect

Overview

Description

- Heart condition in which an opening in the septum between the ventricles allows blood to shunt between the left and right ventricles
- Most common congenital heart disorder
- Also known as *VSD*

Pathophysiology

- The ventricular septum fails to close completely by the 8th week of gestation, as it would normally.
- VSDs are located in the membranous or muscular portion of the ventricular septum and vary in size.
- Some defects close spontaneously; in other defects, the entire septum is absent, creating a single ventricle.
- VSD isn't readily apparent at birth because right and left ventricular pressures are approximately equal, so blood doesn't shunt through the defect.
- As the pulmonary vasculature gradually relaxes, between 4 and 8 weeks after birth, right ventricular pressure decreases, allowing blood to shunt from the left to the right ventricle.

Causes

- Congenital

Risk factors

- Fetal alcohol syndrome
- Coexists with additional birth defects, especially Down syndrome and other autosomal trisomies, renal anomalies, and cardiac defects, such as patent ductus arteriosus and coarctation of the aorta

Incidence

- Affects 2% to 7% of live births
- Slightly more common in females

Common characteristics

- Clinical features of VSD vary with the size of the defect, the effect of the shunting on the pulmonary vasculature, and the infant's age.
- A small VSD may eventually close spontaneously without ever causing symptoms.
- Large VSD shunts eventually cause biventricular heart failure and cyanosis.

Complications

- Heart failure
- Pneumonia

Assessment

History

- Dyspnea
- Cyanosis
- Slow weight gain
- Feeding difficulties
- Rapid grunting respirations

Physical findings

- Prominent anterior chest wall
- Clubbing
- Cyanosis
- With a large VSD, audible murmurs (at least a grade 3 pansystolic), loudest at the fourth intercostal space, usually with a thrill; pulmonic component of S_2 loud and widely split
- With fixed pulmonary hypertension, diastolic murmur possibly audible on auscultation, systolic murmur becoming quieter, and S_2 greatly accentuated
- Displacement of the point of maximal impulse to the left
- Typical murmur associated with a VSD, blowing or rumbling and varying in frequency
- In the neonate, moderately loud early systolic murmur along the lower left sternal border, possibly becoming louder and longer about the second or third day after birth
- In infants, murmur possibly loudest near the base of the heart, which may suggest pulmonary stenosis
- In small VSD, functional murmur or characteristic loud, harsh systolic murmur

Test results

Imaging

- Chest X-rays are normal in small defects; in large VSDs, they show cardiomegaly, left atrial and left ventricular enlargement, and prominent pulmonary vascular markings.
- Echocardiography may detect a large VSD and its location in the septum, estimate the size of a left-to-right shunt, suggest pulmonary hypertension, and identify associated lesions and complications.

Diagnostic procedures

- Electrocardiogram is normal in children with small VSDs; in large VSDs, it shows left and right ventricular hypertrophy, suggesting pulmonary hypertension.
- Cardiac catheterization determines the size and exact location of the VSD, calculates the degree of shunting by comparing the blood oxygen saturation in each ventricle, determines the extent of pulmonary hypertension, and detects associated defects.

Treatment

General

- If the child has other defects and will benefit from delaying surgery, pulmonary artery banding to normalize pressures and flow distal to the band and prevent pulmonary vascular disease
- Low-sodium diet
- Fluid restriction
- Activity as tolerated

Medication

○ Digoxin
○ Diuretics
○ Antibiotics
After surgery
○ Analgesics
○ Antibiotics
○ Vasopressors

Surgery

○ For small defects, simple suture closure
○ For moderate to large defects, insertion of a patch graft using cardiopulmonary bypass

Nursing considerations

Key outcomes

The patient will:
○ maintain adequate ventilation
○ maintain hemodynamic stability
○ remain free from signs and symptoms of infection.

Nursing interventions

○ Provide emotional support.
○ Give prescribed drugs.

Monitoring

○ Vital signs
○ Signs of heart failure
○ Intake and output
○ Respiratory status
After surgery
○ Hemodynamics
○ Cardiac rhythm
○ Oxygenation

Patient teaching

Be sure to cover:
○ preventing complications until the child is scheduled for surgery or the defect closes
○ watching for signs of heart failure, such as poor feeding, sweating, and heavy breathing
○ drug administration, dosage, and possible adverse effects
○ letting the child engage in normal activities
○ the importance of prophylactic antibiotics before and after surgery.

Vesicoureteral reflux

Overview

Description
- A genitourinary condition in which urine flows from the bladder back into the ureters and eventually into the renal pelvis or the parenchyma
- Because the bladder empties poorly, possible urinary tract infection (UTI), which may lead to acute or chronic pyelonephritis with renal damage

Pathophysiology
- Incompetence of the ureterovesical junction and shortening of intravesical ureteral musculature allow backflow of urine into the ureter when the bladder contracts during voiding.

Causes
- Congenital anomalies of the ureters or bladder
- Inadequate detrusor muscle buttress in the bladder, stemming from congenital paraureteral bladder diverticulum
- Acquired diverticulum (from outlet obstruction)
- Flaccid neurogenic bladder
- High intravesical pressure from outlet obstruction
- Cystitis
- Sometimes unknown

Incidence

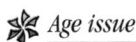 **Age issue**

Most common during infancy in boys and during early childhood (ages 3 to 7) in girls

- Primary vesicoureteral reflux resulting from congenital anomalies most prevalent in females and rare in blacks
- Also shown in up to 25% of asymptomatic siblings of children with diagnosed primary vesicoureteral reflux

Common characteristics
- Signs and symptoms of UTI
- Dark, concentrated urine
- With upper urinary tract involvement: high fever, chills, flank pain, vomiting, and malaise

 Alert

In children, fever, nonspecific abdominal pain, and diarrhea may be the only clinical effects. Rarely, children with minimal symptoms remain undiagnosed until puberty or later, when they begin to exhibit clear signs of renal impairment (anemia, hypertension, and lethargy).

Complications
- Renal impairment
- Urinary tract infections

Assessment

History
- Urinary frequency and urgency
- Burning on urination

Physical findings
- In infants, hematuria or strong-smelling urine
- Hard, thickened bladder (hard mass deep in the pelvis) if posterior urethral valves are causing an obstruction in male infants

Test results
Laboratory
- Clean-catch urinalysis shows a bacterial count greater than 100,000/µl.
- Microscopic examination may reveal white blood cells, red blood cells, and an increased urine pH in the presence of infection. Specific gravity less than 1.010 demonstrates inability to concentrate urine.
- Elevated creatinine levels (more than 1.2 mg/dl) and elevated blood urea nitrogen levels (more than 18 mg/dl) indicate advanced renal dysfunction.

Diagnostic procedures
- Cystoscopy, with instillation of a solution containing methylene blue or indigo carmine dye, may confirm the diagnosis.
- Excretory urography may show dilated lower ureter, ureter visible for its entire length, hydronephrosis, calyceal distortion, and renal scarring.
- Voiding cystourethrography (either fluoroscopic or radionuclide) identifies and determines the degree of reflux and shows when reflux occurs. It may also pinpoint the causative anomaly.
- Nuclear cystography and renal ultrasound may detect reflux.

Other
- Catheterization of the bladder after the patient voids determines the amount of residual urine.

Treatment

General
- Increased fluid intake

Medication
- Antibiotics

Surgery
- UTI that recurs despite adequate prophylactic antibiotic therapy necessitates vesicoureteral reimplantation.
- Bladder outlet obstruction in neurogenic bladder requires surgery only if renal dysfunction is present.

Nursing considerations

Key outcomes

The patient will:
- ◯ return to normal urinary function
- ◯ remain free from infection
- ◯ develop no complications of the disorder.

Nursing interventions

- ◯ Encourage one of the parents to stay with the patient during all procedures.
- ◯ Explain the procedures to the parents and to the child, if he's old enough to understand.
- ◯ Give drug therapy.
- ◯ Make sure catheters are patent and draining well. Maintain sterile technique during catheter care.

Monitoring

- ◯ Intake and output
- ◯ Comfort level
- ◯ Vital signs

Patient teaching

Be sure to cover:
- ◯ utilizing the vesicoureteral reflux to double void (void once and then try to void again in a few minutes)
- ◯ voiding every 2 to 3 hours whether or not the urge exists
- ◯ recognizing and reporting recurring signs of UTI (painful, frequent, burning urination; foul-smelling urine)
- ◯ the importance of completing the prescribed therapy or maintaining low-dose antibiotic prophylaxis.

Discharge planning

- ◯ After surgery, close medical follow-up is necessary even if symptoms haven't recurred.

Vitamin A deficiency

Overview

Description

○ Deficiency of vitamin A in the body possibly resulting in night blindness, decreased color adjustment, keratinization of epithelial tissue, and poor bone growth
○ With therapy, excellent chance of reversing symptoms of night blindness and milder conjunctival changes; with corneal damage, emergency treatment necessary

Pathophysiology

○ A fat-soluble vitamin absorbed in the GI tract, vitamin A maintains epithelial tissue and retinal function.
○ Healthy adults have adequate vitamin A reserves to last up to 1 year; children commonly don't.

Causes

○ Inadequate dietary intake of foods high in vitamin A (liver, kidney, butter, milk, cream, cheese, and fortified margarine) or carotene, a precursor of vitamin A found in dark green leafy vegetables, and yellow or orange fruits and vegetables
○ Malabsorption caused by:
  – Celiac disease
  – Sprue
  – Obstructive jaundice
  – Cystic fibrosis
  – Giardiasis
  – Habitual use of mineral oil as a laxative
○ Massive urinary excretion caused by:
  – Cancer
  – Tuberculosis
  – Pneumonia
  – Nephritis
  – Urinary tract infection
○ Decreased storage and transport of vitamin A from hepatic disease

Incidence

○ Affects more than 80,000 people annually worldwide — mostly children in underdeveloped countries
○ Rare in the United States, although many disadvantaged children have substandard levels of vitamin A

Foods that contain vitamin A

The following foods contain significant amounts of vitamin A.
○ Butternut squash
○ Cantaloupe
○ Carrots
○ Dandelion
○ Kale
○ Mangoes
○ Red peppers
○ Sweet potatoes

Common characteristics

○ Night blindness (nyctalopia)
○ Dry, scaly skin
○ Follicular hyperkeratosis
○ Shrinking and hardening of the mucous membranes
○ Failure to thrive and apathy
○ Corneal changes, which can lead to ulceration and rapid destruction of the cornea (severe deficiency)

Complications

○ Blindness
○ Infections of the eyes and the respiratory or genitourinary tract

Assessment

History

○ Night blindness (nyctalopia)
○ Failure to thrive
○ Apathy

Physical findings

○ Dry, scaly skin
○ Follicular hyperkeratosis
○ Conjunctival changes
○ Shrinking and hardening of the mucous membranes

Test results

Laboratory
○ Carotene levels below 40 µg/dl suggest vitamin A deficiency, but vary with seasonal ingestion of fruits and vegetables.
○ Serum levels of vitamin A below 20 µg/dl are diagnostic.
Other
○ Dietary history and typical ocular lesions suggest vitamin A deficiency.

Treatment

General

○ Increased vitamin A dietary intake
○ Cream-based or petroleum-based products for dry skin
○ Control of underlying condition

Medication

○ Vitamin A replacement
○ Bile salts with biliary obstruction
○ Pancreatin with pancreatic insufficiency

Nursing considerations

Key outcomes

The patient will:
○ improve vitamin levels

- express understanding of dietary changes needed to improve nutritional status
- express understanding of diet high in vitamin A.

Nursing interventions

- Give prescribed oral vitamin A supplements with or after meals or parenterally.
- Provide information on foods high in vitamin A. (See *Foods that contain vitamin A.*)

Monitoring

- Signs of hypercarotenemia (orange coloration of the skin and eyes)
- Signs of hypervitaminosis A (children):
  - Rash
  - Hair loss
  - Anorexia
  - Transient hydrocephalus
  - Vomiting
- Signs of hypervitaminosis A (adults):
  - Bone pain
  - Hepatosplenomegaly
  - Diplopia
  - Irritability

Patient teaching

Be sure to cover:
- signs of hypercarotenemia and hypervitaminosis
- dietary counseling on foods high in vitamin A.

Discharge planning

- Refer the patient for nutritional counseling and, if necessary, to an appropriate community agency.

Vitamin B deficiency

Overview

Description

- Deficiency of vitamin B in the body
- Most common deficiencies: thiamine (B_1), riboflavin (B_2), niacin, pyridoxine (B_6), cobalamin (B_{12})

Pathophysiology

- Vitamin B complex is a group of water-soluble vitamins essential to normal metabolism, cell growth, and blood formation. (See *Recommended daily allowance of B-complex vitamins.*)

Causes

Thiamine deficiency
- Malabsorption
- Inadequate dietary intake of vitamin B_1

Riboflavin deficiency
- Diet deficient in milk, meat, fish, green leafy vegetables, and legumes

Niacin deficiency
- Corn as a dominant staple food
- Carcinoid syndrome
- Hartnup disease

Pyridoxine deficiency
- Destruction of pyridoxine in infant formulas by autoclaving
- Pyridoxine antagonists, such as isoniazid and penicillamine

Cobalamin deficiency
- Absence of intrinsic factor in gastric secretions
- Absence of receptor sites after ileal resection
- Malabsorption syndromes associated with sprue, intestinal worm infestation, regional ileitis, and gluten enteropathy
- Diet low in animal protein
- Pernicious anemia
- Medication

Risk factors

- Chronic alcoholism
- Prolonged diarrhea
- Exposure of milk to sunlight
- Treatment of legumes with baking soda

Incidence

Thiamine deficiency
- Affects males and females equally
- Can occur at any age

Riboflavin deficiency
- Most common nutrient deficiency in the United States

Niacin deficiency
- Usually affects adults

Pyridoxine deficiency
- Can occur at any age
- Rare

Cobalamin deficiency
- Most common in those over age 40

Common characteristics

Thiamine deficiency
- Polyneuritis
- Wernicke's encephalopathy
- Korsakoff's psychosis
- Palpitations
- Tachycardia
- Dyspnea
- Constipation and indigestion

Riboflavin deficiency
- Cheilosis (cracking of the lips and corners of the mouth)
- Sore throat
- Glossitis
- Dermatitis
- Eye disturbances

Niacin deficiency
- Fatigue
- Anorexia
- Muscle weakness
- Headache
- Indigestion
- Mild skin eruptions
- Weight loss
- Dermatitis

Pyridoxine deficiency
- Dermatitis
- Occasional cheilosis or glossitis unresponsive to riboflavin therapy
- Abdominal pain
- Vomiting
- Ataxia
- Seizures

Cobalamin deficiency
- Pernicious anemia, anorexia, weight loss, abdominal discomfort, constipation, diarrhea, and glossitis
- Peripheral neuropathy
- Ataxia, spasticity, and hyperreflexia

Complications

- Cardiomegaly
- Circulatory collapse
- Beriberi
- Pellagra

 Alert

Because of a triad of symptoms, pellagra is sometimes called a "3-D" syndrome — dementia, dermatitis, and diarrhea. If not reversed by therapeutic doses of niacin, pellagra can be fatal.

- Central nervous system disturbances

Recommended daily allowance of B-complex vitamins

Vitamin	Men (23 to 50)	Women (23 to 50)	Infants	Children (1 to 10)
B₁*	1.4 mg	1.4 mg	0.4 mg	0.7 – 12 mg
B₂*	1.6 mg	1.6 mg	0.5 mg	0.8 – 1.4 mg
Niacin*	18 mg	18 mg	5 – 8 mg	9 – 16 mg
B₆	2.2 mg	2.2 mg	0.4 mg	0.9 – 1.6 mg
B₁₂	3 mcg	3 mcg	0.3 mcg	2.0 – 3.0 mcg

*requirements per 1,000 kilocalories of dietary intake

Assessment

History

Thiamine deficiency
- Palpitations
- Dyspnea
- Constipation and indigestion

Riboflavin deficiency
- Burning, itching, light sensitivity, and tearing of the eyes
- Neuropathy
- Signs of mild anemia
- Growth retardation

Niacin deficiency
- Backache
- Sore mouth, tongue, and lips
- Nausea, vomiting, and diarrhea
- Confusion, disorientation, and neuritis — may become severe enough to induce hallucinations and paranoia

Pyridoxine deficiency
- Presence of risk factors
- Fatigue
- Distal limb numbness
- Depression

Cobalamin deficiency
- Pernicious anemia
- Anorexia
- Weight loss
- Constipation, diarrhea
- Glossitis
- Peripheral neuropathy

Physical findings

Thiamine deficiency
- Tachycardia
- Ataxia, nystagmus, and ophthalmoplegia

Riboflavin deficiency
- Seborrheic dermatitis in the nasolabial folds, scrotum, and vulva and, possibly, generalized dermatitis involving the arms, legs, and trunk

Niacin deficiency
- Dark, scaly dermatitis, especially on exposed parts of the body, that makes the patient appear to be severely sunburned
- Red mouth, tongue, and lips

Pyridoxine deficiency
- Weakness
- Confusion
- Glossitis
- Seborrheic dermatitis

Cobalamin deficiency
- Abdominal discomfort
- Peripheral neuropathy
- Ataxia, spasticity, and hyperreflexia

Test results

Laboratory

THIAMINE DEFICIENCY
- Commonly measured as micrograms per deciliter in a 24-hour urine collection

 Age issue

Deficiency levels are age-related.
- *Ages 1 to 3, less than 120 mcg/dl*
- *Ages 4 to 6, less than 85 mcg/dl*
- *Ages 7 to 9, less than 70 mcg/dl*
- *Ages 10 to12, less than 60 mcg/dl*
- *Ages 13 to 15, less than 50 mcg/dl*
- *Adults, less than 27 mcg/dl*

- Pregnant women: less than 23 mcg/dl (second trimester); less than 21 mcg/dl (third trimester)

RIBOFLAVIN DEFICIENCY
- Measured as micrograms per gram of creatinine in a 24-hour urine collection

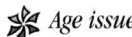

Deficiency levels are age-related.
– *Ages 1 to 3, less than 150 mcg/g*
– *Ages 4 to 6, less than 100 mcg/g*
– *Ages 7 to 9, less than 85 mcg/g*
– *Ages 10 to 15, less than 70 mcg/g*
– *Adults, less than 27 mcg/g*

○ Pregnant women: less than 39 mcg/g (second trimester); less than 30 mcg/g (third trimester)

NIACIN DEFICIENCY
○ Measured by N-methyl nicotinamide in a 24-hour urine collection as micrograms per gram of creatinine
○ Adult deficiency level: less than 0.5 mcg/g
○ Pregnant women: less than 0.5 mcg/g (first trimester); less than 0.6 mcg/g (second trimester); less than 0.8 mcg/g (third trimester)

PYRIDOXINE DEFICIENCY
○ Xanthurenic acid more than 50 mg/day in 24-hour urine collection after administration of 10 g of L-tryptophan
○ Decreased levels of serum and red blood cell transaminases
○ Reduced excretion of pyridoxic acid in urine

COBALAMIN DEFICIENCY
○ Cobalamin serum levels less than 150 pg/ml
○ Schilling test to measure absorption of radioactive cobalamin with and without intrinsic factor
○ Gastric analysis and hemoglobin studies to uncover causation

Treatment

Thiamine deficiency
General
○ High-protein diet, with adequate calorie intake and thiamine rich foods (pork, peas, wheat bran, oatmeal, and liver)
Medication
○ B-complex vitamins
○ Thiamine supplements or thiamine hydrochloride as part of a B-complex concentrate (with alcoholic beriberi)

Riboflavin deficiency
General
○ Diet high in riboflavin foods (meats, enriched flour, milk and dairy products, green leafy vegetables, eggs, and cereal)
Medication
○ Supplemental riboflavin

Niacin deficiency
General
○ Dietary enrichment (meats, fish, peanuts, brewer's yeast, enriched breads, and cereals rich in niacin; milk and eggs, in tryptophan)
Medication
○ Supplemental B-complex vitamins
○ Niacinamide

Pyridoxine deficiency
General
○ Symptomatic
○ Dietary adjustments
○ Increased carbohydrate intake before vigorous exercise
Medication
○ Prophylactic pyridoxine therapy in infants and in children with seizure disorder
○ Supplemental B-complex vitamins

Cobalamin deficiency
General
○ Blood transfusion if severe
○ Diet high in folate
Medication
○ Parenteral cyanocobalamin in patients with reduced gastric secretion of hydrochloric acid, lack of intrinsic factor, some malabsorption syndromes, or ileum resections
○ Folate

Nursing considerations

Key outcomes
The patient will:
○ improve vitamin levels
○ express understanding of dietary adjustments needed to improve nutritional status.

Nursing interventions
○ Administer prescribed supplements.
○ Explain all tests and procedures.

Monitoring
○ Adverse effects from large doses of niacinamide, in patients with niacin deficiency
○ Dietary intake
○ Response to therapy

Patient teaching

Be sure to cover:
- keeping an accurate dietary history
- that prognosis is good with treatment
- importance of adhering strictly to their prescribed treatment for the rest of their lives
- dietary adjustments.

Discharge planning

- Refer the patient to appropriate assistance agencies if his diets are inadequate due to adverse socioeconomic conditions.

Vitamin C deficiency

Overview

Description
○ Deficiency of vitamin C in the body
○ Historically common among sailors and others deprived of fresh fruits and vegetables for long periods of time; uncommon today in the United States, except in alcoholics, people on restricted-residue diets, and

Scurvy's effect on gums and legs

In adults, scurvy causes swollen or bleeding gums and loose teeth.

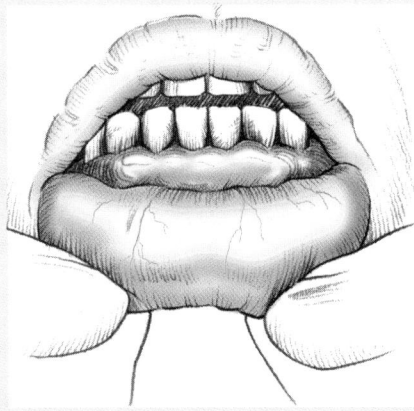

It also causes follicular hyperkeratosis, usually on the legs.

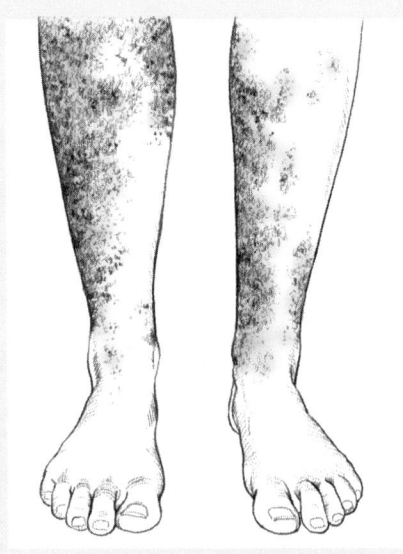

infants weaned from breast milk to cow's milk without a vitamin C supplement
○ Also known as *scurvy*

Pathophysiology
○ Deficiency of vitamin C can lead to scurvy or inadequate production of collagen, an extracellular substance that binds the cells of the teeth, bones, and capillaries.
○ Because the body can't store this water-soluble vitamin in large amounts, the supply needs to be replenished daily.

Causes
○ Diet lacking foods rich in vitamin C, such as citrus fruits, tomatoes, cabbage, broccoli, spinach, and berries
○ Destruction of vitamin C in foods by overexposure to air or by overcooking
○ Excessive ingestion of vitamin C during pregnancy, which causes the neonate to require large amounts of the vitamin after birth
○ Marginal intake of vitamin C during periods of physiologic stress

Incidence
○ Rare in the United States
○ Can occur at any age
○ Can affect males and females

Common characteristics
○ Petechiae
○ Ecchymoses
○ Follicular hyperkeratosis (especially on the buttocks and legs)
○ Signs of anemia
○ Anorexia
○ Limb and joint pain (especially in the knees)
○ Swollen or bleeding gums (see *Scurvy's effect on gums and legs*)
○ Loose teeth
○ Insomnia
○ Poor wound healing
○ Ocular hemorrhages in the bulbar conjunctivae
○ Beading, fractures of the costochondral junctions of the ribs or epiphysis
○ Psychological disturbances such as irritability, depression, hysteria, and hypochondriasis

Complications
○ Sudden death

Assessment

History
○ Anorexia
○ Limb and joint pain (especially in the knees)
○ Insomnia

- ○ Poor wound healing
- ○ Irritability
- ○ Depression
- ○ Hysteria
- ○ Hypochondriasis
- ○ Fatigue

Physical findings

- ○ Pallor
- ○ Petechiae
- ○ Ecchymoses
- ○ Follicular hyperkeratosis (especially on the buttocks and legs)
- ○ Swollen or bleeding gums
- ○ Loose teeth
- ○ Ocular hemorrhages in the bulbar conjunctivae
- ○ Beading, fractures of the costochondral junctions of the ribs or epiphysis

Test results

Laboratory
- ○ Serum ascorbic acid levels are less than 0.2 mg/dl.
- ○ White blood cell ascorbic acid levels are less than 30 mg/dl.

Other
- ○ Dietary history revealing an inadequate intake of ascorbic acid suggests vitamin C deficiency.

Treatment

General

- ○ Diet high in foods rich in vitamin C

Medication

- ○ Vitamin C supplements

Nursing considerations

Key outcomes

The patient will:
- ○ improve vitamin levels
- ○ express understanding of dietary adjustments needed to improve nutritional status.

Nursing interventions

- ○ Give prescribed ascorbic acid orally or by slow I.V. infusion.
- ○ Avoid moving the patient unnecessarily to avoid irritating painful joints and muscles.
- ○ Encourage the patient to consume foods high in vitamin C. (See *Foods that contain vitamin C.*)

Monitoring

- ○ Dietary intake

Foods that contain vitamin C

The following foods contain significant amounts of vitamin C.

○ Blackberries	○ Kiwi
○ Broccoli	○ Lemons
○ Brussels sprouts	○ Oranges
○ Cantaloupe	○ Papaya
○ Green and red peppers	○ Strawberries
○ Guava	○ Peas
○ Kale	○ Tomatoes

Patient teaching

Be sure to cover:
- ○ the importance of supplemental ascorbic acid
- ○ good dietary sources of vitamin C
- ○ not taking too much vitamin C because excessive doses of ascorbic acid may cause nausea, diarrhea, and renal calculi formation and may also interfere with anticoagulant therapy.

Vitamin D deficiency

Overview

Description
○ Deficiency of vitamin D in the body
○ Also known as *rickets*

Pathophysiology
○ Deficiency of vitamin D causes failure of normal bone calcification, which results in rickets in infants and young children and osteomalacia in adults.
○ With treatment, the prognosis is good; however, in rickets, bone deformities usually persist, while in osteomalacia, such deformities may disappear.

Causes
○ Inadequate dietary intake of preformed vitamin D
○ Malabsorption of vitamin D
○ Too little exposure to sunlight
○ Vitamin D-resistant rickets (refractory rickets, familial hypophosphatemia) from an inherited impairment of renal tubular reabsorption of phosphate (from vitamin D insensitivity)
○ Hepatic or renal disease
○ Malfunctioning parathyroid gland (decreased secretion of parathyroid hormone), which contributes to calcium deficiency (normally, absorption of calcium and phosphorus through the intestine controlled by vitamin D) and interferes with activation of vitamin D in the kidneys

---

Recognizing bowlegs

This infant with rickets shows characteristic bowing of the legs.

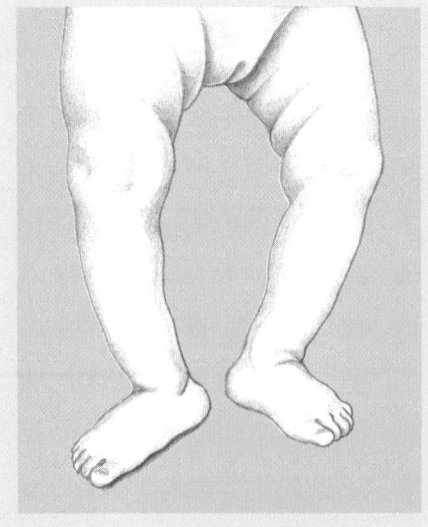

Incidence
○ Once a common childhood disease, now rare in the United States
○ Occasionally appears in breast-fed infants who don't receive vitamin D supplementation and in infants receiving a formula with a nonfortified milk base
○ May also occur in overcrowded, urban areas where smog limits sunlight penetration
○ Highest incidence in black children who, because of their skin color, absorb less sunlight (solar ultraviolet rays irradiate 7-dehydrocholesterol, a precursor of vitamin D, to form calciferol)

Common characteristics
○ Profuse sweating
○ Restlessness
○ Irritability
○ Numerous bone malformations

Complications
○ Spontaneous fractures
○ Abnormal gait
○ Short stature

Assessment

History
○ Spontaneous multiple fractures
○ Pain in the legs and lower back

Physical findings
○ Bowlegs (see *Recognizing bowlegs*)
○ Knock-knees
○ Rachitic rosary (beading of ends of ribs)
○ Enlargement of wrists and ankles
○ Pigeon breast
○ Delayed closing of the fontanels
○ Softening of the skull
○ Bulging of the forehead

Test results
Laboratory
○ Plasma calcium serum levels are less than 7.5 mg/dl.
○ Serum inorganic phosphorus levels are less than 3 mg/dl.
○ Serum citrate levels are less than 2.5 mg/dl.
○ Alkaline phosphatase levels are less than 4 Bodansky units/dl.
Imaging
○ X-rays show characteristic bone deformities and abnormalities such as Looser's zones (pseudofractures).

Treatment

General

○ Sunlight exposure

Medication

○ For osteomalacia and rickets (except when caused by malabsorption), massive oral doses of vitamin D or cod liver oil
○ For rickets refractory to vitamin D or in rickets accompanied by hepatic or renal disease, 25-hydroxy-cholecalciferol, 1,25-dihydroxycholecalciferol, or a synthetic analogue of active vitamin D

Nursing considerations

Key outcomes

The patient will:
○ improve vitamin levels
○ express understanding of dietary adjustments needed to improve nutritional status.

Nursing interventions

○ Obtain a dietary history to assess the patient's current vitamin D intake.
○ Administer supplementary aqueous preparations of vitamin D for chronic fat malabsorption, hydroxylated cholecalciferol for refractory rickets, and supplemental vitamin D for breast-fed infants.

Monitoring

○ Dietary intake
○ Comfort level

Patient teaching

Be sure to cover:
○ watching for signs of vitamin D toxicity (headache, nausea, constipation and, after prolonged use, renal calculi).

Discharge planning

○ If deficiency is due to socioeconomic conditions, refer the patient to an appropriate community agency.

Vitamin E deficiency

Overview

Description

○ Deficiency of vitamin E in the body

Pathophysiology

○ Vitamin E (tocopherol) appears to act primarily as an antioxidant, preventing intracellular oxidation of polyunsaturated fatty acids and other lipids.
○ Deficiency of vitamin E usually manifests as hemolytic anemia in low–birth-weight or premature neonates. With treatment, prognosis is good.

Causes

○ In infants, usually results from consuming formulas high in polyunsaturated fatty acids that are fortified with iron but not vitamin E (Such formulas increase the need for vitamin E because the iron supplement catalyzes the oxidation of red blood cell [RBC] lipids.)
○ Conditions associated with fat malabsorption

Incidence

○ Uncommon in adults but possible in people whose diets are high in polyunsaturated fatty acids, which increase vitamin E requirements, and in people with vitamin E malabsorption, which impairs RBC survival

---

Foods that contain vitamin E

The following foods contain significant amounts of vitamin E.
○ Almonds
○ Almond oil
○ Asparagus
○ Avocadoes
○ Canola oil
○ Corn
○ Corn oil
○ Cottonseed oil
○ Hazelnuts
○ Kiwi
○ Mangoes
○ Nuts
○ Olives
○ Safflower oil
○ Soybeans
○ Soybean oil
○ Sunflower seeds
○ Wheat germ
○ Wheat germ oil

Common characteristics

Infants
○ Edema
○ Skin lesions
Adults
○ Intermittent claudication

Complications

○ Disorders of reproduction
○ Abnormalities of muscle, liver, bone marrow, and brain function
○ Hemolysis of RBC
○ Skeletal muscle dystrophy

Assessment

History

○ Intermittent claudication

Physical findings

○ Edema
○ Skin lesions

Test results

Laboratory
○ Serum alpha-tocopherol levels are below 0.5 mg/dl in adults and below 0.2 mg/dl in infants.
○ Creatinuria, increased creatine kinase levels, hemolytic anemia, and an elevated platelet count support the diagnosis.
Other
○ Dietary and medical histories suggest vitamin E deficiency.

Treatment

General

○ Diet high in foods rich in vitamin E, such as vegetable oils, whole grains, dark green leafy vegetables, nuts, and legumes

Medication

○ Vitamin E supplementation

Nursing considerations

Key outcomes

The patient will:
○ improve vitamin levels
○ express understanding of dietary adjustments needed to improve nutritional status.

Nursing interventions

○ Encourage patient to consume foods high in vitamin E. (See *Foods that contain vitamin E.*)

Monitoring
○ Dietary intake

Patient teaching

Be sure to cover:
○ preventing deficiency by providing vitamin E supplements for low-birth-weight infants receiving formulas not fortified with vitamin E and for adults with vitamin E malabsorption
○ dietary changes.
○ that food manufacturers fortify many products with vitamins and minerals (Read the nutrition facts panel of food labels to find out if a food contains vitamin E.)
○ that most adults in the United States get enough vitamin E from their normal diets to meet current recommendations. (Caution those on low-fat diets that low-fat intake can substantially decrease vitamin E intake if appropriate food choices aren't made.)

Discharge planning
○ If vitamin E deficiency is related to socioeconomic conditions, refer the patient to appropriate community agencies.

Vitamin K deficiency

Overview

Description
○ Deficiency of vitamin K in the body

Pathophysiology
○ Vitamin K is an element necessary for formation of prothrombin and other clotting factors in the liver; deficiency produces abnormal bleeding.
○ If the deficiency is corrected, the prognosis is excellent.
○ Vitamin K is found in specific foods and is also made by the bacteria that line the GI tract.

Causes
○ Prolonged use of drugs, such as the anticoagulant dicumarol and antibiotics that destroy normal intestinal bacteria
○ Obstruction of the bile duct or bile fistula
○ Malabsorption of vitamin K due to sprue, pellagra, bowel resection, ileitis, or ulcerative colitis
○ Chronic hepatic disease
○ Cystic fibrosis

Foods that contain vitamin K

The following foods contain significant amounts of vitamin K.
Breads, cereals, rice, and pasta
○ Oats
○ Wheat bran
○ Whole wheat flour
Fruits
○ Avocados
Vegetables
○ Broccoli
○ Cabbage
○ Cauliflower
○ Endive
○ Kale
○ Lentils (dry)
○ Lettuce (iceberg)
○ Soybeans
○ Spinach
○ Swiss chard
○ Turnip greens
○ Watercress
Organ meats
○ Beef liver
○ Chicken liver
○ Pork liver
Fats, oils, sugars
○ Corn oil
○ Soybean oil

Incidence
○ Vitamin K deficiency is common among neonates in the first few days postpartum due to poor placental transfer of vitamin K and inadequate production of vitamin K-producing intestinal flora.

Common characteristics
○ Abnormal bleeding tendency

Complications
○ Bleeding

Assessment

History
○ Prolonged or easy bleeding

Physical findings
○ Ecchymosis
○ Petechiae

Test results
Laboratory
○ A prothrombin time (PT) that's 25% longer than the normal range of 10 to 20 seconds confirms the diagnosis of vitamin K deficiency after other causes of prolonged PT (such as anticoagulant therapy or hepatic disease) have been ruled out.

Treatment

General
○ Diet rich in foods high in vitamin K, such as green leafy vegetables, cereals, soybeans, and other vegetables. (See *Foods that contain vitamin K.*)

Medication
○ Vitamin K

Nursing considerations

Key outcomes
The patient will:
○ improve vitamin levels
○ show less tendency to bleed easily
○ show improved laboratory values.

Nursing interventions
○ Encourage the patient to consume foods high in vitamin K.
○ Administer vitamin K to newborns and patients with fat malabsorption or with prolonged diarrhea caused by colitis, ileitis, or long-term antibiotic therapy.
Monitoring
○ PT
○ Signs of bleeding

Patient teaching

Be sure to cover:
- ❍ warning against self-medication with or overuse of antibiotics, which destroy the intestinal bacteria necessary to generate significant amounts of vitamin K
- ❍ dietary counseling
- ❍ warning the patient to take safety precautions as vitamin K deficiency can cause increased risk of bruising and bleeding.

Vitiligo

Overview

Description

◯ Hypopigmentation condition of the skin
◯ May cause a serious cosmetic problem
◯ Concurrent risk of other diseases, especially thyroid

Pathophysiology

◯ Destruction of melanocytes and circulating antibodies results in hypopigmented areas.

Causes

◯ Apparently, both genetic and environmental components
◯ In about 30% of patients, first-degree relative with the same disorder
◯ Precipitating factors:
 – Stressful physical or psychological events
 – Chemical agents, such as phenols and catechols
◯ Associated concurrent diseases:
 – Thyroid dysfunction
 – Pernicious anemia
 – Addison's disease
 – Aseptic meningitis
 – Diabetes mellitus

Incidence

◯ Affects about 1% of U.S. population
◯ Onset at any age
◯ About 50% of cases beginning between ages 10 and 30

Recognizing vitiligo

This illustration shows characteristic depigmented skin patches in vitiligo. These patches are usually bilaterally symmetrical, with distinct borders.

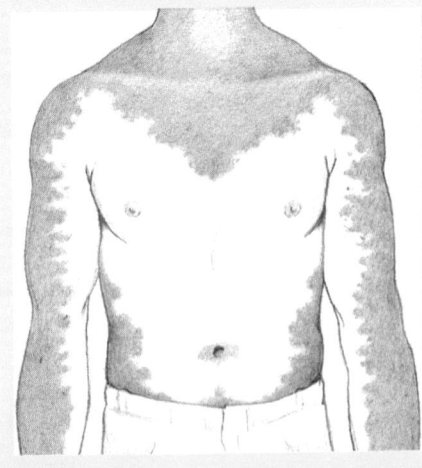

◯ No racial predilection
◯ Males and females about equally affected (Women tend to seek treatment more than men.)

Common characteristics

◯ Loss of pigment
◯ Locally increased sunburn

Complications

◯ Extreme photosensitivity in depigmented areas
◯ Hypersensitivity reactions to therapeutic agents and to dyes or cosmetics used to camouflage lesions

Assessment

History

◯ Familial history of vitiligo

Physical findings

◯ Depigmented or stark-white skin patches; almost imperceptible on fair-skinned whites
◯ Patches usually bilaterally symmetrical, with distinct borders that may be raised and hyperpigmented (see *Recognizing vitiligo*)
◯ Patches most likely over bony prominences, around orifices, within body folds, and at sites of traumatic injury
◯ Hair within lesions also possibly white
◯ Prematurely gray hair
◯ Ocular pigment changes

Test results

Diagnostic procedures
◯ Wood's light examination in a darkened room shows vitiliginous patches in fair-skinned patients.
◯ Skin biopsy result confirms the diagnosis.

Treatment

General

◯ Sunscreens
◯ Cosmetics and skin dyes as cover-ups

Medication

◯ Repigmentation compounds
◯ Depigmentation creams

Surgery

◯ Skin grafting

Nursing considerations

Key outcomes

The patient will:
◯ verbalize understanding of the disorder and treatment
◯ verbalize feelings about changed body image
◯ avoid complications.

Nursing interventions

○ Encourage expression of feelings about appearance.
○ Offer emotional support and reassurance.
○ Reinforce treatment goals.

Monitoring

○ Response to treatment
○ Complications

Patient teaching

Be sure to cover:
○ the disorder, diagnosis, and treatment
○ that exposure to sunlight also darkens normal skin in
  patients undergoing repigmentation therapy
○ the use of sunscreen, sunglasses, and protective
  clothing
○ that results of depigmentation are permanent
○ adverse effects of sunlight.

Discharge planning

○ Refer the patient to the National Vitiligo Foundation.

Volvulus

Overview

Description

- Twisting of the intestine at least 180 degrees on itself
- Marked by sudden onset of severe abdominal pain
- Results in blood vessel compression
- Causes obstruction both proximal and distal to the twisted loop
- Occurs in a bowel segment long enough to twist, most commonly the sigmoid colon (small bowel a common site in children)
- Other common sites: the stomach and cecum

Pathophysiology

- The colon twists on its mesentery.
- A closed loop obstruction occurs, affecting venous drainage and arterial inflow.
- Cecal volvulus is a congenital defect in the peritoneum with inadequate fixation of the cecum. (See *What happens in volvulus.*)

Causes

- Anomaly of bowel rotation in utero
- Ingested foreign body
- Adhesions
- Meconium ileus (in patients with cystic fibrosis)

Risk factors

- Straining at stool
- Pregnancy
- Intestinal malignancy
- Hernia
- High-bulk diet
- History of previous attacks
- Use of chronic neuropsychotropic drugs
- Chronic constipation and laxative abuse

Incidence

- Varies worldwide in cases of volvulus of the large bowel
- Accounts for 1% to 5% of all large-bowel obstructions in advanced Western populations
- Most common sites: sigmoid colon (80%), cecum (15%), transverse colon (3%), and splenic flexure (2%)
- Common in regions of Africa, Southern Asia, and South America
- About 50% of large-bowel obstructions caused by volvulus occurring in the "volvulus belt" of Africa and the Middle East
- Affects men and women equally

Common characteristics

- Severe abdominal pain and distention
- Vomiting
- Constipation

What happens in volvulus

Although volvulus may occur anywhere in a bowel segment long enough to twist, the most common site, as this illustration depicts, is the sigmoid colon, causing edema within the closed loop and obstruction at its proximal and distal ends.

NORMAL BOWEL SEGMENT

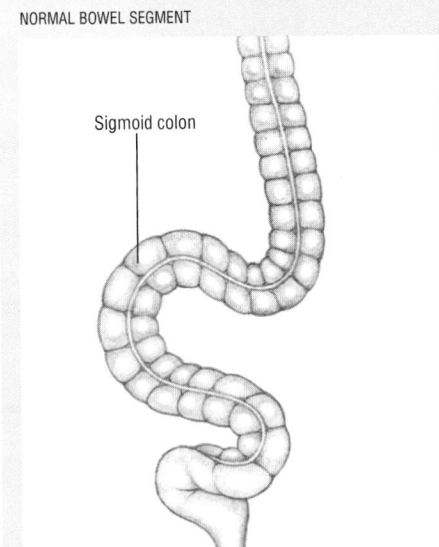

Sigmoid colon

VOLVULUS

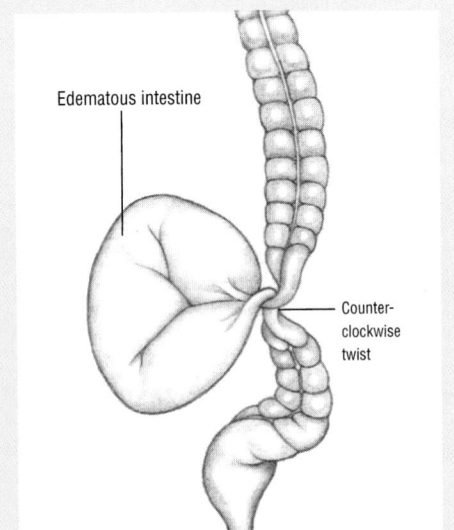

Edematous intestine

Counter-clockwise twist

Complications

○ Strangulation of the twisted bowel loop
○ Bowel ischemia and infarction
○ Bowel perforation

Assessment

History

○ Severe abdominal pain
○ Bilious vomiting
○ Constipation

Physical findings

○ Abdominal distention
○ Palpable abdominal mass

Test results

Laboratory
○ White blood cell count, in strangulation, is greater than 15,000/ml; in bowel infarction, it's greater than 20,000/ml.

Imaging
○ Abdominal X-rays may show multiple distended bowel loops and a large bowel without gas. In midgut volvulus, abdominal X-rays may be normal.
○ Barium enema, in cecal volvulus, shows barium filling the colon distal to the affected section of cecum; in sigmoid volvulus, barium may twist to a point and, in adults, take on an "ace of spades" configuration.

Treatment

General

○ For adults with sigmoid volvulus, nonsurgical treatment: proctoscopy to check for infarction and reduction by careful insertion of a flexible sigmoidoscope to deflate the bowel
○ I.V. therapy
○ Nothing by mouth until condition resolves
○ Bed rest until condition resolves

Medication

○ Antibiotics
○ Analgesics

Surgery

○ For children with midgut volvulus
○ Detorsion (untwisting)
○ Resection and anastomosis

Nursing considerations

Key outcomes

The patient will:
○ express feelings of increased comfort and decreased pain
○ have stable vital signs
○ avoid complications

○ regain normal bowel function
○ express an understanding of the disorder and treatment regimen.

Nursing interventions

○ Encourage verbalization and provide support.
○ Give prescribed drugs.
○ Give prescribed I.V. fluids.

Monitoring

○ Pain control
○ Bowel function
○ Vital signs
○ Fluid and electrolyte balance
○ Nasogastric tube function and drainage
○ Wound site

Patient teaching

Be sure to cover:
○ the disorder, diagnosis, and treatment
○ preoperative teaching
○ drug administration, dosage, and possible adverse effects
○ the signs and symptoms of infection
○ the importance of follow-up care.

von Willebrand's disease

Overview

Description
○ Hereditary bleeding disorder characterized by prolonged bleeding time, moderate deficiency of clotting factor VIII (*antihemophilic factor*), *and impaired platelet function*
○ Also known as *angiohemophilia, pseudohemophilia,* and *vascular hemophilia*

Pathophysiology
○ Mild to moderate deficiency of factor VIII and defective platelet adhesion prolonging coagulation time
○ Results from a deficiency of von Willebrand's factor (factor VIII$_{VWF}$), which appears to occupy the factor VIII molecule and may be necessary for the production of factor VIII and proper platelet function
○ Defective platelet function characterized by decreased agglutination and adhesion at the bleeding site, reduced platelet retention when filtered through a column of packed glass beads, and diminished ristocetin-induced platelet aggregation

Causes
○ Inherited as an autosomal dominant trait
○ Acquired form identified in patients with cancer and immune disorders

Incidence
○ Affects males and females; tends to be more common in males

Common characteristics
○ Bleeding from the skin or mucosal surfaces
○ In females, excessive uterine bleeding

Complications
○ Hemorrhage

Assessment

History
○ Possible familial history of the disease
○ Easy bruising and frequent bleeding from the nose or gums (petechiae rare)
○ Menorrhagia
○ Hemorrhage after a laceration or surgery
○ Possible episodes of GI bleeding

Physical findings
○ Bruises
○ Clinical bleeding

Test results

Laboratory
○ Bleeding time is prolonged to more than 6 minutes.
○ Partial thromboplastin time is slightly prolonged to more than 45 seconds.
○ Factor VIII-related antigen levels are absent or reduced, and factor VIII activity level is low.
○ In vitro platelet aggregation is defective using the ristocetin coagulation factor assay test.
○ Platelet count and clot retraction are normal.

Treatment

General
○ Depends on the symptoms and underlying type of disease
○ Decreasing bleeding time by local measures and replacing factor VIII and, consequently, factor VIII$_{VWF}$
○ Avoidance of aspirin
○ Alternation of activities and rest periods if patient is fatigued after a bleeding episode

Medication
○ Cryoprecipitate (cryoprecipitated antihemophilic factor)
○ Plasma products or vasopressin analogue
○ Factor VIII concentrates

Nursing considerations

Key outcomes
The patient will:
○ experience hemodynamic stability
○ have palpable peripheral pulses
○ maintain normal fluid volume
○ incur no injury
○ exhibit adequate coping skills.

Nursing interventions
○ Provide emotional support as necessary.
○ During a bleeding episode, elevate the area if possible, and apply cold compresses and gentle pressure to the bleeding site. (Pressure is commonly the only treatment necessary.)
○ Give prescribed drugs or transfusions.
○ Prevent potential injury by using an electric razor, keeping the room free from clutter, and providing a cushioned sitting and sleeping surface (such as a convoluted foam mattress).

Monitoring
○ Signs and symptoms of decreased tissue perfusion
○ Vital signs
○ Frequently, for bleeding from the skin, mucous membranes, and wounds
○ After surgery, bleeding time or other clotting procedure for 24 to 48 hours and for signs of new bleeding
○ Adverse reactions to blood products

Patient teaching

Be sure to cover:
- ◯ the disorder, diagnosis, and treatment
- ◯ the need to notify a physician after even minor trauma and before all surgery, including dental procedures, to determine whether replacement of blood components is necessary
- ◯ warnings against using aspirin and other drugs that impair platelet function (how to recognize over-the-counter medications that contain aspirin)
- ◯ special precautions to prevent bleeding episodes
- ◯ the importance of wearing or carrying medical identification
- ◯ measures to control bleeding and how to prevent bleeding, unnecessary trauma, and complications.

Discharge planning

- ◯ Refer parents of an affected child for genetic counseling.

Vulvovaginitis

Overview

Description

- Inflammation of the vulva (vulvitis) and vagina (vaginitis)
- Prognosis good with treatment

Pathophysiology

- Because of the proximity of the vulva and vagina, inflammation of one usually precipitates inflammation of the other.

Causes

Vaginitis
- Protozoan infection (*Trichomonas vaginalis*)
- Fungal infection (*Candida albicans*)
- Bacterial infection (bacterial vaginosis)
- Venereal infection (*Neisseria gonorrhoeae*)
- Viral infection with venereal warts or herpes simplex virus Type 2

Vulvitis
- Parasitic infection (*Phthirus pubis,* crab louse)
- Traumatic injury
- Poor personal hygiene
- Chemical irritations
- Allergic reactions, such as to douches or toilet paper
- Retention of a foreign body such as a tampon

Risk factors

- Pregnancy
- Hormonal contraceptives
- Diabetes mellitus
- Systemic broad-spectrum antibiotics
- Vaginal mucosa and vulval atrophy in menopausal women

Incidence

- Occurs at any age
- Affects most females at some time

Common characteristics

- Vaginal itching in most cases
- Vaginal discharge in many cases

Complications

- Inflammation of the perineum
- Skin breakdown
- Secondary infection
- Dyspareunia
- Dysuria

Assessment

History

Trichomonal vaginitis
- Vaginal irritation and itching
- Urinary symptoms, such as burning and frequency

Candidal vaginitis
- Intense vaginal itching
- Thick, white, cottage cheese-like discharge

Bacterial vaginosis
- Fishy-smelling discharge
- May be asymptomatic

Gonorrhea
- Possibly no symptoms
- Dysuria

Acute vulvitis
- Vulvar burning, pruritus
- Severe dysuria
- Dyspareunia

Physical findings

Trichomonal vaginitis
- Thin, bubbly, green-tinged, and malodorous vaginal discharge

Candidal vaginitis
- Thick, white, cottage cheese-like discharge
- Red, edematous mucous membranes with white flecks on vaginal wall

Bacterial vaginosis
- Gray, foul, fishy-smelling discharge

Gonorrhea
- Profuse and purulent discharge

Acute vulvitis
- Vulvar edema and erythema

Herpesvirus infection
- Ulceration or vesicle formation on the perineum (active phase)
- Severe edema that may involve entire perineum (chronic infection)

Test results

Laboratory
- Wet slide preparation and microscopic examination of vaginal exudates are used in obtaining various test results:
  - Vaginitis diagnosis requires identification of the infectious organism.
  - In trichomonal infections, the presence of motile, flagellated trichomonads confirms the diagnosis.
  - In monilial vaginitis, 10% potassium hydroxide is added to the slide; diagnosis requires identification of *C. albicans* fungus.
  - In bacterial vaginosis, saline wet mount shows the presence of clue cells, giving it a stippled appearance.
  - Gonorrhea requires a culture of vaginal exudate to confirm the diagnosis.
- Diagnosis of vulvitis or a suspected sexually transmitted disease (STD) may require a complete blood

count, urinalysis, cytology screening, biopsy of chronic lesions to rule out cancer, and culture of exudate from acute lesions.

Treatment

General

○ Cold compresses or cool sitz baths to relieve pruritus
○ Warm compresses for severe inflammation
○ Avoidance of drying soaps
○ Loose clothing to promote air circulation
○ For chronic vulvitis, changing problematic environmental factors

Medication

○ Antibacterials
○ Antiprotozoal agents
○ Topical corticosteroids
○ Antipruritics
○ Topical estrogen ointments
○ Antivirals

Nursing considerations

Key outcomes

The patient will:
○ express feelings of increased comfort
○ exhibit no signs of infection
○ express concerns about self-concept, self-esteem, and body image
○ use available counseling or a support group.

Nursing interventions

○ Encourage expression of feelings.
○ Help the patient to develop effective coping strategies.
○ Provide comfort measures.
○ Use meticulous hand-washing technique.
○ Report cases of STDs to the public health authorities.
○ Administer drug therapy.

Monitoring

○ Response to treatment
○ Vaginal discharge
○ Signs and symptoms of secondary infection

Patient teaching

Be sure to cover:
○ the disorder, diagnosis, and treatment
○ the correlation between sexual contact and spread of vaginal infections
○ using condoms to prevent or decrease the spread of sexually transmitted infections
○ notifying sexual partners of the need for treatment
○ abstaining from sexual intercourse until the infection resolves

○ completing prescribed drugs, even if symptoms subside
○ proper application of vaginal ointments and suppositories
○ the need for meticulous hand washing before and after drug administration
○ preventing skin breakdown and secondary infections
○ good hygiene practices
○ wearing all-cotton, white underpants and avoiding tight-fitting pants and panty hose
○ abstaining from alcoholic beverages with metronidazole therapy
○ that metronidazole therapy may turn the urine dark brown.

Warts

Overview

Description
- Common, benign, skin growths
- Prognosis varies, some disappearing readily with treatment, others necessitating more vigorous and prolonged treatment
- Also known as *verrucae*

Pathophysiology
- Warts are small harmless tumors of the skin caused by a virus.
- Most are well defined.
- Mode of transmission is probably through direct contact, but autoinoculation is possible.
- Warts are categorized by location and appearance.

Causes
- Infection with the human papillomavirus, a group of ether-resistant, deoxyribonucleic acid-containing papovaviruses

Incidence
- Highest in children and young adults, but may occur at any age

Common characteristics
- Clinical manifestations depend on the type of wart and its location.

Common (verruca vulgaris)
- Rough, elevated, rounded surface
- Appears most frequently on limbs, particularly hands and fingers
- Most prevalent in children and young adults

Filiform
- Single, thin, threadlike projection
- Commonly occurs around the face and neck

Periungual
- Rough, irregularly shaped, elevated surface
- Occurs around edges of fingernails and toenails
- When severe, may extend under the nail and lift it off the nail bed, causing pain

Flat (juvenile)
- Multiple groupings of up to several hundred slightly raised lesions with smooth, flat, or slightly rounded tops
- Common on the face, neck, chest, knees, dorsa of hands, wrists, and flexor surfaces of the forearms
- Usually in children but can affect adults
- Distribution commonly linear because spreading possible from scratching or shaving

Plantar
- Slightly elevated or flat
- Occur singly or in large clusters (mosaic warts), primarily at pressure points of the feet

Digitate
- Fingerlike, horny projection arising from a pea-shaped base
- On scalp or near hairline

Condyloma acuminatum (moist wart)
- Usually small, pink to red, moist, and soft
- Single or in large cauliflower-like clusters on the penis, scrotum, vulva, or anus
- May be transmitted through sexual contact; not always venereal in origin

Complications
- Scarring
- Recurrence of wart
- Formation of keloid

Assessment

History
- Based on type and location
- Contact with someone who has warts

Physical findings
- Small, hard, flat-to-raised lump or lesion on the skin
- Small, flat lesion on forehead, cheeks, arms, or legs
- Rough, round, painful lesion on sole
- Rough growth around fingernails or toenails

Test results
Diagnostic procedures
- Recurrent anal warts require sigmoidoscopy to rule out internal involvement, which may necessitate surgery.
- Skin biopsy may confirm diagnosis in some cases.

Other
- Visual examination usually confirms the diagnosis.

Treatment

General
- Cryotherapy

Medication
- Acid therapy (primary or adjunctive)
- 25% podophyllin in compound with tincture of benzoin (for venereal warts)
- Carbon dioxide laser therapy

Surgery
- Electrodesiccation and curettage (see *Removing warts by electrosurgery*)

Nursing considerations

Key outcomes
The patient will:
- relate understanding of disorder and treatment

1. Injection of 1% to 2% lidocaine under and around the wart, avoiding the wart itself

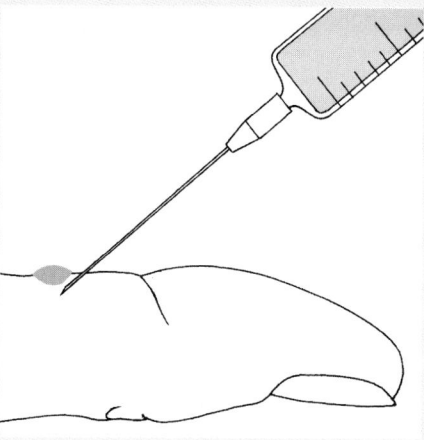

2. Electrodesiccation of the wart

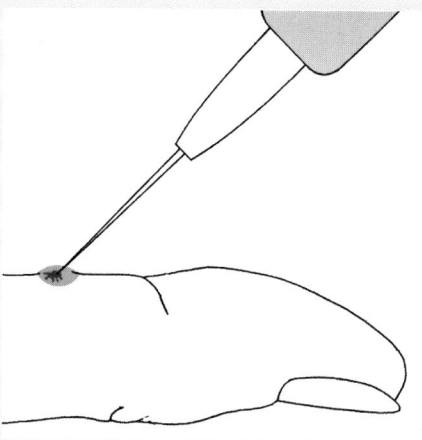

3. Removal of the wart tissue with a curette and curved scissors

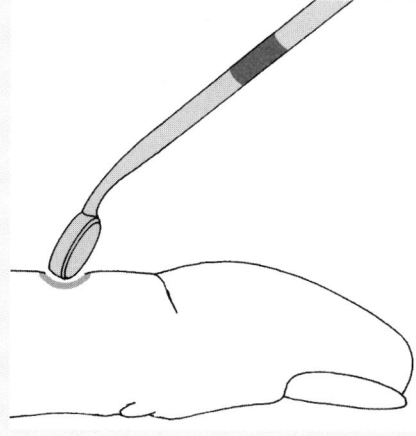

4. Light desiccation of the area to control bleeding and prevent recurrence

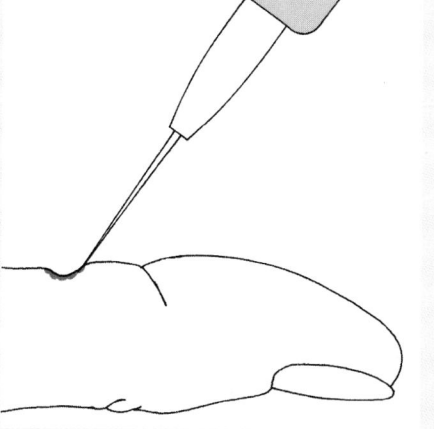

- express feelings about change in body image
- exhibit improved or healed lesions.

Nursing interventions

- During acid or podophyllin therapy, protect the surrounding area with petroleum jelly or sodium bicarbonate (baking soda).

Monitoring

- Response to treatment
- Bleeding
- Lesion healing

Patient teaching

Be sure to cover:
- that conscientious adherence to prescribed therapy is essential
- that the patient's sexual partner may also need treatment
- need to avoid direct contact with warts.

West Nile encephalitis

Overview

Description

- An infectious disease, part of a family of vector-borne diseases that also includes malaria, yellow fever, and Lyme disease
- Mortality rate from 3% to 15%; higher in elderly population
- Ticks infected with the virus found in Africa and Asia only; role of ticks in transmission and maintenance of the virus uncertain
- Also called *West Nile virus*

Pathophysiology

- Virus has an incubation period of 5 to 15 days after exposure.
- Mosquitoes become infected by feeding on birds contaminated with the virus.
- The virus is transmitted to a human by the bite of an infected mosquito (mostly the Culex species).
- Disease primarily causes inflammation or encephalitis of the brain.

Causes

- A flavivirus commonly found in humans, birds, and other vertebrates in Africa, West Asia, and the Middle East

Risk factors

- Recent chemotherapy
- Recent organ transplantation
- Immunocompromised state
- Pregnancy
- Advanced age
- Breast-feeding

Incidence

- In temperate areas, occurs mainly in late summer or early fall
- In milder climates, can occur year-round
- Risk greater in areas with active cases
- Greatest risk in those older than age 50 and those with compromised immune systems

Common characteristics

- Incubation period 5 to 15 days after exposure
- No symptoms in most patients bitten by infected mosquito; only 1 in 300 get sick
- Fever
- Headache
- Myalgia

Complications

- Neurologic impairment
- Seizures
- Death

Assessment

History

- Headache
- Myalgia
- Neck stiffness
- Possible recent exposure to bodies of water, dead birds, or recent mosquito bites
- Decreased appetite
- Nausea
- Vomiting
- Diarrhea

Physical findings

- Fever
- Rash
- Swollen lymph glands
- Stupor and disorientation
- Stiff neck
- Change in mental status

Test results

Laboratory
- White blood cell (WBC) count is normal or increased.
- The enzyme-linked immunosorbent assay (ELISA), the MAC-ELISA, allows a rapid and definitive diagnosis.
- Accurate diagnosis is possible only when serum or cerebrospinal fluid specimens are obtained while the patient is still hospitalized with acute illness and they show an elevated WBC count and protein levels.

Imaging
- Magnetic resonance imaging may show inflammation.

Treatment

General

- No specific treatment
- Respiratory support
- Increased fluid intake
- Rest periods when fatigued

Medication

- Antipyretics

Nursing considerations

Key outcomes

The patient will:
- maintain collateral circulation
- maintain hemodynamic stability
- have adequate cardiac output
- remain afebrile
- have an adequate fluid volume.

Nursing interventions

○ Maintain adequate hydration with I.V. fluids.
○ Give prescribed medications.
○ Provide respiratory support measures when needed.
○ Follow standard precautions when handling blood or other body fluids.
○ Report any suspected cases of West Nile encephalitis to the state department of health.

Monitoring

○ Fluid and electrolyte status
○ Neurologic status
○ Vital signs

Patient teaching

Be sure to cover:
○ the disorder, diagnosis, and treatment
○ the proper use of insect repellants, which can irritate the eyes and mouth, and to avoid applying repellant to the hands of children (shouldn't be applied to children younger than age 3) (see *Preventing West Nile encephalitis*)
○ the expected course and outcomes of the illness
○ the need to drink fluids to avoid dehydration
○ how to stop mosquitoes from breeding by:
  – cleaning out birdbaths and wading pools at least once per week
  – cleaning roof gutters and downspout screens
  – eliminating any standing water
  – not allowing water to collect in trash cans
  – turning over or removing containers in yards where rainwater collects, such as toys and old tires.

Discharge planning

○ Refer the patient to an infectious disease specialist.

Preventing West Nile encephalitis

To reduce the risk of infection with West Nile encephalitis, advise patients to do the following:
○ Stay indoors at dawn and dusk and in early evening when mosquitoes are biting.
○ Wear long-sleeved shirts and long pants when outdoors.
○ Apply insect repellent sparingly to exposed skin. Effective repellents contain 20% to 30% DEET (N,N-diethyltoluamide). DEET in high concentrations (greater than 30%) can cause adverse effects, particularly in children, and should be avoided; adults should apply repellent on children with no more than 10% DEET.
○ Don't place repellent under clothing.
○ Don't apply repellent over cuts, wounds, sunburn, or irritated skin.
○ Wash repellent off daily and reapply as needed.

X-linked infantile hypogamma-globulinemia

Overview

Description

○ A congenital disorder in which all five immunoglobulins (Ig) — IgM, IgG, IgA, IgD, and IgE — and circulating B cells are absent or deficient but T cells are intact
○ Good prognosis with early treatment, except in infants who develop polio or persistent viral infection; usually causes some permanent damage, especially in the neurologic or respiratory system
○ Also called *Bruton's agammaglobulinemia* or *XLA*

Pathophysiology

○ B cells and B-cell precursors may be present in the bone marrow and peripheral blood, but a mutation in the B-cell protein tyrosine kinase causes failure of the B cells to mature and to secrete immunoglobulin.

Causes

○ Congenital

Incidence

○ Affects males almost exclusively
○ Occurs in 1 in 50,000 to 100,000 births

Common characteristics

○ Asymptomatic until age 6 months, when transplacental maternal immunoglobulins that provided immunity have been depleted
○ Recurrent infections such as bacterial otitis media

Complications

○ Hepatitis
○ Enteroviral infections
○ Poliovirus

Assessment

History

○ Recurrent infections:
  – Otitis media
  – Pneumonia
  – Dermatitis
  – Bronchitis
  – Meningitis
  – Conjunctivitis

○ Abnormal dental caries
○ Polyarthritis resembling rheumatoid arthritis

Physical findings

○ Retarded growth
○ Lymphadenopathy and splenomegaly usually absent, despite recurrent infections

Test results

Laboratory

○ Immunoelectrophoresis confirms decreased levels or a total absence of IgM, IgA, and IgG in the serum; however, diagnosis by this method usually isn't possible until the infant is age 9 months.
○ Antigenic stimulation confirms an inability to produce specific antibodies, although cellular immunity remains intact.

Treatment

General

○ Prevention or control of infections
○ Fresh frozen plasma
○ Well-balanced diet

Medication

○ Immune globulin
○ Antibiotics

Nursing considerations

Key outcomes

The patient will:
○ demonstrate an understanding of the disorder
○ prevent infections by limiting exposure
○ report signs and symptoms of infrction promptly.

Nursing interventions

○ Maintain adequate nutrition and hydration.
○ Perform chest physiotherapy if required.

Monitoring

○ Vital signs
○ Intake and output

Patient teaching

Be sure to cover:
○ the disorder, diagnosis, and treatment
○ recognizing early signs of infection and reporting them promptly
○ cleaning cuts and scrapes immediately

○ avoiding crowds and people who have active infections

○ how to meet nutritional and fluid needs during acute infection.

Discharge planning

○ Suggest genetic counseling if parents have questions about the vulnerability of future offspring.

Zinc deficiency

Overview

Description

- Insufficient amounts of zinc, an essential trace element that's a vital component of many enzymes and present in the bones, teeth, hair, skin, testes, liver, and muscles
- Good prognosis with correction of the deficiency

Pathophysiology

- Zinc deficiency causes impairment of synthesis of deoxyribonucleic acid, ribonucleic acid and, ultimately, protein, and alters normal blood concentrations of vitamin A by mobilizing it from the liver.
- About 90% of zinc stores are in bone and skeletal muscle.

Causes

- Excessive intake of foods (containing iron, calcium, vitamin D, and the fiber and phytates in cereals) that bind zinc to form insoluble chelates that prevent its absorption
- Blood loss from parasitism
- Low dietary intake of foods containing zinc

Risk factors

- Alcohol consumption
- Corticosteroids
- Celiac disease

Incidence

- Most common in persons from underdeveloped countries, especially in the Middle East
- Children most susceptible to this deficiency during periods of rapid growth

Common characteristics

- Hepatosplenomegaly
- Sparse hair growth
- Soft, misshapen nails
- Poor wound healing
- Anorexia
- Hypogeusesthesia (decreased taste acuity)

Foods that contain zinc

The following foods contain significant amounts of zinc.
- Beans
- Dairy products
- Fortified breakfast cereals
- Nuts
- Oysters
- Poultry
- Red meat
- Seafood
- Whole grains

- Dysgeusia (unpleasant taste)
- Hyposmia (decreased odor acuity)
- Dysosmia (unpleasant odor in nasopharynx)
- Severe iron deficiency anemia
- Bone deformities

Complications

- Hypogonadism
- Dwarfism
- Hyperpigmentation

Assessment

History

- Weight loss
- Poor appetite
- Growth retardation
- Short stature
- Mental lethargy
- Diarrhea
- Intercurrent infections

Physical findings

- Sparse hair growth
- Rough skin
- Poor wound healing
- Striae
- White spots on fingernails
- Acne

Test results

Laboratory
- Fasting serum zinc levels are below 70 µg/dl.

Treatment

General

- Correction of the underlying cause
- Diet high in zinc

Medication

- Zinc supplementation

Nursing considerations

Key outcomes

The patient will:
- express understanding of dietary needs
- improve zinc levels
- maintain or improve weight
- experience improved skin condition.

Nursing interventions

- Administer drug therapy.
- Provide information about dietary sources of zinc. (See *Foods that contain zinc*.)

Monitoring
○ Response to treatment

Patient teaching

Be sure to cover:
○ taking zinc supplements with milk or meals to prevent gastric distress and vomiting
○ following a balanced diet that includes foods high in zinc
○ correct use of calcium and iron supplements.

Less common diseases

Names	Description	Treatment
Acceleration-deceleration cervical injury (whiplash)	Mild to severe anterior and posterior neck pain resulting from sharp hyperextension and flexion of the neck that damages muscles, ligaments, disks, and nerve tissue	● Mild analgesics are given to relieve neck pain. ● Hot showers or warm compresses to the neck may help relieve pain. ● The neck is immobilized with a soft, padded cervical collar for days or weeks. Physical therapy may be needed in some cases.
Achilles tendon contracture	Shortening of the Achilles tendon that results in foot pain and strain with limited ankle dorsiflexion; may be due to a congenital abnormality, reaction to chronic poor posture, or a paralytic condition	● Conservative treatment includes raising the inside heel of the shoe, lowering the heels of shoes, stretching exercises, support braces, casting, and analgesics. ● Tenectomy may be performed for patients with fixed footdrop.
Actinomycosis (lumpy jaw)	Infection caused by gram-positive anaerobic bacillus *Actinomyces israelii,* resulting in painful swellings of granulomatous, suppurative lesions with abscesses commonly on the head, neck, thorax, or abdomen	● High-dose I.V. penicillin cycline is administered for 1 to 2 months, followed by oral penicillin for 1 to 6 months. ● Lesions are surgically excised and drained.
Adenovirus infection	Acute, self-limiting febrile infection resulting in inflammation of the respiratory or ocular mucous membranes, or both; 35 serotypes cause five major infections; transmitted by direct inoculation into the eye, oral-fecal route, or inhalation of droplets	● Bed rest, antipyretics, and analgesics may be prescribed as needed. ● Ocular infections may require corticosteroid therapy and supervision by an ophthalmologist. ● Hospitalization is required for infants with pneumonia and in epidemic keratoconjunctivitis.
Alpha$_1$-antitrypsin deficiency	Autosomal recessive inherited disorder resulting in emphysema and liver dysfunction problems	● Enzyme replacement therapy is given weekly. ● Smoking cessation and asthma control are promoted to prevent infection and lung problems. ● Vaccination against hepatitis B is given prophylactically. ● Liver and lung function are monitored.
Alport's syndrome	Hereditary nephritis characterized by recurrent gross or microscopic hematuria; associated with deafness, eye defects, albuminuria, and progressive azotemia	● Antihypertensives are given for hypertension. ● Hearing aids, learning sign language, and corrective eyewear or surgical repair of cataracts are employed. ● Dialysis or kidney transplantation may be required for end-stage renal failure.

Names	Description	Treatment
Amyloidosis	A chronic disease resulting in the accumulation of an abnormal fibrillar scleroprotein, which infiltrates body organs and soft tissues, resulting in permanent and usually life-threatening organ damage	• Kidney transplantation is used for renal failure, although the new organ may also develop amyloidosis. • If the heart is affected, diuretics, digoxin, antiarrhythmics, pacemakers, or heart transplantation may be necessary. • In end-stage GI involvement, total parenteral nutrition is used as needed for malnutrition.
Anal stricture (anal stenosis or contracture)	Develops when the lumen of the anus decreases and stenosis prevents dilation of the sphincter and defecation; can result from scarring after surgery, inflammation, laxative abuse, surgical trauma, or congenital abnormality	• Conservative treatment includes laxatives, suppositories, and enemas. • A dilator is used daily. • Anoplasty or excision of eschar is employed with lateral internal sphincterotomy.
Angiofibroma, juvenile	Highly vascular nasopharyngeal tumor made up of fibrous tissue with thin-walled blood vessels that may grow to completely fill the nasopharynx, nose, paranasal sinuses, and the orbit	• Surgery or cryosurgical techniques after embolization decreases vascularization.
Berylliosis	A form of pneumoconiosis resulting from inhalation of beryllium or from its absorption through the skin; characterized by systemic granulomatous disorder with predominant respiratory symptoms that can lead to respiratory failure, cor pulmonale, and death	• Beryllium ulcer requires excision or curettage. Acute berylliosis requires corticosteroid therapy. • Hypoxia may require oxygen; respiratory failure, mechanical ventilation. Other respiratory symptoms may be treated with bronchodilators and chest physiotherapy. • Chronic forms are treated with corticosteroids and immunosuppressants.
Blastocystis hominis infection (blastocystosis)	Parasitic infection resulting in watery or loose stools, diarrhea, abdominal pain, anal itching, weight loss, and flatus; conversely, no symptoms may be present	• Drug therapy includes ketoconazole or itraconazole. • Amphotericin B is required for severe disease.
Celiac disease (sprue, nontropical sprue, gluten intolerance)	Poor food absorption and gluten intolerance from environmental and genetic factors; recurrent diarrhea, steatorrhea, abdominal distention, and anorexia, resulting in malnutrition; hematologic (anemia), musculoskeletal (from vitamin D deficiency), neurologic, dermatologic, and endocrine systems affected	• Gluten (wheat, rye, barley, and oat products, vegetable protein, malt, soy sauce, grain vinegar) should be excluded from the patient's diet for life. • Supplements may be given to correct deficiencies. • Corticosteroids may be required.

Names	Description	Treatment
Chronic granulomatous disease	An inherited disorder in which abnormal neutrophil metabolism impairs phagocytosis, resulting in increased susceptibility to low virulent or nonpathogenic organisms; infections of the skin, lymph nodes, lungs, liver, and bone occur	• Antibiotics are used for early, aggressive treatment.
Chronic mucocutaneous candidiasis	Inherited defect in cell-mediated (T-cell) immune responses leading to recurrent infections with *Candida albicans* and potential for autoimmune-mediated endocrinopathies; usually begins in early childhood with chronic candidal infections; endocrinopathies include hypoparathyroidism (and severe hypocalcemia), hypothyroidism, Addison's disease, diabetes, pernicious anemia; hepatitis	• Topical or oral antifungal agents (miconazole, nystatin, fluconazole) control chronic infection. • Therapy for endocrinopathy is organ-directed, depending on the system affected.
Colorado tick fever (Mountain tick fever, Mountain fever, American Mountain fever)	A benign infection from the bite of a wood tick infected with *Dermacentor andersoni* (Fever begins abruptly after a 3- to 6-day incubation; severe aching of the back, arms, and legs; lethargy; headache with eye movement; photophobia; abdominal pain; nausea; and vomiting.)	• Remove the tick and keep it for identification. • Administer tetanus-diphtheria booster. • Monitor fluid and electrolyte balance. • Antipyretics are given to reduce fever.
Conversion disorder (hysterical neurosis)	A disorder that allows a patient to resolve a psychological conflict through the loss of a specific physical function, such as paralysis or blindness	• Psychotherapy, family therapy, relaxation therapy, behavioral therapy, or hypnosis may be used alone or in combination. • Supportive therapy for affected body part is used to prevent complications.
Cryptosporidiosis	Watery diarrhea, stomach cramps, upset stomach, and slight fever caused by a one-celled parasite, *Cryptosporidium parvum;* life threatening to those with weakened immune systems and transplant recipients	• There's no cure, but paromomycin, atovaquone, nitazoxaine, and azithromycin may reduce symptoms. • Reverse dehydration is used. • Immune status improves with antiviral agents.
Cystinuria	Autosomal recessive disorder resulting from an inborn error of amino acid transport in the kidneys and intestine that allows excessive urinary excretion of cystine and other dibasic amino acids; resulting in recurrent cystine renal calculi	• No effective treatment is available. • Increase fluid intake to 3 L/day. • Sodium bicarbonate or sodium citrate help alkalinize the urine. • Penicillamine is used to increase cystine solubility. • Calculi are removed surgically or through lithotripsy. • Prevent and treat urinary tract infections.
Depersonalization disorder	Recurrent episodes of detachment in which self-awareness is temporarily altered or lost in the entire body or only in a limb; usually caused by severe stress	• Psychotherapy and reality-based coping strategies may be helpful.
Dientamoeba fragilis infection	Loose stools, diarrhea, and abdominal cramping caused by contact with or ingestion of stool, food, or water infected with the parasite *Dientamoeba fragilis*	• Infection can be prevented by prudent hand washing. • Antimicrobial agents are available to treat *Dientamoeba fragilis.*

Names	Description	Treatment
DiGeorge's syndrome (congenital thymic hypoplasia or aplasia)	Fetal thymus fails to develop, leading to partial or total absence of T lymphocytes and cell-mediated immunity; may be linked with maternal alcoholism and fetal alcohol syndrome; increased susceptibility to infections; hypoparathyroidism and cardiac anomalies may also occur	• Early development of life-threatening hypocalcemia is treated immediately with I.V. 10% calcium gluconate infusion. • Fetal thymic transplantation may be required to restore normal cell-mediated immunity.
Dissociative amnesia	Sudden inability to recall important personal information that can't be explained by ordinary forgetfulness; usually caused by severe psychological stress	• Psychotherapy is necessary.
Dissociative fugue	Wandering or traveling while mentally blocking out a traumatic event; a different personality may be assumed and later can't recall what happened; may be related to dissociative identity disorder, narcissistic personality disorder, and sleepwalking	• Psychotherapy is necessary.
Dissociative identity disorder (multiple personality disorder)	Existence of two or more distinct, fully integrated personalities in the same person; cause unknown but some type of abuse may have been experienced	• Psychotherapy may be helpful.
Epidermolysis bullosa (EB)	Blisters occur in response to normally harmless heat and friction and may result in scarring with disfigurement; prognosis depends on severity; may be inherited as an autosomal dominant or recessive disorder and cause multiple complications because skin and mucous membranes are affected	• Avoid skin trauma and high environmental temperatures. • Severe forms may need constant medical attention. • Supportive treatment includes protection of the skin. • Diet therapy helps combat malnutrition and promote healing.
Fallopian tube cancer	Cancer that usually produces a palpable mass, vague abdominal or pelvic complaints, bloating, or pain in the early stages; over time, excessive menstrual bleeding may occur; causes appear to be linked with nulliparity and infertility; more than half of the patients have never given birth	• Total abdominal hysterectomy, bilateral salpingo-oophorectomy, or omentectomy is performed, followed by chemotherapy. • The patient receives external radiation for 5 to 6 weeks.
Fanconi's syndrome (de Toni-Fanconi syndrome)	Hereditary renal disorder producing malfunctions of the proximal renal tubules, leading to electrolyte losses and, eventually, retarded growth and development and rickets	• Symptomatic treatment may be given to replace the patient's specific deficiencies. (Wilson's disease is treated with D-penicillamine; cystinosis is treated with cysteamine.) • Supportive therapy is given by replacing electrolytes, normalizing pH, and giving dietary supplements.
Fever, relapsing (tick, fowl-nest, cabin, or vagabond fever or bilious typhoid)	An acute infectious disease caused by spirochetes of the genus *Borrelia* transmitted by lice or ticks; presents with recurring high fever, prostration, headache, severe myalgia, arthralgia, diarrhea, vomiting, coughing, eye or chest pain, splenomegaly, hepatomegaly, lymphadenopathy, and macular rash	• Tetracycline or erythromycin is given for 4 to 5 days, except during a severe febrile attack because it may cause Jarisch-Herxheimer reaction. • Symptomatic treatment is given; for example, parenteral fluids and electrolytes.

Names	Description	Treatment
Gaucher's disease (glucosylceramide storage disease, GSDI)	Genetic enzyme deficiency that causes abnormal accumulation of glucocerebrosides in reticuloendothelial cells; signs include hepatosplenomegaly and bone lesions	• Long-term therapy includes I.V. replacement of the missing enzyme every 2 weeks. • Gene therapy is an experimental approach, as well as N-butyldeoxynojirimycin (OGT918) to inhibit production of glucocerebroside.
Gender identity disorder (transsexualism)	Persistent feelings of gender discomfort and dissatisfaction from a combination of predisposing factors (chromosomal anomaly, hormonal imbalance, impaired parent-child bonding, and child-rearing practices)	• The patient is referred for psychotherapy to resolve conflict. Individual and family counseling is recommended. • Sex reassignment through surgery and hormonal therapy is used.
Hallux valgus	Lateral deviation of the great toe at the metatarsophalangeal joint, with medial enlargement of the first metatarsal head and painful bunion formation; may be congenital or familial, but is usually acquired from degenerative arthritis or prolonged pressure on the foot, especially from narrow-toed, high-heeled shoes	• In the early stage, proper shoes and good foot care — such as felt pads to protect the bunion, devices to separate the toes at night, and a supportive pad and exercises to strengthen the metatarsal arch — may eliminate the need for bunionectomy. • Surgery to realign the toe or bunionectomy may be ordered.
Hand, foot, and mouth disease (HFMD)	Common disease of infants and children characterized by fever, mouth sores, and a rash with blisters on the hands and soles; caused by coxsackievirus	• Treatment is symptomatic only because disease is self-limiting. • Acetaminophen and salt water mouth rinses (½ teaspoon salt to 1 glass warm water) are used to provide soothing relief.
Herpangina	Acute infection caused by group A coxsackieviruses transmitted by the fecal-oral route, resulting in sore throat, pain on swallowing, headache, and fever that persist for 1 to 4 days and may cause seizures, anorexia, vomiting, malaise, diarrhea, and pain; grayish white papulovesicles appear on the soft palate	• Symptomatic treatment emphasizes measures to prevent seizures (such as antipyretics and and tepid sponge baths), fluids to prevent dehydration, and bed rest. • Provide topical anesthetics for the mouth (benzocaine and xylocaine) as needed. • Provide a non-irritating diet. • Increase fluid intake.
Hydatidiform mole	Chorionic tumor of the placenta that occurs early in pregnancy; may follow death of the embryo and loss of fetal circulation, although in many cases, there is no fetus	• Uterus is evacuated by suction curettage or abdominal hysterectomy. • Supportive treatment is given for postoperative hypovolemia and anemia.
Hypochondriasis (Hypochondria)	The unrealistic misinterpretation of the severity and significance of physical signs or sensations as abnormal and preoccupation with the fear of having a serious disease, which persists despite medical reassurance to the contrary; unlinked to cause, although stress increases the risk; frequently develops in people who have experienced an organic disease or have a relative who has experienced one	• The goal is to help the patient lead a productive life, despite distressing symptoms and fears. Outpatient psychotherapy with behavior modification is the first line of treatment. • Symptoms must be evaluated to rule out medical causes first. • Routine psychiatric appointments, regardless of new symptoms, help as part of psychotherapy.
Iodine deficiency	Insufficient iodine from inadequate intake or thyroid dysfunction; complications range from dental caries to cretinism	• Iodine supplements (potassium iodide [SSKI]) are administered to correct the deficiency. • Increase iodine intake with iodized table salt and iodine-rich foods.

Names	Description	Treatment
Lassa fever	Epidemic hemorrhagic fever caused by the Lassa virus; transmitted to humans by contact with infected rodent urine, feces, and saliva; fever persists for 2 to 3 weeks with exudative pharyngitis, oral ulcers, lymphadenopathy and swelling of the face and neck, purpura, conjunctivitis, and bradycardia; shock and peripheral vascular collapse can occur	• Strict isolation is imposed for at least 3 weeks. • Drug therapy includes antiviral (I.V. ribavirin), I.V. colloids for shock, analgesics for pain, and antipyretics for fever. • Immune plasma from patients who have recovered from Lassa fever is infused.
Leprosy (Hansen's disease)	Chronic, systemic infection with progressive cutaneous lesions caused by *Mycobacterium leprae;* attacks the peripheral nervous system	• Drug regimen includes antimicrobial therapy with dapsone, rifampin, clofazimine, or ethionamide. • Supportive care with aspirin, prednisone, or thalidomide to control inflammation may be used.
Lichen planus	Benign, pruritic skin eruption producing scaling, purple papules with white lines or spots; cause unknown	• Relieve inflammation with topical steroids and suppress immune response. • Antihistamines are used to reduce discomfort. • Viscous lidocaine is used for mouth lesions. • Corticosteroids may be injected into a lesion. • Topical retinoic (vitamin A) cream and other anti-inflammatory or anti-pruritic ointments or creams are used to reduce itching and inflammation. • Ultraviolet light therapy may be used.
Marfan syndrome	Rare inherited, degenerative generalized disease of the connective tissue that causes ocular, skeletal, and cardiovascular anomalies	• Treatment is aimed at relieving the symptoms such as surgical repair of aneurysms and ocular deformities. • Preventive antibiotics are given before dental procedures. • Children shouldn't be involved in maximal exercise programs because of concern of aortic aneurysm.
Mastoiditis	Bacterial infection and inflammation of the air cells of the mastoid antrum resulting in dull ache and tenderness in the area of the mastoid process, low-grade fever, headache, and thick, purulent drainage; meningitis, facial paralysis, brain abscess, and suppurative labyrinthitis may occur	• Intense antibiotic therapy is administered parenterally. • Myringotomy is performed if bone damage is minimal. • Mastoidectomy is performed if the mastoid is chronically inflamed.
Medullary sponge kidney	Inherited disorder, possibly where collecting ducts in renal pyramids dilate and cavities, clefts, and cysts form, producing complications of calcium oxalate stones and infections	• Supportive care focuses on preventing or treating complications caused by stones and infection. Includes increasing fluid intake and monitoring renal function. • Surgery may be required to remove stones during acute obstruction. Nephrectomy is required if serious, uncontrollable infection or hemorrhage occur.

Names	Description	Treatment
Monkeypox	Rare viral disease caused by the monkeypox virus; occurs mainly in the rainforest areas of central and western Africa; symptoms include fever, headache, muscle aches, backache, swollen lymph nodes, and exhaustion; a papular rash develops within 1 to 3 days of the onset of fever (In June 2003, monkeypox was reported in prairie dogs and humans in the United States.)	• There's no specific treatment for monkeypox. • Persons caring for infected individuals should receive a smallpox vaccination.
Motion sickness	Loss of equilibrium associated with nausea and vomiting that result from irregular or rhythmic movements or from the sensation of motion; may follow excessive stimulation of the labyrinthine receptors of the inner ear by certain motions, such as those experienced in a car, boat, plane, or swing; may also be caused by confusion in the cerebellum from conflicting sensory input — for example, a visual stimulus (such as a moving horizon) conflicts with labyrinthine perception	• The best treatment is removal of the stimulus. • If removal isn't possible, the patient will benefit from lying down, closing his eyes, and trying to sleep. • Antiemetics may prevent or relieve symptoms.
Multiple endocrine neoplasia	A hereditary disorder in which two or more endocrine glands develop hyperplasia, adenoma, or carcinoma concurrently or consecutively; symptoms depend on glands affected	• Supportive treatment is dependent on the affected glands. • Tumors are eradicated; subsequent treatment controls symptoms.
Neurofibromatosis	Group of inherited developmental disorders of the nervous system, muscles, bones, and skin that cause formation of multiple, pedunculated, soft tumors and café-au-lait spots	• Intracerebral or intraspinal tumors are removed and kyphoscoliosis is corrected. • Disfiguring or disabling growths are treated with cosmetic surgery. • Annual eye examinations are strongly recommended.
Nocardiosis	Bacterial infection caused by gram-positive species of the genus *Nocardia* and transmitted by inhalation; causes cough, mucopurulent sputum, high fever, chills, night sweats, anorexia, malaise, and weight loss	• Long-term antibiotic treatment with sulfonamides is given. • Abscesses are surgically drained and necrotic tissue is excised. • Bed rest and supportive treatment are ordered.
Orbital cellulitis	Acute infection of the orbital tissues and eyelids that can spread to the cavernous sinus or meninges; produces unilateral eyelid edema, hyperemia, reddened eyelids, and matted lashes	• Hospitalization is required. • Appropriate antibiotics are given. • Supportive therapy includes administration of fluids, application of warm moist compresses, and bed rest. • Surgical drainage may be necessary.
Parainfluenza	Group of respiratory illnesses caused by the parainfluenza virus that affect the upper and lower respiratory tracts; transmitted by direct contact or inhalation of airborne droplets	• Treatment regimen includes bed rest, antipyretics for fever, analgesics for pain, and antitussives for cough. • Specific treatments are available for croup and bronchiolitis.

Names	Description	Treatment
Penile cancer	Malignant, ulcerative or papillary (wartlike, nodular) lesions, which may become quite large before spreading beyond the penis, potentially destroying the glans prepuce and invading the corpora; generally associated with poor personal hygiene and phimosis in uncircumcised men, although the exact cause is unknown	• Depending on the stage of progression, treatment includes surgical resection of the primary tumor and, possibly, chemotherapy (bleomycin) and radiation. • Invasive tumors require partial penectomy (unless contraindicated because of the patient's young age); tumors of the base of the penile shaft require total penectomy and inguinal node dissection. • Radiation therapy may improve treatment effectiveness after resection of localized lesions without metastasis; it may also reduce the size of lymph nodes before nodal resection.
Pilonidal disease	Coccygeal cyst forms in the intergluteal cleft on the posterior surface of the lower sacrum, often becoming infected or developing a fistula; may be congenital or caused by irritation from exercise, heat, perspiration, or constrictive clothing	• Abscesses are incised and drained, protruding hairs are extracted, and sitz baths are ordered. • Entire affected area is excised if infections persist.
Polymyalgia rheumatica	An inflammatory syndrome characterized by significant stiffness and dull aching pain of the proximal muscle groups, weight loss, malaise, and fever; cause unknown, but it predominantly involves whites, tends to run in families, and is possibly associated with HLA-DR4 antigens, all of which suggest a possible genetic predisposition	• Corticosteroids, such as prednisone or prednisolone, are the treatment of choice to help relieve discomfort and stiffness.
Puerperal infection	Inflammation of the birth canal during the postpartum period or after abortion; caused by streptococci, coagulase-negative staphylococci, *Clostridium perfringens, Bacteroides fragilis*, and *Escherichia coli*	• I.V. broad-spectrum antibiotics are ordered to combat infection. • Supportive therapy includes analgesics, anticoagulants, antiemetics, bed rest, administration of I.V. fluids, and prevention of thrombophlebitis (antiembolism stockings).
Rectal polyps	Mass lesions that result from unrestrained cell growth in the upper epithelium and protrude into the intestinal lumen; varying in appearance; include common polypoid adenomas, villous adenomas, polyposis syndromes, juvenile polyps, and focal polypoid hyperplasia; predisposing factors include heredity, age, infection, and diet	• Specific treatment varies according to type and size of the polyps and their location in the colon. • Common polypoid adenomas less than 1 cm require polypectomy, frequently by fulguration (destruction by high-frequency electricity) during endoscopy. For common polypoid adenomas over 4 cm and all invasive villous adenomas, treatment usually consists of abdominoperineal resection or low anterior resection. Transanal excision is performed to remove an adenoma from the rectum. • Depending on large-bowel involvement, hereditary polyposis necessitate restorative proctolectomy, ileoanal anastomosis with temporary ileostomy. • Focal polypoid hyperplasia can be obliterated by a biopsy.

Names	Description	Treatment
Rectal prolapse	Circumferential protrusion of one or more layers of the rectum through the anus caused by straining or conditions that affect the pelvic floor or rectum; patient may also have a feeling of rectal fullness, bloody diarrhea, and pain	• Treat the underlying cause and eliminate predisposing factors (straining, coughing, nutritional disorders). • Manual return of the rectal mucosa may be necessary. • Surgical repair is performed in severe or chronic cases.
Retinitis pigmentosa	Genetically induced progressive destruction of the retinal rods resulting in visual field constriction, cataracts, edema, atrophic maculopathy, and blindness	• No cure exists. • Vitamin A supplementation may be given to slow degeneration. • Advise the use of sunglasses to protect from ultraviolet light.
Throat abscess	Either peritonsillar (quinsy) abscess that forms in the connective tissue space between the tonsil capsule and constrictor muscle of the pharynx or retropharyngeal abscess that forms between the posterior pharyngeal wall and prevertebral fascia (Peritonsillar abscess is a complication of acute tonsillitis, usually after streptococcal or staphylococcal infection. Acute retropharyngeal abscess results from infection in the retropharyngeal lymph glands, which may follow an upper respiratory tract bacterial infection. Chronic retropharyngeal abscess may result from tuberculosis of the cervical spine [Pott's disease].)	• For early-stage peritonsillar abscess, large doses of a broad-spectrum antibiotic are given. • For late-stage peritonsillar abscess with cellulitis of the tonsillar space, primary treatment is incision and drainage under a local anesthetic, followed by antibiotic therapy for 7 to 10 days. • For both stages of peritonsillar abscess, tonsillectomy is recommended after several episodes. It must be scheduled at least 1 month after acute infection. • Incision and drainage of abcesses.
Tinea versicolor (pityriasis versicolor)	Chronic, superficial fungal (yeast) infection producing a multicolored rash or macular or raised scaly lesions, commonly on the upper trunk and caused by *Pityrosporum orbiculare*	• Treat with topical antifungals, such as clotrimazole, ketoconazole, and miconalzole. • Over-the-counter dandruff shampoos applied to the skin for 10 minutes each day in the shower may also eliminate it.
Toxocariasis (ocular larva migrans, visceral larva migrans)	Infection caused by parasitic roundworms in dogs and cats spread by the fecal-oral route and resulting in eye infections that can cause blindness or visceral (rare) symptoms with swelling of body organs or central nervous system	• Infection is treated with mebendazole, albendazole, or diethylcarbamazine. • Preventive measures include treating animals and thorough hand washing.
Trachoma (granular conjunctivitis, Egyptian ophthalmia)	Infection by *Chlamydia trachomatis* that affects the eye but can also localize in the urethra; may cause permanent damage to the cornea and conjunctiva	• Topical or systemic antibiotic therapy with erythromycin or doxycycline is given. • Surgical correction is necessary if severe entropion occurs.
Uveitis (iritis)	Inflammation of one uveal tract producing moderate to severe eye pain, severe ciliary injection, photophobia, tearing, a small nonreactive pupil, and blurred vision; results from allergy, infection, chemicals, trauma, surgery, or systemic diseases or may be idiopathic	• Underlying cause is diagnosed and treated. • Topical cycloplegic and topical corticosteroids are given. • Steroid drops or ointment may be needed. • Oral systemic corticosteroids are given in severe cases.
Vaginismus	Involuntary spastic constriction of the lower vaginal muscles with pain on insertion of any object into the vagina; cause may be physical or psychological	• Maladaptive muscle constriction is eliminated with dilators. • Education, counseling, and behavioral exercises are given. • Kegel exercises to improve voluntary control are ordered.

Names	Description	Treatment
Wilson's disease (hepatolenticular degeneration)	Rare, inherited metabolic disorder characterized by excessive copper retention in the liver, brain, kidneys, and corneas; Kayser-Fleischer rings of the eye are produced, and deposits may lead to tissue necrosis and fibrosis.	• Treatment with pyridoxine in conjunction with penicillamine, a copper-chelating agent that mobilizes copper from the tissues and promotes its excretion in the urine, is life-long. • Copper-containing foods should be avoided as well as tap water (because of copper pipes) and copper cooking utensils. • The patient and his family should receive genetic counseling.
Wiskott-Aldrich syndrome (immunodeficiency with eczema and thrombocytopenia)	X-linked recessive inherited disease characterized by defective B- and T-cell functions (increased susceptibility to infections) and metabolic defects in platelet synthesis (thrombocytopenia) (Male infants develop early bleeding complications [bloody stools, petechiae, and purpura] and by age 6 months develop recurrent systemic infections; by age 1 year, eczema develops, leading to scratching and skin infections; high susceptibility to neoplastic diseases, such as lymphoma and leukemia, occurs. Average life span is 4 years.)	• Bleeding is controlled with platelet transfusions. • Prophylactic or early aggressive therapy with antibiotics is indicated for infections. • Topical steroids help control eczema symptoms. • Bone marrow transplantation may be effective in some patients.

Selected references

Ambrose, J.A., and Martinez, E.E. "A New Paradigm for Plaque Stabilization," *Circulation* 105(16):2000-2004, April 2002.

Angerio, A.D., and Lee, N.D. "Sickle Cell Crisis and Endothelin Antagonist," *Critical Care Nursing Quarterly* 26(3):225-29, July-September 2003.

Atlas of Pathophysiology. Springhouse, Pa.: Springhouse Corp., 2002.

Bender, K., and Thompson, F.E., Jr. "West Nile Virus: A Growing Challenge," *AJN* 103(6):32-40, June 2003.

Berven, S., and Bradford, D. "Neuromuscular Scoliosis: Causes of Deformity and Principles of Evaluation and Management," *Seminars in Neurology* 22(2):167-78, 2002.

Braunwald, E., et al. *Harrison's Principles of Internal Medicine*, 15th ed. New York: McGraw-Hill Book Co., 2001.

Chavez, J., and Brewer, C. "Stopping the Shock Slide," *RN* 65(9):30-35, September 2002.

Degner, L.F., et al. "A New Approach to Eliciting Meaning in the Context of Breast Cancer," *Cancer Nursing* 26(3):169-78, June 2003.

Diagnostic and Statistical Manual of Mental Disorders, Fourth Edition, Text Revision. Washington, D.C.: American Psychiatric Association, 2000.

Evangelista, L., et al. "Compliance Behaviors of Elderly Patients with Advanced Heart Failure," *Journal of Cardiovascular Nursing* 18(3):197-208, July-August 2003.

Fair, J. "Cardiovascular Risk Factor Modification: Is It Effective in Older Adults?" *Journal of Cardiovascular Nursing* 18(3):161-68, July-August 2003.

Faix, R.G. "Immunization During Pregnancy," *Clinical Obstetrics and Gynecology* 45(1):42-58, March 2002.

Ferri, F. *Ferri's Clinical Advisor: Instant Diagnosis and Treatment.* St. Louis: Mosby Year–Book, Inc., 2004.

Fraenkel, L. "Raynaud's Phenomenon: Epidemiology and Risk Factors," *Current Rheumatology Reports* 4(2):123-28. Reviewed April 2002.

Geiter, H., Jr. "Disseminated Intravascular Coagulopathy," *Dimensions of Critical Care* 22(3):108-16, May-June 2003.

Guenter, P., and Silkroski, M. *Tube Feeding: Practical Guidelines and Nursing Procedures.* Gaithersburg, Md.: Aspen Pubs., Inc., 2001.

Halm, M.A., and Denker, J. "Primary Prevention Programs to Reduce Heart Disease Risk in Women," *Clinical Nurse Specialist: The Journal for Advanced Nursing Practice* 17(2):101-11, March 2003.

Haskell, C. *Cancer Treatment,* 5th ed. Philadelphia: W.B. Saunders Co., 2001.

Hedger, A. "Spinal Cord Injury," *Nursing* 32(12):96, December 2002.

Joachim, G. "An Assessment of Social Support in People with Inflammatory Bowel Disease," *Gastroenterology Nursing* 25(6):246-52, November-December 2002.

Johnson, R.M., and Richard, R. "Partial-thickness Burns: Identification and Management," *Advances in Skin and Wound Care: The Journal for Prevention and Healing* 16(4):178-89, July-August 2003.

Joyce, A.M., and Brewer, C. "Recurrent *Clostridium difficile* Colitis: Tackling a Tenacious Nosocomial Infection," *Postgraduate Medicine* 112(5):53-54, November 2002.

Kidd, P.S., and Wagner, K.D. *High Acuity Nursing,* 3rd ed. Upper Saddle River, N.J.: Prentice Hall Health, 2001.

Kriebs, J.M. "The Global Reach of HIV: Preventing Mother-to-Child Transmission," *Journal of Perinatal and Neonatal Nursing* 16(3):1-10, December 2002.

Lane, P., et al. "A Pain Assessment Tool for People with Advanced Alzheimer's and Other Progressive Dementias," *Home Healthcare Nurse* 21(1):32-37, January 2003.

LeJeune, G.M., and Howard-Fain, T. "Nursing Assessment and Management of Patients with Head Injuries," *Dimensions of Critical Care Nursing* 21(6): 226-31, November-December 2002.

London, M.L., et al. *Maternal-Newborn and Child Nursing: Family Centered Care.* Upper Saddle River, N.J.: Prentice Hall Health, 2003.

McCrory, P. "What Advice Should We Give to Athletes Post Concussion?" *British Journal of Sports Medicine* 36(5):316-18, October 2002.

McNally, P. *GI/Liver Secrets,* 2nd ed. Philadelphia: Hanley & Belfus, Inc. 2001.

Mendez-Eastman, S.K. "Skin Grafting: Preoperative, Intraoperative, and Postoperative Care," *Plastic Surgical Nursing* 21(1):49-51, Spring 2001.

Murray, J., and Nadel, J. *Textbook of Respiratory Medicine,* 3rd ed. Philadelphia: W.B. Saunders Co., 2001.

Oman, K., et al. (eds.). *Emergency Nursing Secrets.* Philadelphia: Hanley & Belfus, 2001.

Price, A. "Primary and Secondary Prevention of Colorectal Cancer," *Gastroenterology Nursing* 26(2):73-81, March-April 2003.

Professional Guide to Diseases, 7th ed. Springhouse, Pa.: Springhouse Corp., 2001.

Rakel, R., and Bope, E. *Conn's Current Therapy.* Philadelphia: W.B. Saunders Co., 2004.

Smeltzer, S.C., and Bare, B.G. *Brunner and Suddarth's Textbook of Medical-Surgical Nursing,* 10th ed. Philadelphia: Lippincott Williams & Wilkins, 2004.

Sommers, J., et al. *Diseases and Disorders: A Nursing Therapeutics Manual,* 2nd ed. Philadelphia: F.A. Davis Co., 2002.

Steen. V. "Treatment of Systemic Sclerosis," *American Journal of Clinical Dermatology* 2(5):315-25, 2001.

Tierney, L. et al. *Current Medical Diagnosis and Treatment,* 43rd ed. New York: McGraw-Hill Book Co., 2004.

Timby, B.K. *Fundamental Skills and Concepts in Patient Care,* 7th ed. Philadelphia: Lippincott Williams & Wilkins, 2000.

Veenema, T. "The Smallpox Vaccine Debate," *AJN* 102(9):33-39, September 2002.

VonEssen, L., and Enskar, K. "Important Aspects of Care and Assistance for Siblings of Children Teated for Cancer: A Parent and Nurse Perspective," *Cancer Nursing* 26(3):203-10, June 2003.

Weinstein, S.M. *Plumer's Principles and Practice of Intravenous Therapy,* 7th ed. Philadelphia: Lippincott Williams & Wilkins, 2000.

Wong, D.L., and Hockenberry-Eaton, M. *Wong's Essentials of Pediatric Nursing,* 6th ed. St. Louis: Mosby Year-Book, Inc., 2001.

Woodward, B.G. "Bariatric Surgery Options," *Critical Care Nursing Quarterly* 26(2):89-100, April-June 2001.

Zaima, H., and Koga, M. "Clinical Course of 44 Cases of Localized Type Vitiligo," *Journal of Dermatology* 29(1):15-19, January 2002.

Zucker, D.M., and Miller, B.W. "Assessment of Side Effects in Patients with Chronic Hepatitis C Receiving Combination Therapy," *Gastroenterology Nursing* 24(4):192-96, July-August 2001.

Web resources

Alateen
www.al-ateen.org
Alcoholics Anonymous
www.alcoholics-anonymous.org
Al-Anon
www.al-anon.org
ALS Association
www.alsa.org
American Academy of Allergy, Asthma, and Immunology
www.aaaai.org
American Academy of Dermatology
www.aad.org
American Academy of Neurology
www.aan.com
American Academy of Ophthalmology
www.aao.org
American Academy of Pediatrics
www.aap.org
American Association of Kidney Patients
www.aakp.org
American Burn Association
www.ameriburn.org
American Cancer Society
www.cancer.org
American College of Obstetricians and Gynecologists
www.acog.org
American Heart Association
www.americanheart.com
American Lung Association
www.lungusa.org
American Psychological Association Help Center
www.helping.apa.org
American Society for Reproductive Medicine
www.asrm.org
Arthritis Society
www.arthritis.ca
Asthma and Allergy Foundation of America
www.aafa.org
Autism Society of America
www.autism-society.org
Center for AIDS Prevention Studies
www.caps.ucsf.edu
Centers for Disease Control and Prevention
www.cdc.gov

Dermatology Foundation
www.dermfnd.org
Digestive Disease National Coalition
www.ddnc.org
Emedicine
www.emedicine.com
Harvard Medical School's Consumer Health Information
www.intelihealth.com
Heart Center Online
www.heartcenteronline.com
Hereditary Hemorrhagic Telangiectasia Foundation
www.hht.org
Iron Disorders Institute
www.irondisorders.org
Mayo Clinic
www.mayoclinic.com
NARAL Pro-Choice America (formerly the National Abortion and Reproductive Rights Action League)
www.naral.org
Narcotics Anonymous
www.na.org
National Abortion Federation
www.prochoice.org
National Association of Anorexia Nervosa and Associated Disorders
www.anad.org
National Association for Children of Alcoholics
www.nacoa.net
National Asthma Education and Prevention Program
www.nhlbi.nih.gov/about/naepp
National Cancer Institute
www.cancer.gov
National Center for Infectious Disease
www.cdc.gov/ncidod
National Center for Injury Prevention and Control
www.cdc.gov/ncipc
National Center for Learning Disabilities
www.ncld.org
National Cervical Cancer Coalition
www.nccc-online.org
National Council on Alcoholism and Drug Dependence
www.ncadd.org
National Eye Institute
www.nei.nih.gov

National Health Information Center
www.health.gov/nhic
National Heart, Lung, and Blood Institute
www.nhlbi.nih.gov
National Institute for Occupational Safety and Health
www.cdc.gov/niosh/homepage.html
National Institute of Allergy and Infectious Diseases
www.niaid.nih.gov
National Institute of Arthritis and Musculoskeletal and
Skin Diseases
www.niams.nih.gov
National Institute of Diabetes and Digestive and Kidney
Diseases
www.niddk.nih.gov
National Institute of Neurological Disorders and Stroke
www.ninds.nih.gov
National Lung Health Education Program
www.nlhep.org
National Mental Health Association
www.nmha.org
National Organization for Rare Disorders
www.rarediseases.org
National Women's Health Information Center
www.4woman.gov
Overeaters Anonymous
www.oa.org
Sickle Cell Disease Association of America
www.sicklecelldisease.org
U.S. Food and Drug Administration
www.fda.gov

Index

i refers to an illustration; t refers to a table.

i refers to an illustration; t refers to a table.

i refers to an illustration; t refers to a table.

i refers to an illustration; t refers to a table.

i refers to an illustration; t refers to a table.

i refers to an illustration; t refers to a table.

i refers to an illustration; t refers to a table.

i refers to an illustration; t refers to a table.

i refers to an illustration; t refers to a table.

i refers to an illustration; t refers to a table.

i refers to an illustration; t refers to a table.

i refers to an illustration; t refers to a table.

i refers to an illustration; t refers to a table.